Advanced Techniques in Limb Reconstruction Surgery

Mehmet Kocaoğlu • Hiroyuki Tsuchiya

Levent Eralp

Editors

Advanced Techniques in Limb Reconstruction Surgery

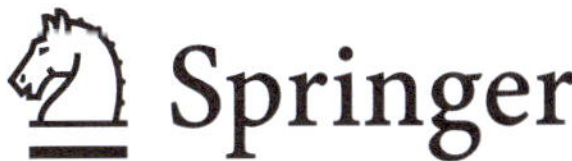

Springer

Editors
Mehmet Kocaoğlu
Department of Orthopaedic
Surgery and Traumatology
Memorial Hospital
Piyalepasa Bulvari, Okmeydani
Istanbul
Turkey

Levent Eralp
Department of Orthopaedic
Surgery and Traumatology
Istanbul University
Istanbul Medical Faculty
Istanbul
Turkey

Hiroyuki Tsuchiya
Department of Orthopaedic Surgery
Kanazawa University Hospital
Kanazawa
Japan

ISBN 978-3-662-50764-3   ISBN 978-3-642-55026-3   (eBook)
DOI 10.1007/978-3-642-55026-3
Springer Heidelberg New York Dordrecht London

Preface

It seems like only yesterday (November 1983) I was introduced to the basic concepts and techniques of limb reconstruction through the pioneering work of Ilizarov. This was only 2 years after Ilizarov first presented his revolutionary ideas to the West on June 12–14, 1981, in Bellagio, Italy. In the 1980s new pioneers from around the world worked through the learning curve of the Ilizarov methods. As we pushed the indications for these original methods, innovation that originated in the Soviet Union during the 1950s, 1960s and 1970s spread across the globe. Treatment barriers that could not be breached before fell before our eyes in synchrony with the fall of the Berlin wall and the great Cold War divide. While a new world order arose so did new treatment obstacles that defied these new techniques and tools. A handful of new surgeon champions arose across the globe and began to solve problems that had not been solved before even by Ilizarov and his coworkers. With fresh ideas, new perspectives, and new and better technologies, advanced limb reconstruction techniques were developed. As Newton noted, we saw farther because we stood on the shoulders of such giants as Ilizarov, Debastiani, Bliskunov, Mueller, Wagner and others. Advanced techniques such as focal dome osteotomy, LON, FAN, superhip, superknee, superankle, Perthes hip distraction, periosteal grafting for CPT, deformity planning by the CORA method, and prediction of LLD by the multiplier method were developed by Paley; caffeine infusion and new innovative bone transport methods for tumor reconstruction by Tsuchiya; fixator assisted locking plates by Rozbruch; patellar knee arthroplasty for tibial hemimelia by Weber; six axis deformity correction using a new circular external fixator by Taylor and Seide; shortening for acute trauma by Lerner; combined techniques for bone defects and osteomyelitis by Cierny, Kocaoglu, and Levent; new implantable limb lengthening methods by Grammont and Guichet, Baumgart, Cole and most recently Green and Paley; improvements in knee arthrodesis methods by Levent; improvements in pelvic support osteotomy by Catagni; and advances in clubfoot management by Herzenberg. All of these next generation advances are presented together in this landmark publication of *Advanced Techniques in Limb Reconstruction Surgery*. While there are many previous publications on the Ilizarov method from basic to advanced applications, this is the first book to focus only on the cutting edge advanced technologies that blossomed from the Ilizarov revolution. As I look back at my own 31-year odyssey, I am amazed to see how far we have come, but even more excited by where we are going. I am proud of my small but significant role in this journey as each of the authors should be proud of their contributions. We are indebted to and congratulate Mehmet Kocaoglu and Levent Erlap, not only for their individual contributions to this field, but to their tireless effort to collect all of these ideas, from a cast of superstar, innovative and brilliant surgeons, and produce this reference tome for all orthopedic surgeons.

West Palm Beach, FL, USA   Dror Paley

Contents

Lengthening over Nails (LON): Femur and Tibia

John E. Herzenberg, Shawn C. Standard, and Janet D. Conway

Contents

J.E. Herzenberg, MD FRCSC (✉)
S.C. Standard, MD • J.D. Conway, MD
International Center for Limb Lengthening,
Rubin Institute for Advanced Orthopedics,
Sinai Hospital of Baltimore, 2401 West Belvedere
Avenue, Baltimore, MD 21215, USA
e-mail: jherzenberg@lifebridgehealth.org,
sstandard@lifebridgehealth.org;
jconway@lifebridgehealth.org

1.1 Femoral LON

1.1.1 Indications

1. Femur LON is indicated for skeletally mature individuals with leg length discrepancy of up to 10 cm in straight bones (no deformity), a reamable intramedullary canal, and no active infection. In selected cases, it is permissible to lengthen over a nail in adolescents, provided a trochanteric entry nail is used, to avoid injury to the blood supply of the femoral head.

   - A stable knee and hip are prerequisite. In the face of moderate knee instability, it is possible to bridge with the external fixator across the knee with a carefully positioned external knee axis hinge that links the femoral frame to a tibial frame, allowing knee flexion and extension but not subluxation. For cases of profound preexisting knee instability, consider preparatory surgery to reconstruct the deficient ligaments.

   - In the face of hip instability or dysplasia, it may be necessary to do a preliminary, staged pelvic/acetabular reorientation procedure, with the goal of obtaining a center-edge angle of at least 20°.

   - Femoral LON is most often done with antegrade nailing, though occasionally retrograde nailing is indicated, as in the case of a distal femoral deformity that requires correction.

2. For select patients, mild to moderate angular or rotational deformities may be acutely corrected with the intramedullary nail.

M. Kocaoğlu et al. (eds.), *Advanced Techniques in Limb Reconstruction Surgery*,
DOI 10.1007/978-3-642-55026-3_1, © Springer Berlin Heidelberg 2015

- Proximal femur deformities (varus, valgus, rotation) can be corrected through a proximal femoral osteotomy that will also function as the lengthening site (Fig. 1.3 A-J). Acute correction may theoretically justify a somewhat longer latency period, as the osteotomy is more traumatic than a classical non-displaced corticotomy. However, acute correction also induces compression at the osteotomy site, which must be overcome with distraction before actual lengthening commences. Therefore, it is usually satisfactory to start lengthening after the usual 5-day latency period in cases of femoral LON.
- Diaphyseal and distal metadiaphyseal deformities may need to undergo preliminary correction and locked nailing, to be followed 6–12 months later (after osteotomy healing) by staged antegrade LON.
- Mild distal femoral metaphyseal angular deformities may be acutely corrected with a nail and the same osteotomy used for lengthening with a retrograde femoral nail. However, if preferred, these two procedures (deformity correction with a nail and lengthening over a nail) may be staged.
- The decision to correct deformities with a nail, often called "fixator-assisted nailing" or FAN, is discussed elsewhere in this book. The osteotomy must be planned to be at a level that will take into account the final position of the end of the nail tip after it has fully retracted at the end of lengthening. The nail tip should be at least 10 cm beyond the lengthening site at the end of lengthening in order to provide sufficient stability in the far fragment. If the deformity is at a level that would not permit this, then the FAN should be staged, rather than simultaneous with the LON. Another alternative technique is "lengthening and then nailing" (LATN). For LATN, an external fixator is used to achieve lengthening, and then a locked nail is inserted after lengthening is achieved to maintain the correction and allow early removal of the fixator. The biggest challenge for LATN is applying a stable external fixator in such a way as not to interfere with subsequent nail insertion.

1.1.2 Examination/Imaging

1. Assess the limb length discrepancy (LLD): Ask the patient to stand, feel the iliac crests, and insert various size lifts under the short limb until the iliac crests are palpable at the same level.
2. Assess joints: The hip, knee, and ankle must all be assessed preoperatively for documentation purposes. Limited knee flexion may be a contraindication to nailing the tibia or retrograde nailing of the femur, if the degree of knee flexion would not permit nail insertion.
3. Assess muscle function: Preoperative documentation of muscle strength and range is essential.
4. Assess the neurovascular status: It is essential to document neurovascular function before surgery. Neuropraxia, particularly of the peroneal nerve, can develop during femoral lengthening. Document sensation of the saphenous nerve (terminal branch of femoral nerve), superficial peroneal nerve, deep peroneal nerve, sural nerve, and medial/lateral plantar nerves. Also, assess for sensation in the upper thigh in the distribution of the lateral femoral cutaneous nerve. If compromised nerve function is preexistent as a result of scarring or trauma, consider simultaneous nerve decompression.
5. Assess the soft tissues: Scar tissue is less compliant than supple skin and may limit joint motion. Scarring around nerves from prior surgery may be asymptomatic but can become problematic under the stress of stretching the nerves and scar during limb lengthening. Consider prophylactic peroneal nerve decompression in such cases. Scarring around muscles and in joints can limit joint mobility and should be addressed. Femoral lengthening should not commence in the presence of a knee flexion contracture, which will only get worse with lengthening. Knee extension contractures can also get worse with lengthening, but may be dealt with 6 months or more after the lengthening with a planned Judet quadricepsplasty or distal quadricepsplasty.
6. Radiographic assessment: Long-leg films with an appropriate size lift under the short leg

are required. The ideal film shows both hip joints, both knee joints, and both ankle joints on the same, long, cassette. A magnification marker should be taped to the leg at the level of the bone for accurate measurement of the LLD.

- Long-leg standing radiographs: Provide information about limb length and frontal plane deformity.
- Long lateral radiographs of the entire limb: Show sagittal plane deformity and sagittal plane malalignment about the knee.

7. Common radiographic angles:
- Lateral distal femoral angle (LDFA): Angle defined by the mechanical axis of the femur and the knee joint reference line. Normal is 85–90°.
- Medial proximal tibial angle (MPTA): Angle defined by the mechanical axis of the tibia and the knee joint reference line. Normal is 85–90°.
- Lateral distal tibial angle (LDTA): Angle defined by the long axis of the tibia in the coronal plane and the distal tibia plafond. Normal is 86–92°.
- Anterior distal tibial angle (ADTA): Angle defined by the long axis of the tibia in the sagittal plane and the distal tibia plafond. Normal is 78–82°.

8. Pearls:
- In the presence of complex deformity of the femur or tibia, do a preliminary operation to straighten the bone, transfix it with a locked IM nail, and then rehabilitate the patient. After healing, you may then unlock the nail distally, apply an external fixator, and perform a corticotomy, at a level other than the original osteotomy, around the nail for LON, being sure to leave sufficient nail beyond the osteotomy at the end of lengthening.
- Corticotomy can be done around an existing nail and is sometimes necessary as a treatment for premature consolidation. Repeat corticotomy around a femoral nail requires one lateral incision and one anterior incision. For the tibia, use one anterior incision (for the medial and lateral cortices) and one posteromedial incision (for the posterior cortices.)

1.1.3 Surgical Anatomy

- The surgeon must be experienced with all aspects of intramedullary nailing and also with the use of external fixators for lengthening. Most of the surgery is very "percutaneous" so the relevant anatomic considerations are fairly straightforward.
- Cutaneous nerves to avoid in femur LON include the lateral femoral cutaneous nerve. Deep nerves to avoid include the femoral nerve and the sciatic nerve.
- Fascia lata: The fascia lata is a thick tendon band linking the pelvis to the proximal tibia. It resists lengthening and, as it tightens, can lead to posterolateral rotary subluxation and lateral patellar mal-tracking. We recommend sectioning the fascia lata at the start of every femoral lengthening. The level of section is the superior pole of the patella. If you do it more proximally, then an unsightly myofascial hernia results.

1.1.4 Positioning

- Place the patient supine on a radiolucent table, with the foot approximately close to the end of the table. Position a bump under the ipsilateral hemisacrum to help maintain the patella forward position and to elevate the femur of the table for femoral lengthening. For femoral lengthening, confirm the ability to obtain orthogonal views of the hip on image intensifier prior to preparing the field and draping the extremity.
- Pearls: Do not place the hip bump under the buttock, as this will compress the sciatic nerve. Instead, position the bump under the bony hemisacrum.

1.1.5 Procedure: Femoral Lengthening

1. Preoperative planning
- Choose a femoral nail, either trochanteric entry or piriformis entry. For normal femoral neck anatomy and a wide canal, piriformis entry (straight nail) is reasonable. For

smaller patients, especially with abnormal anatomy of the proximal femur, trochanteric entry nails are preferable. For example, a short femoral neck is a contraindication for piriformis entry. In skeletally immature patients, always use a trochanteric entry nail, in order to avoid injury to the blood supply to the femoral head, and subsequent avascular necrosis. Plan the placement of the external fixation pins on the sagittal view of the hip. The best place for proximal pin placement is in the lesser trochanter. Some very small individuals may not have enough room for proximal pin placement and therefore are not candidates for femoral LON. Choose the osteotomy level, for most cases without deformity, at a level about 4–5 cm below the lesser trochanter. The level of the osteotomy is chosen in concert with the length of the nail and the desired lengthening amount. At the end of lengthening, there should be at least 10 cm of nail distal to the osteotomy to maintain stability.

2. Step 1: Soft tissue release
   - Release the fascia lata distally at the superior pole of the patella. This is done through a 2 cm longitudinal incision, anterolaterally, under sterile tourniquet control. Elevate the subcutaneous tissue from the fascia lata anteriorly to the midline and laterally to the intermuscular septum (between quads and hamstrings). Make a transverse incision in the fascia lata about 1 cm long with a scalpel and then insert a Metzenbaum scissor to dissect the deep surface of the fascia lata from the vastus lateralis anteriorly to the midline and laterally to the intermuscular septum. Now cut the fascia lata to the midline anteriorly and to the intermuscular septum, including a small amount (~1 cm) of the intermuscular septum as well. Deflate the tourniquet, obtain hemostasis, irrigate, and close the wound.

3. Step 2: Femoral starting point (Fig. 1.1B)
   - Obtain a starting point for the nail under biplanar image intensifier control. Using a 1.8 mm Ilizarov wire as a probe helps to

function as a minimally invasive "try before you buy" technique. Once the ideal starting point and trajectory on the skin has been determined, make a 2.5 cm longitudinal incision and spread with a straight hemostat down to the level of the desired starting point (piriformis or greater trochanter). Next, insert a Steinmann pin (more stable than a Kirschner wire) into the starting point, under careful biplanar image intensifier control, to a depth of about 5 cm. Drill over the Steinman pin with an 8 mm cannulated ACL reamer to broach the cortex. Now insert a beaded guidewire for reaming with a slight prebend in the distal end. Check the position on AP/LAT image intensifier views.
   - Pearls
     - The C-arm (image intensifier) should be positioned with the receiver on the bottom. Obtain a cross-table lateral view by swinging the image intensifier under the table. Placing an extra drape on the surgeon side of the table helps to maintain sterility during this maneuver.
     - The C-arm should be draped not only with a clear plastic sterile pouch but also with a half sheet draped like a skirt around the boom arm. Alternatively, a special drape such as the "C-Armor" (CFI Medical, Fenton, Michigan, USA) may be used.

4. Step 3: Fenestrate the osteotomy site (Fig. 1.1A)
   - At the preoperatively determined osteotomy level, make a 1 cm lateral, longitudinal incision and dissect through the vastus lateralis with a straight hemostat to the lateral aspect of the femur. Insert a small periosteal elevator (5 mm wide) and elevate the periosteum anteriorly and posteriorly, including the linea aspera. Elevating the periosteum helps create a pocket for the bone reamings to accumulate. Now drill transversely with a 4.8 mm solid drill bit bicortically across the osteotomy site. Remember to withdraw the beaded guidewire sufficiently to allow the drill to pass! Through the same entrance drill hole,

angle the drill anteriorly and posteriorly to drill at least two additional exit holes in the far cortex. Fenestrating the osteotomy site decreases the intramedullary pressure during reaming, making fat embolism less likely. It also allows for egress of reamings, which accumulate around the osteotomy and function as a pre-positioned autologous bone graft.

- Pearls: If you use a smaller drill bit than 4.8 mm diameter for fenestration, be careful not to bend the drill while redirecting it, as this may cause it to break. This requires withdrawing the drill bit to the level of the near cortex before reorienting it.

5. Step 4: Femoral reaming (Fig. 1.1C)

- After fenestrating the femoral shaft at the osteotomy level, reinsert the guidewire distally, about 3 cm beyond the planned tip of the length of the chosen nail. Begin reaming with an 8 mm flexible reamer, and increase in size by 0.5 mm increments until you have reamed 2 mm greater than the diameter of the planned nail diameter. For example, for an 8.5 mm nail, ream to 10.5 mm. For a 10.0 mm nail, ream to 12.0 mm.

- Pearls: Ream slowly, and keep the reamer turning always, to prevent incarceration. Back the reamer in and out to help direct the reamings out through the fenestrated osteotomy site. At the end of reaming, you should be able to visualize on the image intensifier a "cloud" of reamings surrounding the osteotomy level. This functions as a pre-positioned bone graft and aids in healing of the regenerate bone. You may also collect the reamings that remain attached to the reamer heads as you retract them from the bone. These reamings can be inserted via a cannula/drill guide into the osteotomy site prior to closing.

6. Step 5: Application of external fixator (Fig. 1.1F)

- This is the most challenging part of the operation. Reinsert a reamer equal to the diameter of the proposed nail, and position it in the canal at the level of the lesser trochanter. This will show you the path of the nail on the lateral view on the image intensifier, so that you can miss it with your external fixation.

- With the image intensifier in the lateral position, visualize the lesser trochanter, and make a 1 cm incision in the skin at that level. Dissect with a straight hemostat to the bone.

- Insert a 1.8 mm wire on the lesser trochanter, perpendicular to the long axis of the femur. Leave enough room to accommodate the insertion of two half pins, and allow sufficient space between the wire and the reamer so that there will be no direct contact between the 6 mm half pin and the intramedullary nail. The distance between the two half pins should be the distance between two holes in the external fixation pin clamp that you select (in case of a monolateral fixator) or the distance between two holes on a Rancho cube (Smith Nephew, Memphis, Tennessee, USA) in the case of an Ilizarov fixator.

- Once the 1.8 mm wire is drilled into place, carefully check its position ("try before you buy"). Once satisfied, ream over it with a 4.8 mm cannulated drill bit, and then insert a 6.0 mm hydroxyapatite-coated stainless steel pin (more stable than titanium pins). Check once again with the image intensifier to make sure that there is no contact between the half pin and the reamer head. Ideally, there should be at least 2–3 mm space between the external fixation half pin and the nail. Repeat this sequence so that there are two parallel pins in the lesser trochanter.

- Next, insert two distal pins in line with the proximal two pins. The position of the two distal pins may be distal to the intended nail length or posterior to where the reamers ended distally. Occasionally, the specific anatomy for a given patient may lead you to place the pins anterior to the nail or in a special anatomic feature, such as old fracture callus.

- It is important to be ready to improvise, both with fixator pin placement and with the fixator itself. For example, it may be necessary to use "sandwich" clamps in monolateral fixators to have the distal pins and the proximal pins at different levels in the sagittal plane.

- In the end, the construct will consist of two proximal pins at the lesser trochanter and two distal pins in the distal metaphysis, all of whom are parallel to each other and perpendicular to the anatomic axis of the femur/intramedullary nail. In cases where a derotational osteotomy was planned, the distal pins would have been inserted at the amount of rotation desired. Lengthening along the anatomic axis is a necessity in femoral LON, but rarely creates clinically significant mechanical axis deviation.

7. Step 6: Osteotomy and nail insertion (Fig. 1.1G-I)

- Withdraw the beaded guidewire to a point just proximal to the fenestration holes that mark the intended site of the osteotomy. Complete the osteotomy with a small osteotome.
- Demonstrate that the osteotomy will translate in two directions, to insure that it is complete. Reinsert the guidewire past the completed osteotomy.
- Load the intramedullary nail onto its insertion jig, and insert it over the guidewire. It should enter the canal relatively easily, without excessive force. Lock proximally. The four half pins that were inserted parallel to each other prior to the osteotomy help to maintain the correct rotational alignment. Once the nail is locked, remove the insertion jig, and mount the external fixator onto the half pins.
- If desired, test the distraction by acutely distracting about 5 mm. Take an image intensifier picture of the osteotomy before and after the test distraction. Undo the distraction.

1.1.6 Postoperative Care

1. Problems

- Infections are common. Most are superficial pin site infections that seldom lead to deep osteomyelitis. Oral antibiotics usually suffice. Serious cases do occur. Toxic shock syndrome and necrotizing fasciitis have been reported. These patients present ill, with loss of appetite, decreased activity, and febrile. A diffuse rash may be present with toxic shock syndrome. Urgent attention is required, with urgent and aggressive resuscitation and initiation of empiric intravenous antibiotics.
- Institute physical therapy for passive knee flexion and extension. Splint the knee in extension at night. Allow "partial weight bearing" (the weight of the leg, which is generally considered as 1/6 of body weight). Consider electrical stimulation of the quadriceps to maintain tone. Supervised physical therapy should be done daily during the week and with the family on weekends.
- Begin distraction after a latency period of 5 days (Fig. 1.1J). Lengthen at a rate of 0.25 mm QID. Later on, this rate may be adjusted up or down depending on bone formation and knee flexion. One strategy to consider is to slightly overlengthen (by up to 1 cm) and then shorten. This compresses the regenerate bone and may speed healing.
- Fixator removal/locking (Fig. 1.1K-L): Once the desired length has been achieved, the patient returns to the operating room for locking of the rod and external fixator removal. It is important to insert the distal interlocking screws *before* removing the external fixator, in order to maintain length. Ideally, preoperative planning included an estimation of where the locking holes in the distal end of the nail would be at the end of lengthening, relative to the external fixator pins. In the operating room, position the patient supine with a bump under the ipsilateral hemisacrum, and bring the image intensifier to the true lateral position, to confirm that you can see "perfect circles" for the distal interlocking sights. If necessary, portions of the external fixator can be modified to provide better visualization and access. For example, the pin trolleys can be locked to the rail, and the compression/distraction rod removed. Such modifications should be

completed before prepping and draping. If the external fixation pins are close by the locking site, it may be advisable to insert the locking screws from the medial side, to avoid surgical proximity to the colonized pin sites. This may be problematic in the diaphysis, due to proximity of the femoral artery. In order to minimize the risk of infection after inserting the locking screws, a meticulous prep and drape procedure is recommended: wash the leg and fixator with antimicrobial soap and then rinse with saline or alcohol.

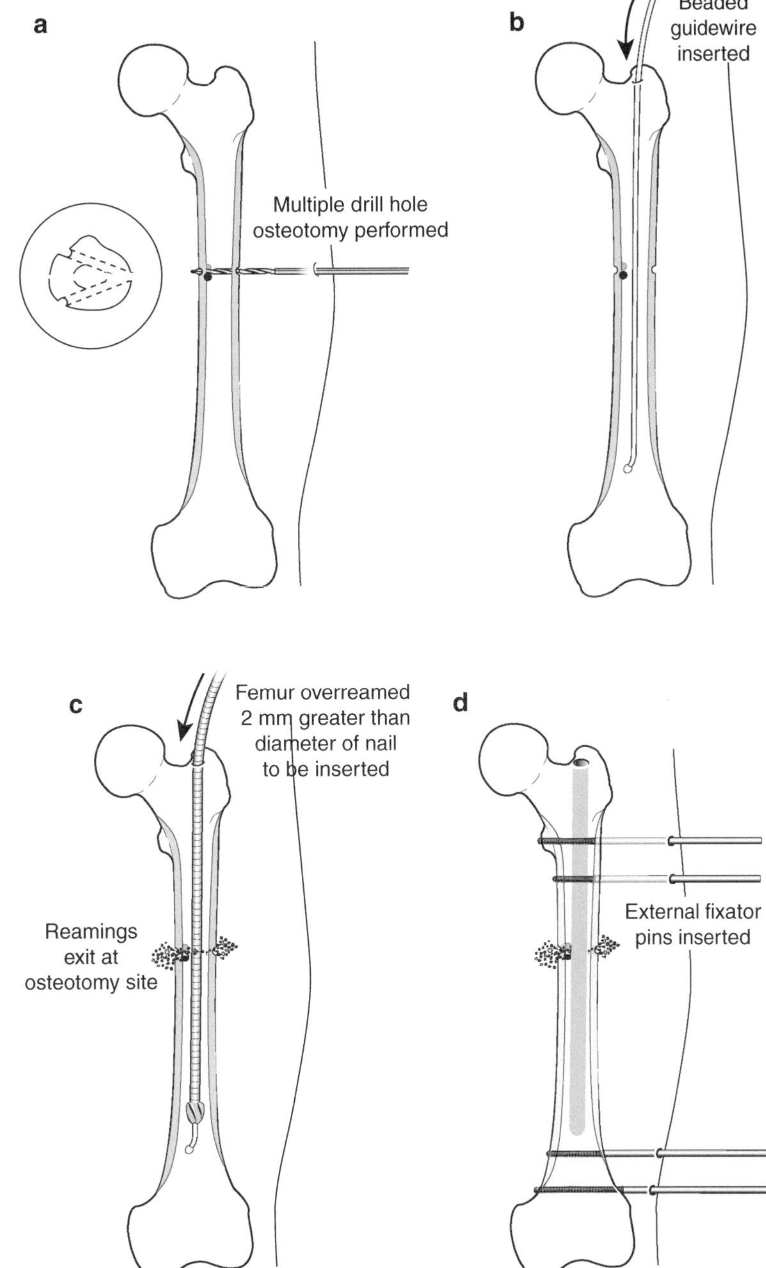

Fig. 1.1 Surgical sequence of femoral LON with a monolateral external fixator. (**a–d**) Initial drilling, reaming, fixator placement. (**e**) Proximal pin placement with wire/cannulated drill/ pin placement at the lesser trochanter. (**f**) Distal pin placement. (**g–j**) Osteotomy, nailing, fixator placement, and lengthening. (**k**) Locking the nail distally after length is achieved. (**l**) External fixator removed (Reprinted with permission from the Rubin Institute for Advanced Orthopedics, Sinai Hospital of Baltimore)

Fig. 1.1 (continued)

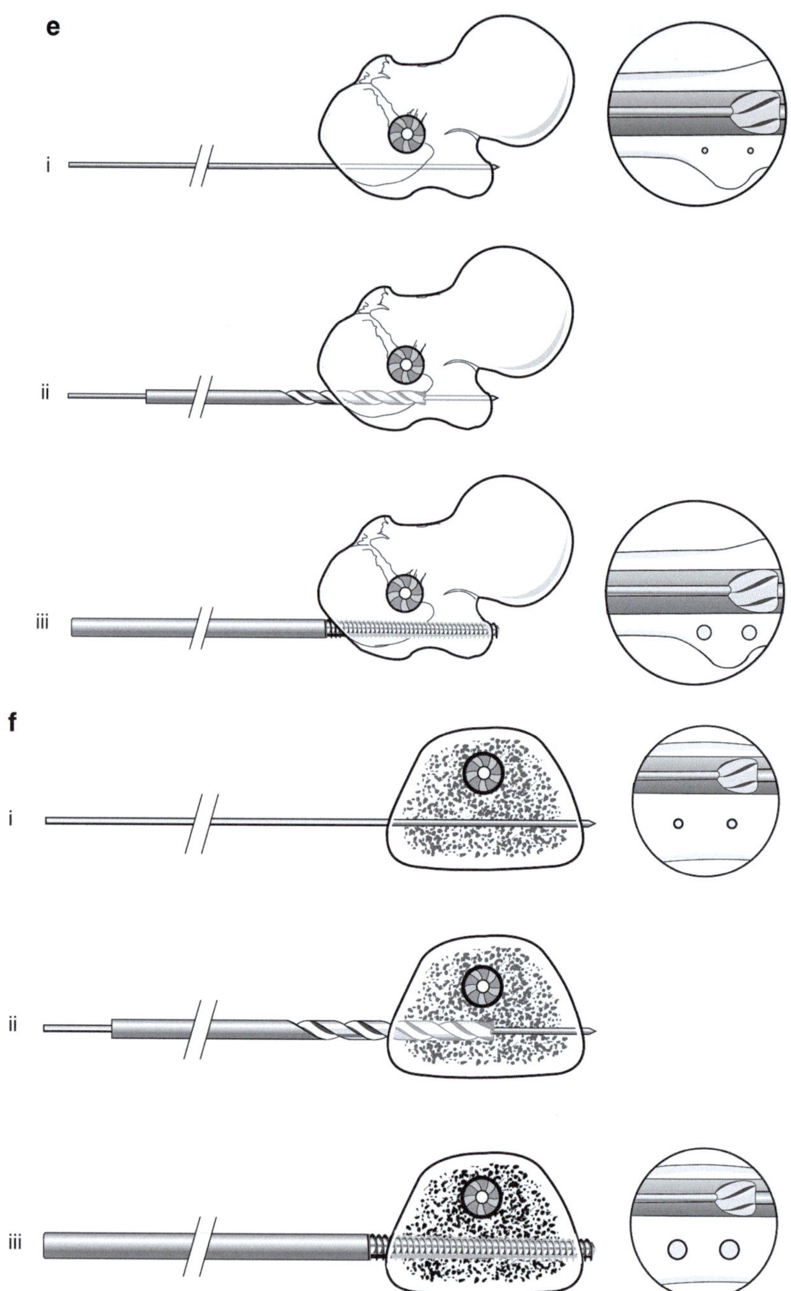

Fig. 1.1 (continued)

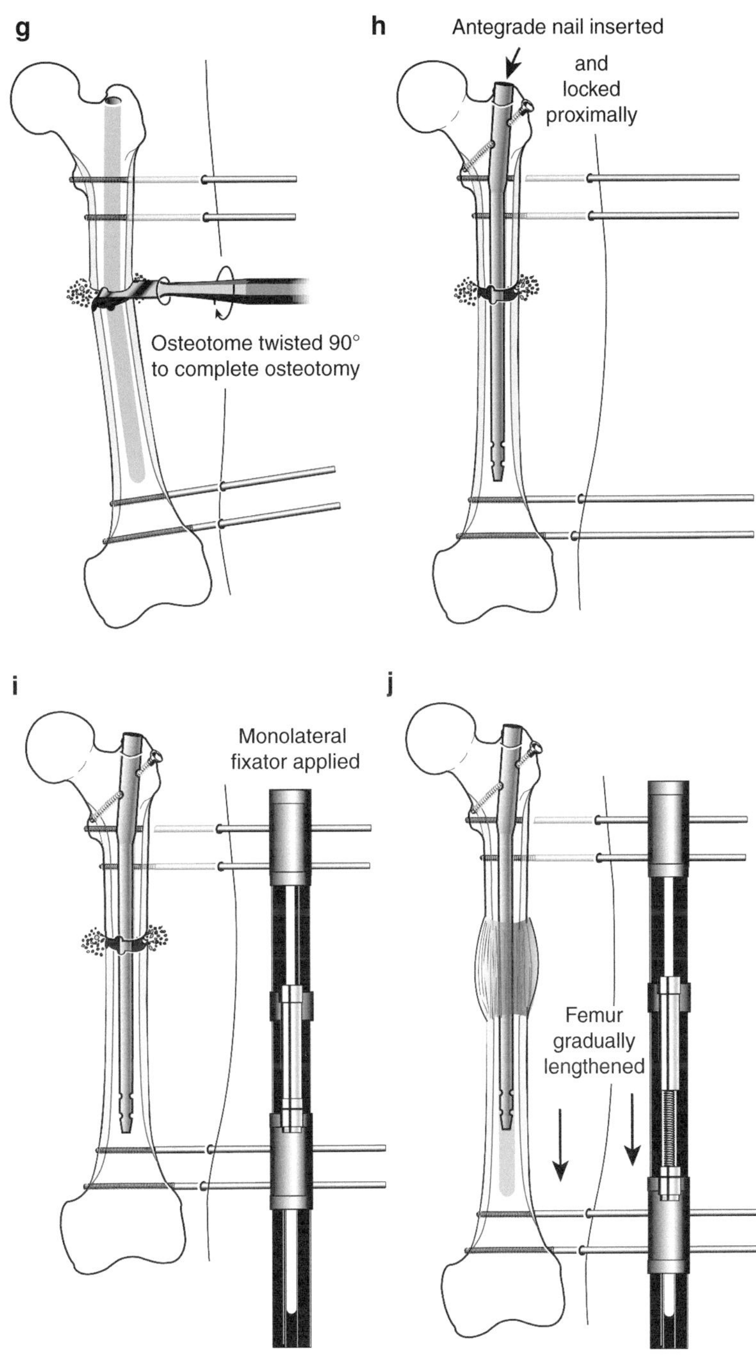

Fig. 1.1 (continued)

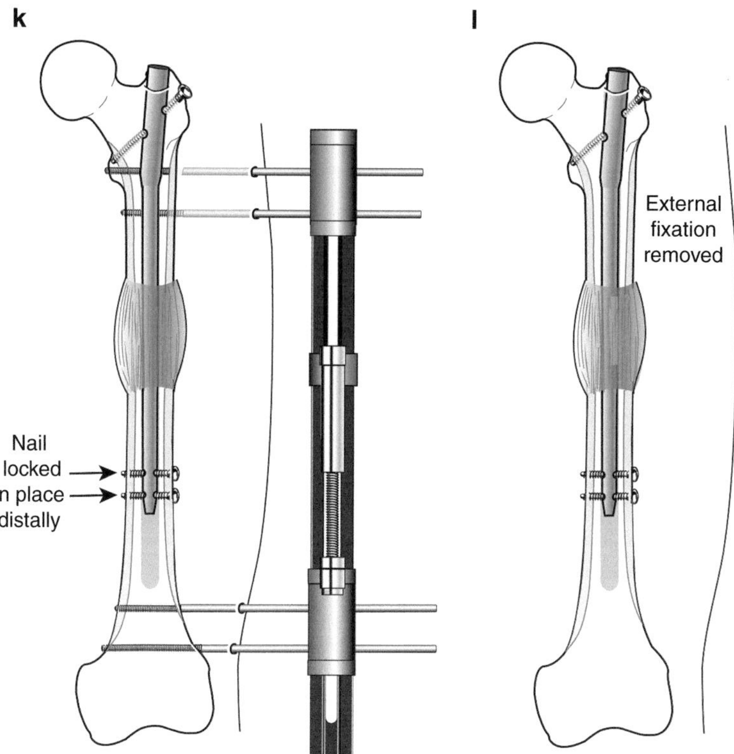

Next, prep the skin and the fixator with an alcohol-based iodine or chlorhexidine solution, painting the pin sites last. Apply sterile drapes, and then take Betadine- or chlorhexidine-moistened sponges and wrap each pin site in them to isolate the contaminated pin-skin interface. Apply sterile towels to those parts of the external fixator that can be covered, minimizing the exposure to less than fully sterile components. Change gloves, and then begin the procedure. Once the interlocking screws are inserted, and the wounds sutured and dressed, the fixator may be removed. Postoperatively, limit weight bearing to 25 % of body weight. Advance to full weight bearing when there is healing in at least two out of four cortices in the AP/LATERAL views of the regenerate bone.

2. Pearls (Fig. 1.2A-F)
   - If regenerate bone formation is poor at the time of distal nail locking and fixator removal, consider concentrated bone marrow injection to the regenerate. Several commercially available systems are present, such as the BioCUE (Biomet, Warsaw, Indiana, USA) or Magellan (Arteriocyte Medical Systems, Hopkinton, Massachusetts, USA).
   - With a monolateral fixator, the femur is sometimes pushed into varus alignment. Once the rod is locked and the fixator removed, all or part of the varus will realign itself, as there is no longer a moment from the fixator pushing the bone into the varus position.
   - Elective removal of the internal rod may take place 1 year later, provided there is healing of all four cortices as seen on AP/LATERAL radiographs. Dynamization can be performed by removing the distal locking screws provided at least two cortices are solidly healed.
   - Deep infection can occur early or late. If early, then use suppressive antibiotics until all the length is achieved. When locking, consider nail exchange for an antibiotic-impregnated cement-coated locked nail. Alternatively,

lock the original nail, with plans to do a nail exchange when the pin sites are well healed. For late infections (defined as infections that present after there is solid healing of at least two cortices of the bone), rod exchange with an antibiotic-impregnated bone cement-coated chest tube nail (with a guidewire core) can be done. When exchanging an infected nail,

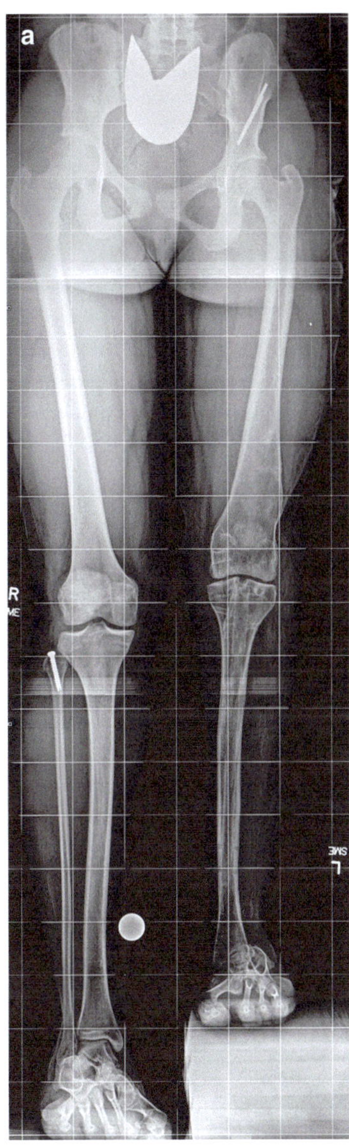
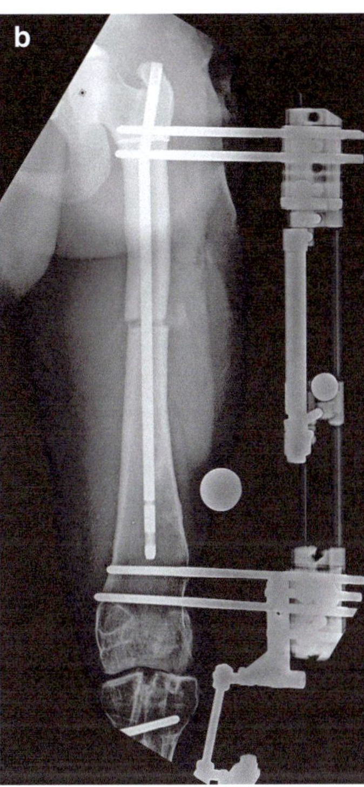
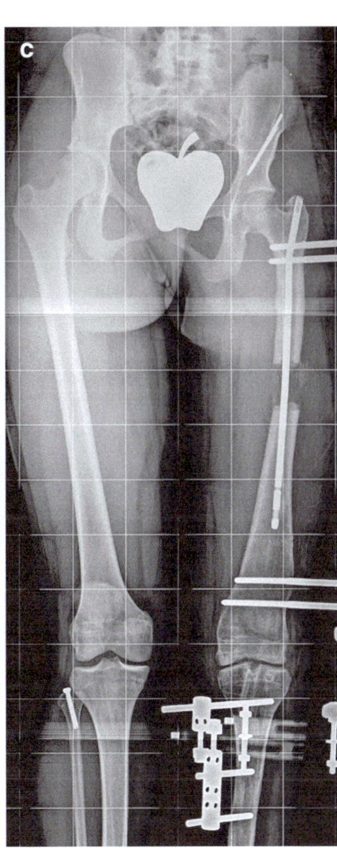

Fig. 1.2 A 15-year-old girl with congenital femoral deficiency who presented with 11 cm discrepancy. She has previously undergone lengthenings and hip and knee reconstructive surgery. (**a**) Preoperative erect legs standing view with 10 cm lift under the short leg. No mechanical axis deviation. (**b**) Immediate postoperative view with nail/fixator in place. Note the fixator bridging across the knee, hinged, to allow joint motion without subluxation. (**c**) After 5 cm lengthening, the nail has risen up but still has sufficient length in the distal segment for stability. (**d**) After nail distal locking and external fixator removal. Concentrated bone marrow was injected into the regenerate bone at the same time. (**e**) Six weeks later, the regenerate bone is much more visible. (**f**) Six months after frame removal, the healing is complete. This patient subsequently underwent tibial LON for final equalization (Reprinted with permission from the Rubin Institute for Advanced Orthopedics, Sinai Hospital of Baltimore)

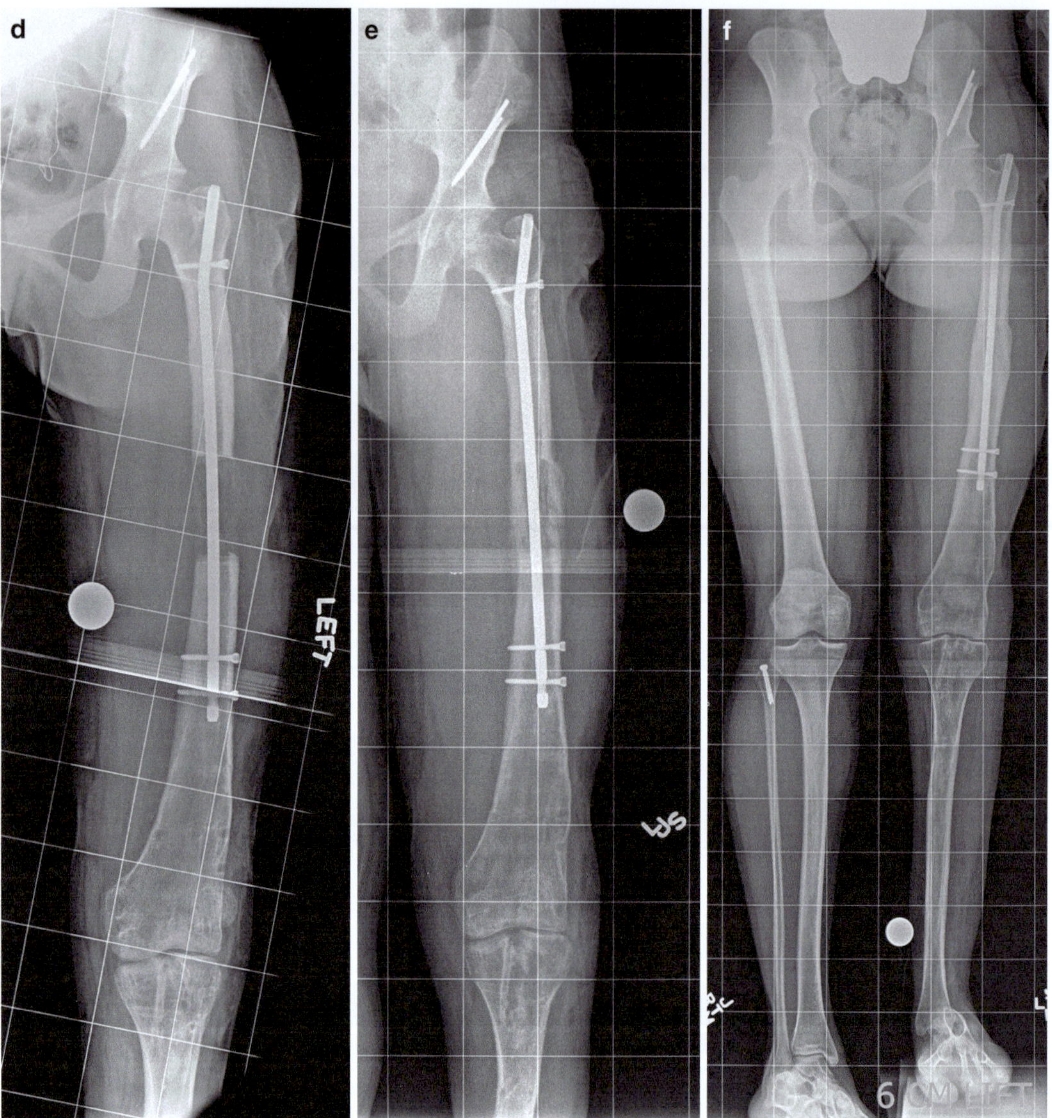

Fig. 1.2 (continued)

thorough reaming of the canal and debridement of sinus tracts is required.

1.2 Tibial LON

1.2.1 Indications

1. Tibial LON is indicated for skeletally mature individuals with leg length discrepancy of up to 10 cm in straight bones (no deformity), a reamable intramedullary canal, and no active infection.
   - A stable knee and ankle are prerequisite. It is possible to bridge with the external fixator across the foot to prevent equinus/subluxation.
   - In the face of knee instability, it may be necessary to do a preliminary, staged ligamentous reconstruction procedure.
   - Tibial LON is almost always done with antegrade nailing. Occasionally, retrograde nailing is indicated, as in the case of a

fused ankle that can be nailed from the bottom up. Simultaneous ankle fusion and diaphyseal tibial lengthening may be accomplished with the LON technique.

2. For select patients, mild to moderate angular or rotational deformities may be acutely corrected with the intramedullary nail.

- Proximal femur deformities of mild severity, less than 10° (varus, valgus, rotation), can be corrected through a proximal tibial osteotomy that will also function as the lengthening site.
- Diaphyseal and distal metadiaphyseal deformities need to undergo preliminary correction and nailing, to be followed 6–12

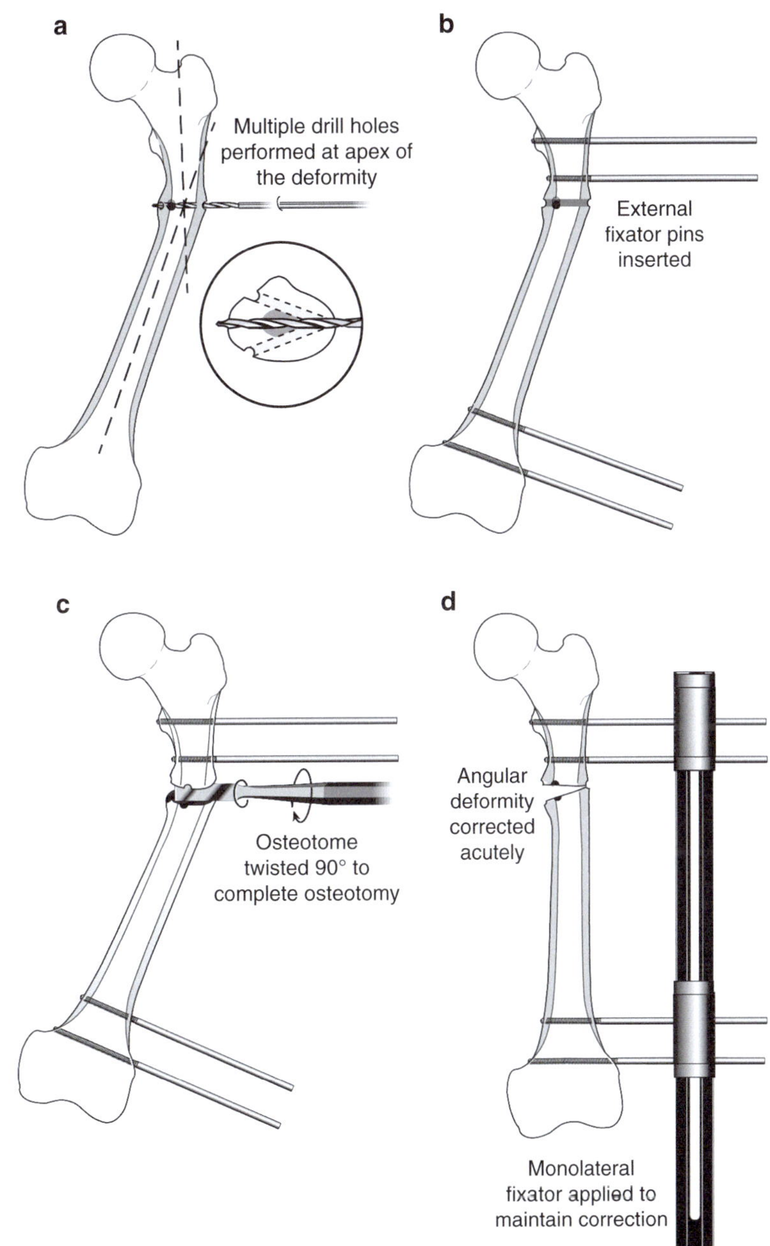

Fig. 1.3 Surgical sequence of femoral LON with simultaneous acute deformity correction (FAN). (**a–d**) Initial drilling, fixator placement, osteotomy, and acute correction. (**e–g**) Guidewire placement, reaming, and nail insertion. (**h**) Lengthening. (**i**) Locking the nail distally after length is achieved. (**j**) External fixation removed (Reprinted with permission from the Rubin Institute for Advanced Orthopedics, Sinai Hospital of Baltimore)

Fig. 1.3 (continued)

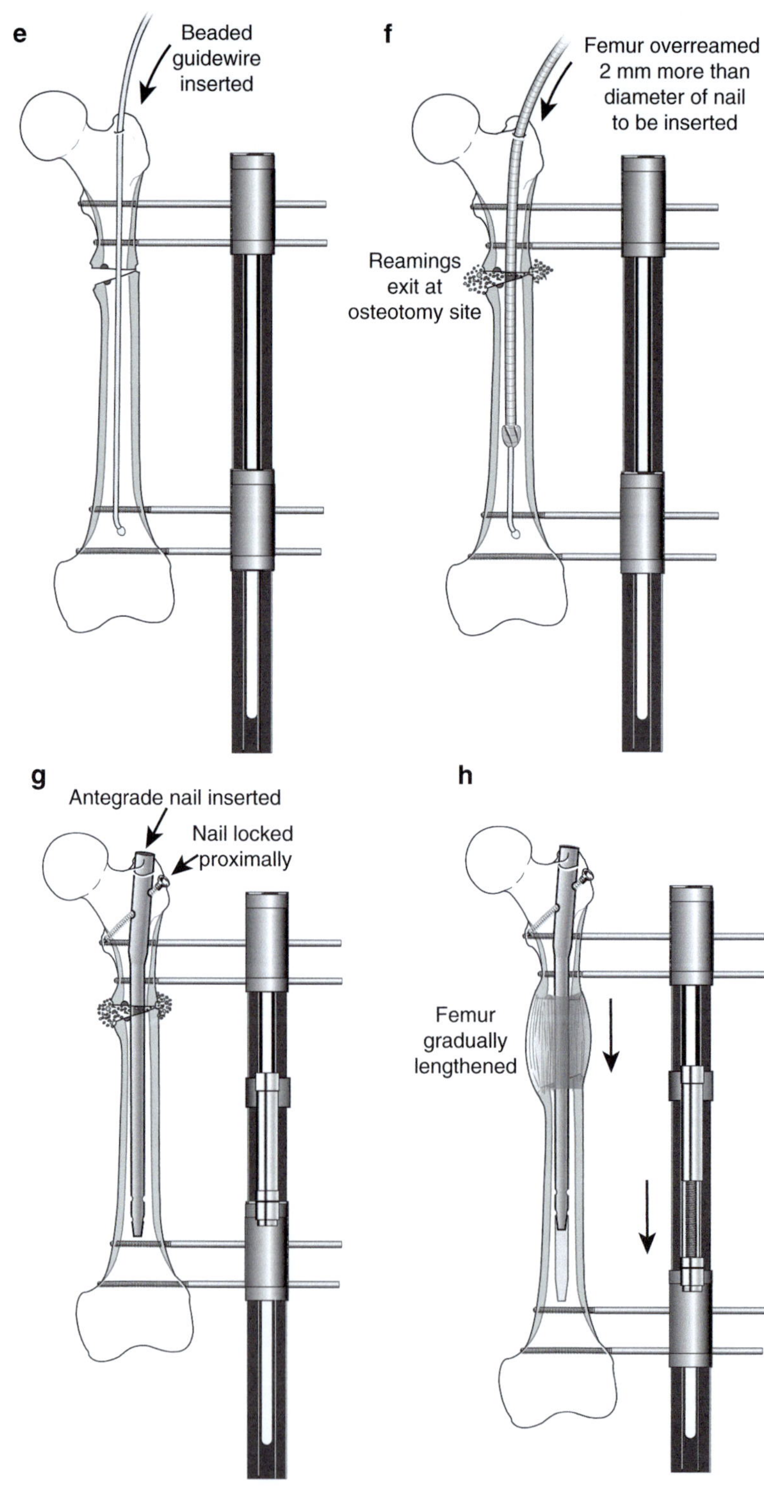

Fig. 1.3 (continued)

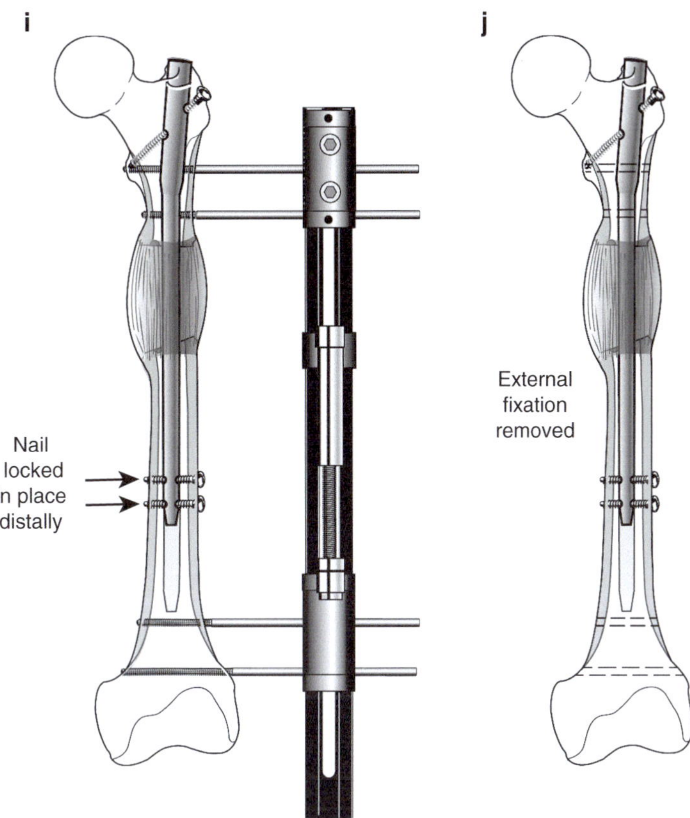

months later by LON. In such cases, once the osteotomy is healed, the nail is unlocked distally, a corticotomy is done around the nail in the proximal metadiaphysis, and external fixator is mounted on the tibia for LON.

- The decision to correct deformities with a nail, often called "fixator-assisted nailing" or FAN, is discussed elsewhere in this book. In some cases, FAN can be combined with simultaneous LON. The osteotomy must be planned to be at a level that will take into account the final position of the end of the nail tip after it has fully retracted at the end of lengthening. The nail tip must be at least 10 cm beyond the lengthening site in order to provide sufficient stability in the far fragment. If the deformity is at a level that would not permit this, then the FAN should be staged, rather than simultaneous with the LON. Another alternative for this is the method known as "lengthening and then nailing" (LATN). For LATN, an external fixator is used to achieve lengthening, and then a locked nail is inserted after lengthening has been achieved to maintain the correction, and allow early removal of the fixator. The biggest challenge for LATN is applying a stable fixator in such a way as not to interfere with subsequent nail insertion.

- Pearl: The primary indication for LATN rather than LON in the tibia is for extensive limb lengthening in dwarfism where the starting length of the bone is very short.

1.2.2 Examination/Imaging

1. Assess the limb length discrepancy (LLD): Ask the patient to stand, feel the iliac crests, and insert various size lifts under the short limb until the iliac crests are palpable at the same level.

2. Assess joints: The hip, knee, and ankle must all be assessed preoperatively for documentation purposes. Limited knee flexion may be a contraindication to nailing the tibia, if the degree of knee flexion would not permit nail insertion. Retropatellar nail insertion may be feasible in cases where knee flexion is limited, provided the surgeon is experienced in retropatellar nailing.

3. Assess muscle function: Preoperative documentation of muscle strength and range is essential.

4. Assess the neurovascular status: It is essential to document neurovascular function before surgery. Neuropraxia, particularly of the peroneal nerve, can develop during tibial lengthening. Document sensation of the saphenous nerve, superficial peroneal nerve, deep peroneal nerve, sural nerve, and medial/lateral plantar nerves. If compromised nerve function is preexistent as a result of scarring or trauma, consider simultaneous nerve decompression (peroneal nerve decompression or tarsal tunnel release).

5. Assess the soft tissues: Scar tissue is less compliant than supple skin and may limit joint motion. Scarring around nerves (as in the tarsal tunnel) from prior surgery may be asymptomatic but can become problematic under the stress of stretching the nerves and scar during limb lengthening. Consider prophylactic tarsal tunnel or peroneal nerve decompression in such cases. Preexisting equinus contracture (less than 10° possible dorsiflexion) of the gastrocsoleus needs to be addressed with a tendon lengthening or recession.

6. Radiographic assessment: Long-leg films with an appropriate size lift under the short leg are required. The ideal film shows both hip joints, both knee joints, and both ankle joints on the same, long, cassette. A magnification marker should be taped to the leg at the level of the bone for accurate measurement of the LLD.
   - Long-leg standing radiographs: Provide information about limb length and frontal plane deformity.
   - Long lateral radiographs of the entire limb: Show sagittal plane deformity and sagittal plane malalignment about the knee.

7. Common radiographic angles:
   - Lateral distal femoral angle (LDFA): Angle defined by the mechanical axis of the femur and the knee joint reference line. Normal is 85–90°.
   - Medial proximal tibial angle (MPTA): Angle defined by the mechanical axis of the tibia and the knee joint reference line. Normal is 85–90°.
   - Lateral distal tibial angle (LDTA): Angle defined by the long axis of the tibia in the coronal plane and the distal tibia plafond. Normal is 86–92°.
   - Anterior distal tibial angle (ADTA): Angle defined by the long axis of the tibia in the sagittal plane and the distal tibia plafond. Normal is 78–82°.

8. Pearls:
   - In the presence of complex deformity of the tibia, do a preliminary operation to straighten the bone, transfix it with a locked IM nail, and then rehabilitate the patient. After healing, you may then unlock the nail distally, apply an external fixator, and perform a corticotomy, at a level other than the original osteotomy, around the nail for LON.
   - Corticotomy can be done around an existing nail and is sometimes necessary as a treatment for premature consolidation. Repeat corticotomy around a tibial nail requires one anterior incision (for the medial and lateral cortices) and one posteromedial incision (for the posterior cortex).

1.2.3 Surgical Anatomy

- The surgeon must be comfortable and familiar with all aspects of intramedullary nailing and also with the use of external fixators for lengthening. Most of the surgery is very "percutaneous" so the relevant anatomic considerations are fairly straightforward.

- Cutaneous nerves to avoid in tibial LON include the peroneal nerve and its branches, the sural nerve, the saphenous nerve, and the posterior tibial nerve.

- Gastrocnemius-soleus complex: These muscles resist ankle equinus and hindfoot valgus correction. Intramuscular lengthening of the gastrocnemius and soleus (as opposed to lengthening of the white tendo Achilles) allows lengthening and minimizes the risk of excessive loss of power. The usual method is the Vulpius approach through either a direct posterior approach or a posteromedial approach. It should be lengthened in most tibial lengthening cases, especially if greater than 3–4 cm is anticipated.

1.2.4 Positioning

- Place the patient supine on a radiolucent table. A triangle leg positioner may be helpful when flexing the knee. Position the image intensifier on the opposite side of the table, and swing under the drapes for cross-table lateral views. Drape the entire extremity.
- Pearls: Consider prophylactic anterior compartment fasciotomy and Vulpius intramuscular gastrocsoleus recession in all tibial lengthenings.

1.2.5 Procedure: Tibial Lengthening

1. Preoperative planning: Choose a standard tibial trauma nail. Use 8.5 mm diameter for small legs and 10.0 mm for larger legs. The starting point is usually via a patellar tendon splitting approach or parapatellar tendon approach. Choose the osteotomy level, for most cases without deformity, at a level about 3–4 cm below the tibial tuberosity. Higher-level osteotomies in the metaphysis may heal better but have a strong tendency to drift into the procurvatum and valgus. The level of the osteotomy is chosen in concert with the length of the nail and the desired lengthening amount. At the end of lengthening, there should be at least 10 cm of nail distal to the osteotomy to maintain stability.

2. Step 1: Soft tissue release
   - Under tourniquet control, perform a Vulpius or other triceps surae recession/lengthening. This is especially recommended if there is underlying preoperative tightness in the ankle. If the ankle has normal dorsiflexion mobility, and the amount of planned tibial lengthening is modest, then this step may be omitted. A prophylactic anterior compartment fasciotomy is simple and can give the surgeon peace of mind when evaluating postoperative pain complaints.
   - Fasciotomy is done through a 2 cm incision one fingerbreadth lateral to the crest of the tibia. Dissect above and below the fascia proximally and distally. Complete the fasciotomy either with a slightly open Metzenbaum scissors or with a fasciotome.
   - At the midpoint of the fasciotomy, release the anterior compartment fascia medially to the tibial crest and laterally to the intermuscular septum.
   - Deflate the tourniquet after completing the fibular osteotomy (see next section), obtain hemostasis, irrigate, and close the wounds.
   - Pearls: If the anterior compartment fasciotomy is too short, then a painful myofascial hernia may develop. If the fibular osteotomy is done too proximal, retraction damage may occur in the branches of the peroneal nerve. If done too distally, the superficial peroneal nerve is at risk.

3. Step 2: Fibular osteotomy and syndesmotic fixation
   - The ideal place for a fibular osteotomy is at the junction of the middle and distal thirds. More proximally risks damaging the nerve to the EHL during retraction. More distally heals more slowly due to less muscle coverage at the osteotomy site.
   - Make a 3–4 cm longitudinal lateral incision, and dissect the interval between the peroneals and the soleus muscles. Lift the peroneals anteriorly with a deep retractor, hugging the fibula. Dissect the fibula subperiosteally over a 1 cm wide path, circumferentially. Apply two small Hohmann retractors around the fibula to isolate it.
   - Make multiple drill holes transversely or obliquely with a 1.8 mm Ilizarov wire. Complete the fibular osteotomy with an osteotome, and demonstrate (with the image intensifier) that the cut fibular ends

can translate. Deflate the tourniquet, obtain hemostasis, irrigate, and close the fibular osteotomy wound. Stabilize the distal tibial-fibular syndesmosis to protect the ankle mortise during lengthening.

- Pass a 1.8 mm from the fibula to the tibia, 1 cm above the ankle joint, parallel to the ankle mortise. Allow the wire to exit medially through the skin. Make a 1 cm incision at that point. Check with the image intensifier in the lateral position to confirm that the 1.8 mm guidewire is truly capturing both the fibula and tibia and not at the edge of either bone.
- Drill retrograde with a 3.2 mm cannulated drill bit through all four cortices. Select a fully threaded solid screw whose thread length will capture all four cortices of the distal tibia/fibula, but will not protrude excessively. The proximal tibial-fibular syndesmosis is less important to stabilize, as descent of the fibular head is not generally problematic for lengthenings of less than 3 cm.
- For lengthenings over 2–3 cm, consider proximal tibial-fibular syndesmosis stabilization. This can be done with a proximal tibial-fibular wire in the head of the fibula or a 4.5 mm bone screw. For screw fixation, it is sufficient to engage three cortices, leaving the lateral head of the fibula unpenetrated. It is best to wait until after the intramedullary nail has been inserted, to delineate the space and corridors available for the screw/wire. Screw fixation starts with passing a wire from the head of the fibula, behind the nail, and out of the medial side of the tibia. Next, make a small medial incision over the wire, and ream with a 3.2 mm cannulated drill bit through the tibia and into the fibular head. Select a solid (non-cannulated) cortical bone screw, 4.5 mm diameter, and insert it from the medial side.
- Pearls:
  - Better not to rely on a wire from the external fixator to stabilize the distal tibial-fibular syndesmosis. Instead, use a fully threaded, solid bone screw which can remain in place after the LON frame has been removed. The regenerate bone of the fibula is under tension, and so removing the distal syndesmotic fixation

(as in a tibial-fibular external fixation wire) prematurely (before solid healing of the fibular osteotomy) can result in the distal fibula migrating proximally, thus disrupting the ankle mortise.
  - The peroneal nerve is at risk during stabilization of the proximal tibial-fibular syndesmosis. Flex the knee slightly to relax the peroneal nerve, so that the peroneal nerve drapes more posteriorly, away from the fibular head during wire insertion.
4. Step 3: Fenestrate the tibial osteotomy site
- At the preoperatively determined osteotomy level, make a 1 cm anterior, longitudinal incision, and dissect down through the anterior periosteum medially and laterally with a small periosteal elevator (5 mm wide). Elevating the periosteum helps create a pocket for the bone reamings to accumulate, which can act as a pre-positioned bone graft.
- Drill anterior to posterior with a 4.8 mm solid drill bit bicortically across the osteotomy site. Through the same entrance drill hole, angle the drill medially and laterally to drill at least two additional exit holes in the far cortex. Clean the drill bit flutes between passes in order to decrease the heat of drilling.
- Pearls: If you use a smaller drill bit than 4.8 mm diameter, be careful not to bend the drill and break it while repositioning for the second and third pass. This requires withdrawing the drill bit all the way to the level of the near cortex before reorienting it.
5. Step 4: Starting point for tibial nail
- This can be done without tourniquet. Incise directly on top of the patella tendon, 3 cm, from the patella downward. Check the position by placing a Steinmann pin over the center of the tibia on the AP image intensifier view. This will tell you if the insertion point should be through the center of the patella tendon or medial/lateral parapatellar. Incise as indicated, spread, and then insert the Steinmann pin into the starting point, under careful biplanar image intensifier control, to a depth of about 5 cm.
- Drill over the Steinman pin with an 8 mm cannulated ACL reamer to broach the cortex.

Now insert a beaded guidewire with a slight prebend in the distal end. Check the position on AP/LAT image intensifier views.

- Pearls: The C-arm (image intensifier) should be positioned with the receiver on the bottom, coming from the opposite side of the table as the leg that is being operated on. Obtain a cross-table lateral view by swinging the image intensifier under the table. The C-arm should be draped not only with a clear plastic sterile pouch but also with a half sheet draped like a skirt around the boom arm. Placing an extra drape on the surgeon side of the table helps to maintain sterility during this maneuver. Alternatively, use a commercially available draping system such as the "C-Armor" (CFI Medical, Fenton, Michigan, USA).

6. Step 5: Reaming
   - After fenestrating the tibial shaft at the osteotomy level, reinsert the guidewire distally, at least 3 cm beyond the planned tip of the length of the chosen nail.
   - Begin reaming with an 8 mm flexible reamer, and increase in size by 0.5 mm increments until you have reamed 2 mm greater than the diameter of the planned nail diameter. For example, for an 8.5 mm nail, ream to 10.5 mm. For a 10 mm nail, ream to 12 mm.
   - Pearls: Ream slowly, and keep the reamer turning always, so as not to get incarcerated. Back the reamer in and out to help force the reamings out through the fenestrated osteotomy site. At the end of reaming, you should be able to visualize a "cloud" of reamings surrounding the osteotomy level. This functions as a pre-positioned bone graft and greatly aids in healing of the regenerate bone. As the reamer heads are swapped out by the surgical technician or scrub nurse, collect any bits of corticocancellous bone that are trapped in the reamer flutes, and place them in a sterile specimen jar. At the end of the procedure, these bits of autologous bone can be inserted around the osteotomy site to act as bone graft.

7. Step 6: Tibial osteotomy and nail insertion
   - Withdraw the beaded guidewire to a point just proximal to the fenestration holes that mark the intended site of the osteotomy. Complete the osteotomy with a small osteotome. This is easiest to do with the knee straight and the leg lying flat on the table. Demonstrate that the osteotomy will translate in two planes, to insure that it is complete.
   - Reduce any displacement and reinsert the guidewire past the completed osteotomy with the knee flexed. Load the intramedullary nail onto its insertion jig, test the locking guides, and insert the tibial nail over the guidewire. Lock proximally with two locking screws. Once the nail is locked, remove the insertion jig.

8. Step 7: Tibial external fixator application
   - Straighten the knee and apply a prebuilt circular external fixator to the tibia. This should consist of three rings: one proximal at the level just above the tibial tubercle, one distal at the level about 2 cm above the ankle, and a third in the mid diaphysis. The middle ring will be "empty," containing no fixation wires or half pins. It serves as a force transmitter and makes the lengthening rods shorter and thus more stable. Consider where the tip of the nail will start in the distal tibia and where it will end up after lengthening. Ideally the middle ring should not overly the final position of the distal few centimeters of the nail, so that eventual distal locking will not be impeded by the middle ring. The distal two rings are connected by an anterior and posterior threaded rod. The proximal and distal rings are connected by two lengthening rods (either thread rods or graduated telescopic rods). Later on, after the fixation points on the rings have been determined, two additional rods are added proximally and distally, for a total of four vertical elements at each segment.
   - Start by passing a 1.8 mm wire transverse wire behind the nail, perpendicular to it. Tension this wire on the proximal ring. The wire should not touch the intramedullary nail. On the AP view, the lengthening members (rods) should be parallel to the tibial rod.
   - Next, insert a distal transverse tibial wire, distal to the nail tip, and perpendicular to the long axis of the tibia (nail). The length of the fixator may be adjusted to match the wire. Flex and extend the external fixator on the proximal tensioned wire until the fixator

lengthening members become parallel to the rod on the lateral image intensifier view, and fix the wire to the ring in that position.

- Add a second 1.8 mm tensioned wire to the distal ring, either parallel to the medial face of the tibia or as a tibiofibular wire. Add a half pin to the proximal ring, suspended off of a cube.
- The "wire/cannulated drill" technique can be used for accurate placement to avoid contact between the proximal half pin and the intramedullary rod, similar to the technique described for half-pin placement in the section above on femoral LON.
- If desired, test the distraction by acutely distracting about 5 mm. Take an image intensifier picture before and after the test distraction. Undo the distraction.

- Pearls: An alternative approach is to use a monolateral fixator from the medial side instead of a circular fixator. The advantage is that the monolateral fixator is less bulky. The disadvantage is that it is trickier to apply correctly. Four medial half pins, two proximal (behind the nail) and two distal to the nail, are inserted. They should be 6 mm stainless steel pins (titanium pins are not sufficiently stiff). Monolateral fixators tend to push the tibia into a valgus position during lengthening, but this generally bounces back after locking the nail and removing the fixator. Blocking screws (pollard screws) in the proximal metaphysis may be inserted to prevent valgus (Figs. 1.4, 1.5, and 1.6).

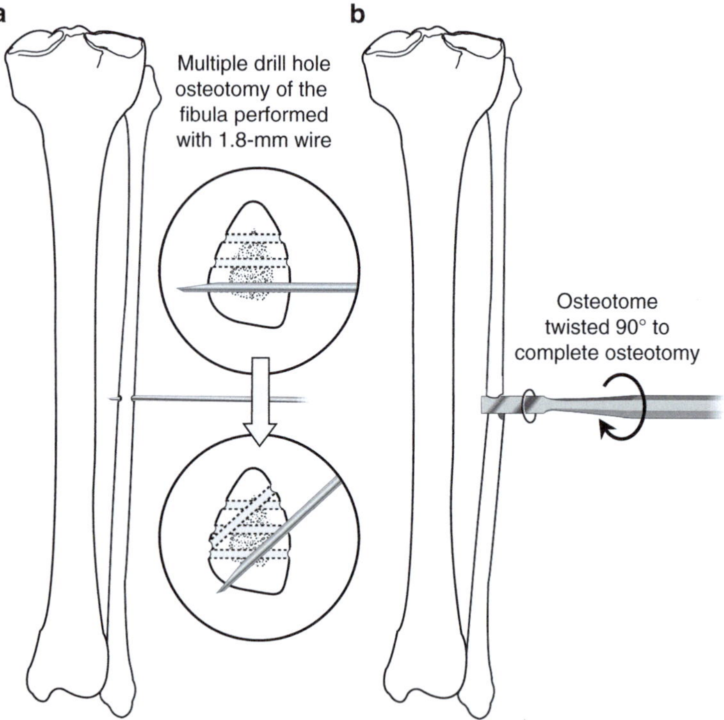

Fig. 1.4 Surgical sequence of tibial LON. (a, b) Initial drilling of osteotomy site. (c) Proximal tibial-fibular fixation with wire followed by cannulated drill followed by fully threaded solid bone screw. This is generally done after the nail is inserted. (d) Same sequence as in "c" for distal tibial-fibular syndesmosis. (e) Reaming, with bone and marrow fragments exiting through the drill holes in the tibia osteotomy site. (f) Cross-sectional view of drill holes made at tibial osteotomy site prior to reaming. (g) After reaming, the osteotomy is completed with an osteotome. (h) Completing the osteotomy by rotating the osteotome. (i) Nail insertion, locking proximally. (j) External fixator applied (see text for details). (k) Cross section of proximal tibia showing half pin placement and tibial-fibular syndesmosis screw placement. (l) Same as "k" but with wire transfixation of tibial-fibular syndesmosis instead of bone screw. (m) Lengthening. (n) Locking the nail distally after length achieved. (o) External fixator removed, but syndesmotic screws left in place to prevent proximal and distal migration of fibula (Reprinted with permission from the Rubin Institute for Advanced Orthopedics, Sinai Hospital of Baltimore)

Fig. 1.4 (continued)

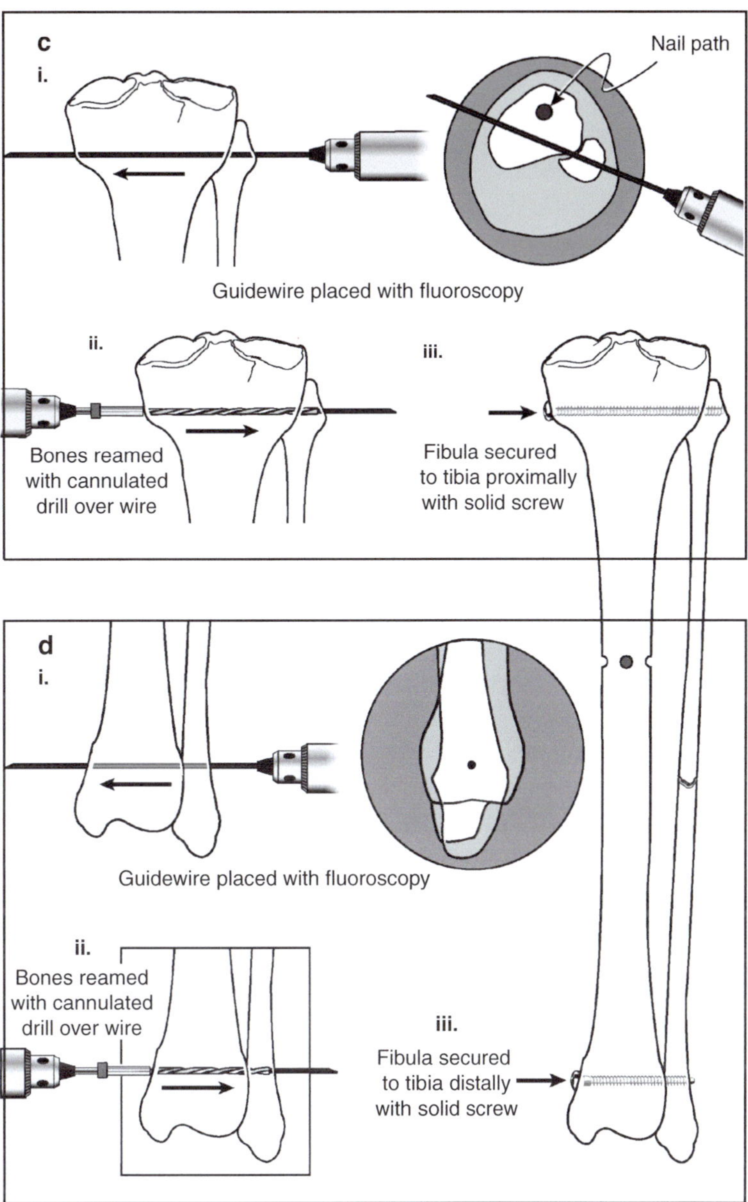

Fig. 1.4 (continued)

e

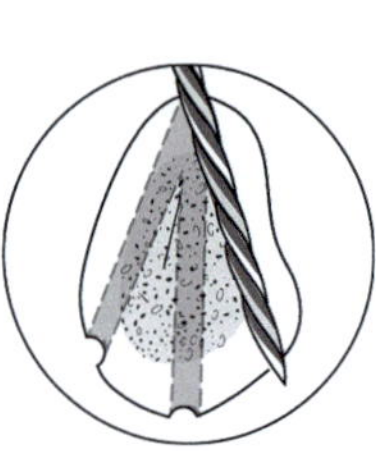

Tibial multiple
drill hole osteotomy
performed
anterior to posterior

f

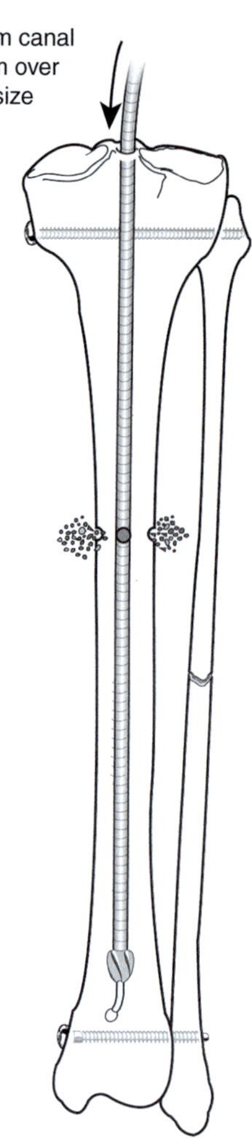

Fig. 1.4 (continued)

g

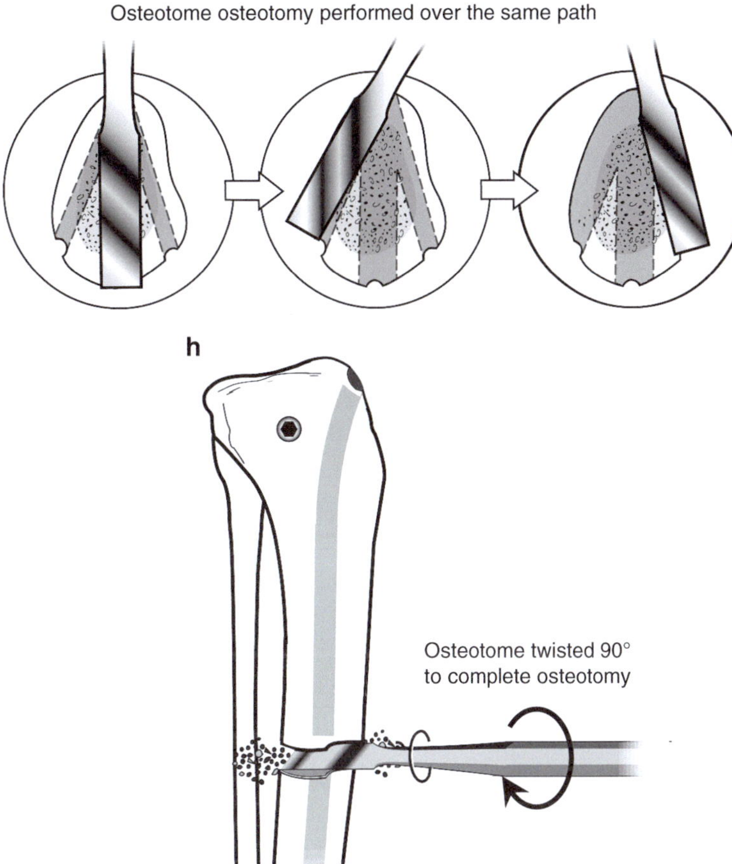

h

Fig. 1.4 (continued)

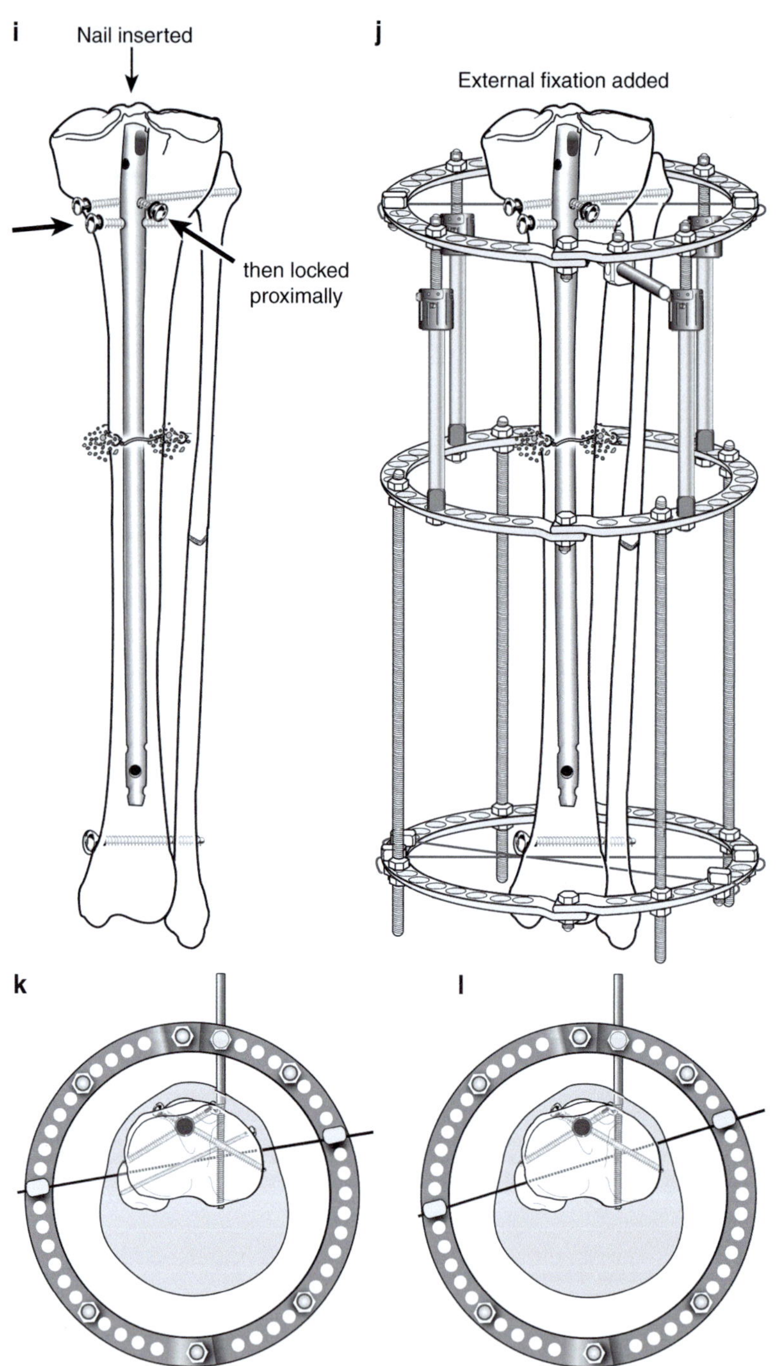

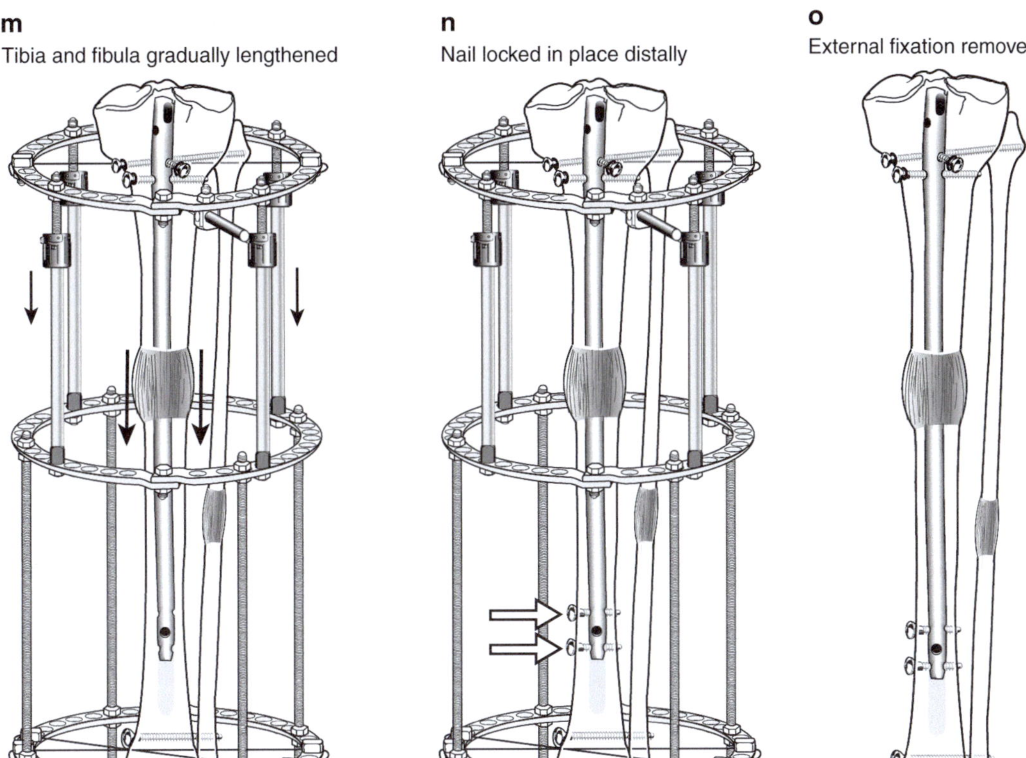

Fig. 1.4 (continued)

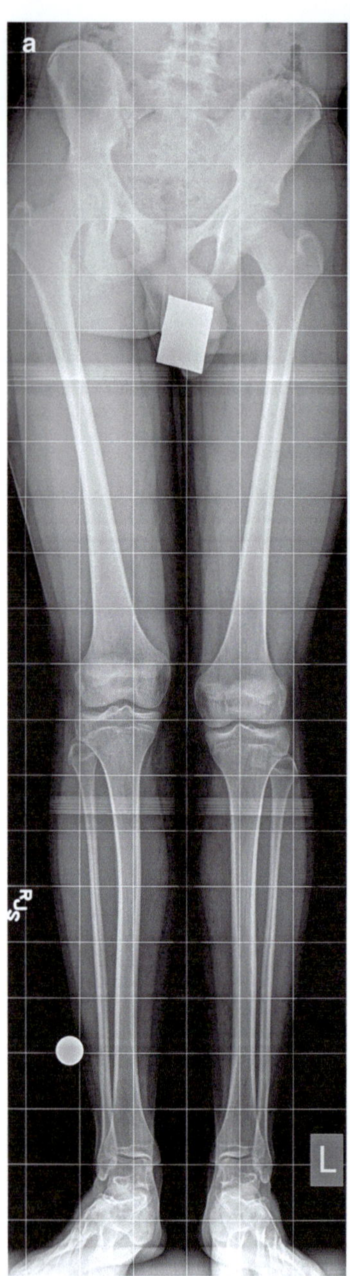
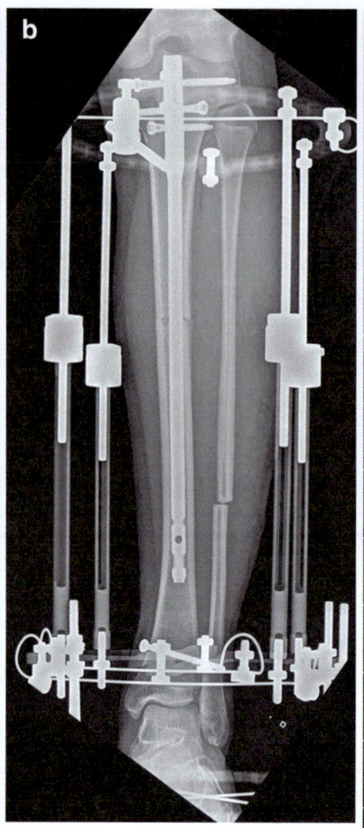
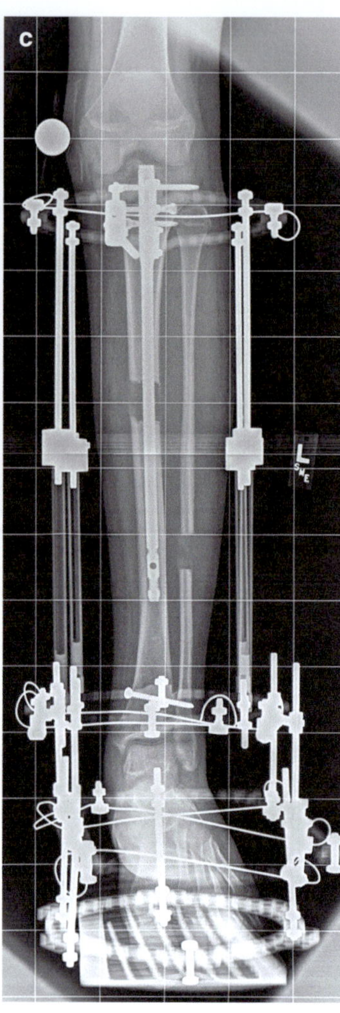

Fig. 1.5 A 17-year-old boy with 3 cm tibial discrepancy on the basis of clubfoot pathology. (**a**) Preoperative erect legs standing view (no lift). (**b**) Immediate postoperative view with nail/fixator in place, spanning across the ankle to prevent equinus. The distal tibial-fibular syndesmosis is transfixed with a bone screw. (**c**) After 3 cm lengthening, the nail has risen up but still has sufficient length in the distal segment for stability. (**d**) After nail distal locking and external fixator removal. The distal tibial-fibular screw prevents the distal fibula from riding up. (**e**) Standing film 4 months after locking, showing complete healing. (**f**) Standing film after hardware removal (Reprinted with permission from the Rubin Institute for Advanced Orthopedics, Sinai Hospital of Baltimore)

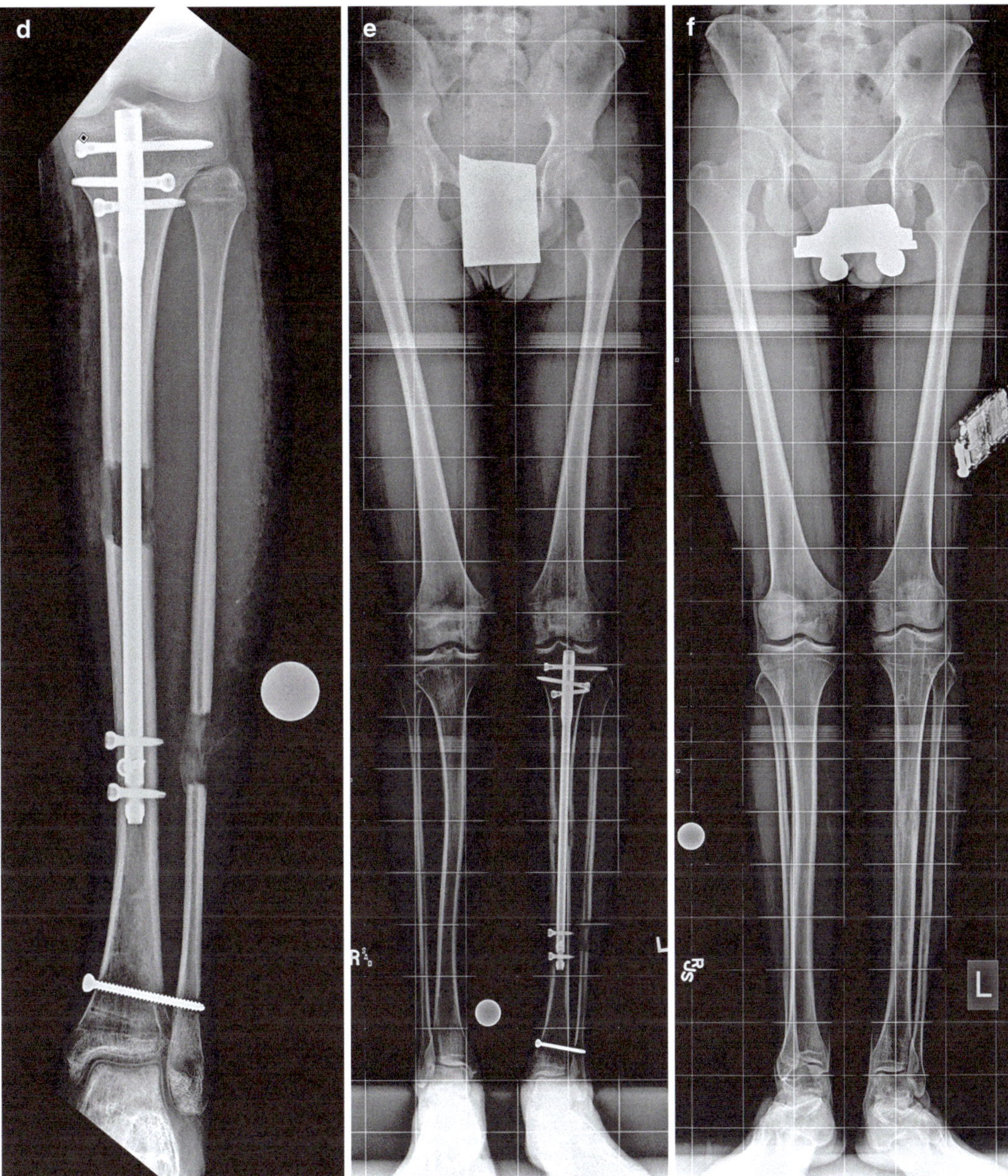

Fig. 1.5 (continued)

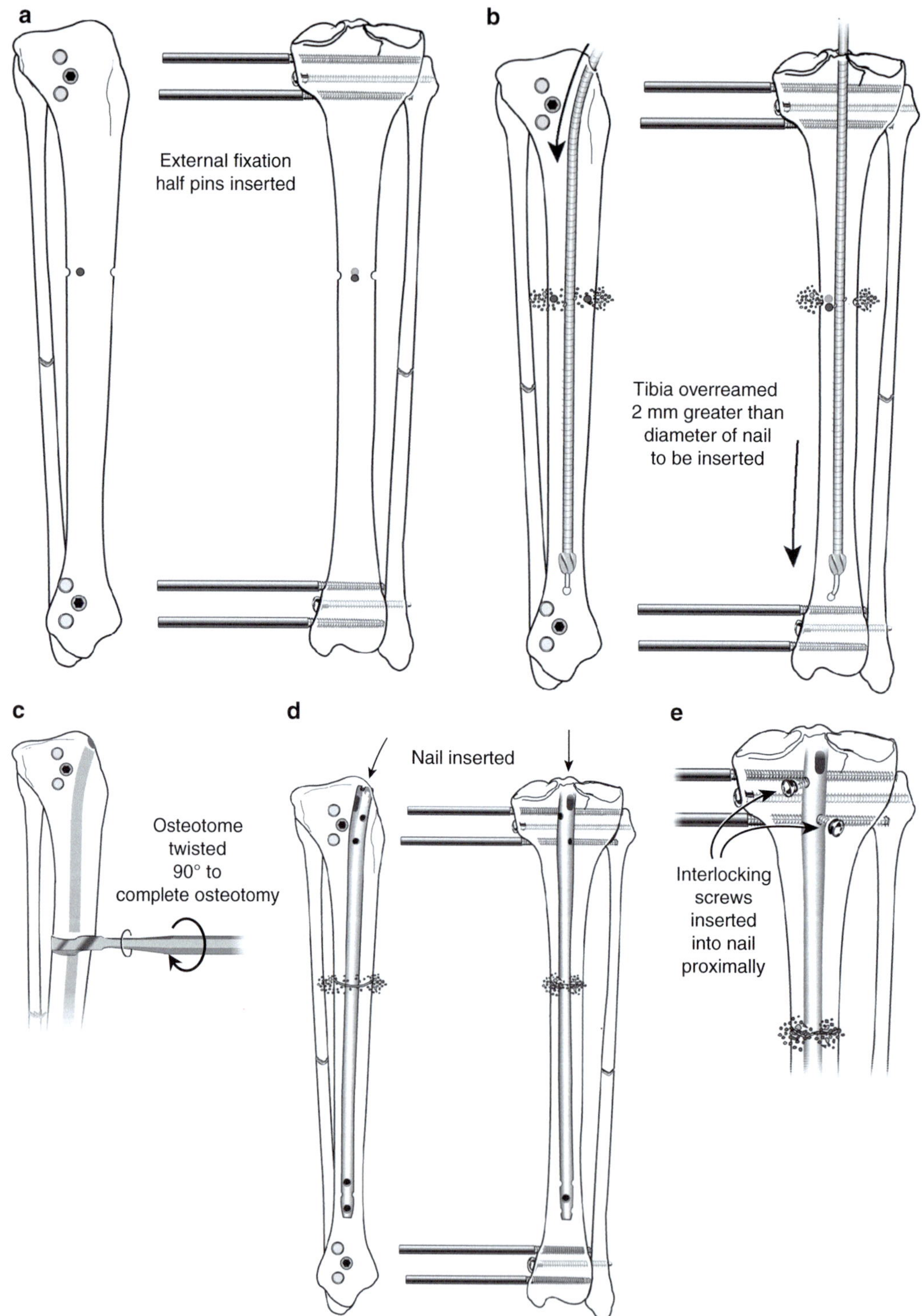

Fig. 1.6 Surgical sequence of tibial LON with monolateral external fixator. (**a**) Initial drilling of osteotomy site, proximal and distal tibial-fibular transfixation, and external fixation half pins inserted (two proximal and two distal). (**b**) Reaming, showing reamings exiting through drill holes. (**c**) Osteotomy completed with an osteotome. (**d**) Nail insertion. (**e**) Locking the nail proximally. (**f**) External fixator applied. (**g**) After lengthening. (**h**) Locking screws applied distally in the nail. (**i**) External fixator removed (Reprinted with permission from the Rubin Institute for Advanced Orthopedics, Sinai Hospital of Baltimore)

Fig. 1.6 (continued)

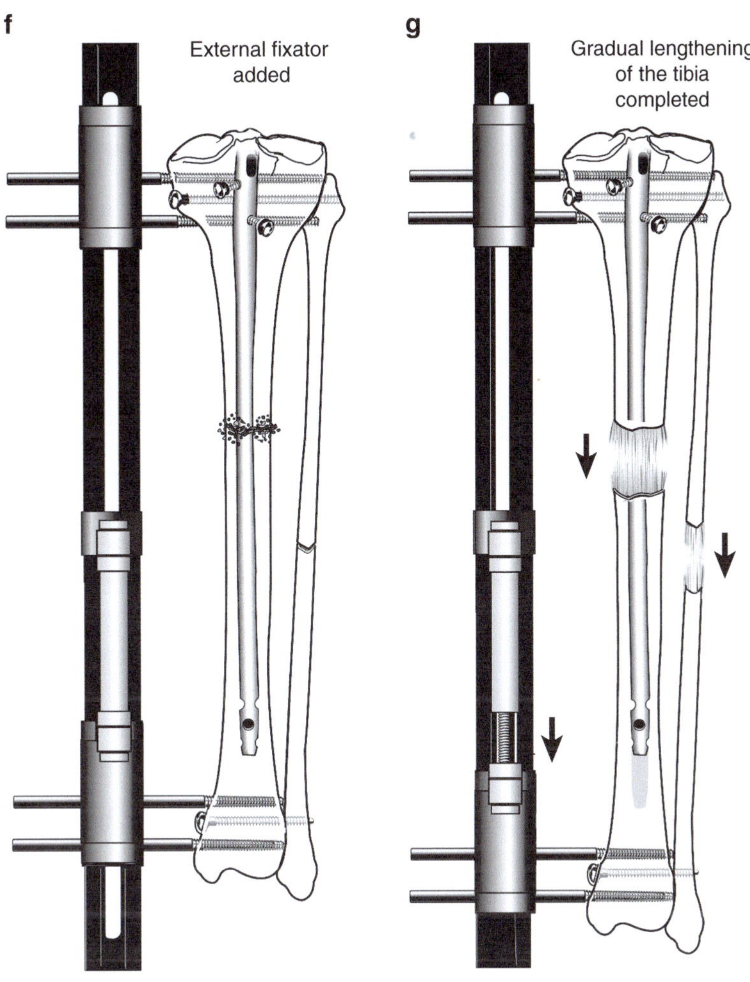

Fig. 1.6 (continued)

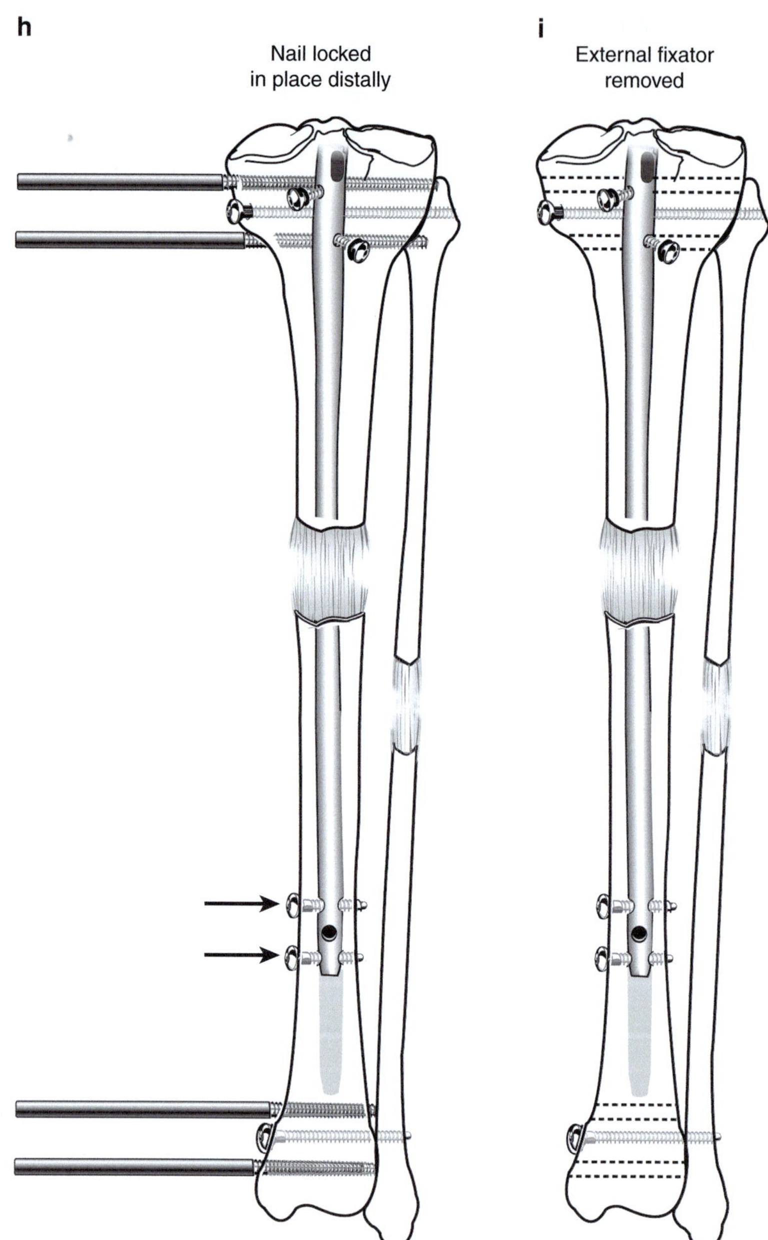

1.2.6 Postoperative Care

1. Problems
   - Infections are common. Most are pin site infections that seldom become osteomyelitis. Oral antibiotics usually suffice. Serious cases do occur. Toxic shock syndrome and necrotizing fasciitis have been reported. These patients present ill, with loss of appetite, decreased activity, and febrile. A diffuse rash may be present with toxic shock syndrome. Urgent attention is required, with urgent and aggressive resuscitation and initiation of empiric intravenous antibiotics.
   - Equinus contractures and knee flexion contractures can occur with tibial lengthening due to stretch on the gastrocsoleus mus-

cles. The foot should be prophylactically splinted in a neutral position. At night, the knee should be positioned in full extension by placing a pillow under the *distal* ring of the external fixator.

- Pearl: An alternate method of foot splinting is to extend the external fixator to the foot by adding a foot ring or heel half ring to the distal part of the tibial frame. Foot fixation may consist of two counter opposed tensioned 1.8 mm olive wires on the calcaneus and a forefoot 1.8 mm tensioned wire.

- Distraction typically begins on postoperative day 7 at a rate of 0.25 mm TID-QID. Follow-up radiographs should be made every 10–14 days, and the rate of distraction adjusted up or down based on the appearance of regenerate bone. One strategy to consider is to slightly overlengthen (by 1 cm) and then shorten, to compress the regenerate bone and speed healing.

- Institute physical therapy the day after surgery for passive knee and ankle flexion and extension. The toes should also be stretched. Allow "touchdown weight bearing" (the weight of the leg, not the body weight). Ideally, supervised physical therapy should be done daily during the week and with the family on weekends.

- Fixator removal/locking: Once the desired length has been achieved, the patient returns to the operating room for locking of the rod and external fixator removal. It is important to insert the two distal interlocking screws *before* removing the external fixator, in order to maintain length. Ideally, preoperative planning included an estimation of where the locking holes in the distal end of the nail would be at the end of lengthening relative to the middle ring. In the operating room, position the patient supine with a bump under the ipsilateral hemisacrum, and bring the image intensifier to the true lateral position, to confirm that you can see "perfect circles" for the distal interlocking sights. If necessary, one or two threaded rods of the external fixator can be removed to provide better visualization and surgical access. Such modifications should be completed before prepping and draping. In order to minimize the risk of infection after inserting the locking screws, a meticulous prep and drape procedure is recommended: wash the leg and fixator with antimicrobial soap, then rinse with saline or alcohol. Next, prep the skin and the fixator with an alcohol-based iodine or chlorhexidine solution, painting the pin sites last. Apply sterile drapes, and then take Betadine- or chlorhexidine-moistened sponges and wrap each pin site in them to isolate the contaminated pin-skin interface. Apply sterile towels to those parts of the external fixator that can be covered, minimizing the exposure to less than fully sterile components. Change gloves, and then begin the procedure. Once the interlocking screws are inserted, and the wounds sutured and dressed, the fixator may be removed. Postoperatively, limit weight bearing to 25 % of body weight. Advance to full weight bearing when there is healing in at least two out of four cortices in the regenerate bone. A fully healed fibula counts as a "cortex."

- If the fibula was transfixed distally by a screw, leave that screw in place until the fibular osteotomy has fully healed. If the fibula was transfixed by an external fixator wire only, then a "permanent" internal tibial-fibular syndesmosis screw should be inserted before removing the distal fibular wire.

2. Pearls
- If regenerate bone formation is noted to be poor at the time of distal nail locking and fixator removal, consider concentrated bone marrow injection to the regenerate.

- After fixator removal, allow partial weight bearing. Progress to full weight bearing when there are two cortices of healed tibia noted on radiographs. A solidly healed fibula "counts" as one cortex. Dynamization by removing the distal locking screws can be done if desired, when there are two cortices intact. For persistent defects in one or two tibial cortices ("partial healing"), consider bone grafting with autologous bone graft. For absent bone formation, the entire volume of tibia around the nail must be grafted.

- One year later, the intramedullary nail can be removed, provided there is healing of all four cortices. The syndesmosis screws can be removed provided the fibula has healed. Nonunion of the fibular osteotomy can be treated with open reduction, bone grafting, and plate fixation.

Bibliography

Bilen FE, Kocaoglu M, Eralp L, Balci HI (2010) Fixator-assisted nailing and consecutive lengthening over an intramedullary nail for the correction of tibial deformity. J Bone Joint Surg Br 92(1):146–152

Chen D, Chen J, Jiang Y, Liu F (2011) Tibial lengthening over humeral and tibial intramedullary nails in patients with sequelae of poliomyelitis: a comparative study. Int Orthop 35(6):935–940

Gordon JE, Goldfarb CA, Luhmann SJ, Lyons D, Schoenecker PL (2002) Femoral lengthening over a humeral intramedullary nail in preadolescent children. J Bone Joint Surg Am 84-A(6):930–937

Guo Q, Zhang T, Zheng Y, Feng S, Ma X, Zhao F (2012) Tibial lengthening over an intramedullary nail in patients with short stature or leg-length discrepancy: a comparative study. Int Orthop 36(1):179–184

Jain S, Harwood P (2012) Does the use of an intramedullary nail alter the duration of external fixation and rate of consolidation in tibial lengthening procedures? A systematic review. Strategies Trauma Limb Reconstr 7(3):113–121

Kim SJ, Mandar A, Song SH, Song HR (2012) Pitfalls of lengthening over an intramedullary nail in tibia: a consecutive case series. Arch Orthop Trauma Surg 132(2):185–191

Kocaoglu M, Eralp L, Kilicoglu O, Burc H, Cakmak M (2004) Complications encountered during lengthening over an intramedullary nail. J Bone Joint Surg Am 86-A(11):2406–2411

Kocaoglu M, Eralp L, Bilen FE, Balci HI (2009) Fixator-assisted acute femoral deformity correction and consecutive lengthening over an intramedullary nail. J Bone Joint Surg Am 91(1):152–159

Kristiansen LP, Steen H (1999) Lengthening of the tibia over an intramedullary nail, using the Ilizarov external fixator. Major complications and slow consolidation in 9 lengthenings. Acta Orthop Scand 70(3):271–274

Lin CC, Huang SC, Liu TK, Chapman MW (1996) Limb lengthening over an intramedullary nail. An animal study and clinical report. Clin Orthop Relat Res 330:208–216

Mahboubian S, Seah M, Fragomen AT, Rozbruch SR (2012) Femoral lengthening with lengthening over a nail has fewer complications than intramedullary skeletal kinetic distraction. Clin Orthop Relat Res 470(4):1221–1231

Min WK, Min BG, Oh CW, Song HR, Oh JK, Ahn HS, Park BC, Kim PT (2007) Biomechanical advantage of lengthening of the femur with an external fixator over an intramedullary nail. J Pediatr Orthop B 16(1):39–43

Paley D, Herzenberg JE (2002) Intramedullary infections treated with antibiotic cement rods: preliminary results in nine cases. J Orthop Trauma 16(10):723–729

Paley D, Herzenberg JE, Paremain G, Bhave A (1997) Femoral lengthening over an intramedullary nail. A matched-case comparison with Ilizarov femoral lengthening. J Bone Joint Surg Am 79(10):1464–1480

Park HW, Yang KH, Lee KS, Joo SY, Kwak YH, Kim HW (2008) Tibial lengthening over an intramedullary nail with use of the Ilizarov external fixator for idiopathic short stature. J Bone Joint Surg Am 90(9):1970–1978

Rozbruch SR, Kleinman D, Fragomen AT, Ilizarov S (2008) Limb lengthening and then insertion of an intramedullary nail: a case-matched comparison. Clin Orthop Relat Res 466(12):2923–2932

Simpson AH, Cole AS, Kenwright J (1999) Leg lengthening over an intramedullary nail. J Bone Joint Surg Br 81(6):1041–1045

Song HR, Oh CW, Mattoo R, Park BC, Kim SJ, Park IH, Jeon IH, Ihn JC (2005) Femoral lengthening over an intramedullary nail using the external fixator: risk of infection and knee problems in 22 patients with a follow-up of 2 years or more. Acta Orthop 76(2):245–252

Watanabe K, Tsuchiya H, Sakurakichi K, Yamamoto N, Kabata T, Tomita K (2005) Tibial lengthening over an intramedullary nail. J Orthop Sci 10(5):480–485

Combined Technique: Correction of Long Bone Deformities Using Fixator-Assisted Nailing

2

Dror Paley, Mehmet Kocaoğlu, and F. Erkal Bilen

Contents

D. Paley, MD, FRCSC (✉)
Paley Advanced Limb Lengthening Institute,
Kimmel Building 901 45th St.,
West Palm Beach, FL 33407, USA
e-mail: drorpaley@gmail.com,
dpaley@lengthening.us

M. Kocaoğlu, MD
Orthopedic Surgery Department,
Istanbul Memorial Hospital, Piyalepasa Bulvari,
Okmeydani, Istanbul 34385, Turkey
e-mail: drmehmetkocaoglu@gmail.com

F.E. Bilen
Istanbul Memorial Hospital,
Piyalepasa Bulvari, Okmeydani,
Istanbul 34385, Turkey
e-mail: bilenfe@gmail.com

2.1 Introduction

Deviation of the mechanical axis (MAD) results primarily in deformities of the long bones, which result in the development of secondary osteoarthritis of the hip, knee, and/or ankle joints (Tetsworth and Paley 1994b; Chao et al. 1994; Sharma et al. 2001). Orthopedic surgeons have utilized many different procedures to correct these deformities to prevent secondary osteoarthritis. However, these techniques generally result in low patient comfort and lack accuracy. A comprehensive technique termed "fixator-assisted nailing" (FAN) was developed by Dror Paley in 1993 and was first described by Paley et al. in 1997 (Paley et al. 1997a). Its goal was to combine the accuracy and minimal invasiveness of external fixation with the convenience of internal fixation. Internal fixation prevents the recurrence of the deformity and allows early mobilization of joints and quicker rehabilitation.

2.2 Indications and Contraindications

Indications include the following:

- Metabolic bone disease with multilevel, complex deformities (Fig. 2.1)
- Congenital deformities around the knee joint
- Acquired posttraumatic deformities (malunions)
- Acquired hypertrophic nonunions with deformities

M. Kocaoğlu et al. (eds.), *Advanced Techniques in Limb Reconstruction Surgery*,
DOI 10.1007/978-3-642-55026-3_2, © Springer Berlin Heidelberg 2015

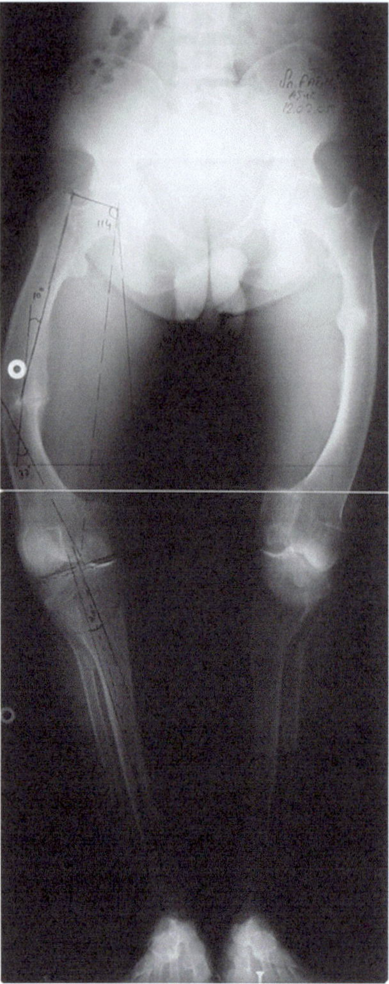

Fig. 2.1 A patients orthoroentgenogram showing multi-apical deformities in the lower extremities

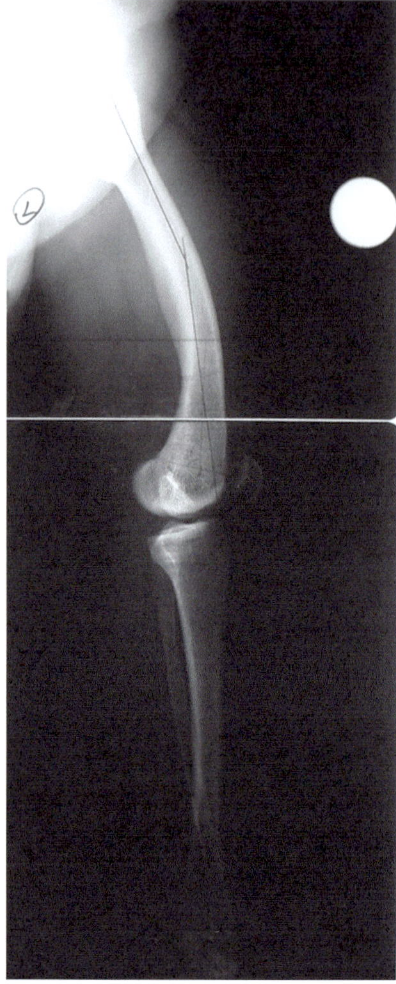

Fig. 2.2 A sagittal standing orthoroentgenogram showing long bowing deformity at the femur

- Sequelae of poliomyelitis
  Contraindications include the following:
- Presence or a history of infection
- Deformities in the pediatric age (before physeal closure)
- Long bones that are sclerotic and/or are narrow (medullary canal <7 mm)

2.3 Examination

Physical examination should include documentation of the range of motion of the adjacent joints, muscle strength, and neurologic status. Clinical length alignment and discrepancies should be noted and then measured radiographically.

2.4 Imaging Studies

- An orthoroentgenogram in both planes should be obtained according to the following guidelines (Fig. 2.2):
  - The knee should be at maximum extension, especially in the lateral view.
  - The x-ray beam should be level with the knee joint and taken from a distance of 10 ft away (3 m) so as to minimize magnification.
  - One-centimeter blocks should be used to level the pelvis in the AP view.
  - A magnification marker is used to determine the size and diameter of the IM nail and to determine the number and level of the osteotomy(ies) (Fig. 2.3).

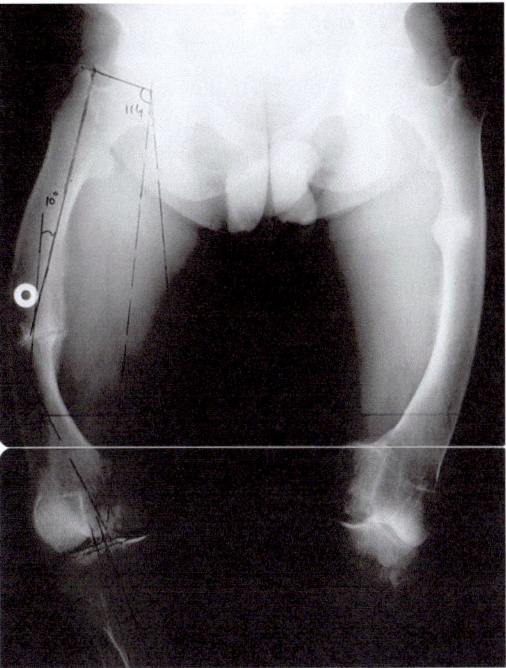

Fig. 2.3 Deformity analysis is performed on the x-ray of the right femur. A metallic marker is placed to predict the size of the IM nail

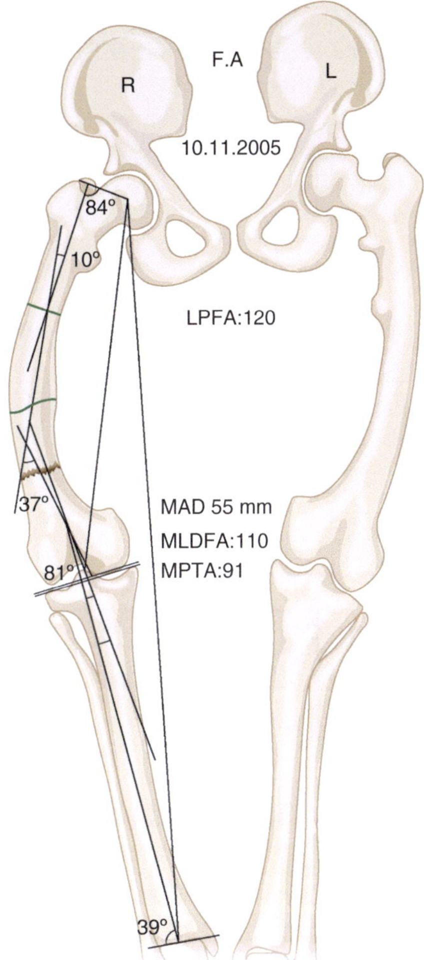

Fig. 2.4 Paper-tracing according to deformity analysis prior to correction

2.5 Preoperative Planning

- Deformity analysis should be performed according to the deformity planning guidelines given by Paley et al. (CORA planning method using joint orientation lines) (Paley and Tetsworth 1992; Paley et al. 1994) (Fig. 2.3).
- Determination of the level(s) of the osteotomy(ies) should be conducted.
- If the deformity is at the distal femoral metaphysis, retrograde IM nail insertion should be performed through the intercondylar notch.
- The diameter and size of the IM nail should be determined based on the scaled AP and lateral x-rays of the affected bone segment(s).
- Digital or paper tracing should be performed to simulate the surgery and to determine the provisional and final position of the bone segment, according to the following factors (Figs. 2.4 and 2.5):
  - The location of the extra, custom-made hole(s) on the IM nail should be determined.
  - The location and the number of interference screws (polar) should be determined

in a manner that increases the stability of the construct (Fig. 2.5).
  - The incision at the entry point of the IM nail and the osteotomy levels should be mapped out (Paley and Tetsworth 1994; Eralp et al. 2004; Kocaoglu et al. 2009).

2.6 Surgical Technique

2.6.1 Equipment

- Radiolucent table
- Radiolucent knee support or a rolled, sterile towel
- Large-field fluoroscopy
- Flexible intramedullary reaming system

- 6-mm conical Schanz screws
- Unilateral external fixator (EBI Monorail System or Orthofix LRS)
- 1.8-mm Kirschner wires (bayonette type)
- 3.5-mm cannulated drill bits
- Intramedullary nail

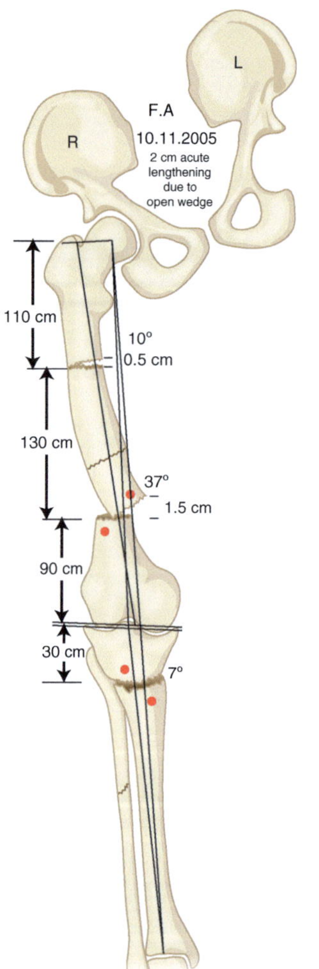

Fig. 2.5 Paper-tracing depicting the planned deformity correction. Note the placement of interference screws

2.6.2 Positioning

- The patient is placed in the supine position on the radiolucent table, and the affected hip should be slightly elevated using a silicone bag under the buttock to provide a lateral view of the femoral deformities (Fig. 2.6).
- Fluoroscopy from the hip to the ankle joint should be accessible (Fig. 2.7).
- If a long grid is available, it is placed under the matress of the patient.
- Sterile preparation should be used prior to draping the entire lower extremity beginning at the anterosuperior iliac spine

2.6.3 FAN for Femoral Deformity

For distal femoral deformity corrections, retrograde intramedullary nailing is preferred. For more proximal deformities, antegrade intramedullary nailing is more suitable.

In the presence of severe distal femoral valgus deformities (greater than 15°), the authors recommend prophylactic peroneal nerve release.

Two pairs of 6-mm half pins that are perpendicular to the anatomic axis of the femur (5–7° to the diaphysis, and 8–10° to the knee joint line) are inserted proximally and distally, respectively (Figs. 2.8 and 2.9). In the sagittal plane, it is crucial that the pins avoid any contact with the intramedullary nail (Figs. 2.10 and 2.11). Since the nail enters posteriorly, the distal half pins should be based anteriorly. Proximally, the nail is located anteriorly. The half pins should be located posteriorly at the level of the lesser trochanter.

In the presence of a rotational deformity, the distal and proximal pairs of pins are inserted in different rotational planes to each other.

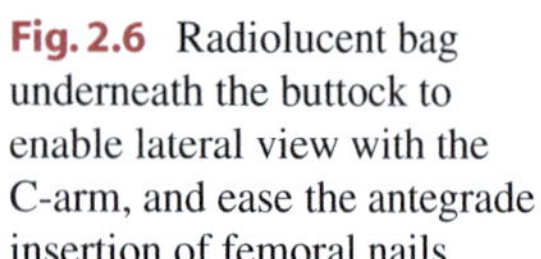

Fig. 2.6 Radiolucent bag underneath the buttock to enable lateral view with the C-arm, and ease the antegrade insertion of femoral nails

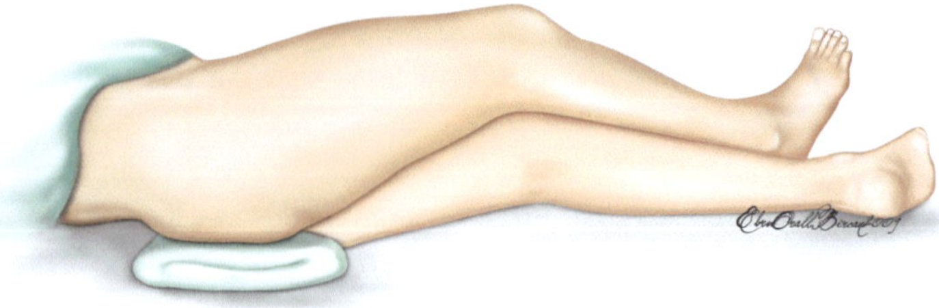

Fig. 2.7 Preoperative checking with the C-arm from hip to the ankle

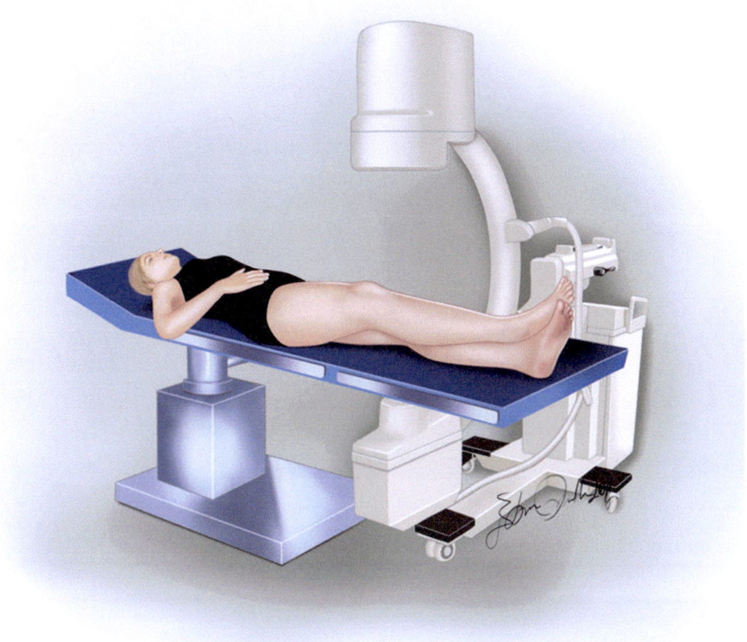

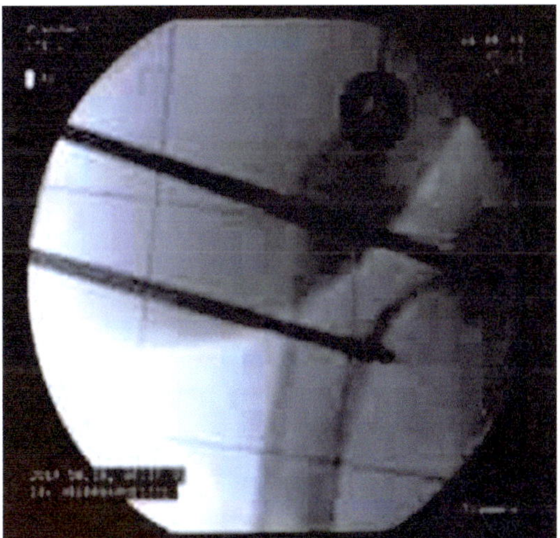

Fig. 2.8 AP view of the Schanz screws perpendicular to the anatomic axis of proximal femur

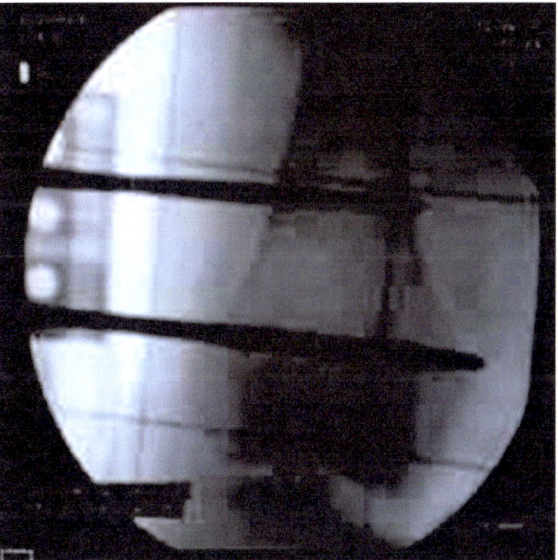

Fig. 2.9 AP view of the Schanz screws perpendicular to the anatomic axis of distal femur

A sterile inclinometer or even a smart phone in a sterile bag (Graham et al. 2013) can be used to measure the rotation angle between the proximal and distal pins. During the insertion of the distal Schanz screws, the patella should be centered, facing forward to capture the true AP view (Fig. 2.12). Determining the true sagittal plane of the proximal portion of the femur is not clear; however, a rotational arc and a lateral view using the C-arm may help in estimating the true proximal sagittal plane. Preoperative prone clinical rotation measurements are used to determine the correct rotation position of the upper femur relative to the knee joint. CT scan measurements can also be used to determine the rotation angle to correct.

Osteotomies are performed percutaneously from the lateral side of the femur. Either multiple

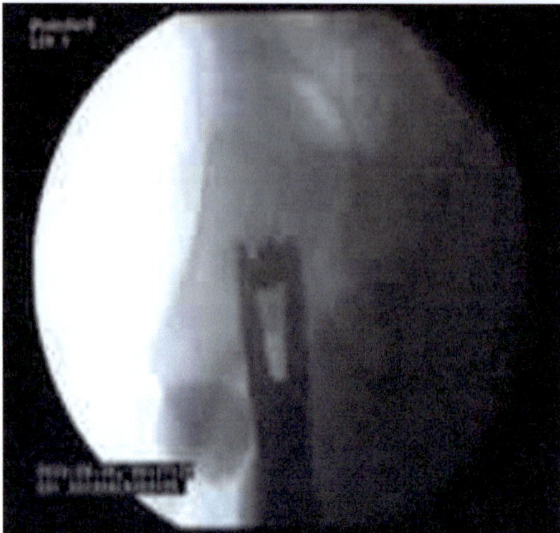

Fig. 2.10 Posterior placement of the Schanz screws at the proximal femur to allow insertion of the IM nail

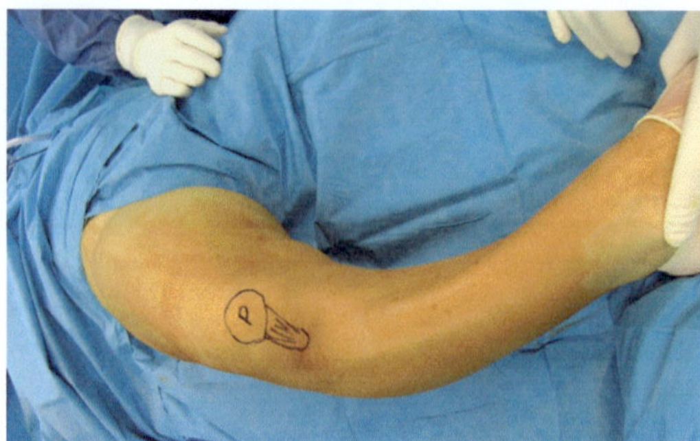

Fig. 2.12 Patella should face forward to establish the true AP view

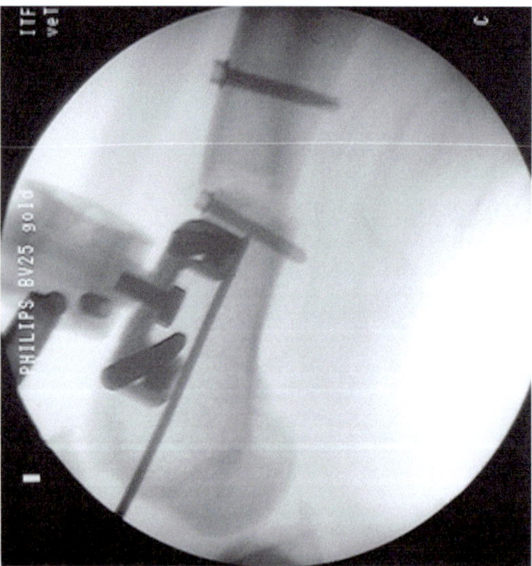

Fig. 2.11 Anterior placement of the Schanz screws at the distal femur to allow space for the IM nail

drill holes followed by an osteotome or Paley's focal dome drill guide technique can be used (Paley et al. 1997b; Paley and Herzenberg 2002). The medial and the lateral edges of the osteotomy are completed by an osteotome. If translation is needed at the osteotomy site, the osteotome is inserted into the center of the osteotomy site and twisted such that the desired translation is produced. Alternatively, half pins can be used as a joystick to produce the translation manually (Fig. 2.13).

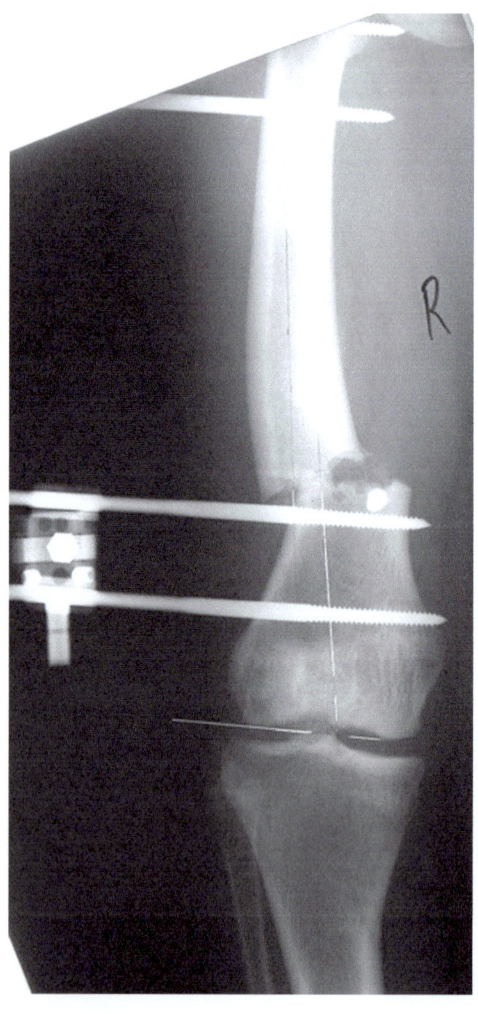

Fig. 2.13 Translation and correction are shown in this AP view x-ray, which is maintained by the unilateral external fixator

Angular correction is performed by accurately using an external fixator. The accuracy of the correction is verified by intraoperative x-rays of both the anteroposterior and the lateral views (Tetsworth and Paley 1994a). If the correction is not successful, the steps are repeated until the intraoperative x-rays dictate accurate correction.

Before reaming, some authors prefer to insert interference (blocking) screws to guide the intramedullary drill and to prevent loss of the correction (Kocaoglu et al. 2009; Bilen et al. 2010). With more three-dimensional locking hole patterns in third-generation locking nails, this may not be needed. Conventional entry points are used during the insertion of the intramedullary nail both proximally or distally. Intramedullary reaming produces an internal grafting effect on the osteotomy site.

After the correction is achieved with the external fixator, the alignment should be checked before insertion of the nail. This can be accomplished by several ways. If a grid was inserted under the patient, the grid lines can be used to draw a virtual mechanical axis that can be visualized intraoperatively. If the goal is a zero mechanical axis deviation, then the grid line is centered over the hip and ankle joints and should be also centered at the knee joint to form a collinear Mikulicz line. If no grid is available, the cautery cord can be used in the same manner. Alternatively, an intraoperative radiograph of the femur can be taken and the joint orientation angle of the distal femur measured. The fixator can be readjusted according to the x-ray findings until the desired correction is achieved. This gives the correction the same accuracy as with external fixation.

The nail is then inserted and locked statically (proximally and distally). To avoid creating a sagittal plane flexion deformity, a nail without a bend is used for retrograde nailing. However, if a distal sagittal plane deformity (e.g., pro- or recurvatum) has to be corrected, then a supracondylar nail with a bend or tibial nail can be used, and the bent end of the nail inserted so as to extend or flex the distal fragment (Kocaoglu et al. 2009) (Fig. 2.14).

If needed, additional interference screws may be inserted to increase stability.

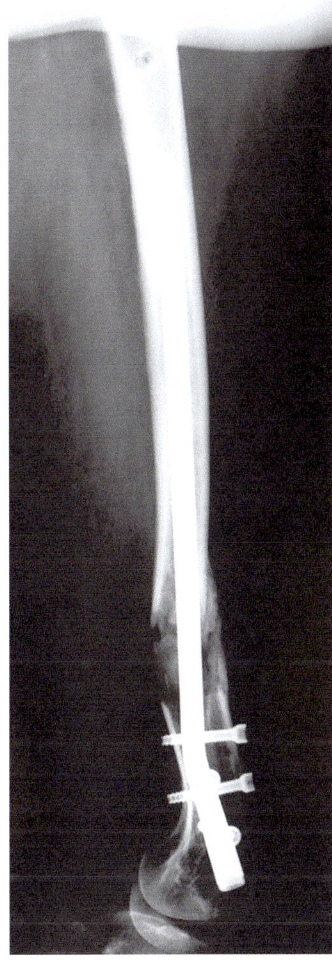

Fig. 2.14 Lateral x-ray of a femur following FAN procedure depicting usage of a tibial nail to help correct sagittal plane deformity

The external fixator is removed at the end of the surgery, and the incisions are closed primarily.

2.6.4 FAN for Tibial Deformity

Two pairs of half pins perpendicular to the anatomic axis of the tibia are inserted distally and proximally (Figs. 2.15 and 2.16). In the sagittal plane, it is crucial that the Schanz screws avoid any contact with the intramedullary nail. The pins should be at the posterior aspect of the tibia on the sagittal plane to leave enough space for the nail (Figs. 2.17 and 2.18).

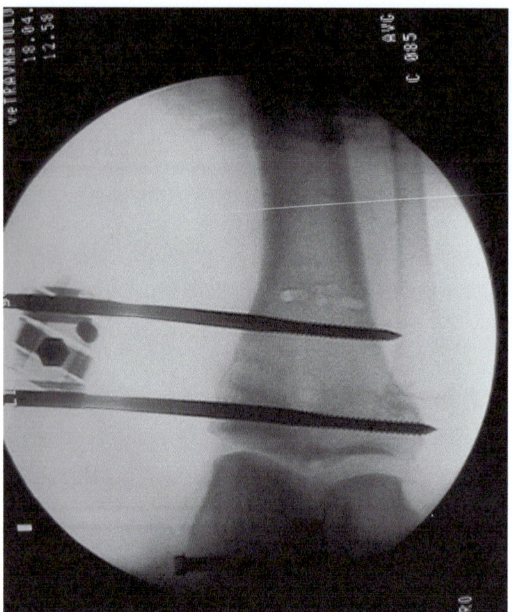

Fig. 2.15 AP view showing placement of the proximal Schanz screws parallel to the knee joint

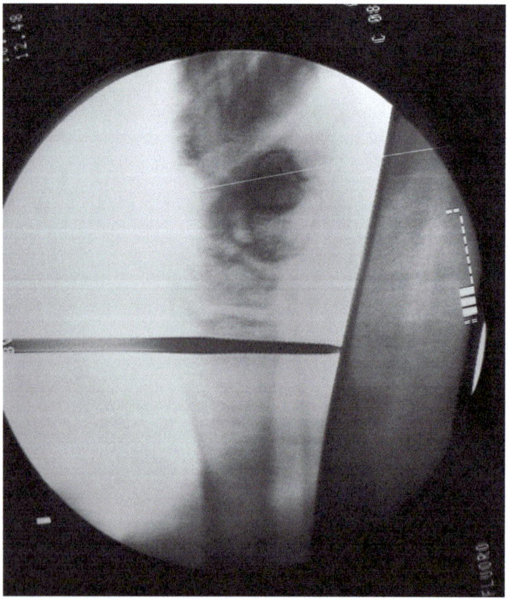

Fig. 2.16 AP view showing placement of the first distal Schanz screw parallel to the ankle joint

As opposed to acute femoral deformity correction, for acute rotation or valgus correction of the tibia, the authors recommend prophylactic peroneal nerve release (Slawski et al. 1994). If

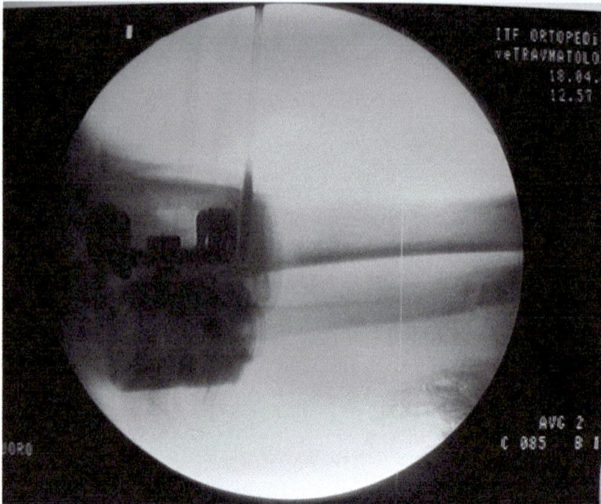

Fig. 2.17 Schanz screws are placed posteriorly at the proximal tibia to allow insertion of the IM nail

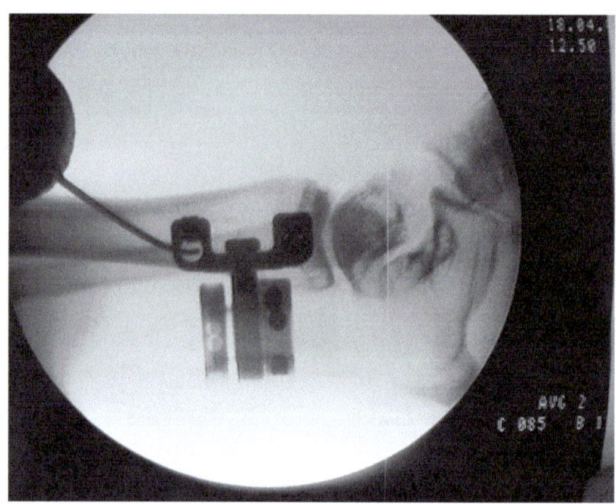

Fig. 2.18 Schanz screws are placed posteriorly at the distal tibia to allow space for the IM nail

this is performed, the fibular osteotomy can be performed at the same level since the nerve is protected and the osteotomy is performed under direct vision of the nerve.

For FAN of the tibia, the fibula is osteotomized at the mid-diaphyseal level through a small posterolateral incision (Fig. 2.19).

Percutaneous tibial osteotomy can be performed through a mini incision using either multiple drill holes or Paley's focal dome drill guide (Fig. 2.20). With an osteotome, the completeness of the osteotomy is verified as described previously.

The osteotome is inserted into the center of the osteotomy and twisted to create the desired amount

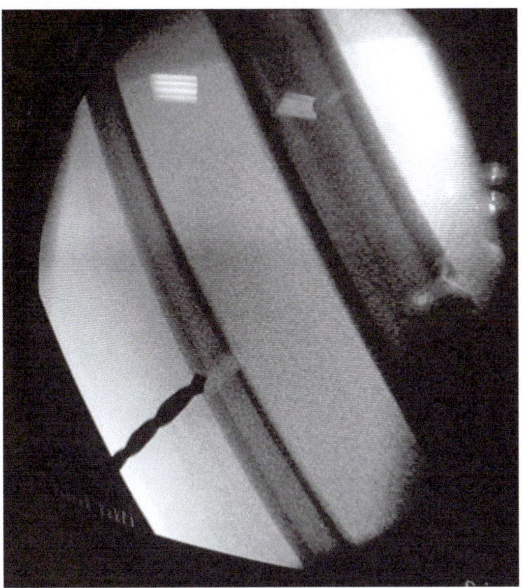

Fig. 2.19 The fibular osteotomy at the mid-diaphyseal level

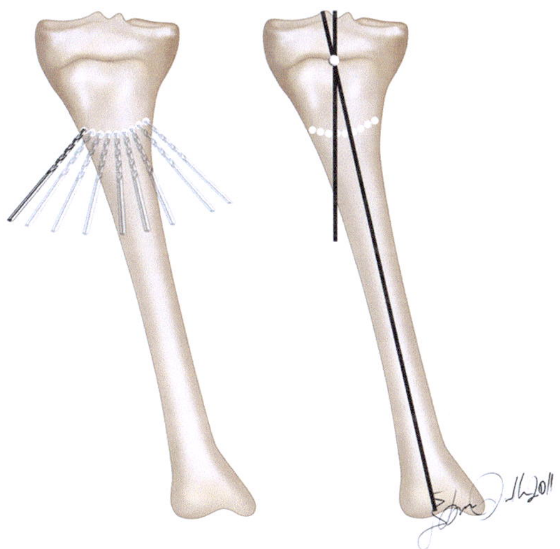

Fig. 2.20 Schematic drawing of the multiple drill hole osteotomy technique

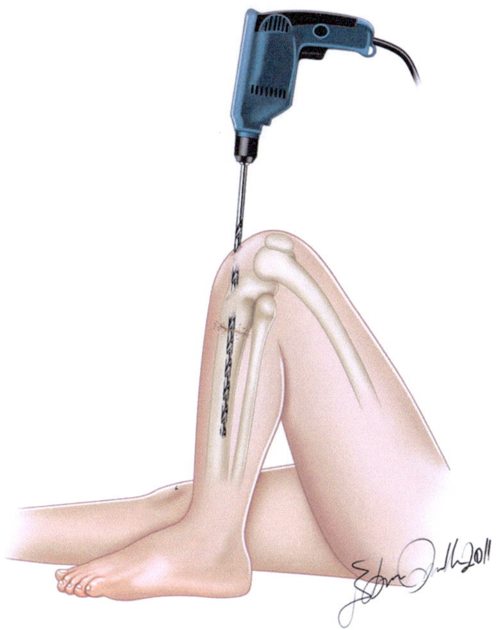

Fig. 2.21 Drilling of the medulla creates internal grafting effect

The reaming produces an internal grafting effect (Fig. 2.21). Percutaneous fasciotomy of the anterior compartment is recommended in most cases. The nail is inserted and locked statically. If needed, additional interference (blocking) screws can be inserted to increase stability.

The external fixator is removed and the incisions are closed primarily.

2.7   Postoperative Period and Follow-Up

The patients are mobilized at the first postoperative day with weight bearing as tolerated. For approximately 3 weeks, ice is applied to prevent synovitis at the knee joint; the ice also has analgesic properties. Muscle strengthening and range of motion exercises are initiated immediately.

The patients are followed clinically and radiologically on a monthly basis until bone healing is established. Clinical and radiologic pictures of a patient with severe lower extremi-

of translation. The angular correction is maintained through the application of a unilateral fixator. Intraoperative x-rays of the two planes are required to verify if the desired correction has been achieved. Adjustment of the fixator and repeat x-rays are performed as needed to fine-tune the correction.

Antegrade reaming over a guide wire is performed conventionally through a mini incision.

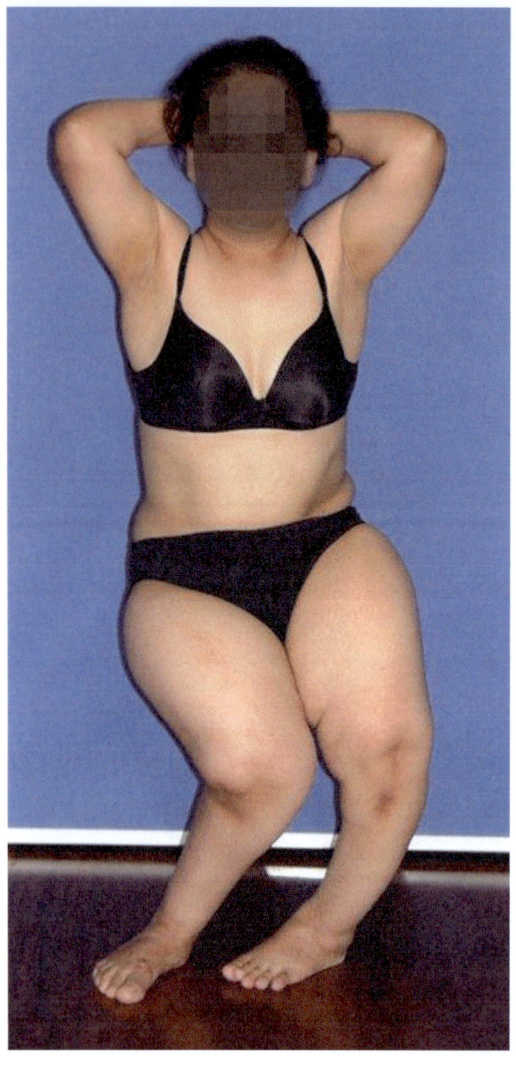

Fig. 2.22 A patient with windswept deformity (frontal picture)

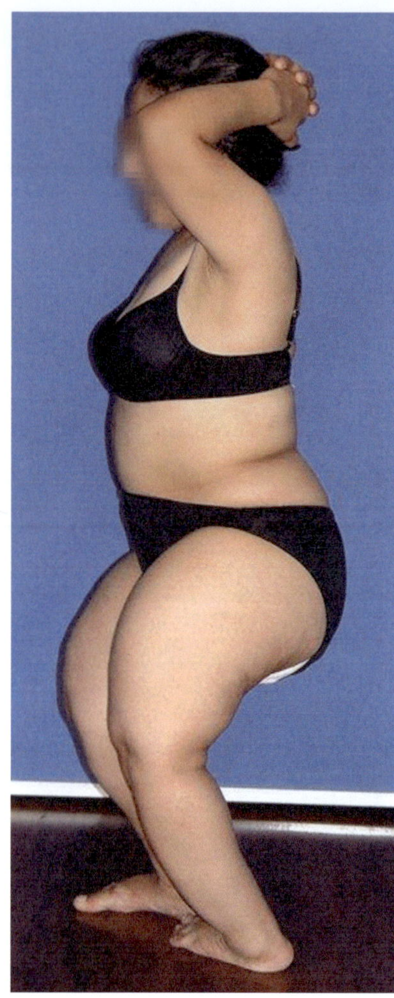

Fig. 2.23 Same patient from the side

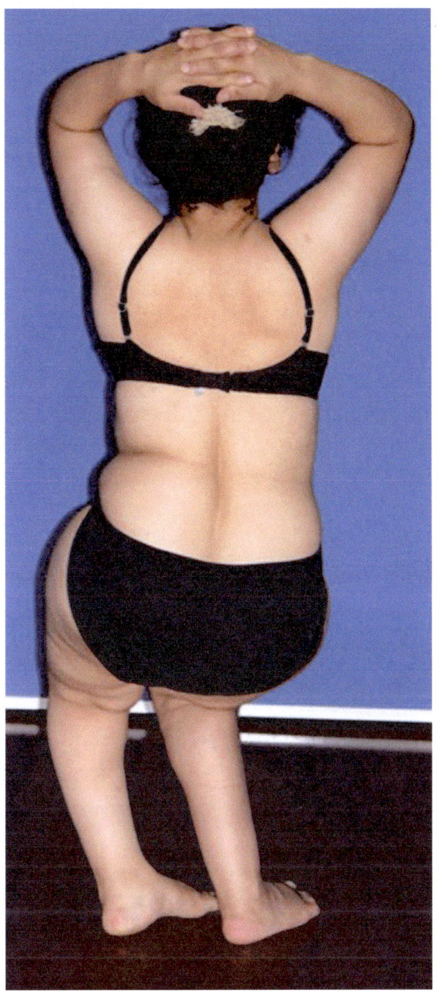

Fig. 2.24 Same patient from the back

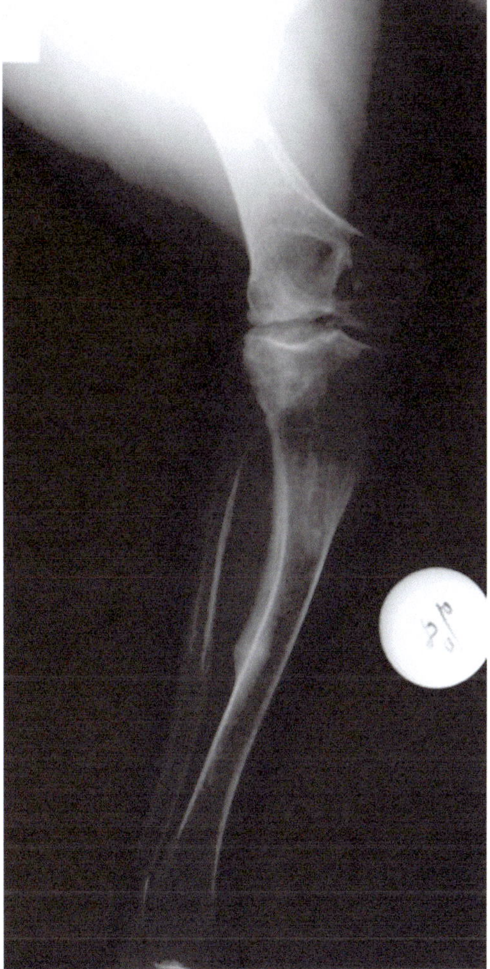

Fig. 2.25 AP x-ray of the right tibia showing severe genu valgum. Note that the lower extremities of this patient wouldn't fit into a single orthoroentgenogram

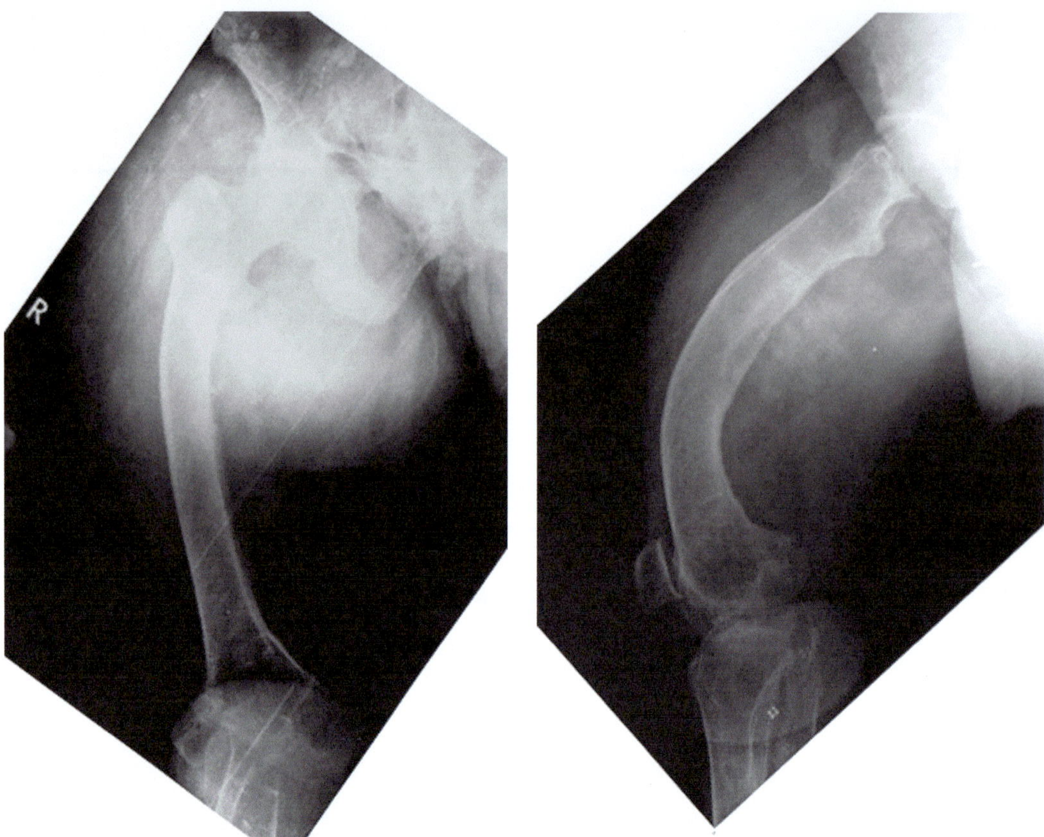

Fig. 2.26 AP x-ray of the right femur showing long bowing deformity

Fig. 2.27 Lateral x-ray of the right femur showing the severity of the deformity

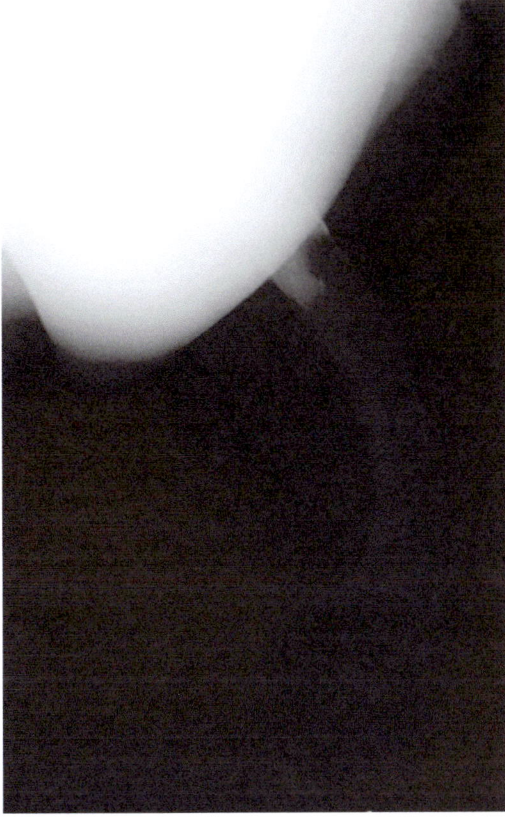

Fig. 2.28 This is the lateral view of the proximal femur and AP view of the distal femur: there is associated rotational deformity

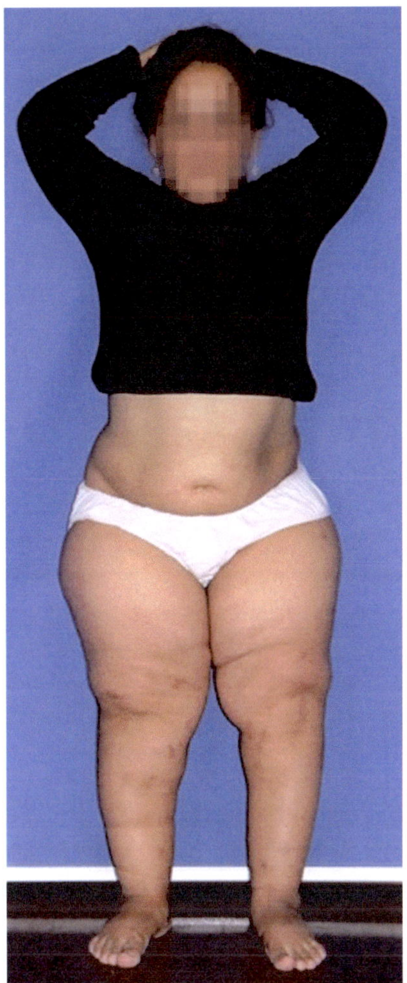

Fig. 2.29 Clinical picture following deformity correction by FAN procedure (frontal picture)

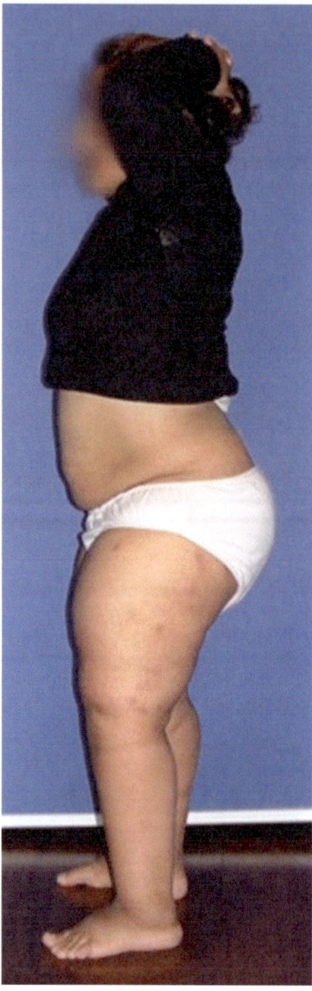

Fig. 2.30 Same patient from the side after deformity correction

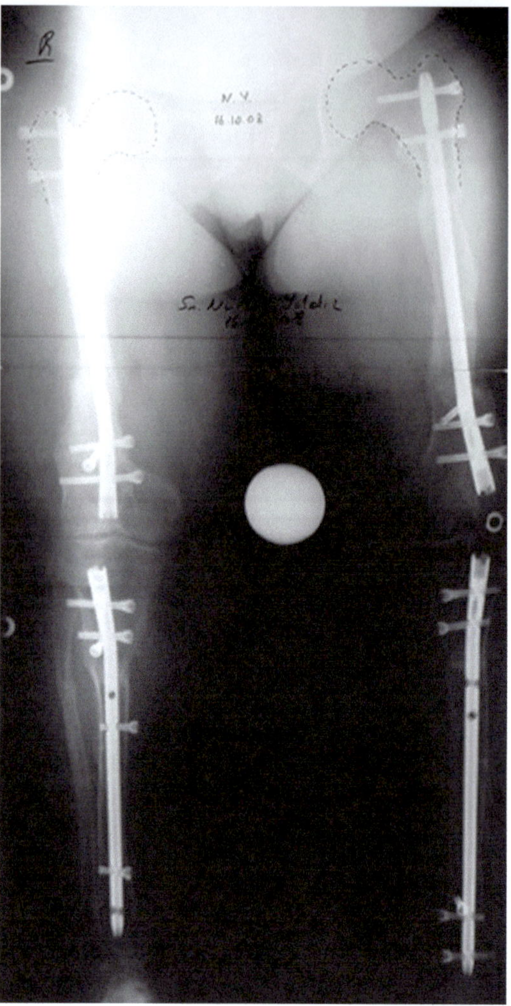

Fig. 2.31 AP orthoroentgenogram after deformity correction

ties prior and after FAN procedure are shown in Figs. 2.22, 2.23, 2.24, 2.25, 2.26, 2.27, 2.28, 2.29, 2.30 and 2.31.

References

Bilen FE, Kocaoglu M, Eralp L et al (2010) Fixator-assisted nailing and consecutive lengthening over an intramedullary nail for the correction of tibial deformity. J Bone Joint Surg Br 92:146–152

Chao EYS, Neluheni EVD, Hsu WW et al (1994) Biomechanics of malalignment. Orthop Clin North Am 25:379–386

Eralp L, Kocaoglu M, Cakmak M et al (2004) A correction of windswept deformity by fixator assisted nailing. A report of two cases. J Bone Joint Surg Br 86:1065–1068

Graham D, Suzuki A, Reitz C et al (2013) Measurement of rotational deformity: using a smart phone application is more accurate then conventional methods. ANZ J Surg 83(12):937–941

Kocaoglu M, Eralp L, Bilen FE et al (2009) Fixator-assisted acute femoral deformity correction and consecutive lengthening over an intramedullary nail. J Bone Joint Surg Am 91:152–159

Paley D, Herzenberg JE (eds) (2002) Hardware and osteotomy consideration, in Principles of Deformity Correction. Springer, Berlin, pp 291–410

Paley D, Tetsworth K (1992) Mechanical axis deviation of the lower limbs. Preoperative planning of multiapical frontal plane angular and bowing deformities of the femur and tibia. Clin Orthop 280:65–71

Paley D, Herzenberg JE, Tetsworth K et al (1994) Deformity planning for frontal and sagittal plane corrective osteotomies. Orthop Clin North Am 25:425–465

Paley D, Herzenberg JE, Bor N (1997a) Fixator-assisted nailing of femoral and tibial deformities. Tech Orthop 12:260–275

Paley D, Herzenberg JE, Paremain G et al (1997b) Femoral lengthening over an intramedullary nail. A matched-case comparison with Ilizarov femoral lengthening. J Bone Joint Surg Am 79:1464–1480

Sharma L, Song J, Felson DT et al (2001) The role of knee alignment in disease progression and functional decline in knee osteoarthritis. JAMA 286:188–195

Slawski DP, Schoenecker PL, Rich MM (1994) Peroneal nerve injury as a complication of pediatric tibial osteotomies: a review of 255 osteotomies. J Pediatr Orthop 14:166–172

Tetsworth K, Paley D (1994a) Accuracy of correction of complex lower-extremity deformities by the Ilizarov method. Clin Orthop 301:102–110

Tetsworth K, Paley D (1994b) Malalignment and degenerative arthropathy. Orthop Clin North Am 25:367–378

Mehmet Kocaoğlu and F. Erkal Bilen

Contents

M. Kocaoğlu, MD (✉)
Orthopedic Surgery Department,
Istanbul Memorial Hospital, Istanbul, Turkey
e-mail: drmehmetkocaoglu@gmail.com

F.E. Bilen, MD, FEBOT
Orthopedic Surgery Department, Istanbul Memorial
Hospital, Istanbul, Turkey
e-mail: bilenfe@gmail.com

3.1   Introduction

The management of patients with multi-apical deformities is complicated, especially if these deformities are associated with a limb-length discrepancy (Paley and Tetsworth 1991; Paley et al. 1989). Multi-apical deformities are generally due to metabolic bone diseases, and they usually result in bowing of the entire long bone. More than one osteotomy is often needed to correct these deformities to produce a straight bone and to avoid creating secondary iatrogenic deformities (Paley and Tetsworth 1991) (Fig. 3.1a, b). Correction of all deformities with an Ilizarov-type external fixator during a single operation can cause considerable discomfort (Bilen et al. 2010), but it allows for postoperative adjustments and prevents inequality of limb length.

However, Ilizarov-type external fixators have disadvantages, such as pin-track infections, discomfort, and bulkiness (Bilen et al. 2010). Internal fixation provides better patient comfort but requires substantial technical skill and expertise (Paley et al. 1997a, b).

Two techniques, fixator-assisted nailing and lengthening over a nail, have been combined for the treatment of cases of femoral deformity associated with limb-length discrepancy (Bilen et al. 2010; Kocaoglu et al. 2009; Paley and Herzenberg 2002).

The standard treatment for this group of patients has been external fixation alone. With the combined technique, we capitalized on the

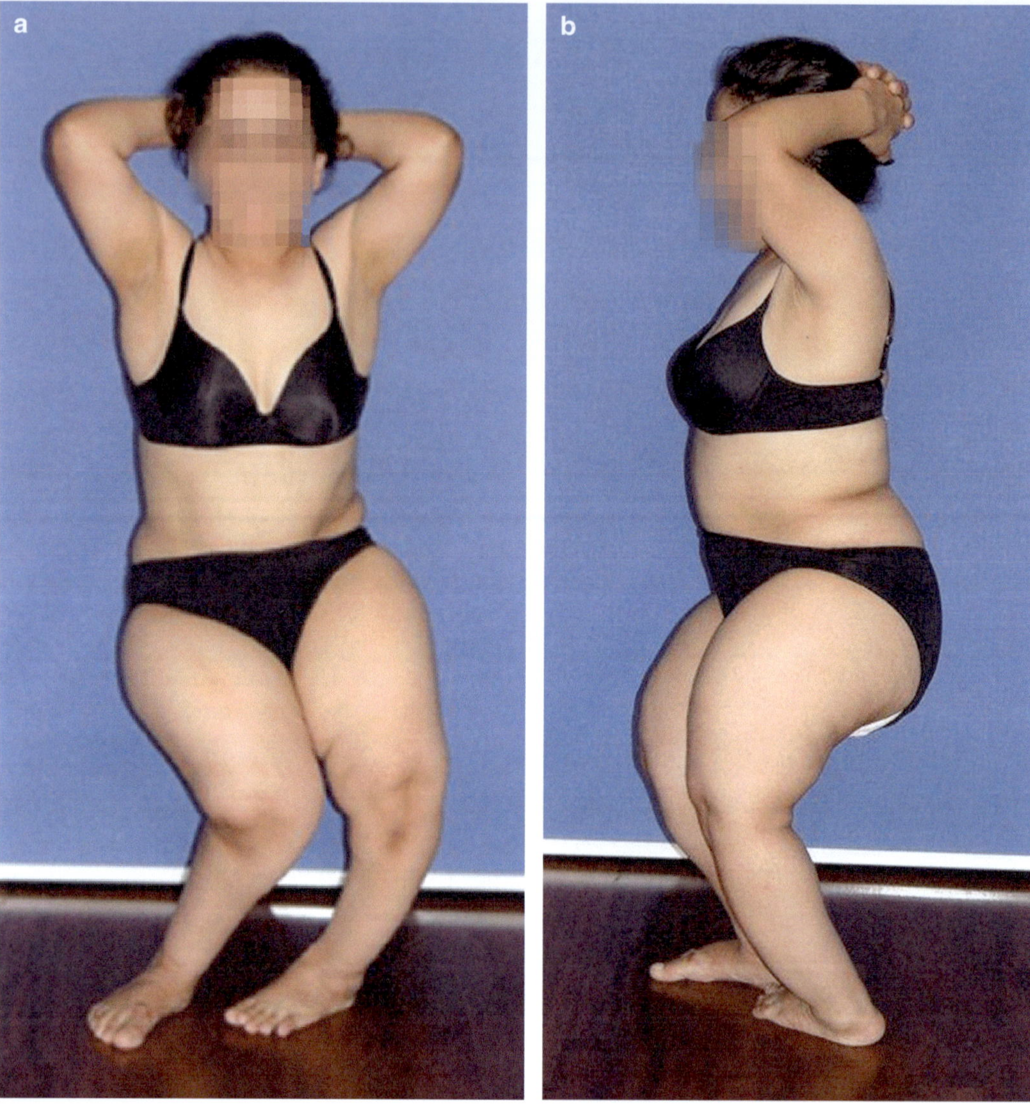

Fig. 3.1 A patient's preoperative photographic documentation displaying long bowing deformities in the lower extremities (**a**, front view; **b**, side view)

advantages of both individual techniques (Bilen et al. 2010; Kocaoglu et al. 2009; Paley and Herzenberg 2002). However, the combination of fixator-assisted acute deformity correction and consecutive lengthening over an intramedullary nail requires careful analysis of the deformity and extensive preoperative preparation (Paley and Herzenberg 2002; Paley and Tetsworth 1992). The surgeon must be familiar with both intramedullary nailing and external fixation techniques, as the two techniques both have steep learning curves (Eralp et al. 2004).

In this chapter, we describe the technical details and tips and tricks.

3.2 Femoral FAN-LON

3.2.1 Indications

3.2.1.1 Congenital Deformities
- PFFD Paley type 1 (congenital short femur with distal valgus deformity)
- Short stature with deformities due to bone dysplasias (achondroplasia, hypochondroplasia, spondyloepiphyseal dysplasia, multiple epiphyseal dysplasia, etc.)
- Hemihypertrophy (Beckwith-Wiedemann syndrome)

3.2.1.2 Acquired Deformities
- Posttraumatic defect nonunions associated with deformities (Paley B3) (Paley et al. 1989)
- Deformity with LLD due to posttraumatic or postinfectious epiphyseal damage
- Postinfectious defect stage 1 nonunions created by the surgeon (Kocaoglu et al. 2006)
- LLDs and deformities due to bone tumors (including postsurgical iatrogenic defects and sequelae)
- Multi-apical deformities and constitutional short stature due to metabolic bone disease (rickets, hypophosphatemic rickets, etc.)

3.2.2 Examination

The physical examination should include the following:
- ROM of the hip, knee, and ankle joints bilaterally.
- Measurement of the real (distance between the anterior superior iliac spine [ASIS] and medial malleolus) and apparent LLD (distance between the umbilicus and medial malleolus).
- Determination of the number of blocks (each 1 cm) under the shortened extremity to provide a level pelvis (Fig. 3.2a, b).
- Photographic documentation of the patient, initially and at the end of the treatment.

- Evaluation for joint contractures.
- Careful evaluation of neurologic and vascular status.
- In the presence of a history of thromboembolism, Doppler ultrasound examination should be performed, and prophylaxis should be started.

3.2.3 Imaging Studies

- Plain x-rays in both planes (true AP and lateral)
- Orthoroentgenogram in both planes (Fig. 3.3a, b)
  - The knee should be in maximum extension, especially in the lateral view.
  - One-centimeter blocks should be used to level the pelvis in the AP view (Fig. 3.4).
- Scaled AP and lateral x-rays of the affected bone segment are necessary to obtain the size and the diameter of the IM nail and to determine the numbers and levels of the osteotomy/osteotomies.
- A computed tomography (CT) scan or even a magnetic resonance imaging (MRI) study provides useful information in cases of articular pathologies (Fig. 3.5).

3.2.4 Preoperative Planning

- All data obtained via clinical examination and imaging studies should be carefully evaluated.
- The deformity should be analyzed according to deformity planning guidelines outlined by Paley (Paley and Tetsworth 1992) (Fig. 3.6).
- The level(s) of the osteotomy/osteotomies in the affected bone segment should be determined according to anatomic axis planning (Paley and Herzenberg 2002).
- If there is a deformity at the distal femoral metaphysis, retrograde IM nail insertion should be performed through the intercondylar notch.

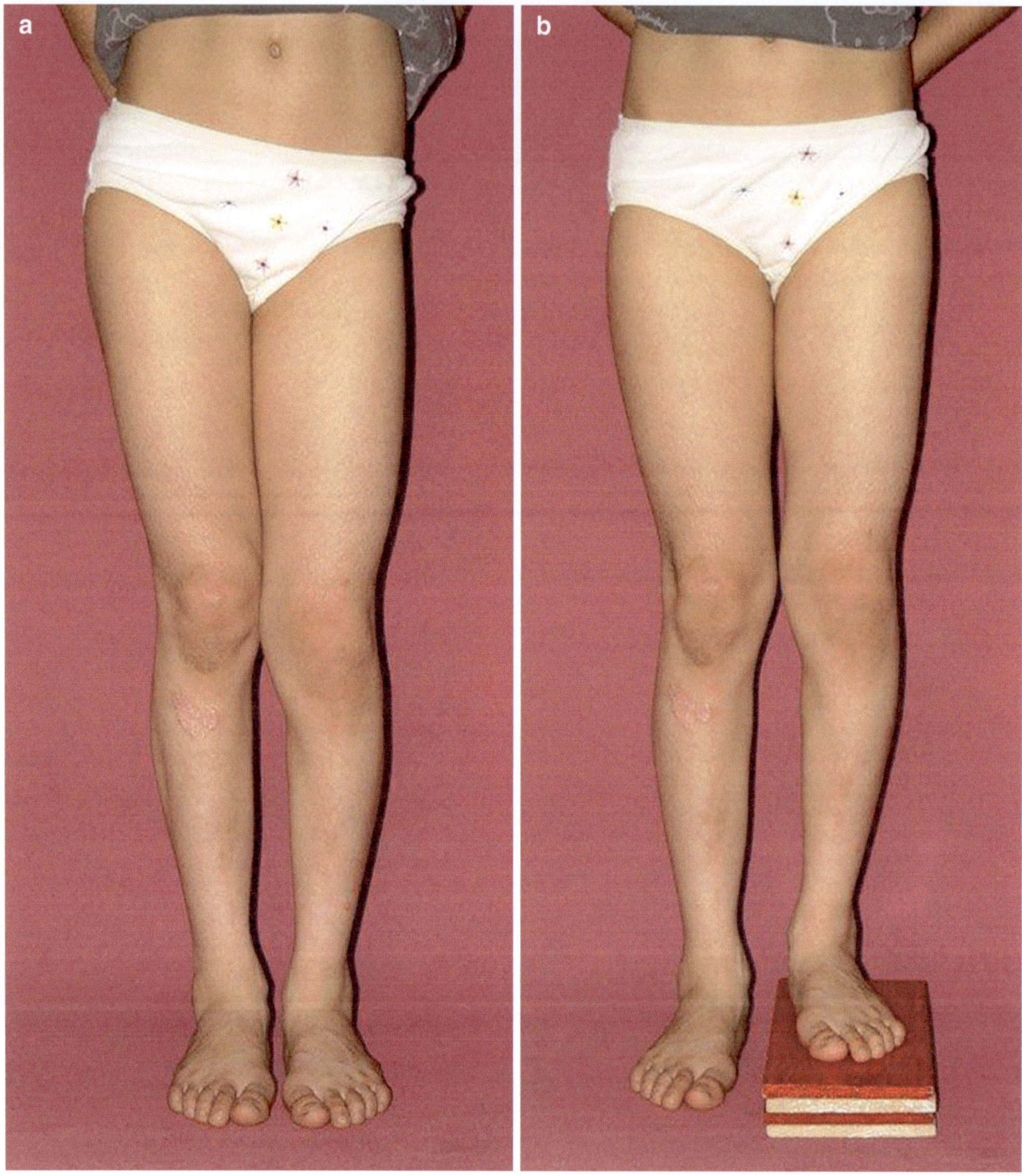

Fig. 3.2 A patient with limb length discrepancy displays pelvic asymmetry (**a**), which diminishes using blocks under the shortened extremity (**b**)

- If there is an additional proximal metaphyseal deformity, then the length of the IM nail chosen should be longer than the femur. The amount of the nail length outside of the femur should be as long as the planned amount of the lengthening (Figs. 3.7a, b and 3.8).

- If there is only a proximal metaphyseal deformity of the femur, then an antegrade IM nail can be chosen.

- The diameter and the size of the IM nail should be determined based on the scaled AP and lateral x-rays of the affected bone segment(s) (Fig. 3.9a, b).

Fig. 3.3 Preoperative orthoroentgenograms, AP (**a**) and lateral (**b**)

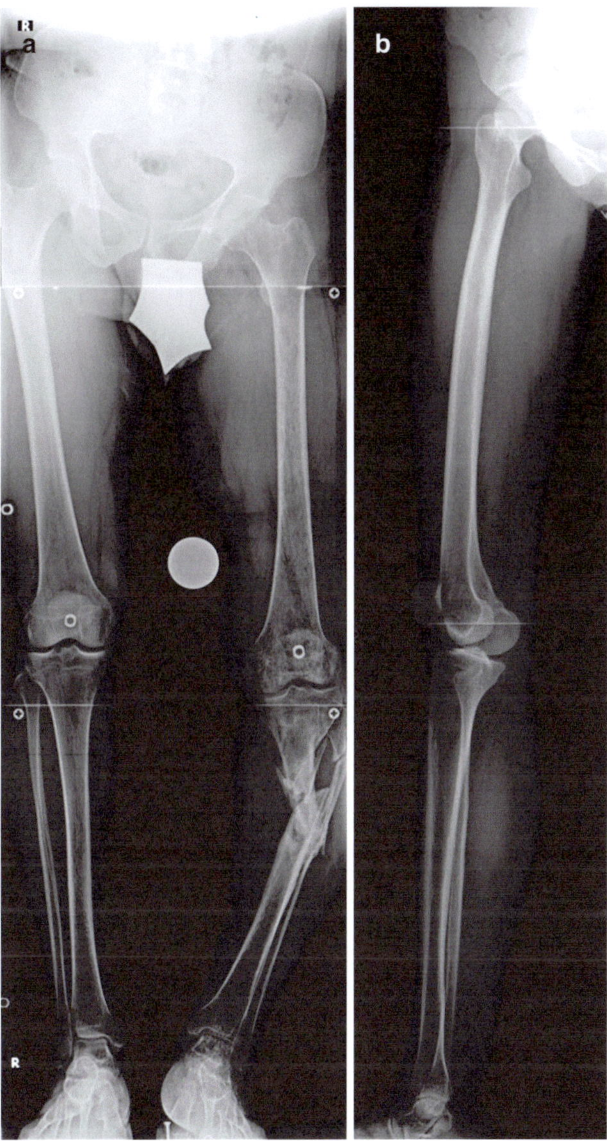

- Paper tracing should be performed to simulate the surgery and to determine the provisional final position of the bone segment(s) (Fig. 3.10).
  - The extra custom-made hole(s) on the IM nail should be determined (Fig. 3.11).
  - The location and number of the interference (poller) screws should be assigned to increase the stability of the reconstruction (Fig. 3.12) (Krettek et al. 1999a, b; Seligson 2000).

  - The incision of the entry point of the IM nail and the osteotomy levels should be determined.

3.2.5   Equipment

1. Radiolucent table
2. Radiolucent knee support or rolled sterile towel
3. Large-field fluoroscopy

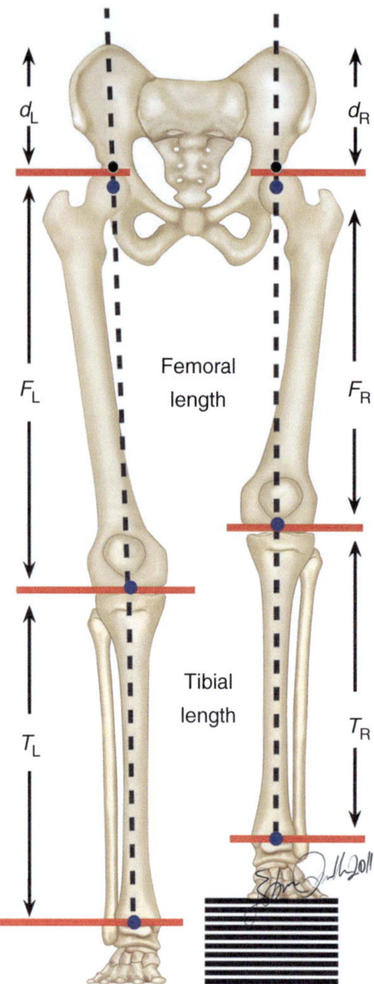

Fig. 3.4 A drawing displaying one-centimeter blocks under the shortened extremity to provide a level pelvis

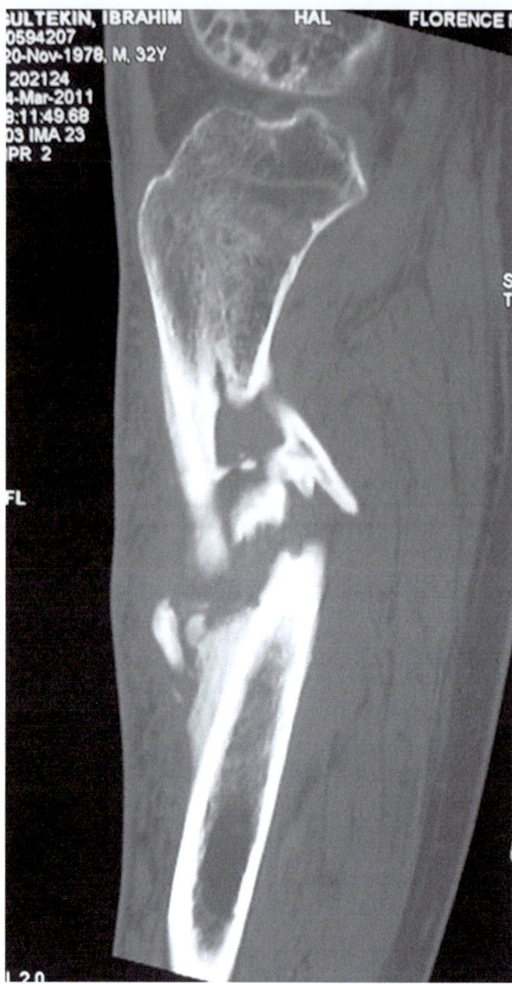

Fig. 3.5 A computerized scan (CT) displaying a non-union of the tibia associated with shortening

4. Six-millimeter conical hydroxyapatite-coated Schanz screws
5. Unilateral external fixator (Orthofix LRS, Bussolengo, Italy, or EBI Monorail Fixation System, Biomet, Parsippany, NJ, USA) (Fig. 3.13)
6. Flexible intramedullary reaming system
7. Kirschner wires (bayonet tip), 1.8 mm
8. Cannulated drill bits, 3.5 mm
9. Intramedullary nail (the authors prefer Ortopro Retrograde 4G Nails, Istanbul, Turkey) (Fig. 3.11)

3.2.6 Positioning

• The patient is placed supine on the radiolucent table with the affected hip slightly elevated, using a silicone bag under the buttock to facilitate the lateral view (Fig. 3.14).
• The region from the hip to the ankle joint is checked by fluoroscopy in both planes before sterile preparation.
• The entire lower extremity is sterile prepared and draped, starting from the ASIS.

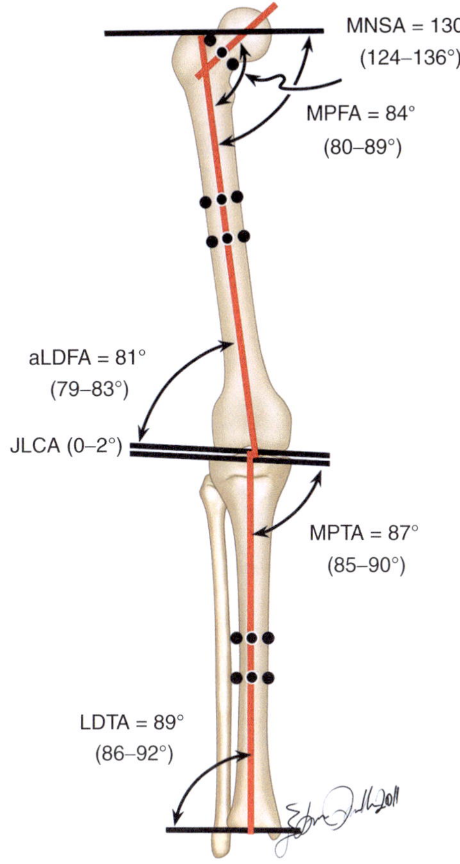

Fig. 3.6 Normal values of deformity planning analysis of the lower extremities

The reason behind the choice for a transverse incision is that it leads to less scarring, thus making it cosmetically more acceptable (Fig. 3.16). However, the paratenon and the patellar ligament are split longitudinally (Fig. 3.15 right). Before the acute correction of valgus deformities around the knee of more than 20°, prophylactic peroneal nerve release must be performed (Paley 1990) (Fig. 3.17).

- Schanz screws are placed perpendicular to the anatomic axis of each segment, proximally and distally (and at the middle segment, when present) with the cannulated drill technique (Figs. 3.18 and 3.19) (Paley and Herzenberg 2002).
  - The Schanz screws should be placed posteriorly to leave enough space for the IM nail (Fig. 3.20).
  - There should be at least 1 mm of space between the IM nail and the Schanz screws to avoid spreading any pin-track infection into the medullary space (Fig. 3.21).
  - Schanz screws are placed parallel to the axial plane of each fragment. Thus, once the Schanz screws are secured to the external fixator following the osteotomy/osteotomies, the rotational deformities have been corrected (Fig. 3.22a, b).
  - To correct sagittal plane deformities, the Schanz screws need to be placed parallel to the sagittal plane axis of each fragment (Figs. 3.23a, b).
- Using 3.5-mm drill bits, multiple drill holes are created percutaneously at the osteotomy level(s).
  - An obligatory translation is necessary at the osteotomy level, especially in the metaphyseal area if the center of rotation of angulation (CORA) is at a different level (Fig. 3.24).
  - The maximum contact at the translated osteotomy level can be obtained with a dome-shaped osteotomy (Fig. 3.25).
  - The creation of a dome osteotomy is technically demanding, whereas a transverse-shaped osteotomy is easier to create; however, after translation and angulation,

- Prophylactic antibiotherapy is initiated (first-generation cephalosporin, cephamezine 4 × 1 g IV for 3 days).

3.2.7 Surgical Technique

3.2.7.1 Exposure/Incision

Osteotomies in the long bones can be executed percutaneously through limited incisions, by either the Gigli saw technique or the multiple drill hole technique (Paley and Tetsworth 1991). The placement of the intramedullary nail also can be performed through a 2-cm transverse incision over the patellar ligament (Fig. 3.15 left).

Fig. 3.7 The intramedullary nail is longer than the femur and lies outside of the bone proximally (**a**). At the end of lengthening, the entire nail lies within the bone and is locked statically at the proximal femur (**b**)

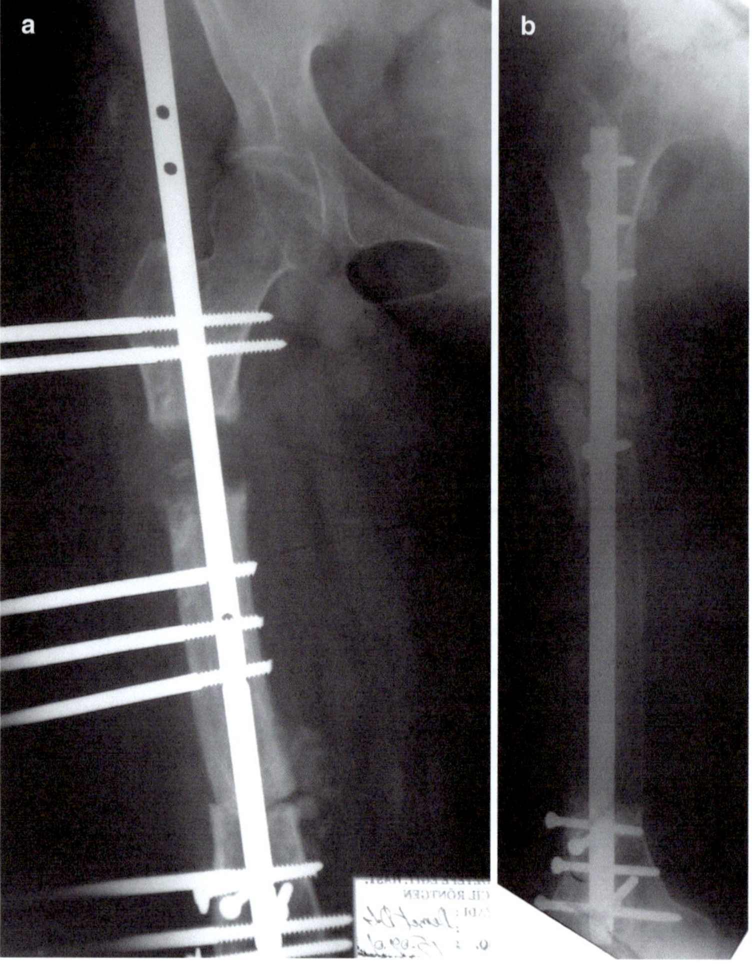

Fig. 3.8 Schematic drawing of a femoral FAN-LON procedure. Initially the IM nail is longer than the bone; however, it lies entirely within the bone at the end of lengthening

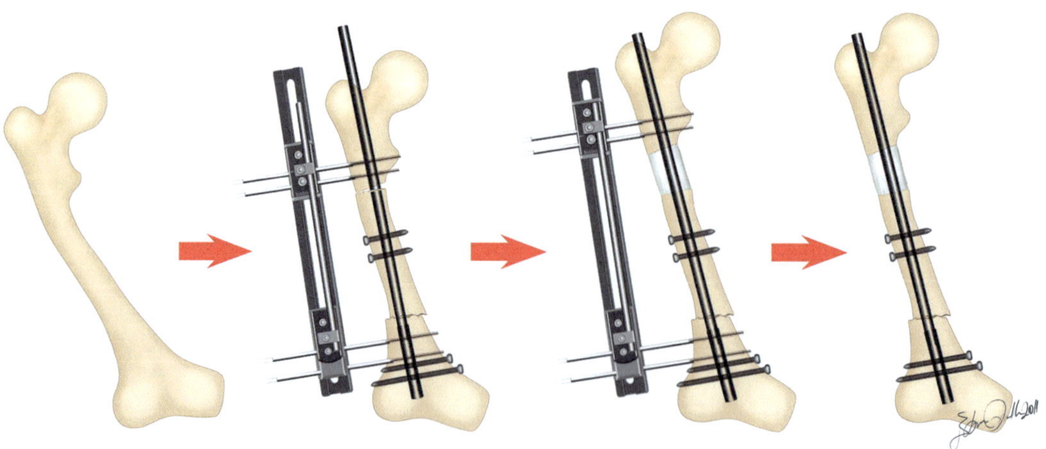

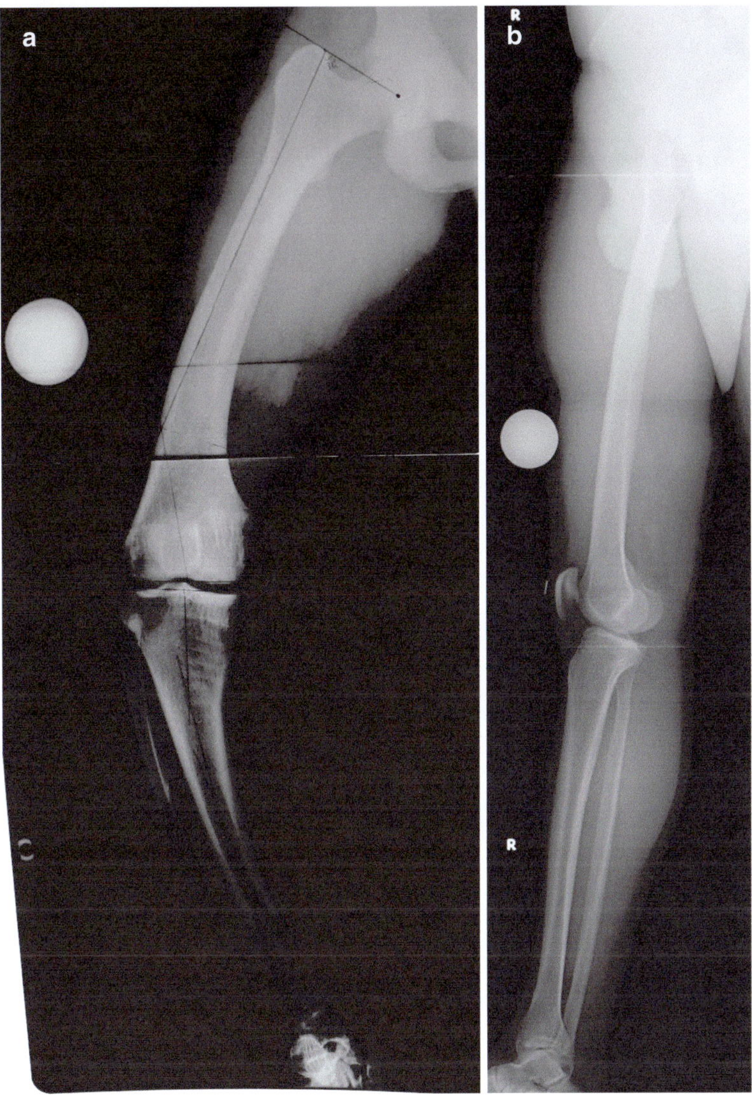

Fig. 3.9 On AP (**a**) and lateral (**b**) x-rays, marked with a 2.5-cm radius circle, the length and the size of the IM nail can be determined

the contact between the two fragments remains only at the edge of the fragment (Fig. 3.26).

- The level of lengthening osteotomy and the length of the IM nail are chosen to ensure that at least 8 cm of the nail lies above the distraction gap at the end of the lengthening procedure (Fig. 3.27) (Paley et al. 1997a, b).

- The deformity is corrected acutely using an LRS-type external fixator (Orthofix, Bussolengo, Italy) or an EBI Monorail Fixation System (Biomet, Parsippany, NJ, USA) (Fig. 3.28).

- Using swivel clamps, small amounts of adjustment (up to 10°) are possible in the frontal plane.

- As mentioned above, axial and sagittal plane deformities are corrected spontaneously after securing the Schanz screws with the external fixator, if the Schanz screws are placed appropriately, as described previously.

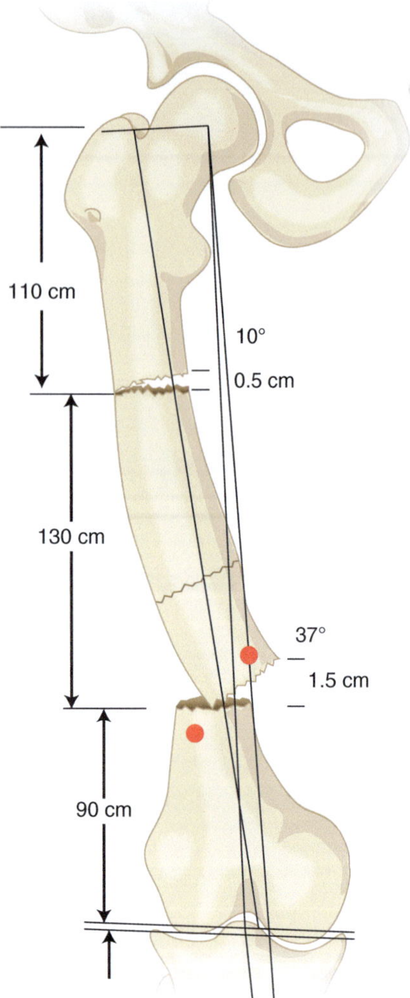

Fig. 3.10 Paper tracing to stimulate a femoral procedure

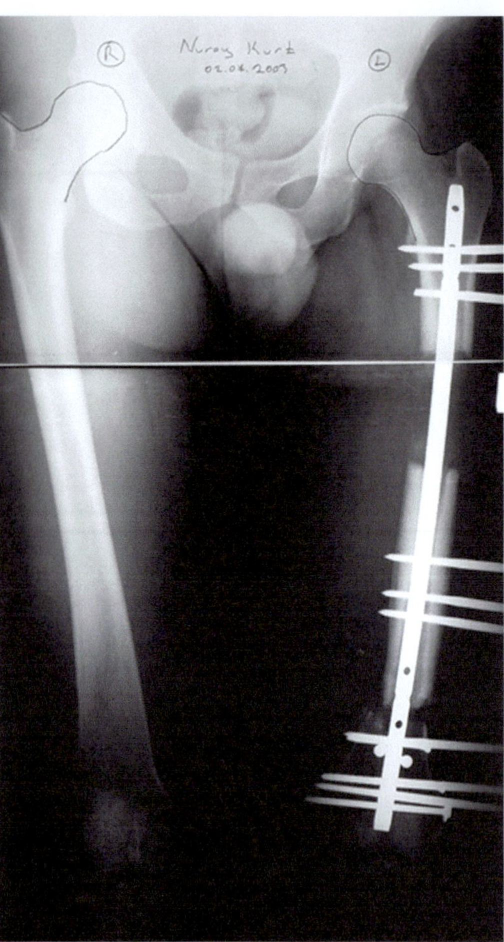

Fig. 3.12 Two poller screws distally provide extra stability around the IM nail distally at the metaphyseal level

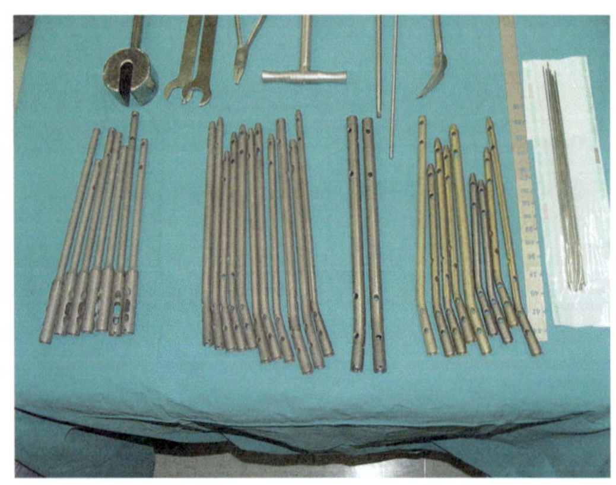

Fig. 3.11 A set of IM nails of different types with custom-made extra holes

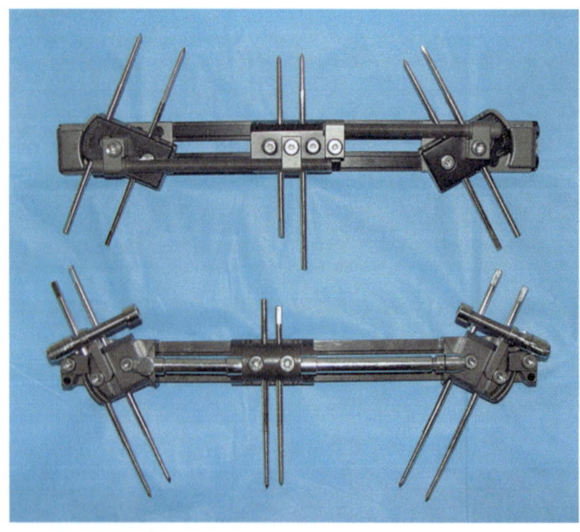

Fig. 3.13 Unilateral external fixators to be used in FANLON cases: Orthofix LRS, Bussolengo, Italy (*above*), and EBI Monorail Fixation System, Biomet, Parsippany, NJ, USA (*below*)

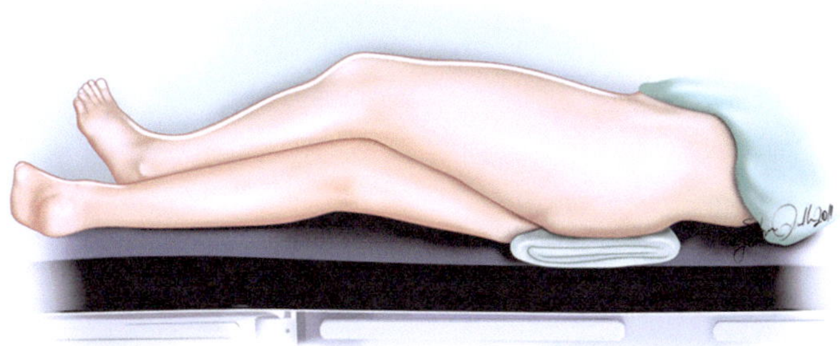

Fig. 3.14 Positioning of the lower extremity on a radiolucent table, with a silicon bag underneath the buttock to facilitate lateral view

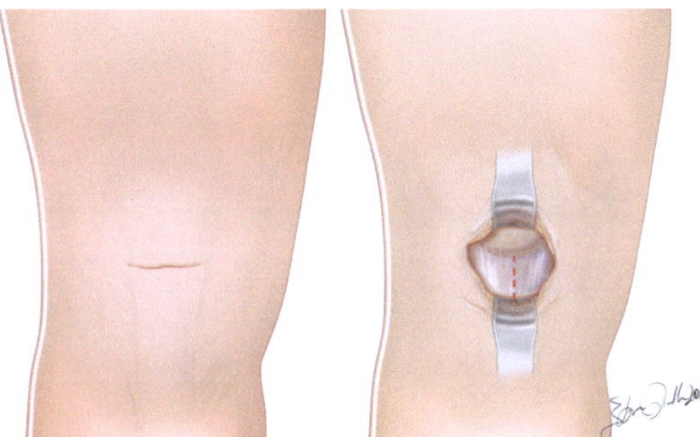

Fig. 3.15 A transverse skin incision (*left*) is used over the patellar ligament, then the paratenon and the (*red*) dotted line depicts the longitudinal split of the patellar ligament (*right*)

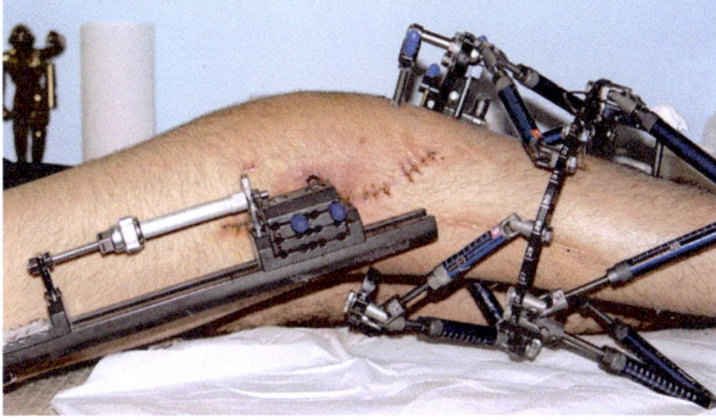

Fig. 3.17 A patient's photograph who underwent prophylactic peroneal release

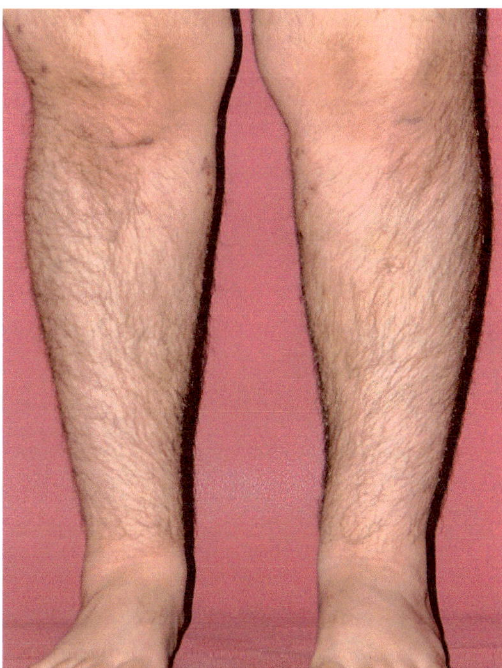

Fig. 3.16 A much better cosmetic healing can be obtained using transverse incision

- An intraoperative control x-ray is taken (AP and lateral).
  - The x-ray should simulate the preoperative paper tracing.
  - If the desired correction is not achieved, the ex-fix is readjusted, and additional radiographs are made.
- Once the satisfactory correction is achieved, interference screws (poller screws) are inserted in the frontal plane and/or the sagittal plane to maintain the necessary amount of translation and to narrow the medullary canal, especially in the metaphyseal area (Fig. 3.26) (Krettek et al. 1999a, b; Seligson 2000).
- An intramedullary guide is then inserted percutaneously through the intercondylar notch (retrograde insertion) or through the piriformis fossa (antegrade insertion) (Fig. 3.29).
- The authors recommend using a long, rigid, 6-mm drill bit to create a straight femoral canal before inserting the intramedullary guide (Fig. 3.30).

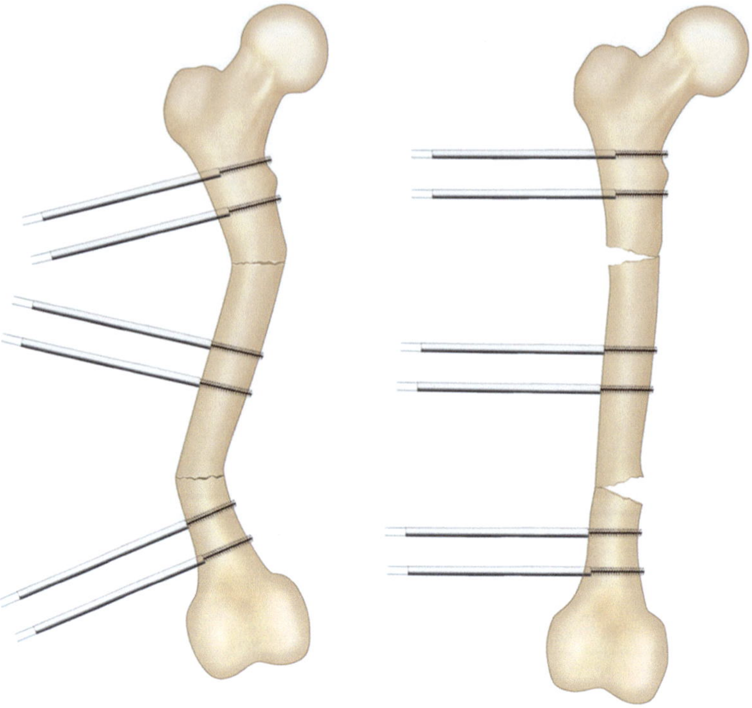

Fig. 3.18 Correction of a femoral deformity using perpendicular (to the anatomic axis of each segment) Schanz screws

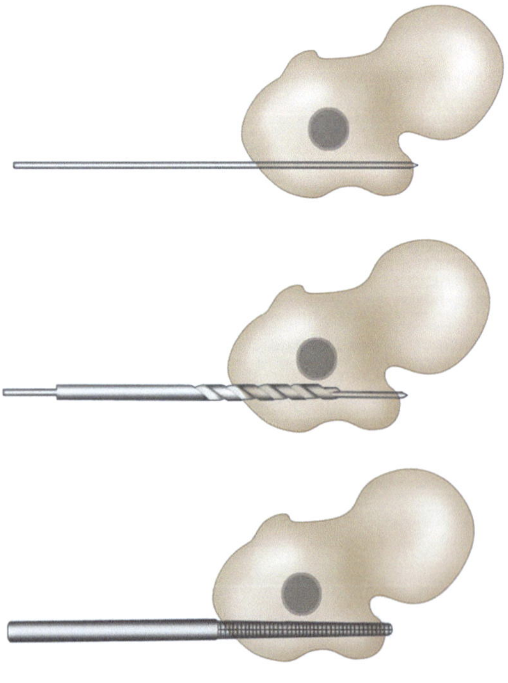

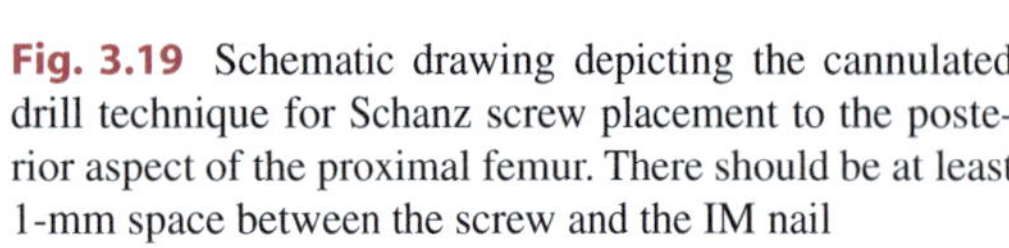

Fig. 3.19 Schematic drawing depicting the cannulated drill technique for Schanz screw placement to the posterior aspect of the proximal femur. There should be at least 1-mm space between the screw and the IM nail

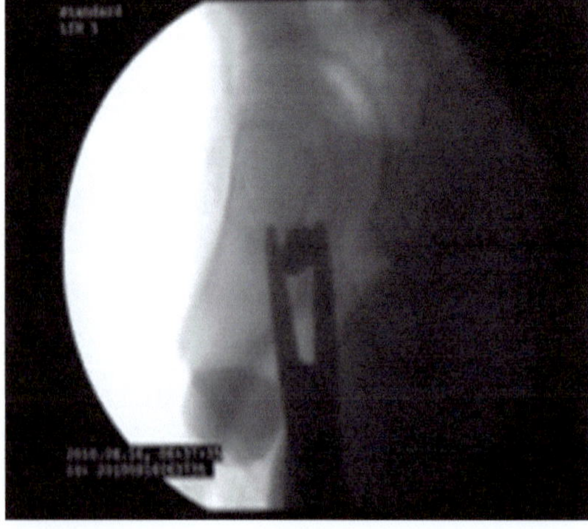

Fig. 3.20 Enough space should be left for the IM nail at the posterior aspect of the proximal femur

- The medullary canal is overreamed by 1.5 mm (in 0.5-mm increments) more than the diameter of the intramedullary nail to be used to allow sliding of the nail for lengthening (Fig. 3.8).
  - The osteotomies are excellent venting holes to avoid high pressure within the medullary canal during reaming, protecting it from fat embolisms.
  - The reaming material acts as an osteoinductive and osteoconductive substance (internal grafting) (Figs. 3.30 and 3.31).

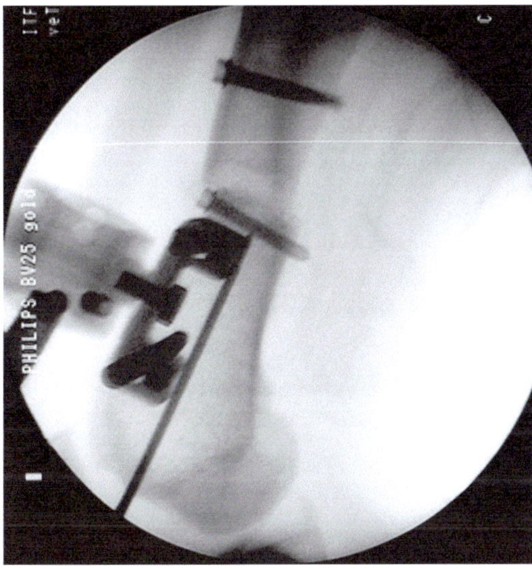

Fig. 3.21 Enough space should be left for the IM nail at the posterior aspect of the distal femur

- The nail is then inserted slowly.
  - As the medullary canal has been overreamed to 1.5 mm larger than the IM nail, the nail is inserted easily by hand, without the need for forceful maneuvers or hammer slaps.
  - We prefer regular tibial nails for retrograde femoral nailing because their curves help to correct any sagittal deformities present (Fig. 3.32).
- Interlocking screws are inserted distally (retrograde nail) or proximally (antegrade nail), whereas the proximal/distal interlocking screws are not placed until lengthening has been completed. The nail is locked only at one side of the osteotomy so that the nail slides at the other side during distraction through the osteotomy site.
- An image intensifier is used to check all Schanz screws to ensure that they are not in contact with the IM nail (Fig. 3.33a, b).
- Distraction testing (0.5 cm) is performed with the ex-fix to confirm that the distraction occurs at the lengthening osteotomy level.
  - After a successful distraction test, the gap is compressed to the original position.
  - If the distraction test is unsuccessful, extract the nail and then overream the canal to 2 mm larger than the nail; repeat the steps.
- Epidural analgesia is preferred for a comfortable postoperative period.

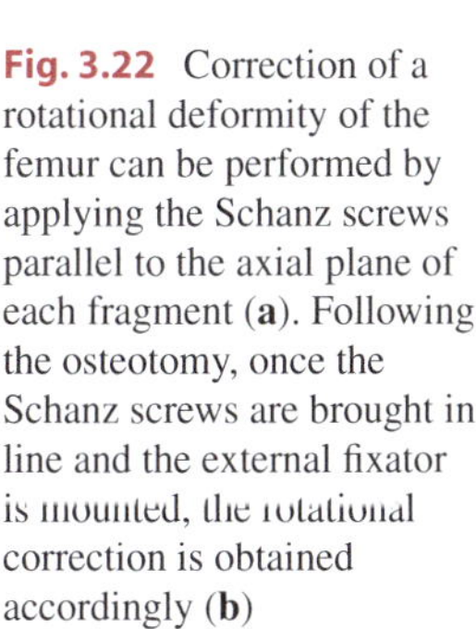
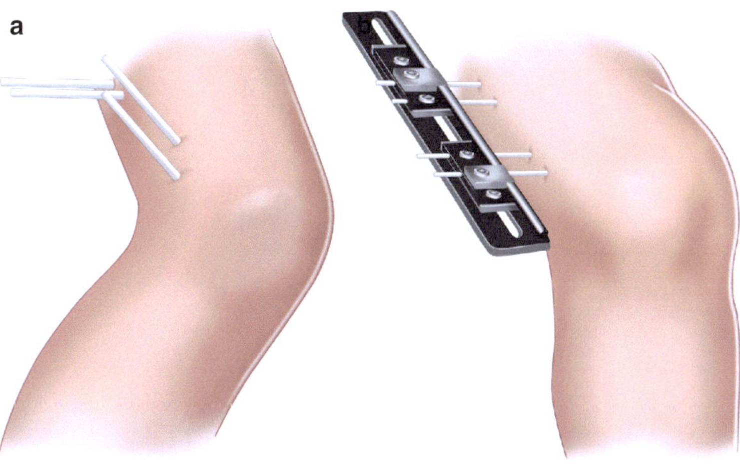

Fig. 3.22 Correction of a rotational deformity of the femur can be performed by applying the Schanz screws parallel to the axial plane of each fragment (**a**). Following the osteotomy, once the Schanz screws are brought in line and the external fixator is mounted, the rotational correction is obtained accordingly (**b**)

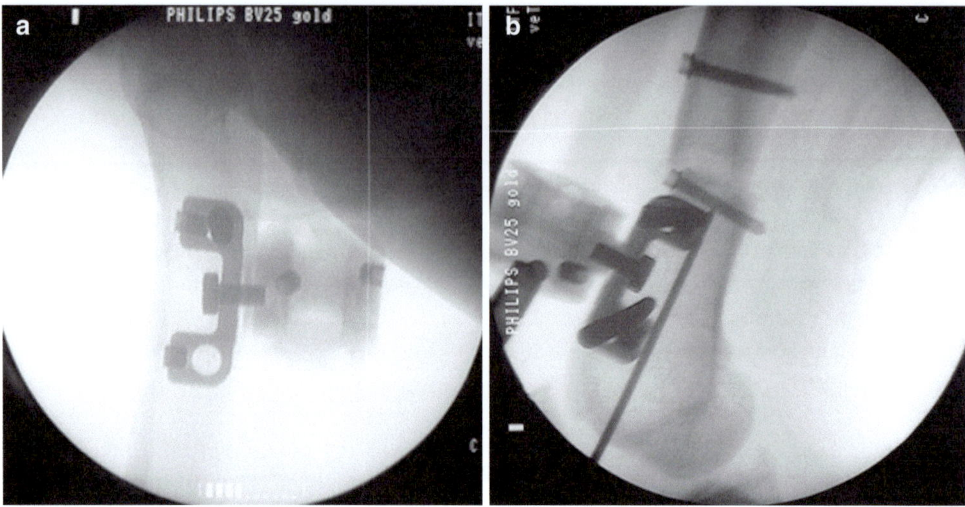

Fig. 3.23 Sagittal plane deformities can be corrected by placement of the Schanz screws parallel to the sagittal plane axis of each fragment proximally (**a**) and distally (**b**)

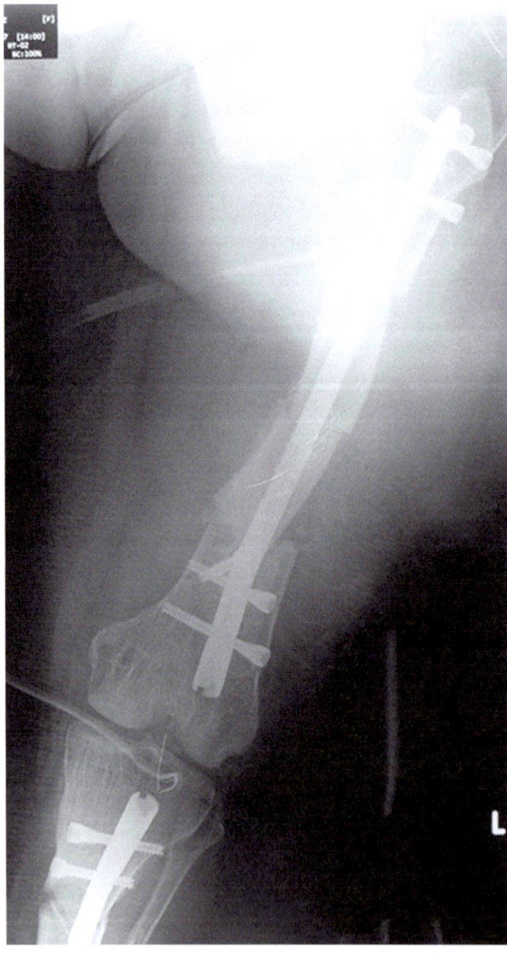

Fig. 3.24 X-ray of a patient displaying an obligatory translation due to the osteotomy (because the level of the osteotomy is different than the CORA)

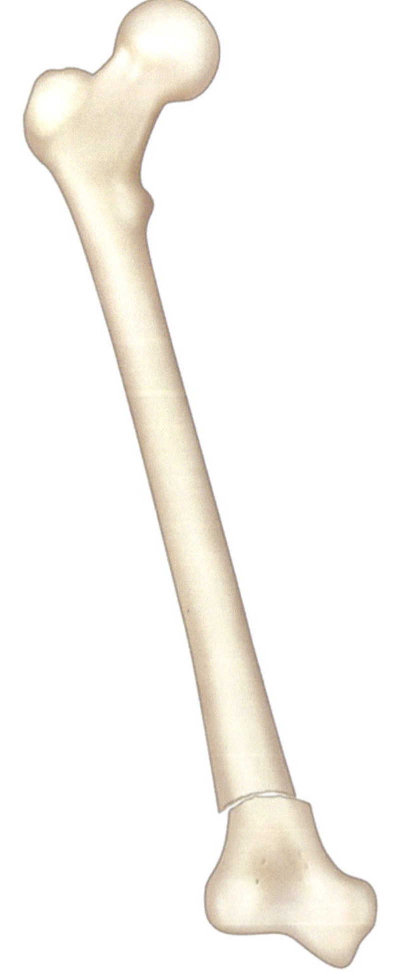

Fig. 3.25 Schematic drawing of a dome-shaped osteotomy providing a large contact area

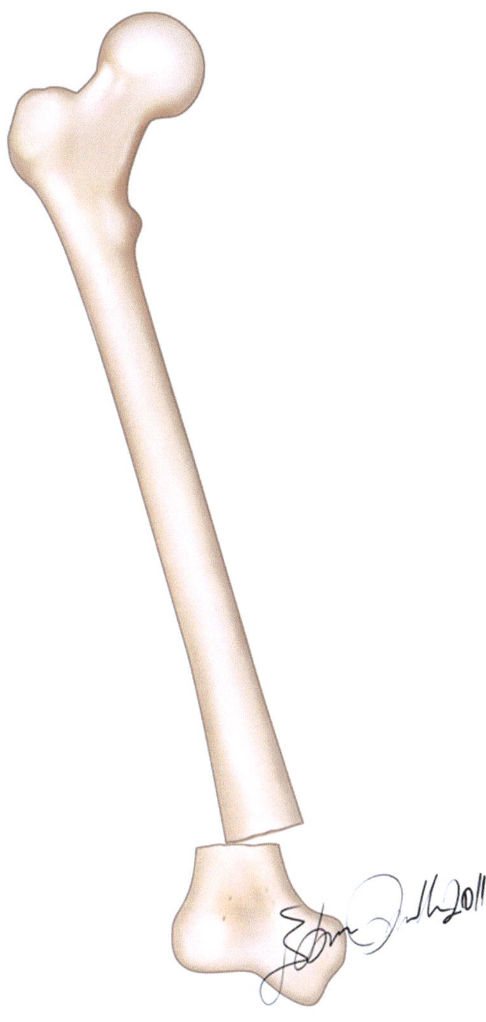

Fig. 3.26 Schematic drawing of a transverse osteotomy leading to a point contact between the fragments

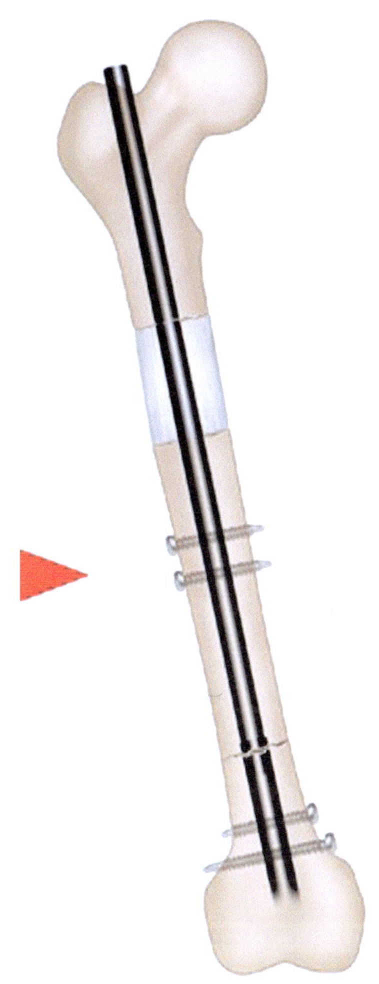

Fig. 3.27 Schematic drawing of a femoral FAN-LON procedure at the end of the treatment. The length of the IM nail must extend at least 8 cm above to the level of the distraction gap

- Additionally, epidural analgesia also decreases the risk of postoperative DVT.
- However, epidural analgesia might mask the signs of compartment syndrome, but the risk of compartment syndrome in a femoral application is quite low (Tornero et al. 2010).

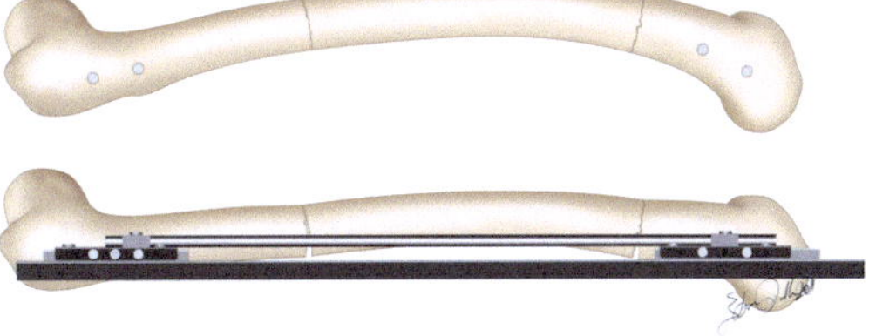

Fig. 3.28 Correction of a sagittal deformity using an external fixator. The Schanz screws are placed parallel to the sagittal axis of each fragment

3.2.8 Postoperative Period

- Dressing changes begin during the first 48 h. We prefer gentle, normal saline cleansing around the pin sites and nonocclusive dressings every 3rd day.

- On the day of the operation, isometric quadriceps and knee range of motion exercises are initiated.

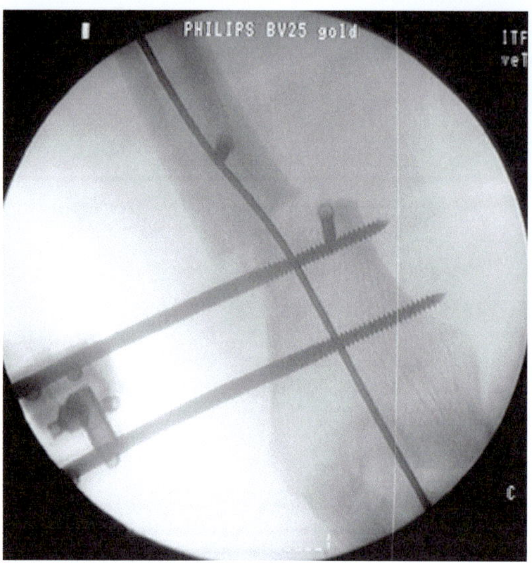

Fig. 3.29 Placement of a retrograde guidewire through in the intercondylar notch of the femur

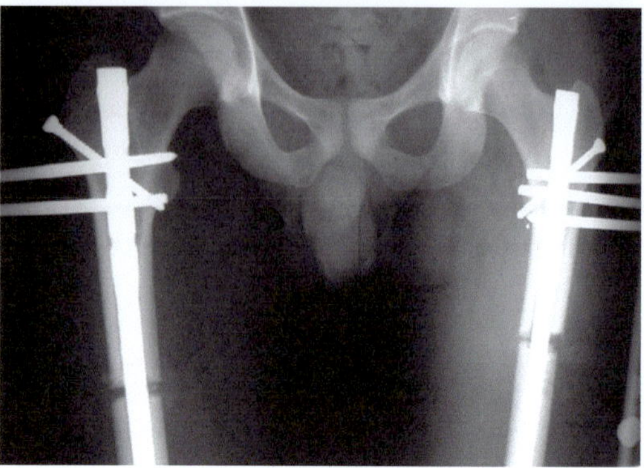

Fig. 3.31 The reaming material acts as internal grafting at the osteotomy level

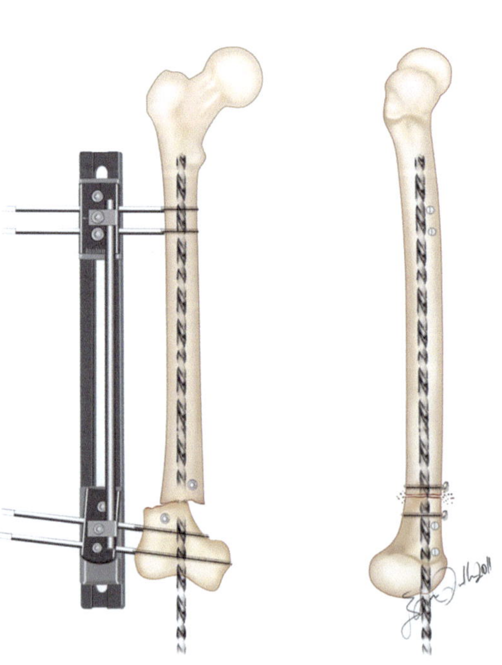

Fig. 3.30 Long, rigid, 6-mm drill bit is used to create a straight femoral canal

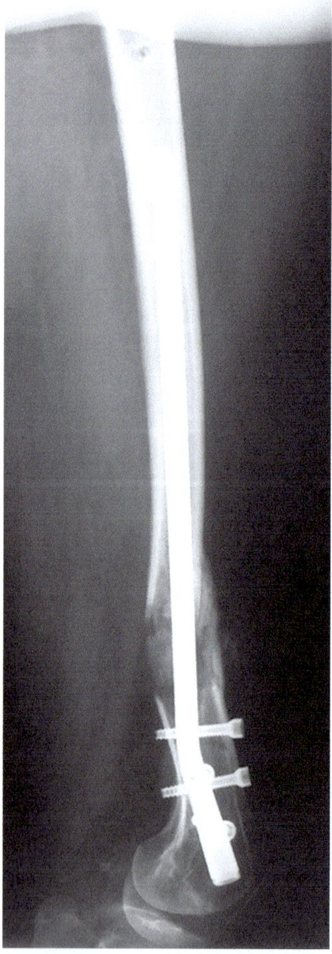

Fig. 3.32 X-ray of a patient, in which a tibial nail was used to correct sagittal deformity (extension effect was obtained)

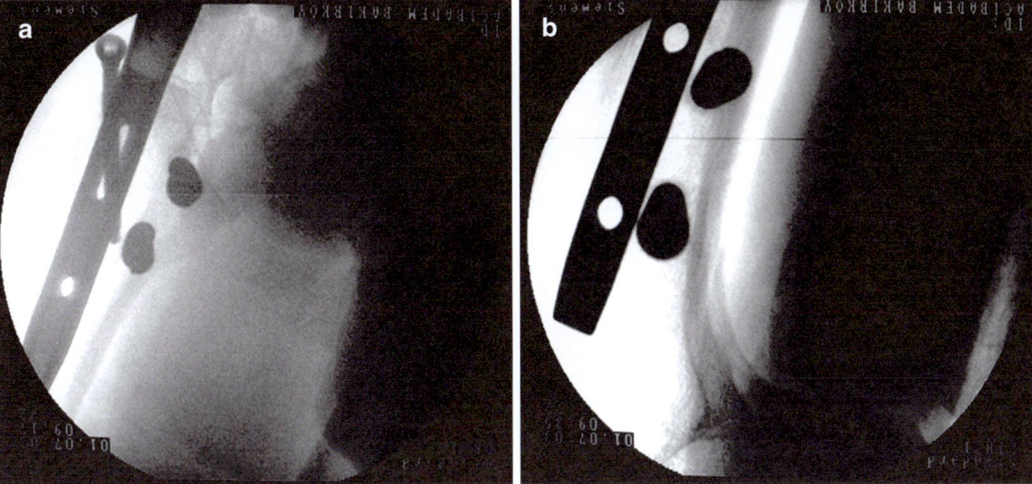

Fig. 3.33 There should be at least 1-mm clear space between the IM nail and the Schanz screws both proximally (**a**) and distally (**b**)

- In retrograde insertion cases, ice application is recommended over the knee joint for 3 weeks (20-min periods, four times a day).
- On the first postoperative day, full weight bearing with two crutches is allowed.
- The patient is discharged from the hospital on the second or third postoperative day if he or she is able to walk independently with two crutches and if the active range of motion of the hip and the knee joint is not limited.
- The authors recommend daily physical therapy after discharge from the hospital until the end of the treatment period.
- Distraction begins 7 days postoperatively (the so-called latency period) at a rate of 0.25 mm four times a day (=1 mm per day).
- During the lengthening period, we recommend radiographs be made every 2 weeks to monitor the distraction progress (the amount of lengthening, the quality of the regenerate formation, and the presence of any mechanical failure and/or osteolysis around the Schanz screws). At each visit, the patient is evaluated for ROM of the hip and the knee joints, pin site status, stability of the external fixator, and neurovascular status (clinically, especially for the presence of drop foot).

3.2.9 Removal of the External Fixator

When the desired of amount of lengthening has been achieved, the patient undergoes the second stage of surgical treatment.

- In the supine position on the radiolucent table, the empty holes of the IM nail are checked with an image intensifier in both planes prior to sterile preparation.
- Prophylactic antibiotics are initiated (cephamezine 4×1 g IV for 3 days).
- The patient is prepared from the hip to the toes, as in the first procedure.
- After preparation of the entire extremity, the external fixator is cleansed again with Betadine solution and is then wrapped with towels.
- Interlocking of the empty holes on the IM nail is performed utilizing the cannulated drill technique (Fig. 3.34).

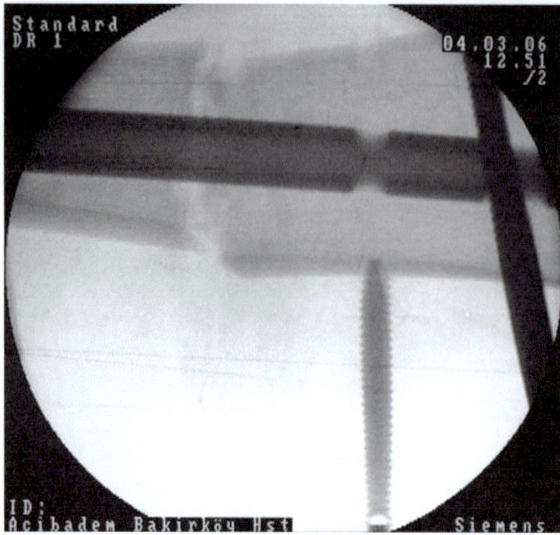

Fig. 3.34 The empty holes of the IM nail are locked using cannulated drill technique

- The external fixator is removed once the IM nail has been locked statically and secured mechanically (with interference screws if necessary).
- This step is usually performed as an outpatient procedure.

3.2.10 Follow-Up After the Second Procedure

- The patient is allowed to bear full weight with two crutches until full consolidation of the regeneration takes place.
- The first visit following discharge from the hospital is on the 7th day postoperatively. At this visit, the wounds are checked for any problems. No x-rays are needed at this point.
- Follow-up of the consolidation of the regeneration and healing of the osteotomy/osteotomies for deformity correction are checked with AP and lateral x-rays at monthly intervals (Fig. 3.35). At this visit, the ROM of the hip and the knee joint and muscle strength are also assessed.
- In cases that develop loss of knee joint ROM, we prefer using custom braces, along with physical therapy.

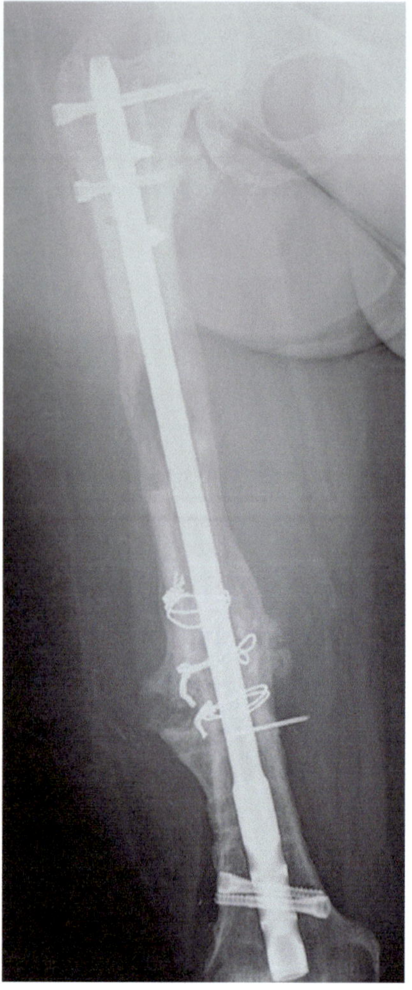

Fig. 3.35 A patient's x-ray at displaying good consolidation of the regenerate

3.3 Tibial FAN-LON

3.3.1 Indications

3.3.1.1 Congenital Deformities
- Fibular hemimelia with LLD and deformities (Achterman and Kalamchi classification types 1A and 1B) (Figs. 3.36 and 3.37)
- Short stature with deformities due to bone dysplasias (achondroplasia, hypochondroplasia, spondyloepiphyseal dysplasia, multiple epiphyseal dysplasia, etc.)
- Hemihypertrophy (Beckwith-Wiedemann syndrome)

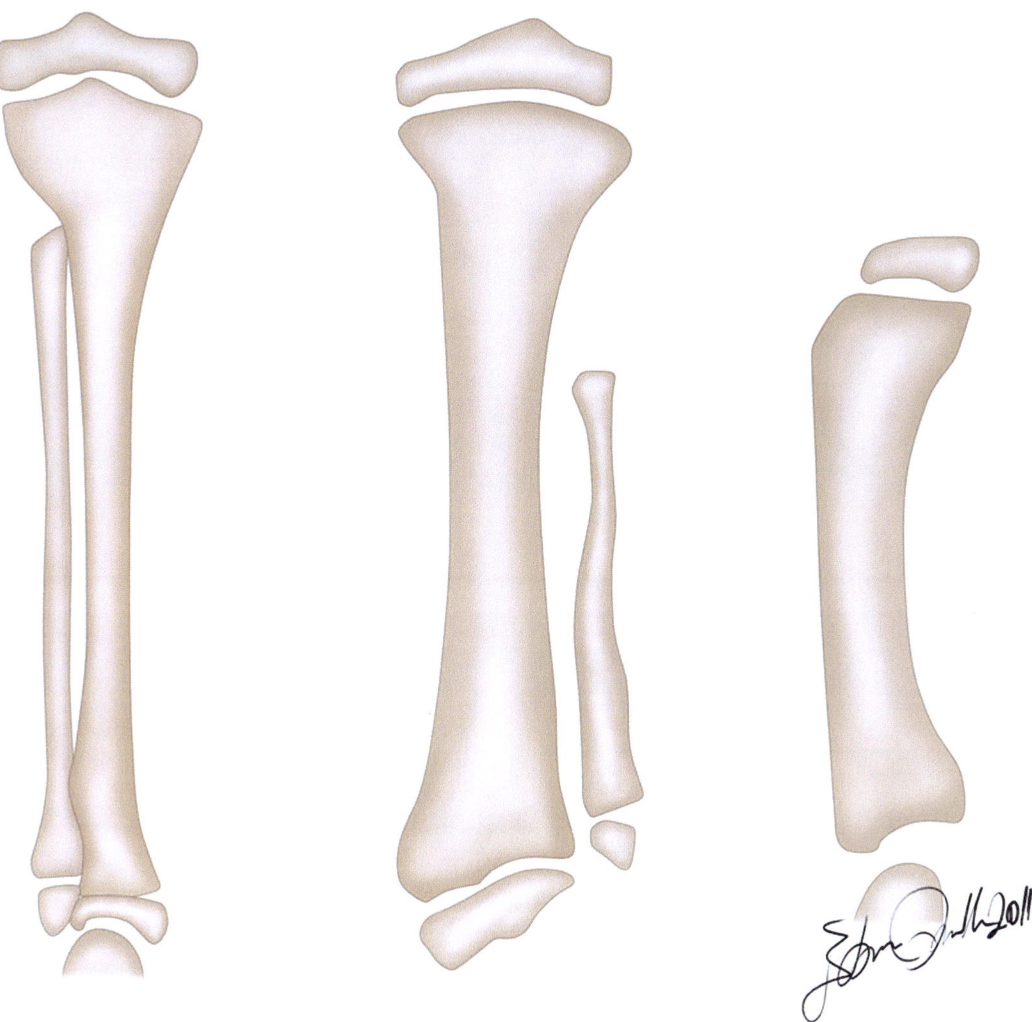

Fig. 3.36 Achterman and Kalamchi classification for fibular hemimelia

3.3.1.2 Acquired Deformities

- Posttraumatic defect nonunions associated with deformities (Paley type B3) (Paley et al. 1989) (Figs. 3.38 and 3.39)
- Deformity with LLD due to posttraumatic or postinfectious epiphyseal damage
- Postinfectious defect stage 1 nonunions created by the surgeon (Kocaoglu et al. 2006) (Fig. 3.40)
- LLDs and deformities due to bone tumors (including postsurgical iatrogenic defects and sequelae)

- Multi-apical deformities and constitutional short stature due to metabolic bone disease (rickets, hypophosphatemic rickets, etc.) (Fig. 3.41)

3.3.2 Examination

- A thorough physical examination of the lower extremities should again be conducted, as described for femoral FAN-LON cases.

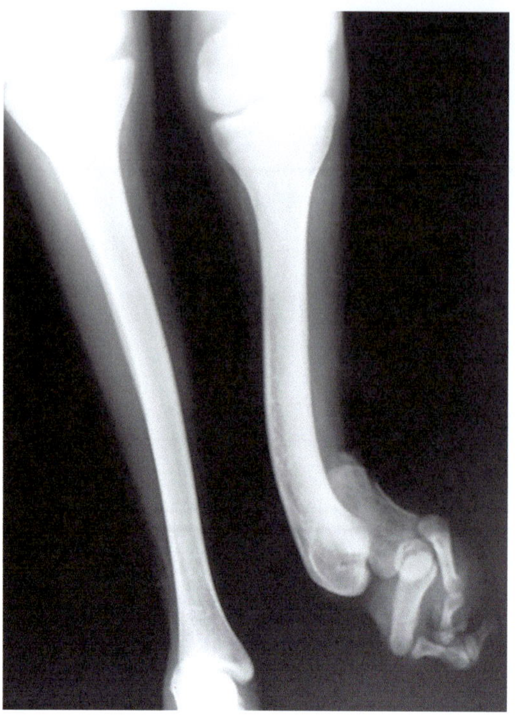

Fig. 3.37 A patient's x-ray with fibular hemimelia

3.3.3 Imaging Studies

- A complete imaging series of the lower extremities must be obtained, as for femoral FAN-LON cases.

3.3.4 Preoperative Planning

- All data obtained via clinical examination and imaging studies should be carefully evaluated.
- The deformity should be analyzed according to the deformity planning guidelines outlined by Paley (Paley and Tetsworth 1992).
- The levels of the osteotomy/osteotomies in the affected bone segment(s) should be determined according to anatomic/mechanical axis planning (Paley and Herzenberg 2002).
- The diameter and the size of the IM nail should be determined based on the scaled AP and lateral x-rays of the affected bone segment(s).
- Paper tracing should be performed to simulate the surgery and to determine the provisional final position of the bone segment (Figs. 3.42 and 3.43).
  - The extra custom-made hole(s) on the IM nail should be determined.
  - The location and number of the interference (poller) screws should be assigned to increase the stability of the reconstruction (Fig. 3.43).
  - The incision of the entry point of the IM nail and the osteotomy levels should be determined.

3.3.5 Equipment

- The same equipment is needed as for femoral FAN-LON cases. Additionally, a tibial intramedullary nail (the authors prefer Ortopro Tibial 4G Nails, Istanbul, Turkey) and a circular-type external fixator (Tasarim Med, Istanbul, Turkey) are required.
- Custom-made extra holes for locking screws are made in the nails if necessary (Fig. 3.44).

3.3.6 Positioning

- The patient is placed supine on the radiolucent table.
- The region from the hip to the ankle joint in both planes is checked by fluoroscopy before sterile preparation (Fig. 3.45a, b).
- The entire lower extremity starting from the ASIS is sterile prepared and draped.
- Prophylactic antibiotics are initiated (cephamezine 4 × 1 g IV for 3 days).

Fig. 3.38 Paley's classification of pseudarthrosis. Type B3 depicts shortening with bone loss (*bottom right*)

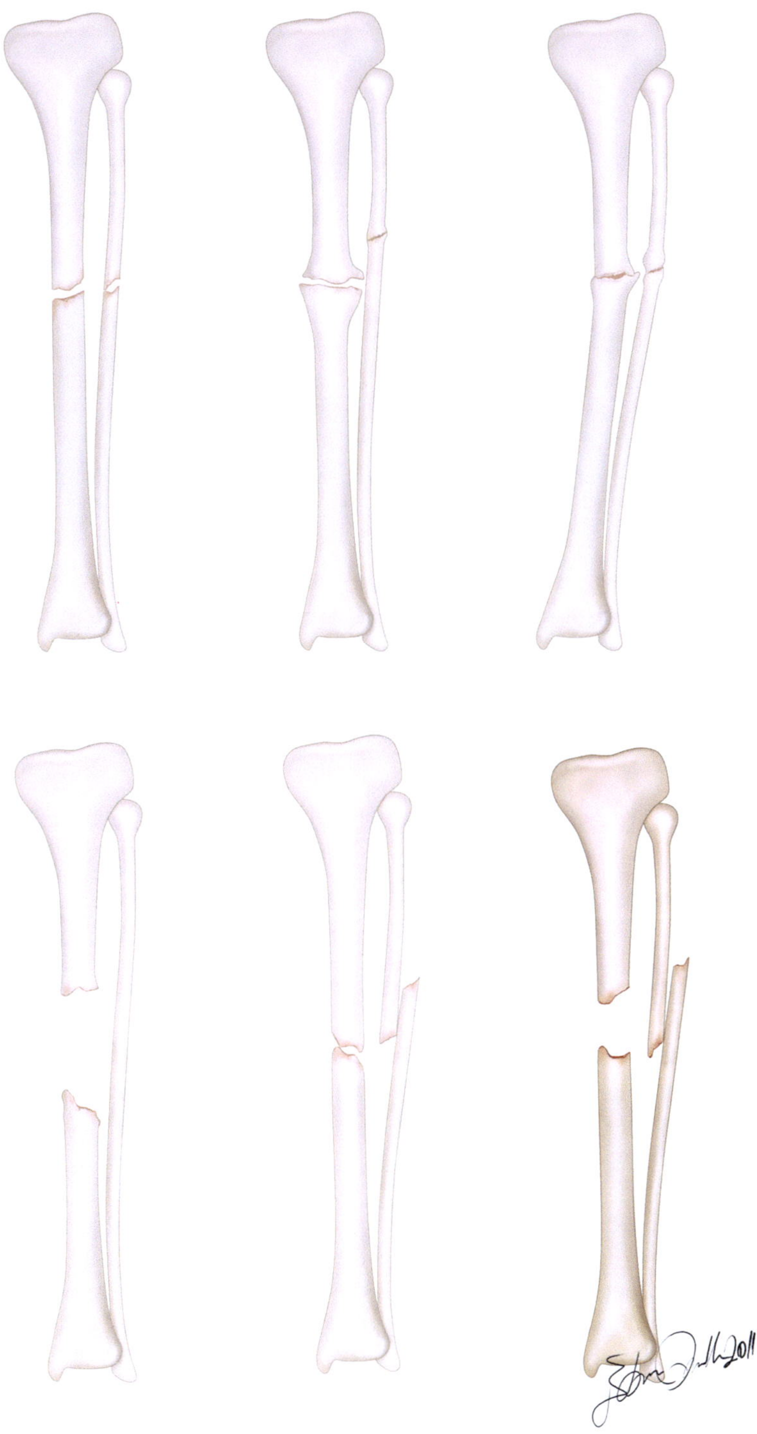

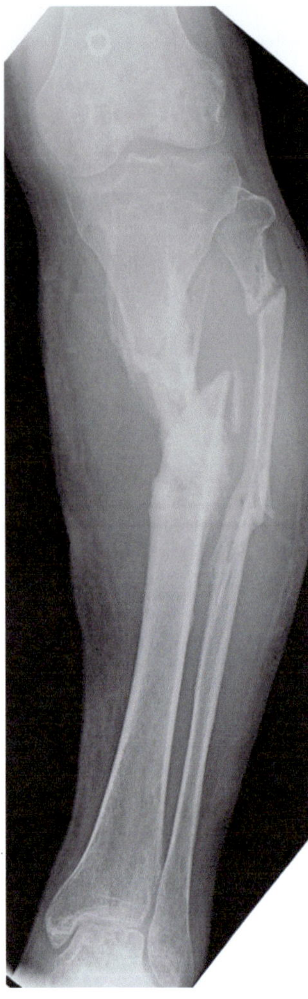

Fig. 3.39 A patient's x-ray with tibial shortening associated with bone loss

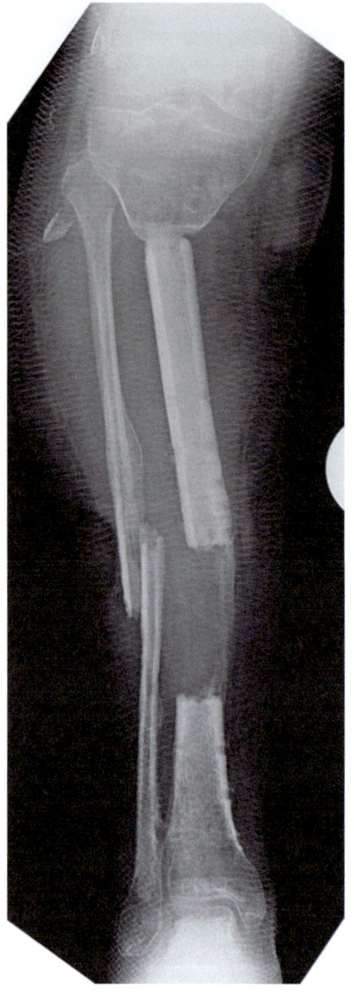

Fig. 3.40 A patient's x-ray with postinfectious bone loss of the tibia

3.3.7 Surgical Technique

3.3.7.1 Exposure/Incision

Again, the tibial intramedullary nail can be inserted through a 2-cm transverse incision over the patellar ligament (Fig. 3.15).

Before the acute correction of valgus deformities around the knee of more than 20°, prophylactic peroneal nerve release must be performed (Paley 1990).

- Schanz screws are placed perpendicular to the anatomic/mechanical axes (which are parallel, almost identical, in the tibia) of each segment proximally and distally (and at the middle segment when present) with the cannulated drill technique (Fig. 3.46).
- The Schanz screws should be placed posteriorly to leave enough space for the IM nail (Fig. 3.47a, b).
- There should be at least 1 mm of space between the IM nail and the Schanz screws to avoid spreading any pin-track infection into the medullary space (Fig. 3.48).

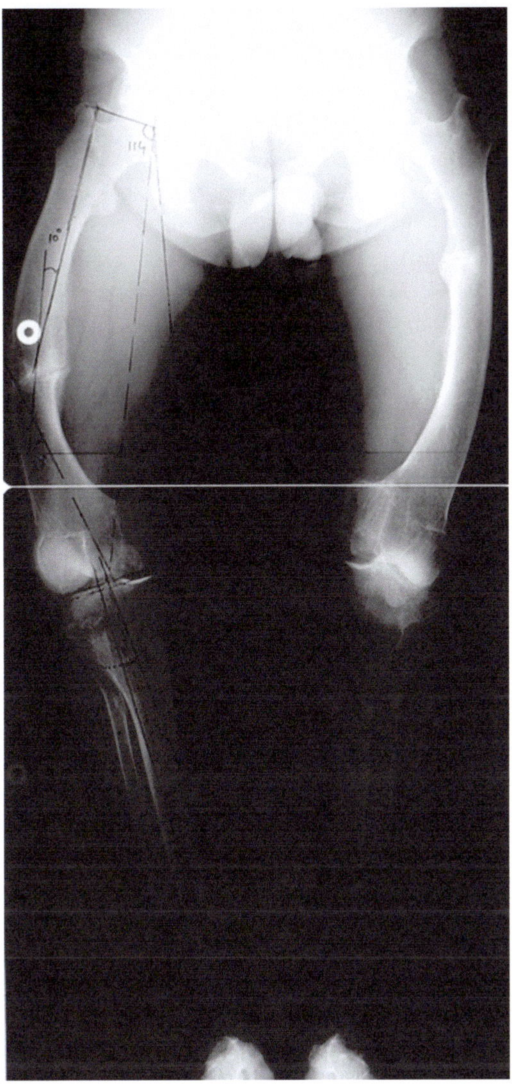

Fig. 3.41 A patient's x-ray with rickets displaying long bowing deformities

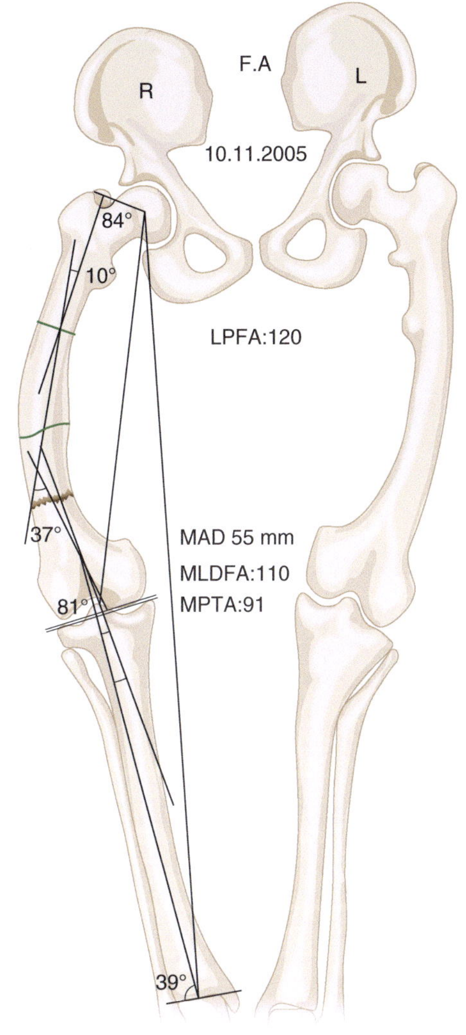

Fig. 3.42 Paper tracing for analysis of the deformity

- Schanz screws are placed parallel to the axial plane of each fragment. Thus, once the Schanz screws are secured to the external fixator following the osteotomy/osteotomies, the rotational deformities have been corrected (Fig. 3.49a, b).
- To correct sagittal plane deformities, the Schanz screws need to be placed parallel to sagittal plane axis of each fragment (Fig. 3.50a, b).

- To correct and/or maintain the rotational alignment of the tibia, the proximal screws are inserted horizontally once a true lateral view of the knee is obtained using the image intensifier. The distal Schanz screws are inserted horizontally once a true lateral view of the ankle is obtained in the same manner (Fig. 3.47a, b).

- The tibial osteotomy can be performed either proximally or distally using either the multiple drill hole technique or the Gigli saw. Multiple drill hole technique:

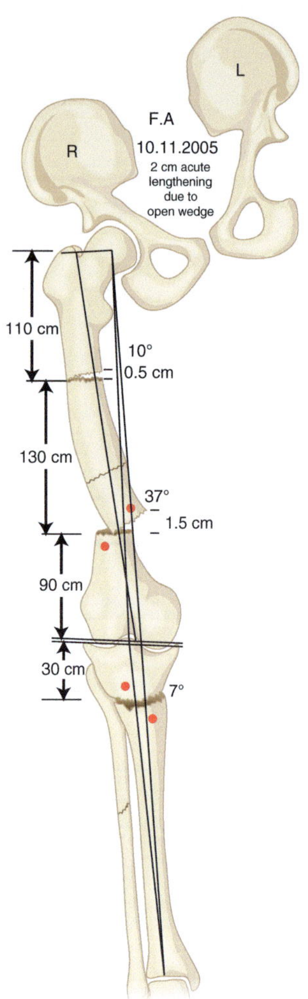

Fig. 3.43 Paper tracing to stimulate the surgical procedure

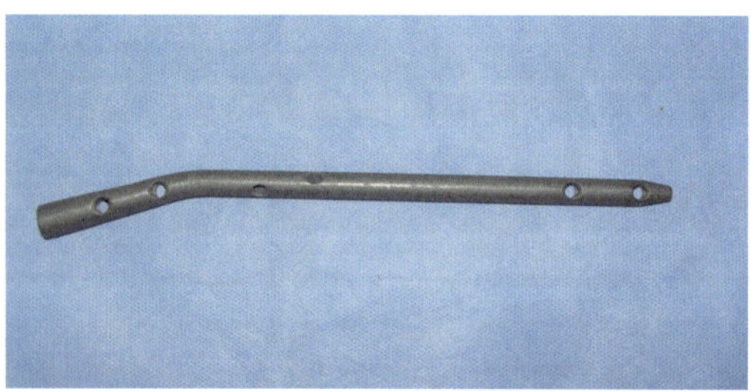

Fig. 3.44 A custom-made tibial intramedullary nail containing extra custom-made holes

– Using 3.5-mm drill bits, multiple drill holes are created percutaneously at the osteotomy level(s) (Fig. 3.51) (Paley and Tetsworth 1991).

Gigli saw technique:

– Performed through a small, 0.5-cm incision over the anterior tibial crest in the proximal metaphyseal area (Fig. 3.52).
– A tiny periosteal elevator is introduced subperiosteally to the lateral border of the tibia until the posterior edge. (During this maneuver, the sound created by the vacuum effect is heard.) Through this tunnel created on the lateral tibial wall, a right-angle clamp is inserted (Fig. 3.53).
– Through a second 0.5-mm incision at the posteromedial corner of the tibia (at the same level as the first incision), the periosteal elevator is again introduced subperiosteally until it touches the right-angle clamp. This position is confirmed with the motion of the handle of the right-angle clamp (Fig. 3.54).
– A heavy no. 5 suture is fixed at the tip of a right-angle clamp, passed through the posteromedial (second) incision, and introduced until the posterolateral border. A hemostatic clamp is introduced through the anterolateral (first) incision, and the suture at the tip of the right-angle clamp is grasped and pulled out (Fig. 3.55).
– The heavy suture is tied to the Gigli saw, and the saw is then passed around the tibia (Figs. 3.56 and 3.57). Alternatively, a vascular clamp can be modified by flattening the radius of curvature near the tip of the clamp, as this shape is much more suitable for passing the clamp around the bone and exiting at the site of the other incision (Paktiss and Gross 1993).
– An obligatory translation is necessary at the osteotomy level, especially in the metaphyseal area, if the center of rotation of angulation (CORA) is at a different level (Fig. 3.58).

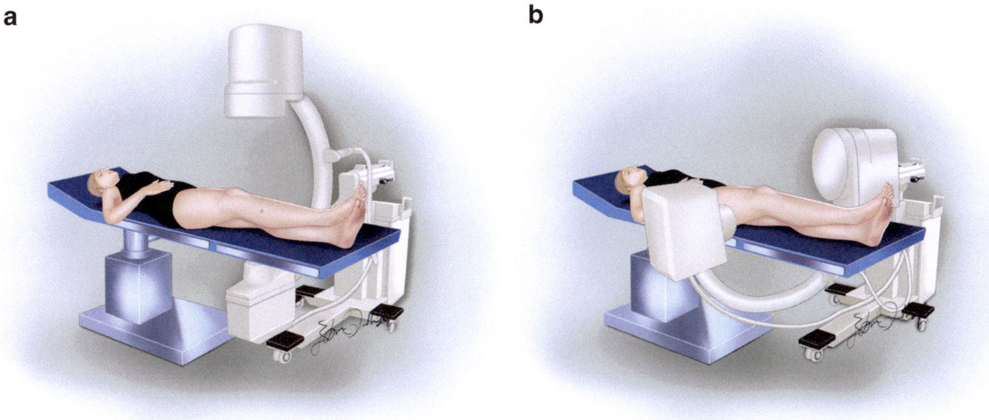

Fig. 3.45 Fluoroscopic visualization of the entire lower extremity on both planes, AP (**a**) and lateral (**b**)

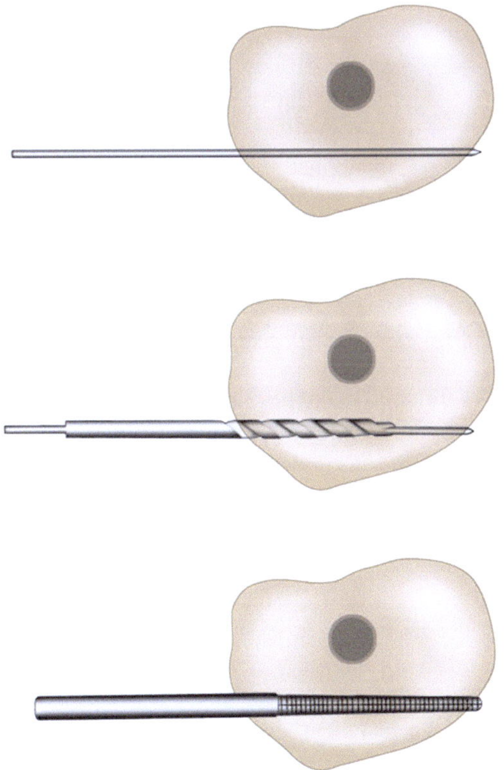

Fig. 3.46 Schanz screw placement to the proximal posterior aspect of the tibia using cannulated drill bit technique

- The maximum contact at the translated osteotomy level can be obtained with a reverse dome-shaped osteotomy (Fig. 3.59).
- Creating a dome osteotomy is technically demanding, whereas a transverse-shaped osteotomy is easier; however, after translation and angulation, the contact between the two fragments remains only at the edge of the fragment (Fig. 3.60).
- The level of the lengthening osteotomy and the length of the IM nail are chosen to ensure that at least 6 cm of the nail lies above the distraction gap at the end of the lengthening procedure (Fig. 3.61).
- The fibula is osteotomized at the mid-diaphyseal level through a small incision.
  - If there is another deformity close to the distal tibial metaphysis, then the authors prefer a second distal fibular osteotomy approximately four fingerbreadths proximal to the ankle joint (Fig. 3.62).
- The deformity is corrected acutely using an LRS-type external fixator (Orthofix, Bussolengo, Italy) or an EBI Monorail Fixation System (Biomet, NJ, USA).

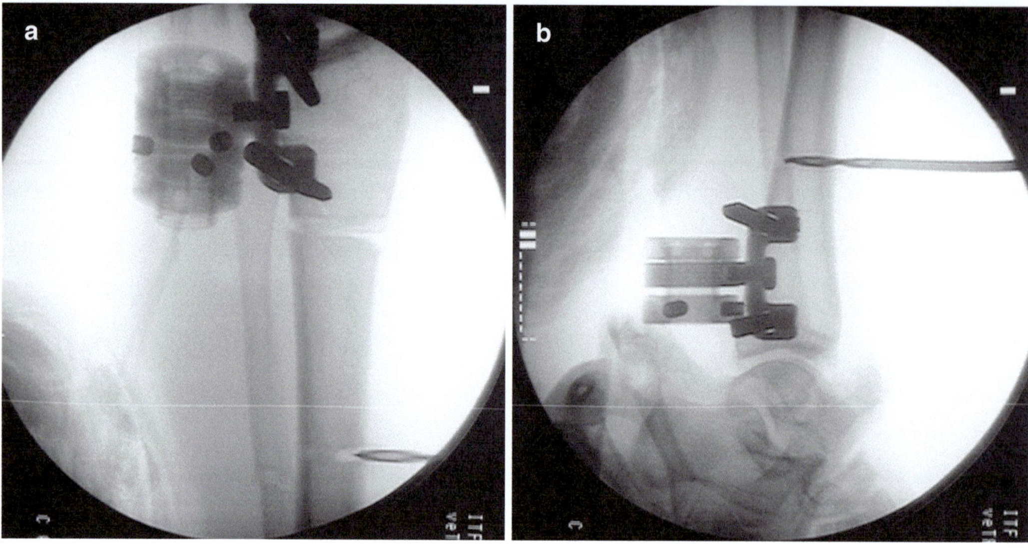

Fig. 3.47 Schanz screws are placed posteriorly to leave enough space to the IM nail proximally (**a**) and distally (**b**)

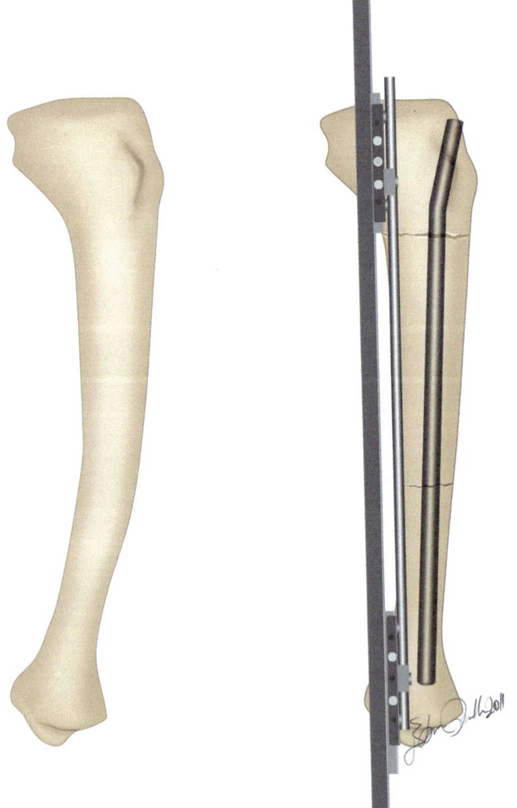

Fig. 3.48 There should be at least 1-mm clear space between the IM nail and the Schanz screws

- Using swivel clamps, a small amount of adjustment (up to 10°) is possible in the frontal plane.
- As mentioned above, axial and sagittal plane deformities are corrected spontaneously after securing the Schanz screws with the external fixator if the Schanz screws are placed appropriately.
- An intraoperative control x-ray is taken (AP and lateral).
  - The x-ray should simulate the preoperative paper tracing.
  - If the desired correction is not achieved, the ex-fix is readjusted, and additional radiographs are made.
- Once satisfactory correction is achieved, interference screws (poller screws) are inserted in the frontal plane and/or the sagittal plane to maintain the necessary amount of translation and to narrow the medullary canal, especially in the metaphyseal area (Fig. 3.63) (Krettek et al. 1999a, b; Seligson 2000).
- The insertion of the IM reaming guide is the same as that for other IM nailing procedures.
- The authors recommend using a long, rigid, 6-mm drill bit to create a straight tibial canal before inserting the IM guide.

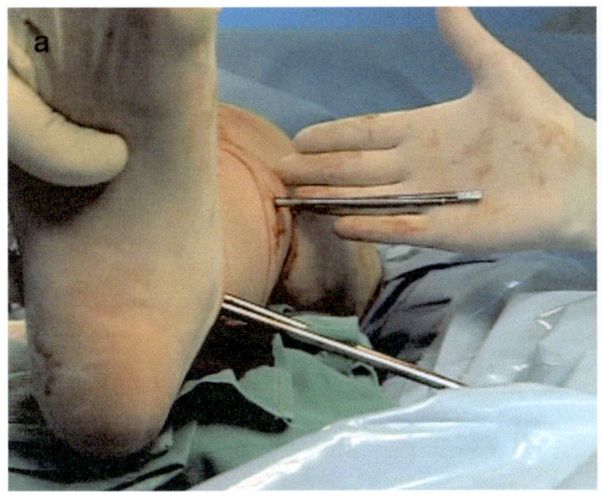

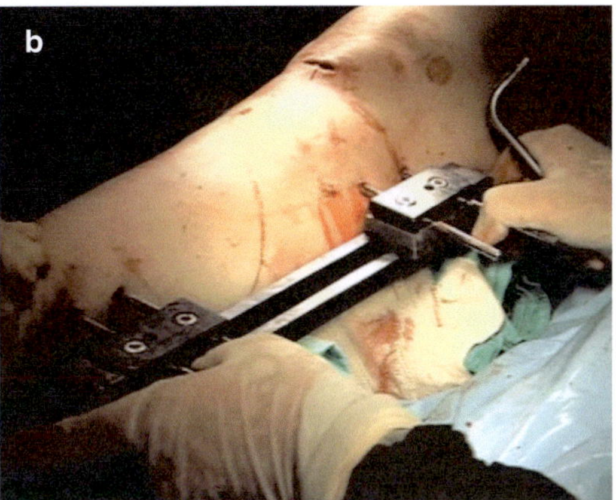

Fig. 3.49 In presence of tibial rotational deformity, the Schanz screws are placed provisionally according to the axial plane (**a**) so that following the osteotomy and rotational correction, all Schanz screws come to a line and are fixed with the external fixator (**b**)

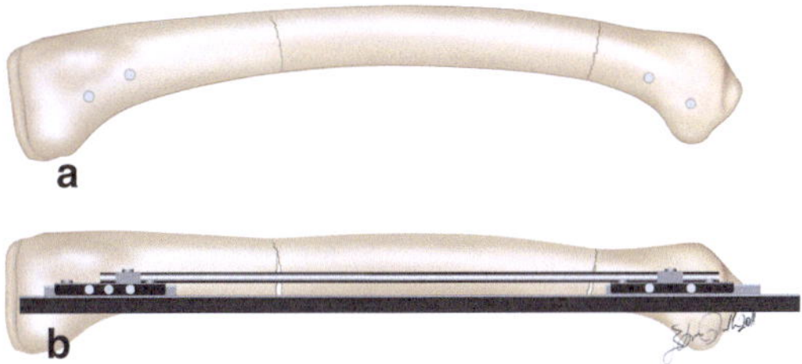

Fig. 3.50 To correct the sagittal deformity, Schanz screws are placed parallel to the sagittal axis of the corresponding segment (**a**), and following osteotomy and derotation of the fragments, all Schanz screws come in line and are fixed with an external fixator (**b**)

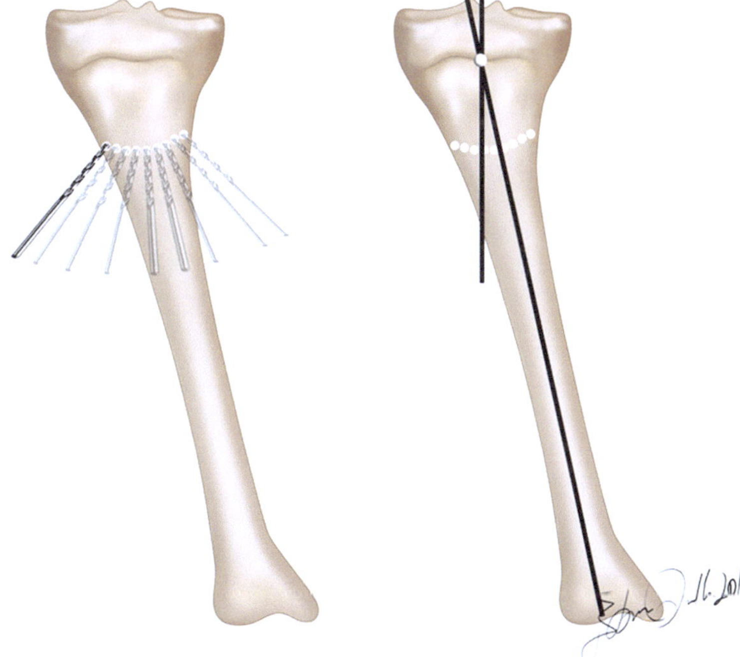

Fig. 3.51 Schematic drawing depicting multiple drill hole technique creating a reverse dome-shaped osteotomy to the tibia

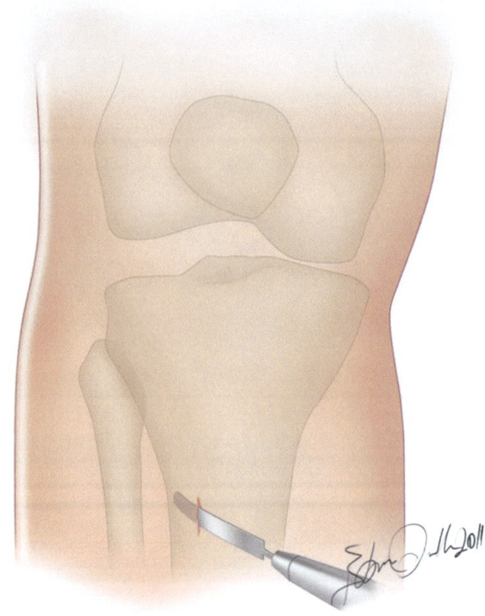

Fig. 3.52 Anterolateral incision over the anterior tibial crest for Gigli osteotomy technique

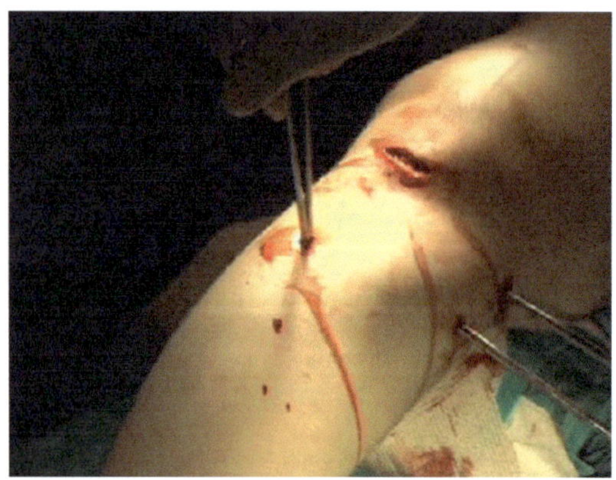

Fig. 3.53 A right-angle clamp is inserted subperiosteally

- The medullary canal is overreamed by 1.5 mm (0.5-mm increments) more than the diameter of the intramedullary nail to be used to allow sliding of the nail for lengthening (Fig. 3.61).
    - The osteotomies are excellent venting holes to avoid high pressure within the medullary canal during reaming, protecting it from the fat embolisms (Fig. 3.64).

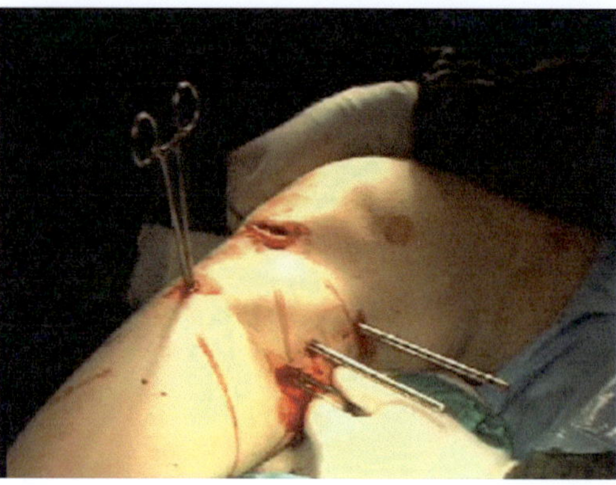

Fig. 3.54 A second right-angle clamp is introduced through the posteromedial incision subperiosteally until it reaches the first clamp, and the correct positioning is confirmed with the motion of the first clamp

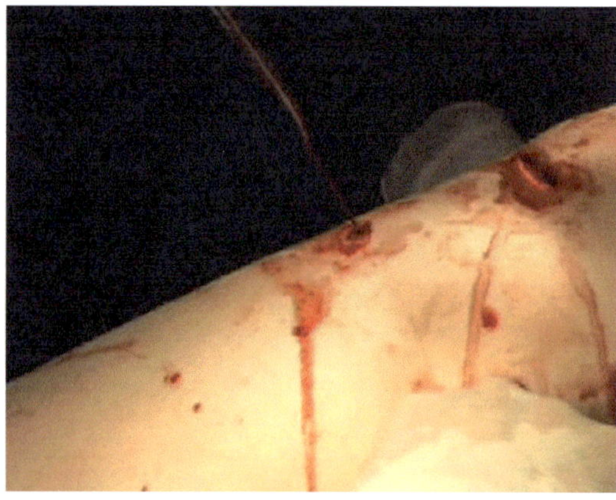

Fig. 3.55 A heavy suture is introduced through the first incision and grasped and pulled out through the second incision

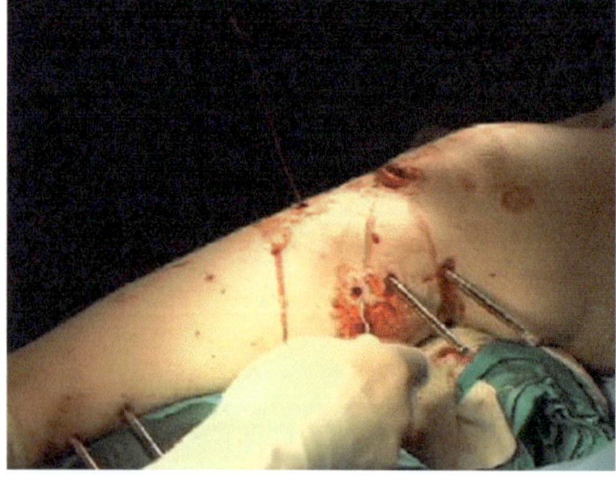

Fig. 3.56 The heavy suture is tied with the Gigli saw, and then the Gigli saw is passed around the tibia

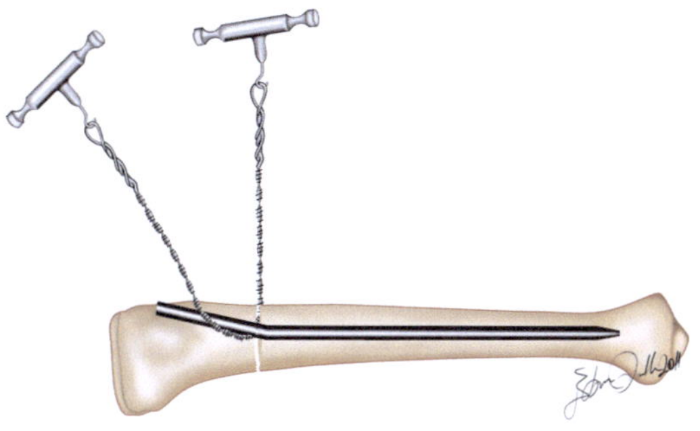

Fig. 3.57 Schematic drawing depicting usage of the Gigli saw to perform a tibial osteotomy

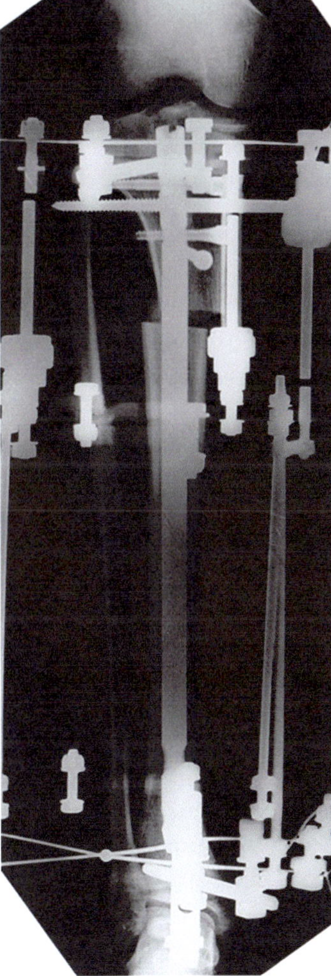

Fig. 3.58 A patient's x-ray displaying obligatory translation at the osteotomy level

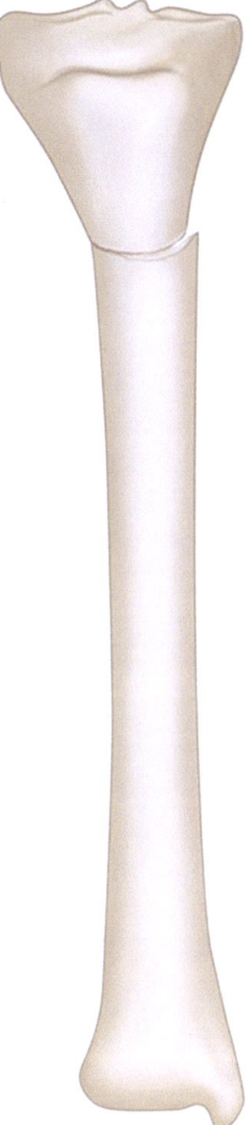

Fig. 3.59 Schematic drawing of a dome-shaped osteotomy providing a large contact area

- The reaming material acts as an osteoinductive and osteoconductive substance (internal grafting).
- The nail is then inserted slowly.
  - As the medullary canal has been over-reamed by 1.5 mm larger than the IM nail, the nail is inserted easily by hand, without the need for forceful maneuvers or hammer slaps.
- Interlocking screws are inserted proximally, whereas the distal interlocking screws are not

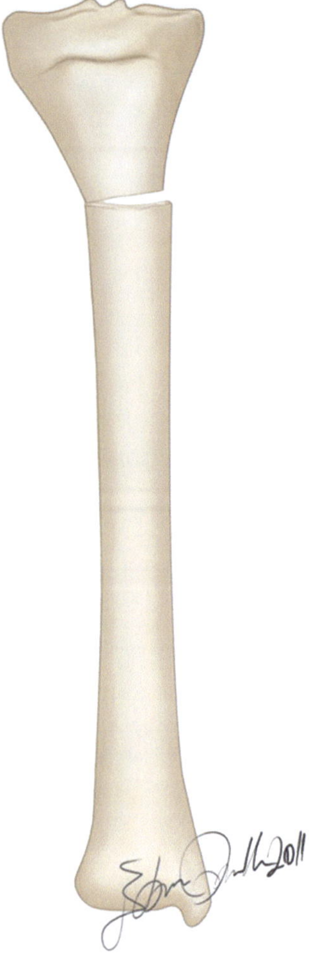

Fig. 3.60 Schematic drawing of a transverse osteotomy leading to point contact of the fragments

placed until lengthening has been completed. The nail is locked only at the proximal side of the osteotomy so that the nail slides during distraction through the osteotomy site.

- All the Schanz screws are now removed, along with the unilateral fixator, exchanging it for a circular external fixator consisting of three rings.
  - The middle ring (so-called dummy ring) adds stability but is not used for fixation (Fig. 3.65).
- To prevent dislocation of the tibiofibular joints during lengthening, a Schanz screw is used proximally to secure the fibula to the tibia, with purchase only on the medial cortex to prevent discomfort and skin problems

(Fig. 3.66), and an olive K-wire is used distally (Fig. 3.67).

- Using an image intensifier, all Schanz screws and K-wires are checked to ensure that they are not in contact with the IM nail.
- The image intensifier is then used to check that the long axis of the circular external fixator is parallel to the IM nail on both planes (AP and lateral) (Fig. 3.68a, b). This step ensures a smooth slide of the nail during distraction.
- The distraction testing (0.5 cm) is performed with ex-fix to confirm that the distraction is occurring at the lengthening osteotomy level.
  - After a successful distraction test, the gap to the original position can be compressed.
  - If the distraction test is unsuccessful, extract the nail and then overream the canal to 2 mm larger than the nail; repeat the steps.
- Epidural analgesia is not preferred because it may mask the signs of compartment syndrome (Tornero et al. 2010). The authors prefer IV analgesia.

3.3.8 Postoperative Period

- Dressing changes begin during the first 48 h. We prefer gentle normal saline cleansing around the pin sites and nonocclusive dressings every 3rd day.
- On the day of the operation, isometric quadriceps and knee range of motion exercises are initiated.
- Ice application is recommended over the knee joint for 3 weeks (20-min periods, four times a day).
- On the first postoperative day, full weight bearing with two crutches is allowed.
- The patient is discharged from the hospital on the second or third postoperative day if he or she is able to walk independently with two crutches and if the active range of motion of the hip and the knee joint is not limited.
- The authors recommend daily physical therapy after discharge from the hospital until the end of the treatment period.
- Distraction begins 7 days postoperatively (the so-called latency period) at a rate of 0.25 mm four times a day (=1 mm per day).

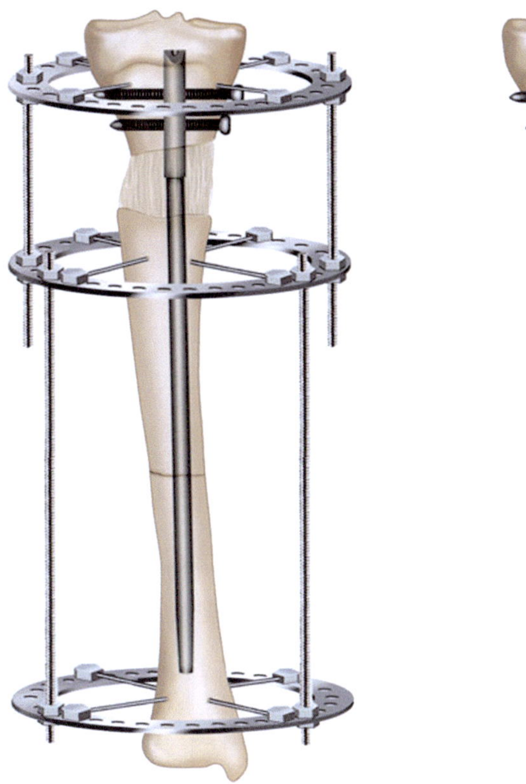

Fig. 3.61 The IM nail should extend at least 6 cm beyond the distraction gap in tibial lengthening cases

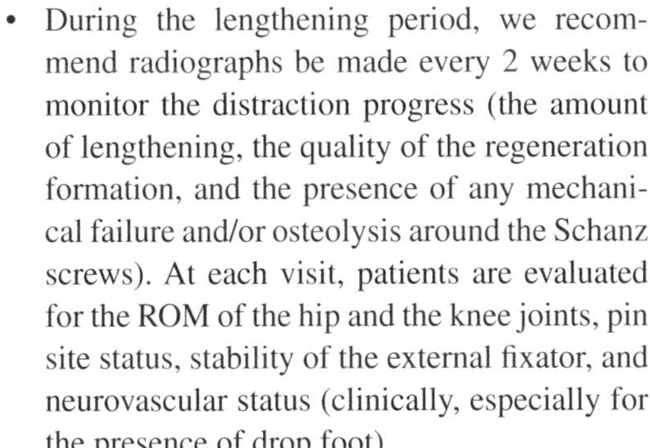

- During the lengthening period, we recommend radiographs be made every 2 weeks to monitor the distraction progress (the amount of lengthening, the quality of the regeneration formation, and the presence of any mechanical failure and/or osteolysis around the Schanz screws). At each visit, patients are evaluated for the ROM of the hip and the knee joints, pin site status, stability of the external fixator, and neurovascular status (clinically, especially for the presence of drop foot).

3.3.9   Removal of the External Fixator

When the desired of amount of lengthening has been achieved, the patient undergoes the second stage of surgical treatment.

- In a supine position on the radiolucent table, check the empty holes of the IM nail with an image intensifier in both planes prior to sterile preparation.
- The patient is prepared from the hip to the toes, as in the first procedure.
- After preparation of the entire extremity, the external fixator is cleansed again with Betadine solution and is then wrapped with towels.
- Interlocking of the empty holes on the IM nail is performed utilizing the cannulated drill technique.
- The external fixator is then removed once the IM nail has been locked statically and secured mechanically (with interference screws if necessary).
- This step is usually performed as an outpatient procedure.

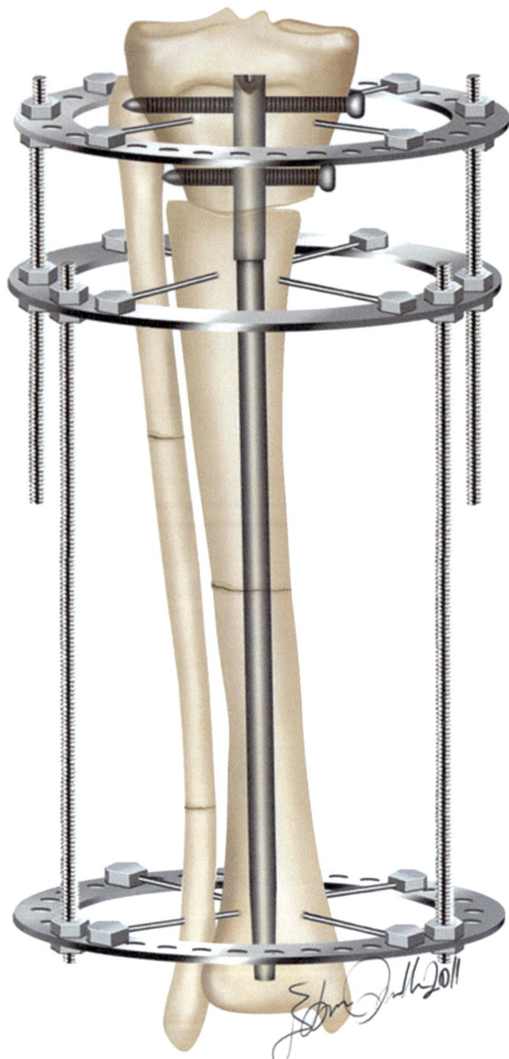

Fig. 3.62 Schematic drawing of a tibial FAN-LON case requiring a second fibular osteotomy to prevent fibular malalignment following correction

3.3.10 Follow-Up After the Second Procedure

- The patient is allowed to bear full weight with two crutches until full consolidation of the regenerate takes place.
- The first visit following discharge from the hospital is on the 7th day postoperatively. At

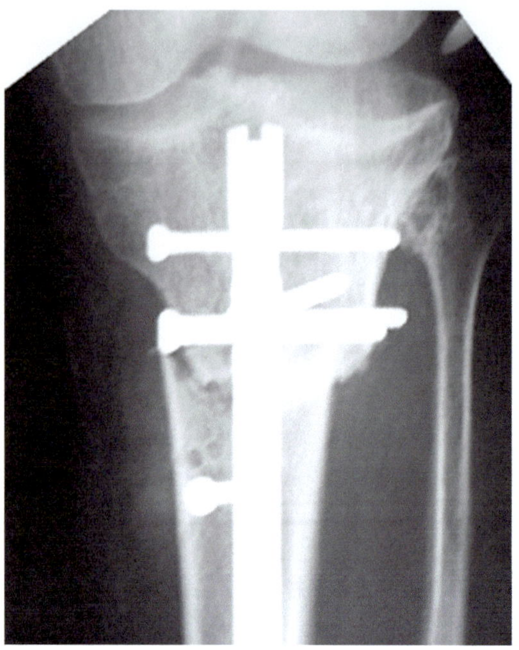

Fig. 3.63 Poller screws are recommended to narrow the medullary canal for enhanced stability especially in the metaphyseal region

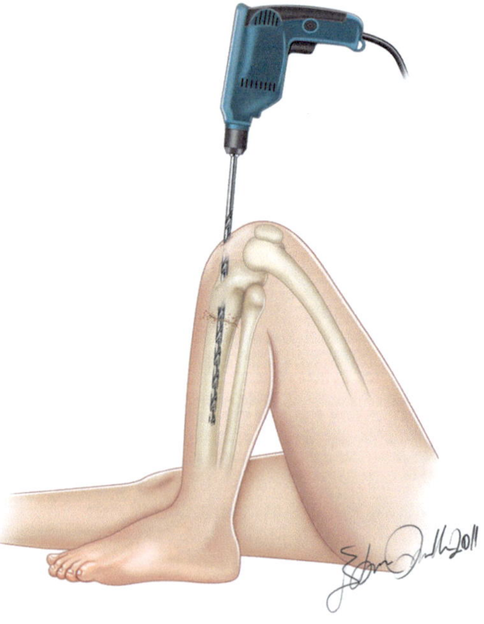

Fig. 3.64 The osteotomies act as venting holes during reaming to avoid fat embolism

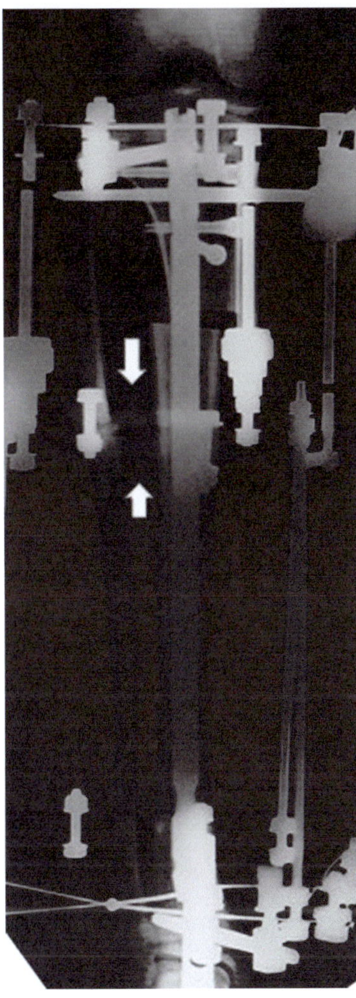

Fig. 3.65 Dummy ring is depicted by the *arrows*, which is not used for fixation but just to increase the stability of the frame

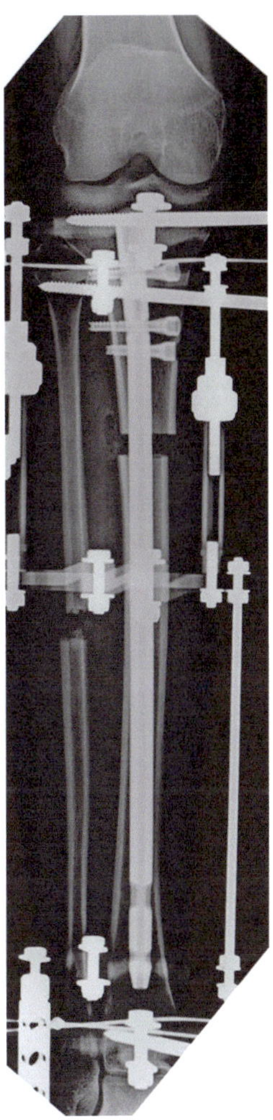

Fig. 3.66 Proximal tibiofibular joint is secured with a Schanz screw without purchasing the lateral cortex of the fibula to prevent skin problems and discomfort

this visit, the wounds are checked for any problems. No x-rays are needed at this point.
- Follow-up of the consolidation of the regenerate and of the healing of the osteotomy/ osteotomies for deformity correction is checked with AP and lateral x-rays at monthly intervals. At this visit, the ROM of the hip and the knee joint and muscle strength are also assessed.

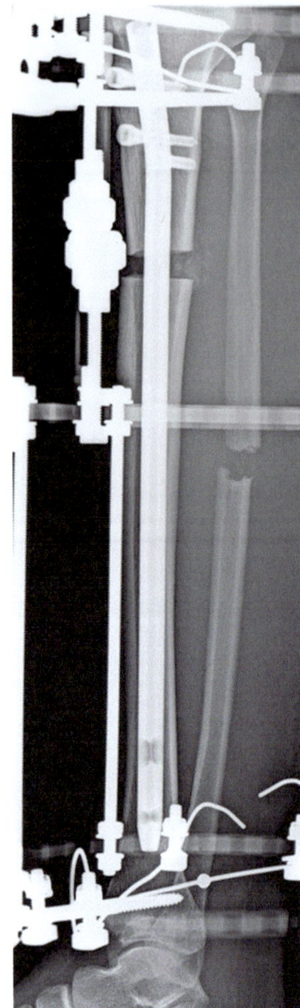

Fig. 3.67 Distal tibiofibular joint is secured with an olive K-wire

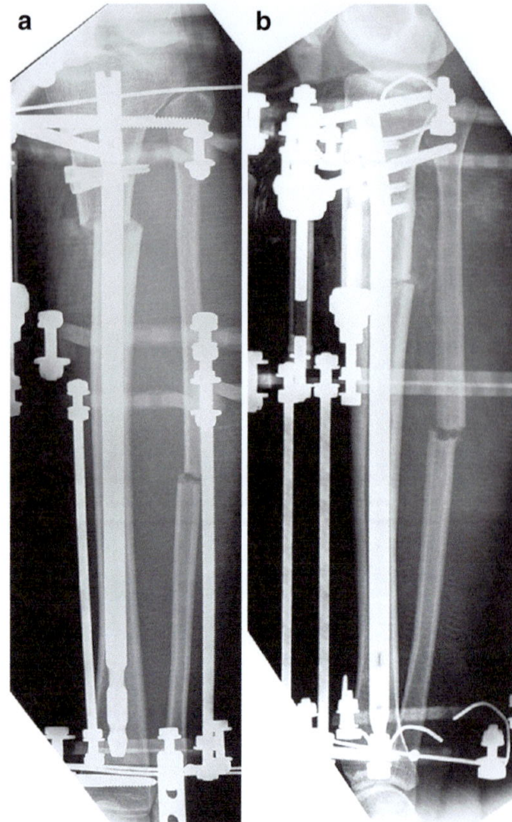

Fig. 3.68 The long axis of the IM nail must be parallel with the long axis of the external fixator on both planes AP (a) and lateral (b) to allow sliding during distraction

Pearls

- Complete routine imaging on the radiolucent table preoperatively.
- Do not use sterile nylon drapes to avoid wrapping them around the screws, drills, and pins.
- Pay attention to avoid any iatrogenic rotational deformity.
- Always confirm the correction with intraoperative x-rays on both planes before concluding the surgical procedure. Image intensifier views may be misleading.
- Always use the cannulated drill bit technique for the Schanz screw placement.

Pitfalls

- The sandbag under the affected buttock may mislead to a rotational deformity.

References

Bilen FE, Kocaoglu M, Eralp L et al (2010) Fixator-assisted nailing and consecutive lengthening over an intramedullary nail for the correction of tibial deformity. J Bone Joint Surg Br 92:146–152

Eralp L, Kocaoglu M (2008) Distal tibial reconstruction with use of a circular external fixator and an intramedullary nail. Surgical technique. J Bone Joint Surg Am 90: Suppl 2 pt 2: 181–194

Eralp L, Kocaoglu M, Cakmak M et al (2004) A correction of windswept deformity by fixator assisted nailing. A report of two cases. J Bone Joint Surg Br 86:1065–1068

Herzenberg JE, Paley D (1997) Tibial lengthening over nails (LON). Tech Orthop 12:250–259

Kocaoglu M, Eralp L, Rashid HU et al (2006) Reconstruction of segmental bone defects due to chronic osteomyelitis with use of an external fixator and an intramedullary nail. J Bone Joint Surg Am 88:2137–2145

Kocaoglu M, Eralp IL, Bilen FE et al (2009) Fixator assisted acute femoral deformity correction and consecutive lengthening over an intramedullary nail. J Bone Joint Surg Am 91:152–159

Krettek C, Miclau T, Schandelmaier P et al (1999a) The mechanical effect of blocking screws ("Poller screws") in stabilizing tibia fractures with short proximal or distal fragments after insertion of small-diameter intramedullary nails. J Orthop Trauma 13(8):550–553

Krettek C, Stephan C, Schandelmaier P et al (1999b) The use of Poller screws as blocking screws in stabilising tibial fractures treated with small diameter intramedullary nails. J Bone Joint Surg Br 81(6):963–968

Paktiss AS, Gross RH (1993) Afghan percutaneous osteotomy. J Pediatr Orthop 13(4):531–533

Paley D (1990) Problems, obstacles, and complications of limb lengthening by the Ilizarov technique. Clin Orthop 250:81–104

Paley D, Herzenberg JE (2002) Hardware and osteotomy considerations. In: Paley D, Herzenberg JE (eds) Principles of deformity correction. Springer, Berlin

Paley D, Tetsworth K (1991) Percutaneous osteotomies. Osteotome and Gigli saw techniques. Orthop Clin North Am 22(4):613–624

Paley D, Tetsworth K (1992) Mechanical axis deviation of the lower limbs. Preoperative planning of multiapical frontal plane angular and bowing deformities of the femur and tibia. Clin Orthop 280:65–71

Paley D, Catagni MA, Argnani F et al (1989) Ilizarov treatment of tibial nonunions with bone loss. Clin Orthop 241:146

Paley D, Herzenberg JE, Bor N (1997a) Fixator-assisted nailing of femoral and tibial deformities. Techn Orthop 12:260–275

Paley D, Herzenberg JE, Paremain G et al (1997b) Femoral lengthening over an intramedullary nail. A matched-case comparison with Ilizarov femoral lengthening. J Bone Joint Surg Am 79:1464–1480

Seligson D (2000) Poller screws. J Orthop Trauma 14(6):454

Tornero EF, Martínez IG, Tonal BG et al (2010) Comparison of hemostatic markers under different techniques for anesthesia-analgesia in total hip or knee replacement. Rev Esp Anestesiol Reanim 57(6):333–340

Hybrid Lengthening Techniques: Lengthening and Then Nailing (LATN) and Lengthening and Then Plating (LAP)

4

S. Robert Rozbruch and Austin T. Fragomen

Contents

S.R. Rozbruch, MD (✉) • A.T. Fragomen, MD
Limb Lengthening and Complex Reconstruction
Service, Hospital for Special Surgery, Weill Medical
College of Cornell University, New York, NY, USA
e-mail: rozbruchsr@hss.edu

4.1   Introduction

Distraction osteogenesis by the Ilizarov method is a widely used technique for leg lengthening (Fischgrund et al. 1994; Ilizarov 1990, 1992), deformity correction (Pinzur 2009; Pugh and Rozbruch 2005; Rozbruch et al. 2005b, 2006a, 2009), and reconstruction of nonunion and bone defects (Nho et al. 2006; Pugh and Rozbruch 2005; Rozbruch et al. 2005a, 2006b, 2008b). The overall process is comprised of two stages, distraction and consolidation (Ilizarov 1990; Paley et al. 1997), which takes place successively. External fixation has generally been considered necessary for both stages.

Limb lengthening in skeletally mature patients has unique issues. Adult patients have closed growth plates, have longer and wider bones, and typically take longer to achieve bony union than children. In the adult patient, the consolidation phase can be prolonged, often estimated to be 2 months per cm of lengthening (Fischgrund et al. 1994). This prolonged time in a frame confers several disadvantages. First, there is a greater chance of health-related complications including pin tract infection and decreased range of motion in the surrounding joints. Second, the process can affect the patient psychologically, increasing frustration and decreasing compliance. Finally, when the frame is removed, there is a risk for fracture of the regenerated bone due to the lack of any internal stabilization. O'Carrigan et al. (2007) reported an 8 % fracture rate after frame removal in a review of 650 patients with 986

M. Kocaoğlu et al. (eds.), *Advanced Techniques in Limb Reconstruction Surgery*,
DOI 10.1007/978-3-642-55026-3_4, © Springer Berlin Heidelberg 2015

lengthening segments. Simpson and Kenwright (Simpson and Kenwright 2000) reported a fracture rate of 9.4 % in a series of 180 lengthening segments.

With closed growth plates and larger bones in adults comes the opportunity to use hybrid techniques that include both external and internal fixation such as intramedullary rods and plates. Methods of lengthening that minimize the time in external fixation and protect against refracture include lengthening and then nailing (LATN) (Rozbruch et al. 2008a) and lengthening and then plating (LAP) Harbechuski et al. (2012).

4.2 Lengthening and Then Nailing (LATN)

We introduced a novel technique called lengthening and then nailing (LATN) (Fig. 4.1). External fixation is used for lengthening during the distraction phase. The external fixator is applied so that an intramedullary nail (IMN) can be inserted while the frame is in place, however, without contact between the internal fixation and the external fixation pins and wires. Once length has been achieved, a reamed locked IMN is inserted across the regenerate bone and the frame is removed. The IMN supports the bone during the consolidation phase allowing removal of the external fixator after the distraction phase of lengthening. Advantages of this technique include a significant decrease in time wearing the external fixator and protection against refracture (Rozbruch et al. 2008a). The benefits of LATN over lengthening over a nail (LON) include the ability to gradually correct deformity while lengthening and to insert a large diameter full length IMN after distraction (Fig. 4.2). In addition, bony healing is hastened likely due to reaming across the regenerate bone and/or the increased stability of a large diameter full length IMN. Furthermore, with LATN the time when both internal and external fixation are simultaneously applied to the bone is minimized (Rozbruch et al. 2008a).

4.2.1 LATN: Clinical Experience

We published a retrospective case-matched comparison (Rozbruch et al. 2008a) of patients lengthened with LATN (39 limbs in 27 patients) vs. the classic technique (34 limbs in 27 patients). The LATN group wore the external fixator for less time (12 versus 29 weeks) and had a lower external fixation index (EFI) (0.5 versus 1.9) and a lower bone healing index (BHI) (0.8 versus 1.9) than the classic group (Fig. 4.3). One deep infection developed in the LATN group after the regenerate was fully united. This was successfully treated by removing the IMN and administering antibiotics. We concluded that LATN confers advantages over the classic method including shorter times needed in external fixation, quicker bone healing, and protection against refracture. There are also advantages over the lengthening over a nail (LON) and internal lengthening nail techniques.

4.2.2 LATN of Tibia: Surgical Technique

4.2.2.1 Tibia and Fibula Osteotomy

The fibula osteotomy is performed using a multiple-drill-hole technique with a 1.8-mm wire and then completed with an osteotome. A three-ring Taylor Spatial Frame (TSF) (Smith and Nephew, Inc, Memphis, TN) is applied using a rings-first method (Rozbruch et al. 2006a; Taylor 2007). The proximal ring is stabilized with a 1.8-mm tensioned transverse wire, a 1.8-mm tibia-fibula wire, an anteromedial half pin, and an anterolateral half pin. The configuration of this proximal ring fixation is unique in that the bone fixation is placed peripherally within the proximal tibia to allow future insertion of an IMN avoiding any contact with the external fixation pins (Fig. 4.1a). The 1.8-mm wires are placed more posterior in the tibia than is typical. The half pins are inserted using a cannulated wire technique for precision. The anteromedial half pin is peripheral and runs in an anterior to

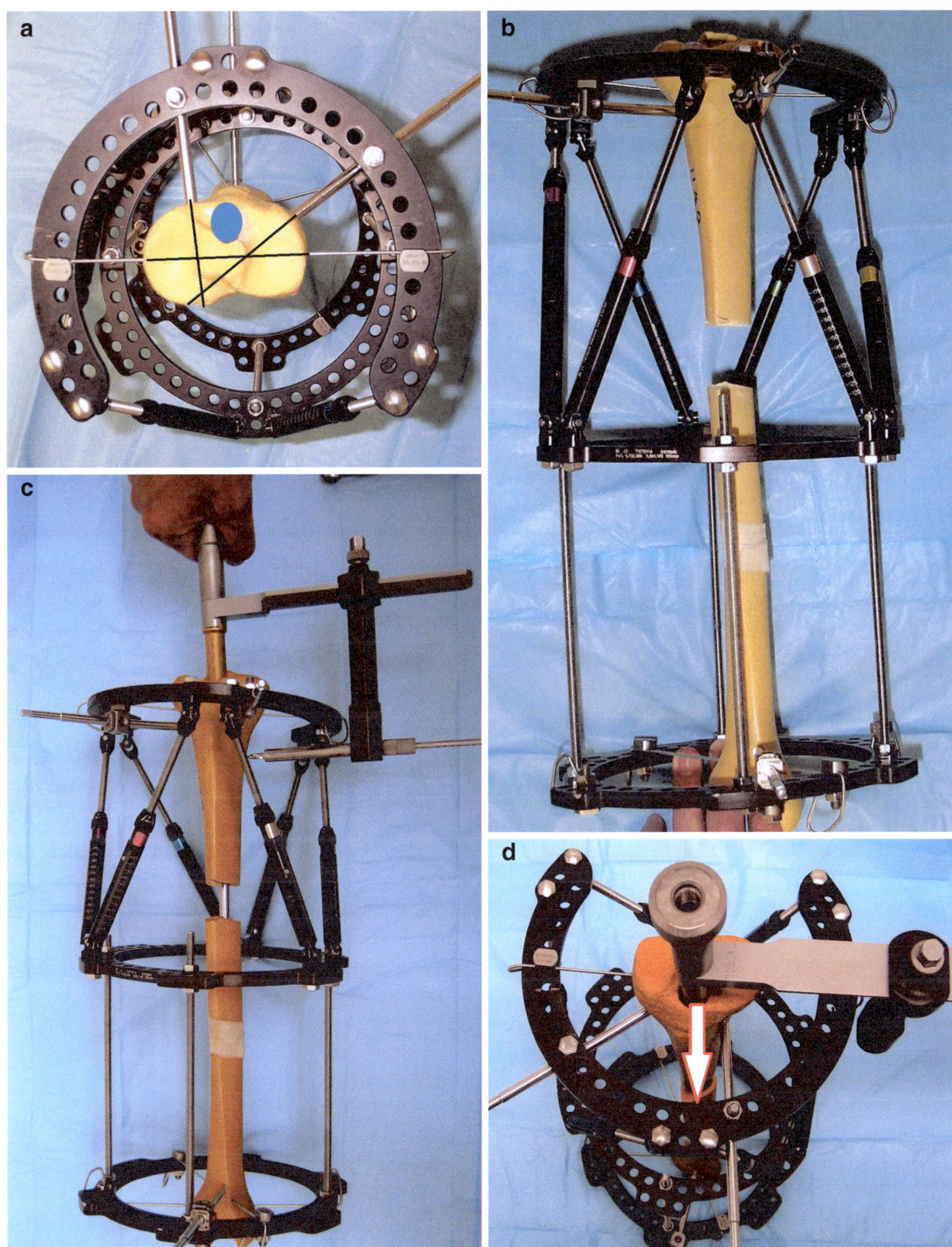

Fig. 4.1 Saw bone model demonstration of LATN. (**a**) Axial view showing that external fixation is peripherally placed in order to avoid contact with the IMN. The *black lines* depict the course of the external fixation pins > the *blue dot* depicts the future IMN location. (**b**) The TSF may be used to optimally align the bone fragments. (**c**) The IMN is inserted while the frame is in place. (**d**) Contact between internal and external fixation is avoided

posterior direction. The anterolateral half pin is peripheral and runs in an anterolateral to posterior central direction. The proximal ring is the reference ring and TSF mounting parameters (Taylor 2007) are measured in relation to this ring. The origin (Taylor 2007) is placed at the level of deformity within the diaphysis. When there is no deformity, we assign the origin to the center of the bone at the level of osteotomy 10 to 12 cm distal to the knee joint. Next, a ring block consisting of two rings connected with four rods is applied to the mid-distal tibia orthogonal to the tibial diaphysis. The distal ring is stabilized with a transverse 1.8-mm wire 1.5 cm proximal

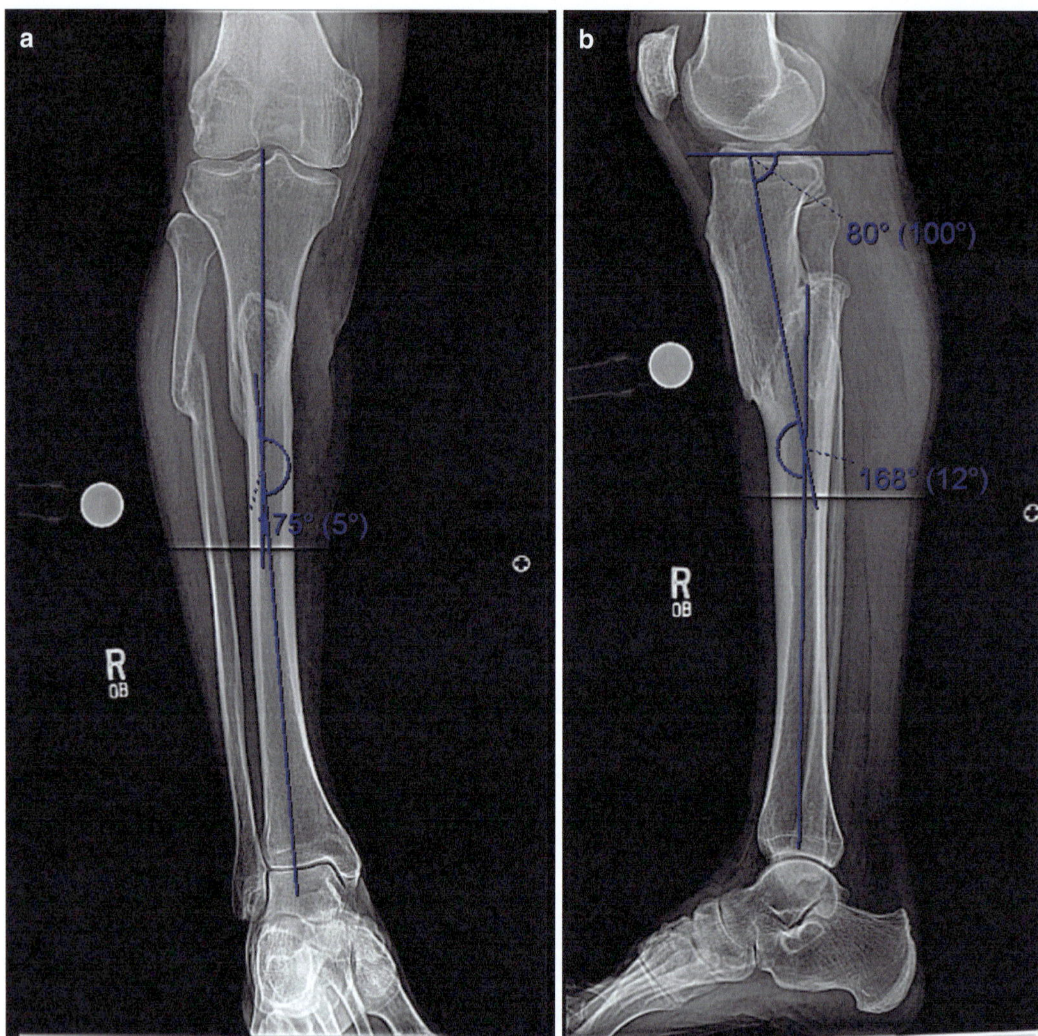

Fig. 4.2 A 48-year-old male with malunion consisting of varus, recurvatum, and shortening that was treated with LATN. (**a**) AP x-ray showing 5° of varus deformity. (**b**) Lateral x-ray showing 12° of recurvatum (apex posterior) deformity. (**c**) Erect leg radiograph showing right leg shortening of 24 mm. (**d**) Clinical photo at end of distraction. (**e**) AP x-ray at end of distraction showing lengthening and correction of deformity. (**f**) Lateral x-ray showing the same. (**g**) Erect leg x-ray showing the same. (**h**) Clinical photo 4 months after IMN insertion. (**i**) AP x-ray showing the same. (**j**) Lateral x-ray showing the same

Fig. 4.2 (continued)

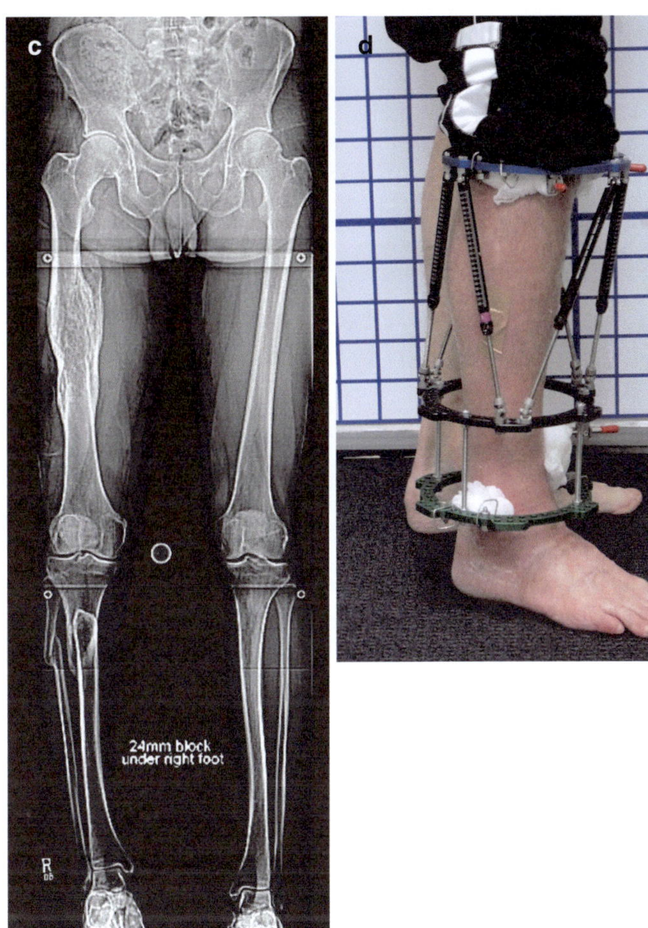

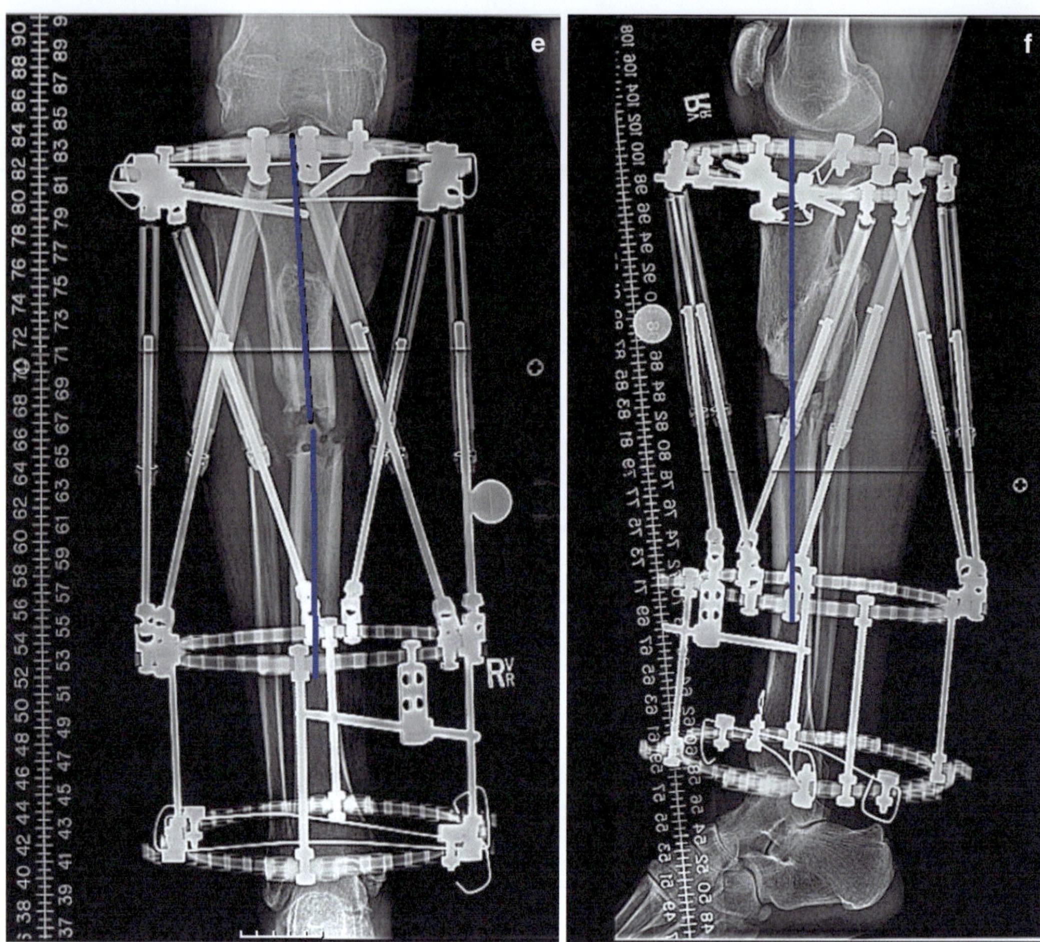

Fig. 4.2 (continued)

Fig. 4.2 (continued)

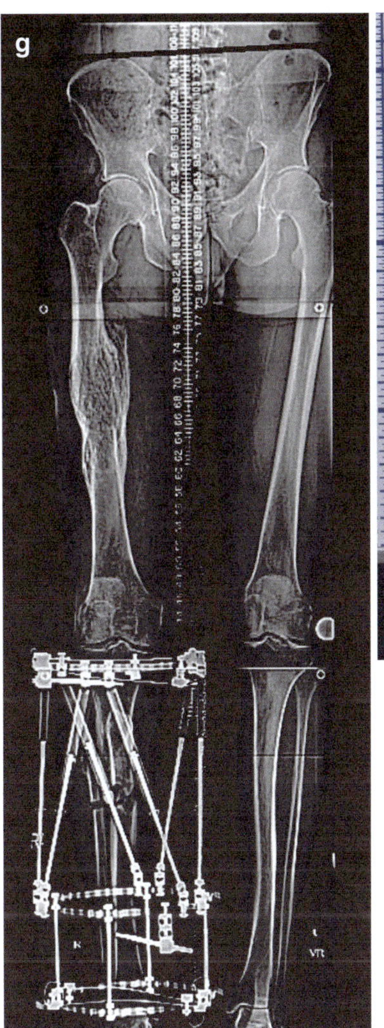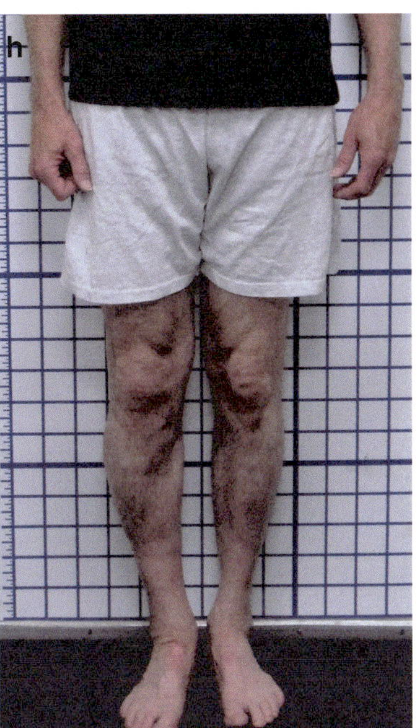

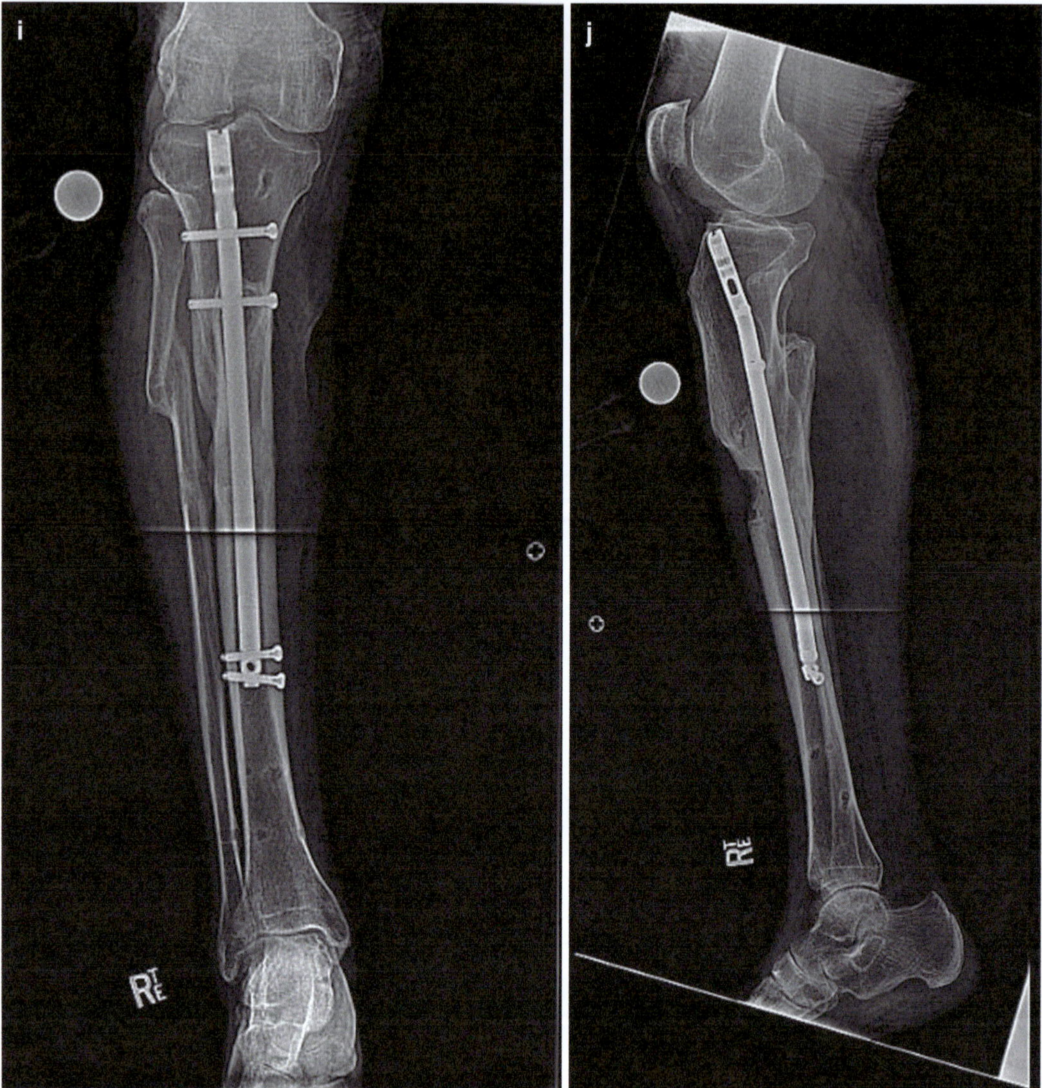

Fig. 4.2 (continued)

to the ankle joint, a 1.8-mm tibia-fibula wire 2 cm proximal to the ankle joint, and an antero-medial to posterolateral 6-mm half pin. The middle ring is typically left with no fixation. In cases where there is deformity correction, we may insert a wire or half pin off the middle ring to achieve optimal leverage during the correction. The proximal and middle rings are then connected with six TSF struts whose lengths are recorded (Fig. 4.1b). The struts are then removed for the tibial osteotomy.

The tibial osteotomy is performed in a percutaneous fashion using a multiple-drill-hole technique. Distraction is started on postoperative days 7–10. The distraction schedule is made using the TSF Internet-based software using the total residual method (Smith and Nephew, Inc, Memphis, TN). Care is taken to correct all

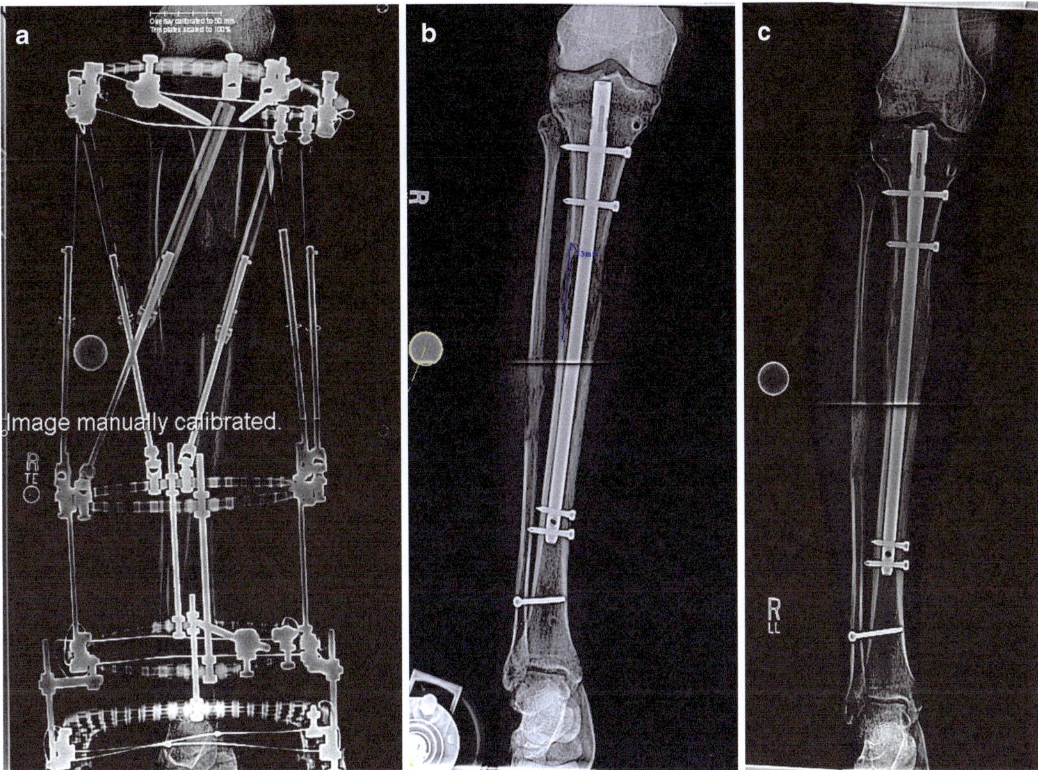

Fig. 4.3 Tibia lengthening of 7 cm in a 28-year-old man. (**a**) At the end of distraction. (**b**) Six weeks after IMN insertion. (**c**) Six months after IMN insertion

deformity at the osteotomy site prior to nail insertion.

4.2.2.2 Insertion of Intramedullary Nail and Removal of Frame

Once length and deformity correction are achieved, the second-stage surgery is performed without the use of a tourniquet. The external fixator is prepped into the surgical field, and betadine-soaked sponges are placed around all pin sites. The frame is covered with sterile towels. To prevent proximal migration of the fibula, we insert a 4.5-mm solid syndesmosis screw 1 cm proximal to the distal tibia pin fixation. An IMN with an extra hole 8 cm from the proximal end is used in order to be able to insert two proximal interlocking screws. A minimal incision technique for IM nail insertion is used. A guidewire was passed across the regenerate and into the distal fragment ending at the syndesmosis screw. Serial reaming is performed until cortical chatter is achieved, and a nail 1 mm smaller than the last reamer used is inserted. We do not open the regenerate site and we do not remove any reaming particles. The IMN is locked with two screws in both the proximal and distal fragments. The external fixator is then removed without risk of tibial displacement or shortening (Fig. 4.1c). The pin sites were irrigated but not curettaged and are not closed. While in some cases, we use a full length IMN, there are situations where we use a short custom-made IMN. Such situations include an abnormal intramedullary canal in the distal bone or a multilevel reconstruction. In all circumstances, there is no contact between internal and external fixation in order to minimize the chance of developing infection (Figs. 4.2 and 4.3).

4.3 Lengthening and Then Plating (LAP)

The lengthening and then plating (LAP) technique Harbechuski et al. (2012) (Figs. 4.4 and 4.5) was developed to decrease the time in the frame when the osteotomy is in close proximity to a joint such as in a periarticular deformity with shortening. External fixation is used for lengthening during the distraction phase. The external fixator is applied so that a plate can be inserted while the frame is in place, however, without contact between the internal fixation and the external fixation pins and wires. After length and deformity correction have been achieved, a locked plate is inserted across the regenerate bone and the frame is removed (Fig. 4.4). The plate supports the bone during the consolidation phase allowing removal of the external fixator before complete bone healing. This technique is an alternative to LATN when it was necessary for the osteotomy location to be in the proximal tibia

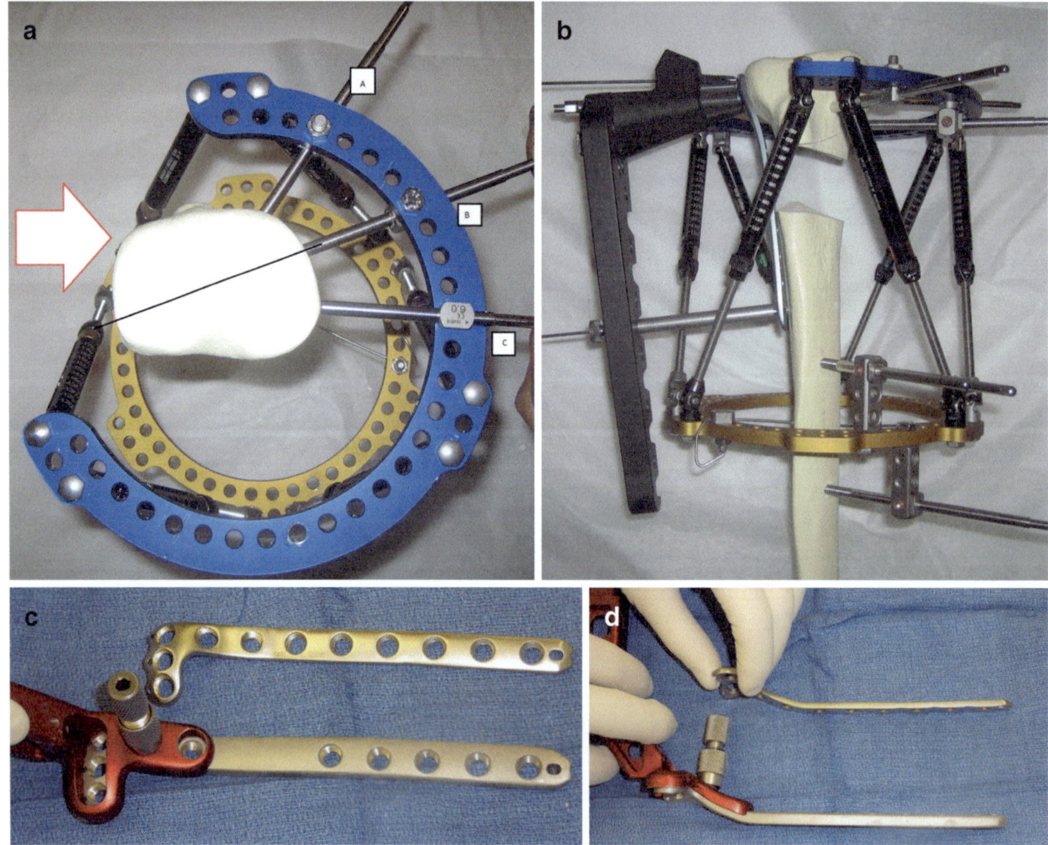

Fig. 4.4 Saw bone model demonstration of the LAP technique. (**a**) Axial view showing that external fixation is placed from the medial side leaving the lateral side free for future plate placement. The 2/3 ring is positioned open on the lateral side (*arrow*) to allow access for plate inser-tion. Pin B is used to capture the fibula head (note the trajectory shown with *black line*). (**b**) Insertion of plate after lengthening from the lateral side. (**c**) Front view of the thicker custom plate that also lacks unnecessary screw holes. (**d**) Side view of the same

or distal femur. The proximal tibial osteotomy location may be necessary because that is the location of the apex of deformity such as in genu varum and shortening. Alternatively, the treatment may be bifocal with nonunion repair or ankle fusion taking place in the distal tibia while lengthening takes place in the proximal tibia (Fig. 4.5). Of note, we have also used LAP in the distal tibia location.

4.3.1 LAP: Clinical Experience

We performed a retrospective case-matched comparison of our LAP and classic lengthening patients Harbechuski et al. (2012). The groups had 27 extremities each and were matched for age, etiology, amount of lengthening, preoperative mechanical axis deviation (MAD), and tibia/femur distribution. The following data was compared:

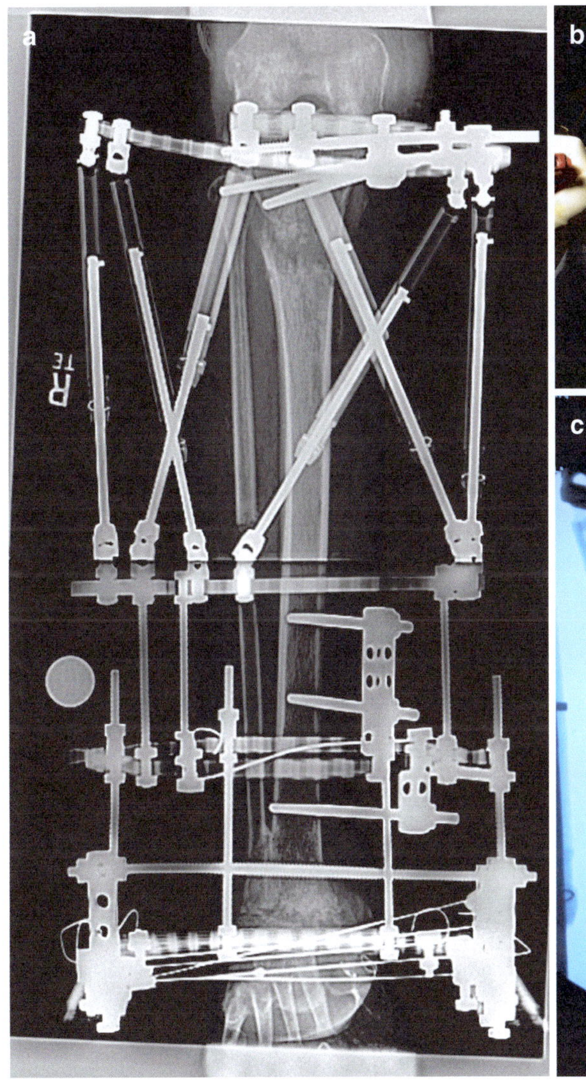

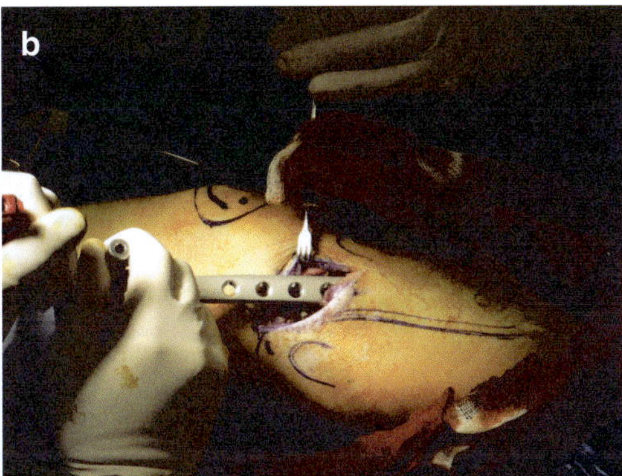

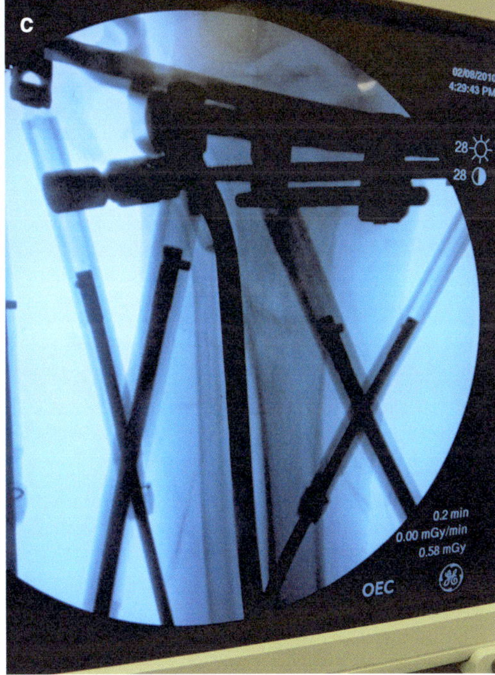

Fig. 4.5 A 55-year-old woman who underwent proximal tibial lengthening (LAP technique) along with tibiocalcaneal fusion. (**a**) AP x-ray at the end of distraction. (**b**) Frame is prepped into the field and maximally covered for plate insertion. Plate is inserted through small lateral incision in an antegrade fashion. (**c**) AP fluoroscopy image used to confirm direction of plate. (**d**) Lateral fluoroscopy image used to confirm direction of plate. (**e**) The jig is attached for percutaneous screw insertion. (**f**) Same. (**g**) After removal of frame. Bone marrow aspirate concentrate is percutaneously inserted into the bony regenerate. (**h**) AP x-ray 3 months later. (**i**) Lateral x-ray 3 months later

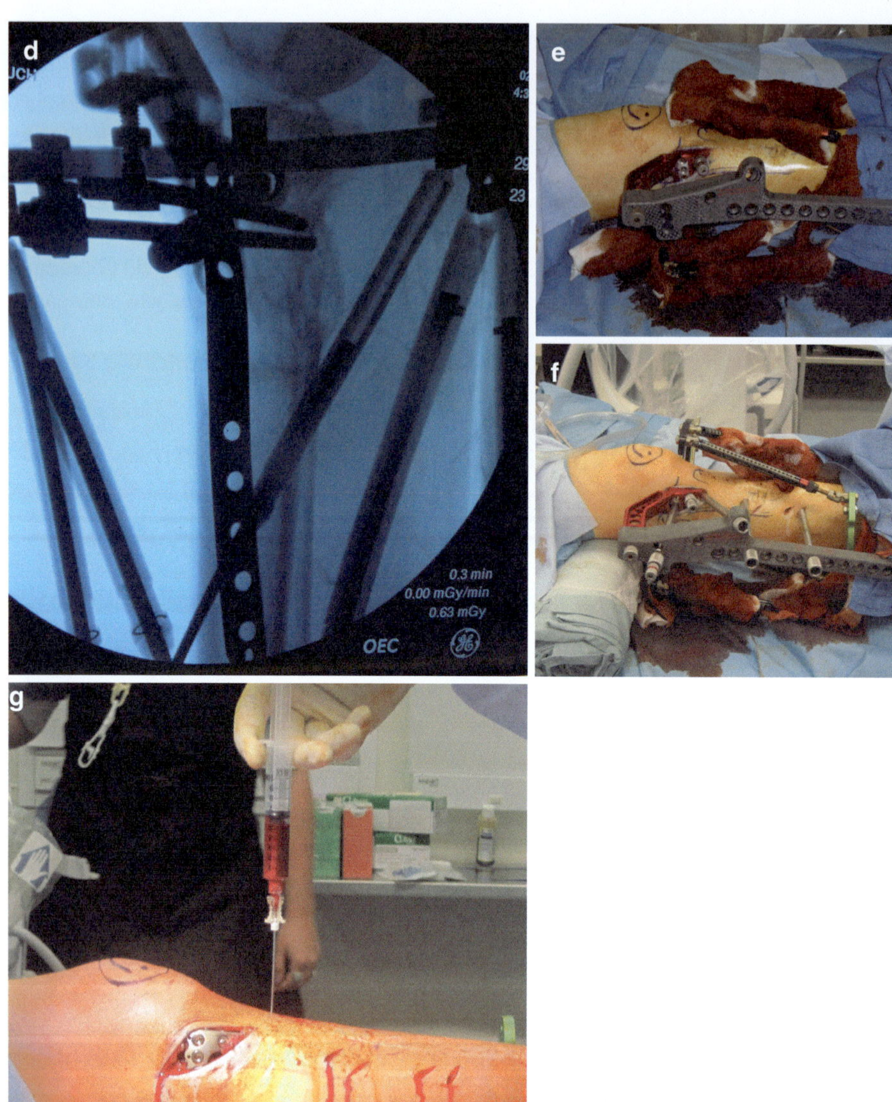

Fig. 4.5 (continued)

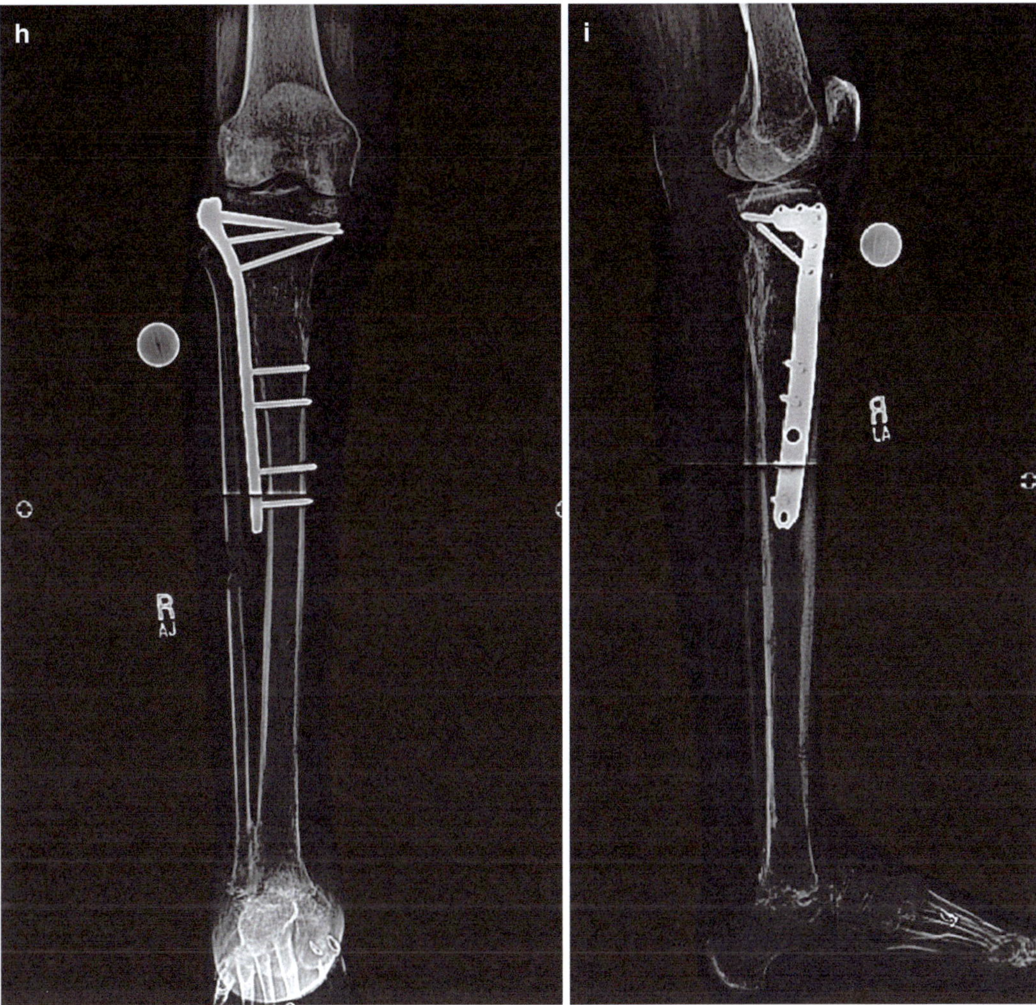

Fig. 4.5 (continued)

time in the frame, bone healing index (BHI), external fixation index (EFI), adjacent joint range of motion (ROM), alignment, and complications.

The time in external fixation was 4.4 months in LAP group vs. 6.3 months in the classic group. EFI in LAP group was 1.5 vs. 2.0 in the classic group. BHI was similar in both cohorts: 2.1 in LAP group and 2.2 in classic group. Deviation from normal alignment on latest x-rays was found in 7 patients in LAP and 5 in classic group ($p = 0.32$). Varus malalignment in 2 LAP patients was associated with the plate breakage at the level of immature regenerate. Incidence of pin tract infection was higher in classic group: 12 patients vs. 2 patients in LAP group ($p = 0.0001$).

We concluded that the LAP technique shortens the time in external fixation, and this may explain the decreased risk of pin tract infection. Lateral plate insertion seems to protect against valgus malalignment in the end but conventional plates may not be strong enough to prevent varus deformity.

We believe that LAP seems to be a safe and effective procedure for limb lengthening and deformity correction (Fig. 4.5). The use of LAP shortens the patient's time in external fixation by substituting a plate for all or part of the consolidation phase. This technique also helps protect against refracture after frame removal. The distal femur plates are quite strong and this allows insertion of the plate soon after the end of distraction. The tibial plates are less strong requiring more advanced bony healing prior to plate insertion. At this time, we use LAP of the tibia as a way to moderately decrease the time in frame and prevent refracture. We do not substitute the plate immediately at the end of the distraction phase. We wait until the regenerate healing has progressed to a reasonable degree. In addition, we have begun to use a custom-made proximal tibial plate that is both 2 mm wider and thicker in the region of previous plate failure (Fig. 4.4c, d).

4.3.2 LAP of the Tibia: Surgical Technique

4.3.2.1 Tibia and Fibula Osteotomy

A fibula osteotomy is performed. A three-ring Taylor Spatial Frame (TSF) (Smith and Nephew, Inc, Memphis, TN) was applied using a rings-first method. The unique features of the technique relate to the orientation of and pin placement for the proximal ring (Fig. 4.4a). We use a 2/3 ring at the proximal tibia with the opening of the ring facing lateral. The pin fixation is placed from the medial side leaving the lateral approach undisturbed. Using cannulated wire technique, the reference pin is placed from medial to lateral perpendicular to the proximal mechanical axis. The second pin is directed anteromedial to posterolateral and sets the ring in both the coronal and sagittal planes. The third pin is anteromedial to posterolateral and captures the fibula head. This is placed using a cannulated wire technique. First the 1.8-mm wire is directed from the proximal fibula in an anteromedial direction. Then a cube is placed on the ring at the location of the wire. A cannulated 4.8-mm drill is directed from anteromedial to posterolateral ending in the fibula head. A 6-mm pin is then inserted. The distal ring is applied so that the pin fixation will be distal to the future plating. At the plate insertion, it is desirable to place 3–4 locking screws into the distal fragment.

4.3.2.2 Insertion of Plate and Frame Removal

After the lengthening is complete, the plate is inserted with the TSF in place (Fig. 4.4b–d). Pin sites are covered with betadine-soaked sponges and the frame is prepped into the field. The frame should be maximally covered with towels to minimize contact and contamination (Fig. 4.5). The plate is inserted through a minimal incision approach at the proximal lateral tibia (Fig. 4.5b). The iliotibial band insertion on Gerdy's tubercle is released and a split in the anterior fascia is made as a portal for the plate. A locked plate is inserted along the lateral aspect of the tibia in an antegrade direction. Biplanar fluoroscopy is helpful for optimal positioning of the plate (Figs. 4.5c, d). The plate targeting device is attached and is used for locking screw insertion (Figs. 4.5e, f). Care is taken not to deform the plate as the distal plate is often translated off the bone. Typically, we insert 4 screws in both the proximal and distal segments, and then the frame is removed. Care is taken to avoid contact between the internal and external fixation. We usually take the opportunity while in the operating room to inject mesenchymal stem cells from bone marrow aspirate concentrate into the still unhealed regenerate. We believe this stimulates quicker bony union (Fig. 4.5g–i)

4.4 Choice of Technique

I prefer to use LATN whenever possible for tibial lengthening because of the IMN stability and enhancement of bony healing. The osteotomy should be at least 10 cm distal to the knee joint to get adequate stability from the IMN. If the apex of the deformity is close to the joint, then I will use the LAP technique. Both techniques allow gradual correction of deformity as well as lengthening prior to insertion of the internal fixation. I have expanded my indications for LATN over LAP by utilizing a custom-made short IMN in situations where middle tibia external fixation pins are necessary (such as a simultaneous ankle fusion).

In the femur, we prefer to use LON whenever possible. Although the LATN has theoretical advantages (increased nail length and diameter, reaming across the regenerate), I have found it difficult to control the femur position during lengthening without the IMN already in place. If there is distal femur deformity, then standard LON cannot be used. In this case, I would use either LAP of the femur or LON using a retrograde IMN. With the advent of new motorized intramedullary nails that can be used to lengthen bone in a reliable fashion, the use of these hybrid techniques will decrease Rozbruch et al. (2014).

References

Fischgrund J, Paley D, Suter C (1994) Variables affecting time to bone healing during limb lengthening. Clin Orthop Relat Res 301:31–37

Ilizarov GA (1990) Clinical application of the tension-stress effect for limb lengthening. Clin Orthop Relat Res 250:8–26

Ilizarov GA (1992) Tranosseous osteosynthesis, 1st edn. Springer, Berlin

Harbechuski R, Fragomen AT, Rozbruch SR: Does lengthening and Then Plating (LAP) Shorten Duration of External Fixation? Clin Orthop Rel Res (2012) 470:1771–1781

Nho SJ, Helfet DL, Rozbruch SR (2006) Temporary intentional leg shortening and deformation to facilitate wound closure using the Ilizarov/Taylor spatial frame. J Orthop Trauma 20:419–424

O'Carrigan T, Paley D, Herzenberg JE (2007) Obstacles in limb lengthening: fractures. In: Rozbruch SR, Ilizarov S (eds) Limb lengthening and reconstruction surgery, 1st edn. Informa Healthcare, New York, pp 675–679

Paley D, Herzenberg JE, Paremain G, Bhave A (1997) Femoral lengthening over an intramedullary nail. A matched-case comparison with Ilizarov femoral lengthening. J Bone Joint Surg Am 79:1464–1480

Pinzur MS (2009) Use of platelet-rich concentrate and bone marrow aspirate in high-risk patients with charcot arthropathy of the foot. Foot Ankle Int 30:124–127

Pugh K, Rozbruch SR (2005) Nonunions and malunions. In: Baumgaertner MR, Tornetta P (eds) Orthopaedic knowledge update trauma 3, 3rd edn. American Academy of Orthopaedic Surgeons, Rosemont, IL pp 115–130

Rozbruch SR, Ilizarov S, Blyakher A (2005a) Knee arthrodesis with simultaneous lengthening using the Ilizarov method. J Orthop Trauma 19:171–179

Rozbruch SR, Paley D, Bhave A, Herzenberg JE (2005b) Ilizarov hip reconstruction for the late sequelae of infantile hip infection. J Bone Joint Surg Am 87:1007–1018

Rozbruch SR, Fragomen AT, Ilizarov S (2006a) Correction of tibial deformity with use of the Ilizarov-Taylor spatial frame. J Bone Joint Surg Am 88(Suppl 4):156–174

Rozbruch SR, Weitzman AM, Watson JT et al (2006b) Simultaneous treatment of tibial bone and soft-tissue defects with the Ilizarov method. J Orthop Trauma 20:197–205

Rozbruch SR, Kleinman D, Fragomen AT, Ilizarov S (2008a) Limb lengthening and then insertion of an intramedullary nail: a case-matched comparison. Clin Orthop Relat Res 466:2923–2932

Rozbruch SR, Pugsley JS, Fragomen AT, Ilizarov S (2008b) Repair of tibial nonunions and bone defects with the Taylor Spatial Frame. J Orthop Trauma 22:88–95

Rozbruch SR, Segal K, Ilizarov S, Fragomen AT, Ilizarov G (2010) Does the Taylor Spatial Frame accurately correct tibial deformities? Clin Orthop Relat Res 468(5):1352–1361

Rozbruch SR, Birch JG, Dahl MT, Herzenberg JE (2014) Motorized Intramedullary Nail for Treatment of Limb Length Discrepancy and Deformity. JAAOS 22: 403–409

Simpson AH, Kenwright J (2000) Fracture after distraction osteogenesis. J Bone Joint Surg Br 82:659–665

Taylor JC (2007) Taylor spatial frame. In: Rozbruch SR, Ilizarov S (eds) Limb lengthening and reconstruction surgery, 1st edn. Informa, New York, pp 613–637

Levent Eralp and İlker Eren

Contents

L. Eralp (✉)
Department of Orthopaedics and Traumatology,
Istanbul Universtiy, Istanbul, Turkey
e-mail: drleventeralp@gmail.com

İ. Eren
Department of Orthopaedics and Traumatology,
School of Medicine, Koc University, Istanbul, Turkey
e-mail: ilker.eren@gmail.com

Abbreviations

CRP   C-reactive protein
ESR   Erythrocyte sedimentation rate

5.1   Introduction

Arthrodesis of the knee is a well-known treatment option for pain and instability due to advanced osteoarthritis, posttraumatic arthritis, infectious arthritis, Charcot arthropathy, poliomyelitis, and reconstruction following tumor resection since the early 1900s (Charnley 1960). The number of knee arthrodesis performed has decreased significantly due to modern knee arthroplasty techniques. Currently, the most common indication for knee arthrodesis is an unreconstructable knee following an infection at the site of knee arthroplasty (Hanssen et al. 1995). Arthrodesis by internal fixation by either a plate or an intramedullary nail provides rigid fixation. Intramedullary nailing has the advantage of allowing early weight bearing and has a high rate of fusion ranging from 88 to 100 % (Arroyo et al. 1997). But it is crucial to apply it after infection has been successfully treated which may take up to 40 wccks, and still there is a risk of dissemination of latent infection (Vlasak et al. 1995). On the other hand, external fixation offers possible progressive adjustment to stimulate the bony fusion and to correct malalignment, and there is a considerably lower risk of intramedullary dissemination of the infection, and easy removal of the hardware is possible (Manzotti et al. 2001;

M. Kocaoğlu et al. (eds.), *Advanced Techniques in Limb Reconstruction Surgery*,
DOI 10.1007/978-3-642-55026-3_5, © Springer Berlin Heidelberg 2015

Eralp et al. 2004). The purpose of this study is to describe the indications, surgical technique, common pitfalls, and key points of the technique used for arthrodesis of the knee by using uniplanar external fixators.

5.2 Indications

- Infected primary and revision total knee arthroplasty (Fig. 5.1).
- Multiple revised knees may have a large amount of bone loss, which would otherwise require massive allografts for arthroplasty.

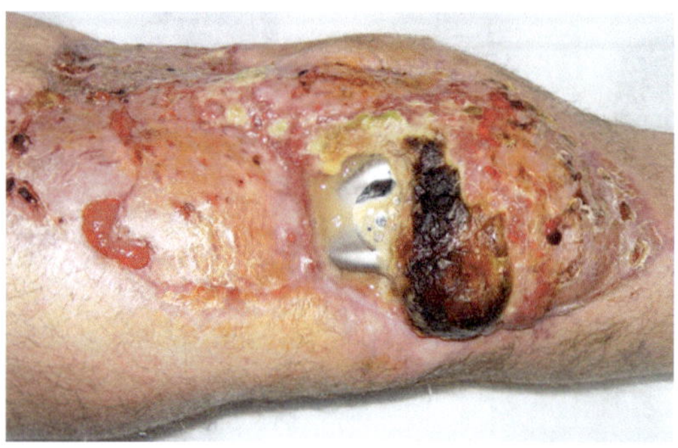

Fig. 5.1 An infected, exposed tumor prosthesis with extensive skin necrosis

- Patients who are candidate for skin breakdown like with rheumatologic problems (rheumatoid arthritis, vasculitis, etc.) and dermatologic disorders or have skin problems due to a previous incident.
- Patients using immunosuppressive agents like methotrexate have a tendency towards nonunion (who require gradual compression for solid union).
- Recurrent infection of young, active patients.
- Osteoporotic bone which will require a period of gradual compression for union.
- Vascular problems which would render extensive exposures for a two-stage revision difficult or inapplicable.
- Arthrodesis with an intramedullary nail or with other internal implants is not suggested if there is rigorous infection, especially for a Cierny–Mader host B or C patients.
- Arthrodesis with external fixation is an alternative for patients with high risk of fat embolism which makes reaming contraindicated.
- Unrepairable extensor mechanism problem with gross instability of the knee which is not possible to reconstruct (Fig. 5.2).

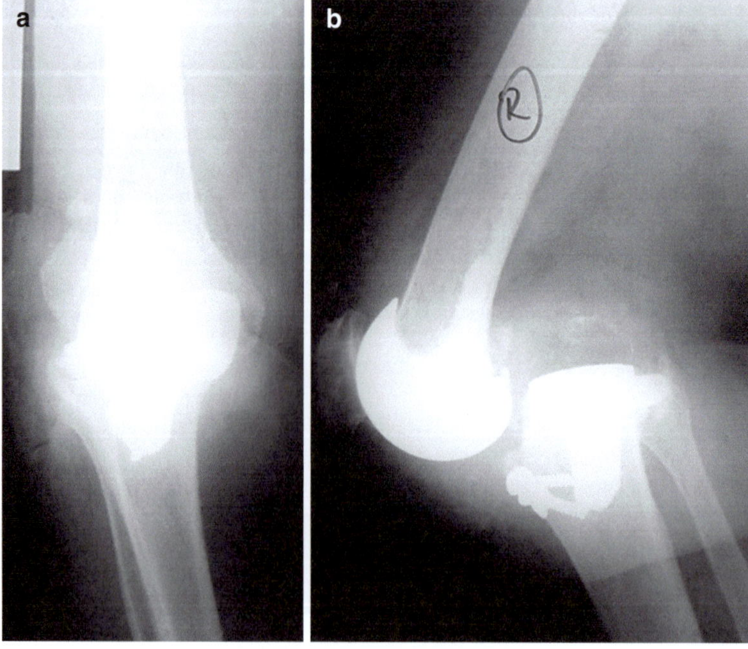

Fig. 5.2 A patient with a gross instability. (**a**) Anteroposterior and (**b**) lateral X-rays

5.3   Examination/Imaging

- A patient has to be examined for the extent of the infection. Cardinal findings of infection have to be noted for postoperative follow-up.
- The condition of the soft tissue is one of the most important issues. Debridement may cause soft tissue defects necessitating local or free flaps. Too much skin tension also may lead to skin necrosis. Thus, any soft tissue reconstruction has to be planned carefully preoperatively.
- Plain anteroposterior and lateral X-rays, including an orthoroentgenogram, are required for preoperative planning. Femoral and tibial cuts have to be planned preoperatively, relative to current shortening. The limb has to be 1 cm shorter than the site with a mobile knee, but any shortening exceeding 1 cm requires support.
- Most of the uncontrolled infections cause fistulae. Its tract has to be removed with debridement. Preoperative fistulography with radiopaque contrast will state its extent.
- In case there is marked bone loss, a computerized tomography will display the amount and location of the defect.

- Widespread osteomyelitis will require an extended bone debridement, even resection. Magnetic resonance imaging is a sensitive method to state the extent of infection (Fig. 5.3).
- In case there is doubt for infected arthroplasty, an indium-labeled leukocyte bone scan is a sensitive and specific technique for diagnosis.

5.4   Surgical Anatomy

5.4.1   Structures at Risk

- The preferred application direction of the Schanz screws is in the sagittal plane.
- The anterior half of the femur is a safe zone and far from neurovascular structures.
- For the tibia, care is required not to miss the medial wall, as the anterior edge of the tibia makes an acute angle with the lateral wall. It is safe to check every Schanz screw at the AP view.
- The application of the fixator does not jeopardize neurovascular structures around the popliteal region, but during debridement and cuts, especially if posterior capsulotomy is being performed, care must be taken.

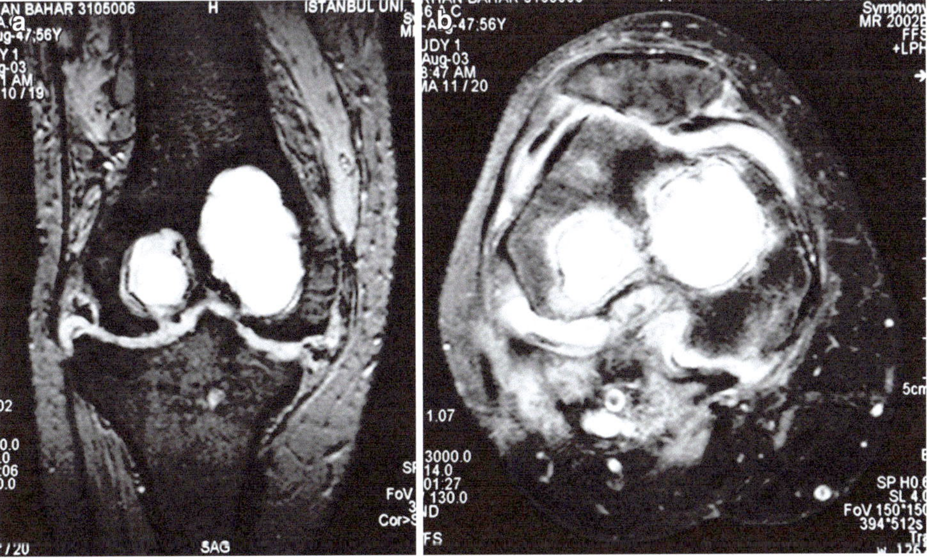

Fig. 5.3 (**a, b**) Magnetic resonance scan reveals osteomyelitis sequela with huge bone defect

5.5 Positioning

- Supine position with a sandbag under the ipsilateral buttock is required to overcome external rotation of the limb.
- For initial debridement, knee flexion over 90° is required.
- After debridement and resection, limb alignment should be checked in extension to 5° of flexion in anteroposterior and lateral planes with image guidance. If required, additional resection can be done.
- The limb is supported with folded sheets in full length for external fixator application.
- Fluoroscopy guidance is mandatory for this procedure. The device should be a C-arm and able to turn for lateral view.
- A radiolucent operating table is required.

5.6 Exposures

- There are various methods to access the knee joint. However, patients will have a previous knee replacement surgery incision, which may be used multipl times for debridements or revisions. Using it including deep planes facilitates skin healing and reduces the risk of skin necrosis.
- If there is a fistula, incision should center it with fistulectomy.
- In case the patient had a soft tissue reconstruction surgery (like free or local flaps), care must be taken not to damage the pedicle of the flap. If necessary, perform a preoperative ultrasound scan of the flap and mark the pedicle.

5.7 Procedure

5.7.1 Phase 1: Implant Removal and Antibiotic Spacer

- Although the procedure does not include implants, we suggest fusing the knee in two stages.
- While removing the implant, make sure it detaches from the bone–cement interface and does not cause additional bone loss.

- Remove any cement residue.
- Culture-specific antibiotics can be loaded into the cement (2,000 mg teicoplanin per 40 g cement powder).
- The second stage is performed when there is no laboratory or clinical evidence of active infection, checked by the erythrocyte sedimentation rate (ESR) and C-reactive protein (CRP) levels every 2 weeks.

5.7.2 Phase 2: Knee Arthrodesis

5.7.2.1 Step 1: Debridement, Spacer Removal, and Cuts

- A sterile, above-knee tourniquet can be applied during debridement.
- Care must be taken not to detach the skin from subcutaneous tissue, and unnecessary dissection should be avoided.
- Bone quality will be poor just under the spacer. The metaphyseal, bleeding bone must be exposed to achieve union. Usually, bone cuts are sufficient for this; occasionally it may be required to remove more bone (Fig. 5.4).
- It is possible to use knee arthroplasty tray's cutting blocks. This ensures a smooth cut surface, with anatomical inclination in the frontal plane.
- It is suggested to fuse the knee joint at 7±5° valgus and 7±5° flexion.
- Avoid removing unnecessary bone. The extremity with a fused knee requires slight shortening (~1 cm), to successfully advance the extremity at the swing phase of the gait. Above 1–2 cm, shortening compensation will be required. Also excessive cut will lead to reduced fusion interface as the proximal tibia and distal femur have a conical shape.
- In case there is excessive flexion contracture, even after bone cuts, it may not be possible to extend the knee. Consider posterior capsulotomy if required.
- Due to previous surgeries and infection, soft tissues and bones will slightly alter biologic activity which may lead to nonunion. It is wise to refer bone grafts to facilitate union. Considering the bone loss, structural auto- or

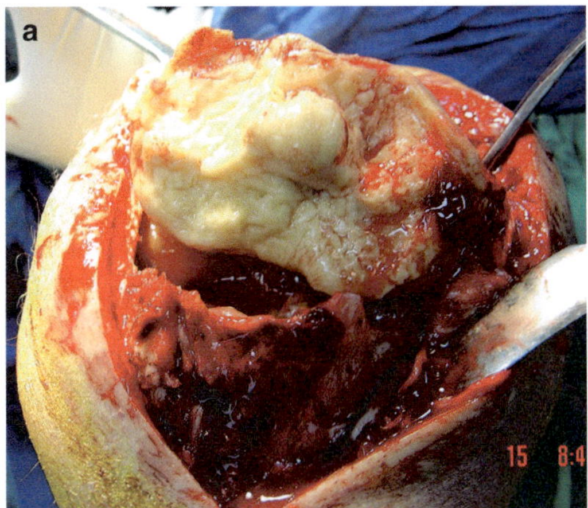

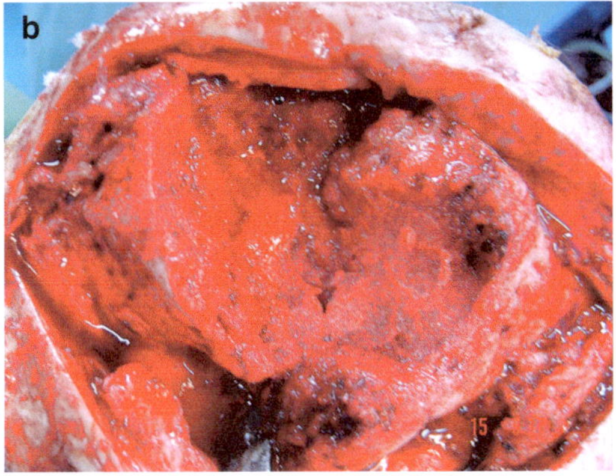

Fig. 5.4 (**a**) Removal of cement spacer. (**b**) Filling bone defects by antibiotic-loaded demineralized bone matrix

allografts, morselized allografts, demineralized bone matrix, and bone morphogenic protein can be utilized.
- It is possible to mix culture-specific antibiotics to the graft for continuing local antimicrobial effect.

5.7.2.2 Step 2: Fixator Application
- With temporary K wires, arthrodesis position can be maintained (Fig. 5.5).
- Once the knee position is stabilized in the desired alignment, the wound is closed before the application of the external fixator, using monofilamentous surgical threads (Prolene) in order to decrease the risk of infection.
- The application of the external fixator is started in the sagittal plane. Hydroxyapatite-coated Schanz screws of 6 mm diameter are used.

- The first Schanz screw is applied in the distal part of the femur; it should be centralized to the bone in the frontal plane and perpendicular to the anatomical axis of the femur in the sagittal plane.
- The frame of the external fixator (Orthofix LRS®, Bussolengo, Italy) is connected to the Schanz screw, with temporary application of two Steinmann pins to the most proximal and most distal holes in the clamps of the fixator to maintain the alignment of the fixator during application of the rest of the Schanz screws.
- Generally, four Schanz screws are applied in each bone segment (Fig. 5.6).
- The application of a Schanz screw medially in the frontal plane to the proximal one third of the tibia and connecting it to the fixator using an arch or a plate from the Ilizarov system can also increase the stability of the fixation when needed (unilateral and multiplanar application) (Fig. 5.7).
- Once the frame is applied, the K wires are removed, and intraoperative compression of the bone ends is done under guidance of an image intensifier. Two millimeters of additional compression is suggested, after full contact of the bone ends.

5.8 Postoperative Care and Expected Outcomes

- Postoperative compression is carried on by the external fixator at a rate of one quarter of 1 mm every 12 h for 1–2 weeks.
- The patient is mobilized on the second day postoperatively by using crutches. Full weight bearing is allowed immediately.
- Provide shortening compensation if required.
- Administer adequate antibiotherapy according to preoperative cultures. C-reactive protein and erythrocyte sedimentation levels are monitored during follow-ups. Unexpected elevation may point to osteomyelitis relapse.
- Postoperative radiography was evaluated for evidence of bony fusion. This was detected by

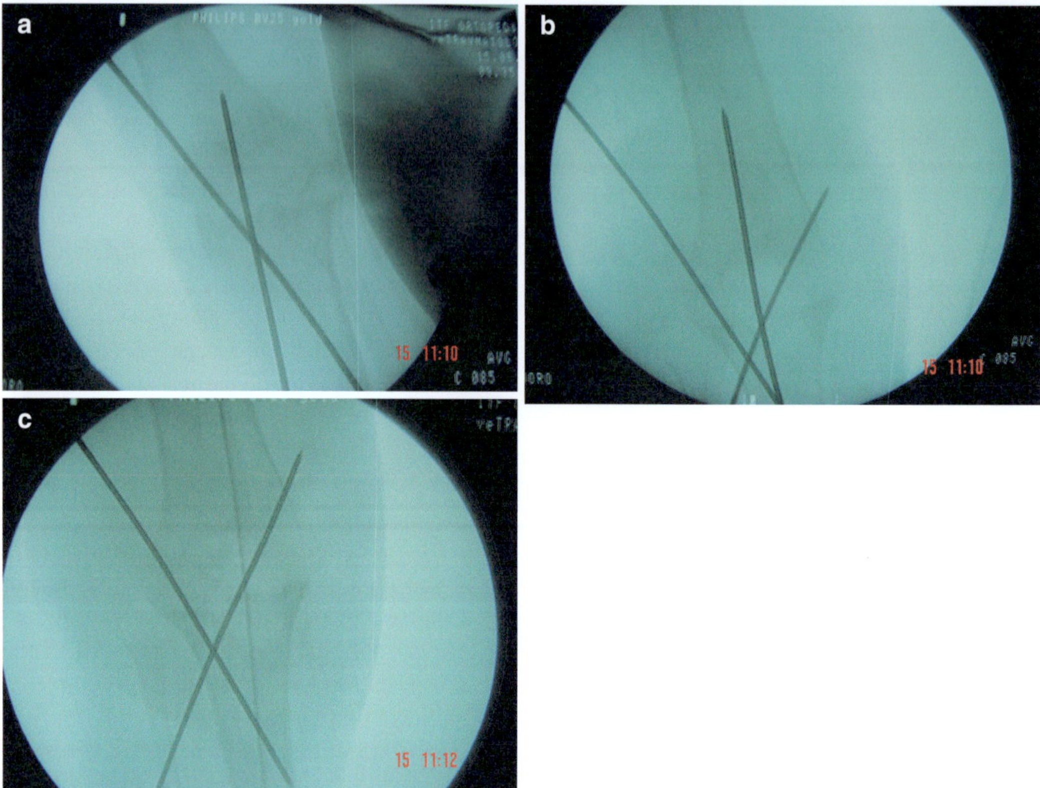

Fig. 5.5 (**a**, **b**) Temporary fixation of the position of knee arthrodesis by two crossed K wires. (**c**) Checking the mechanical axis of the limb using an electrocautery cord stretched from the center of the femoral head to the center of the ankle joint

trabecular bridging between the tibia and femur. Radiographic evidence of fusion coupled with no evidence of motion on clinical examination after removal of the fixator was the criteria for successful arthrodesis. It usually takes 8–12 months for sufficient union.

- Progressive pain may point to nonunion or infection relapse. In case there is a relapse, consider redebridement (Fig. 5.9).

Fig. 5.6 (**a**) Application of the first Schanz screw into the central part of the distal femur in the frontal plane. (**b**) Steinmann pins were used in the most proximal and distal holes, to check the placement of the fixator. Middle screws are introduced when the placement is comfirmed. Finally steinman pins are converted to schanz screws

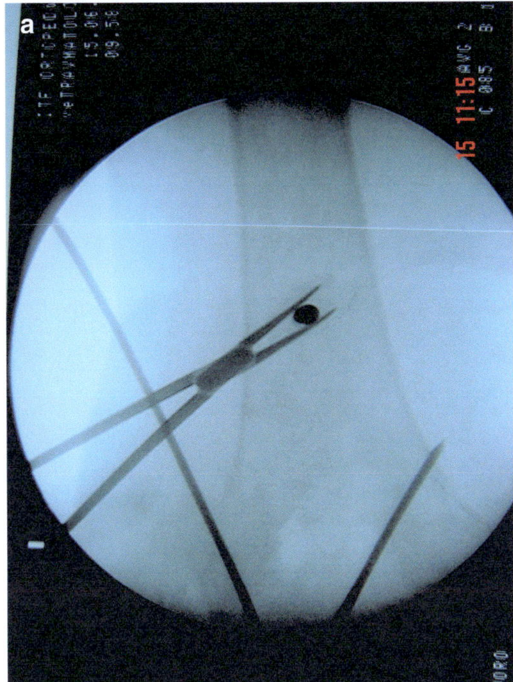

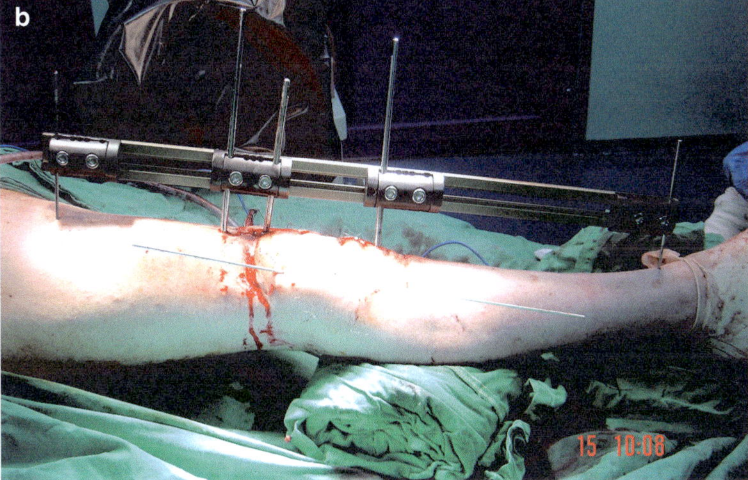

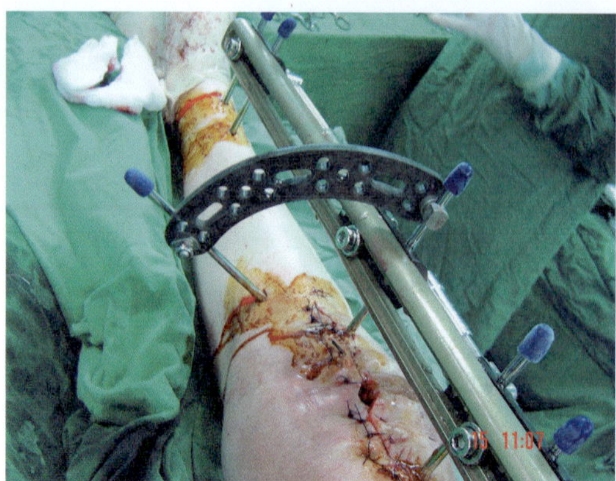

Fig. 5.7 Schanz screw applied to the medial surface of the proximal one third of the tibia and connected to the frame of the external fixator by an arch from the Ilizarov system

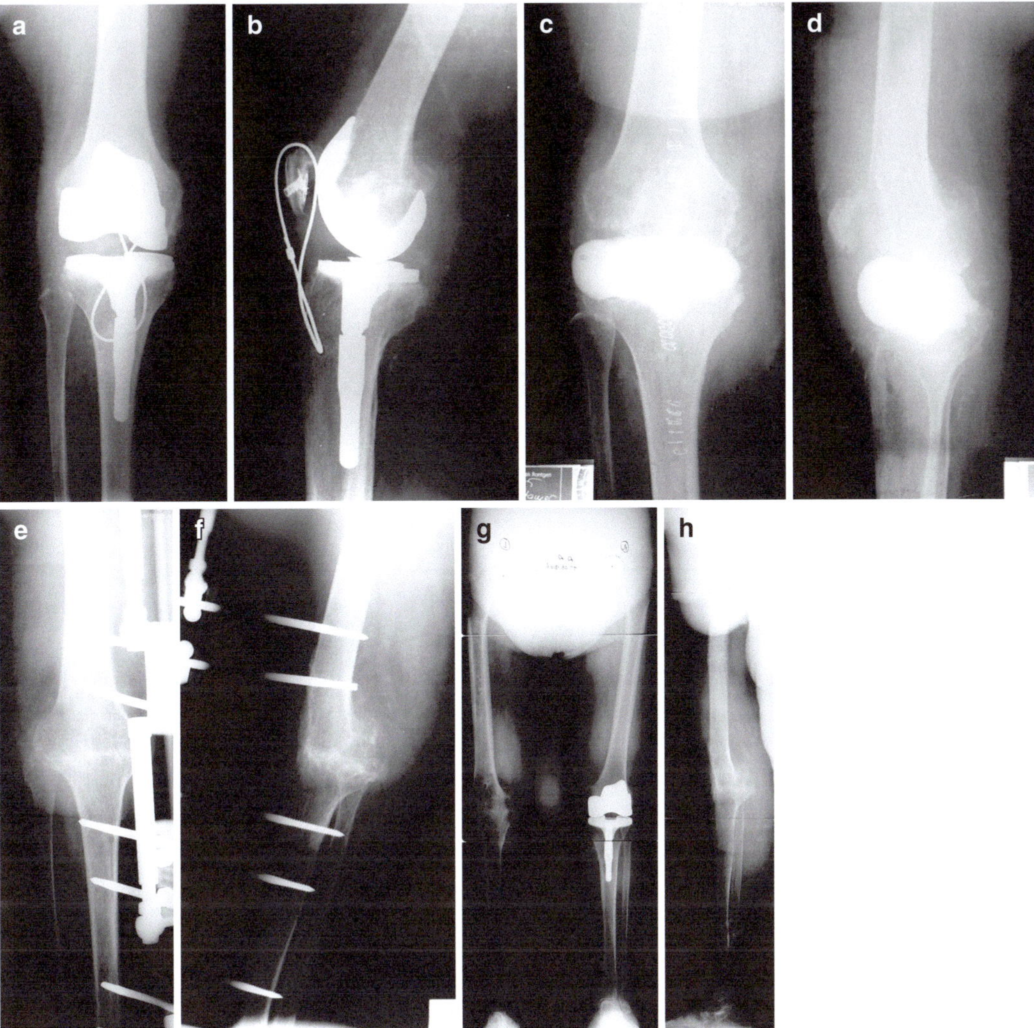

Fig. 5.8 (**a**, **b**) Failed knee arthroplasty with patellar tendon disruption and gross infection. (**c**, **d**) First phase: debridement and antibiotic-impregnated spacer. (**e**, **f**) Knee arthrodesis performed with unilateral external fixation. (**g**, **h**) Successful union

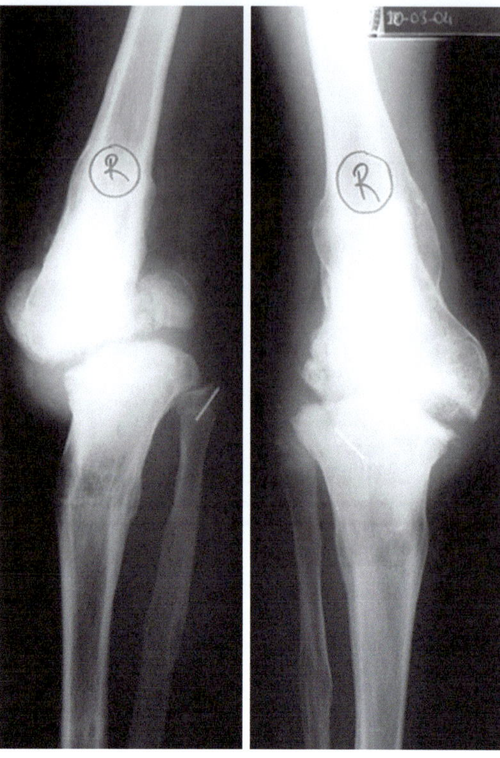

Fig. 5.9 Failed previous knee arthrodesis

is applied in the frontal plane, with two Schanz screws in each bone segment to obtain stable fixation.

- Hydroxyapatite Schanz screws improve bone–screw integration and prevent osteolysis.

Pitfalls

- Inappropriate Schanz screw orientation and bone cuts will lead to malalignment. Thus, meticulous attention is required for these steps. Do not neglect checking alignment with image intensifier often, in both AP and lateral views.

Pearls

- Knee position is checked by doing intraoperative malalignment test using the wire of the electrocautery device under image intensifier
- If there is marked osteoporosis or bone loss, another monolateral external fixator

References

Arroyo JS, Garvin KL, Neff JR (1997) Arthrodesis of the knee with a modular titanium intramedullary nail. J Bone Joint Surg Am 79(1):26–35

Charnley J (1960) Arthrodesis of the knee. Clin Orthop Relat Res 18:37–42

Eralp L, Kocaoglu M, Tuncay İ, Bilen FE, Samir SE (2004) Knee arthrodesis using a unilateral external fixator for the treatment of infectious sequelae. Acta Orthop Traumatol Turc 2:84–89

Hanssen AD, Trousdale RT, Osmon DR (1995) Patient outcome with reinfection following reimplantation for the infected total knee arthroplasty. Clin Orthop Relat Res 321:55

Manzotti A, Pullen C, Deromedis B, Catagni MA (2001) Knee arthrodesis after infected total knee arthroplasty using the İlizarov method. Clin Orthop Relat Res 389:143

Vlasak R, Gearen PF, Petty W (1995) Knee arthrodesis in the treatment of failed total knee replacement. Clin Orthop Relat Res 321:138

Acute Temporary Malpositioning for Dealing with Extensive Tissue Loss After Severe High-Energy Trauma to Extremities

6

Alexander Lerner, Lucian Fodor, and Yehuda Ullmann

Contents

A. Lerner, MD, PhD (✉)
Department of Orthopaedic Surgery,
Ziv Medical Center, 1 Rambam Street, Zefat, Israel

Faculty of Medicine, Bar-Ilan University,
Ramat Gan, Israel
e-mail: alex_lerner@yahoo.com

L. Fodor, MD
Department of Plastic and Reconstructive Surgery,
Emergency District Hospital, Cluj-Napoca, Romania

University of Medicine and Pharmacy "Iuliu Hatieganu",
Cluj-Napoca, Romania
e-mail: lucifodor@yahoo.com

Y. Ullmann, MD
Plastic and Reconstructive Surgery Department,
Rambam Health Care Campus, Haifa, Israel
e-mail: y_ullmann@rambam.health.gov.il

6.1 Introduction

High-energy complex limb injuries, especially with significant and extensive post-traumatic tissue damage or loss, pose a challenge for orthopedic, plastic, and vascular surgeons (Sherman et al. 2006; Bernstein and Chung 2007; Ullmann et al. 2006; Lerner et al. 2006). The classic, widely accepted treatment protocol for such patients usually includes a radical debridement procedure followed by bone fragment realignment, fixation, and limb length reconstruction as soon as possible. Immediate fracture stabilization in patients suffering from high-energy trauma is usually performed using unilateral tubular external fixation frames, providing a quick and minimally invasive approach, in accordance with the "orthopedic damage control" principles (Lerner et al. 2009). An external fixation frame applied at a site distant to the injury zone does not interfere with wound management. Temporary trans-articular bridging of the injured limb is indicated in the treatment of patients suffering from complex periarticular fractures.

Once this is accomplished, the surgeon is faced with large gaping wounds (resulting from the primary trauma itself and the surgical debridement procedure), where the exposed bone fragments and fracture site are at risk of infection.

6.2 Soft Tissue Management

Open limb fractures do not heal without adequate coverage of the fracture area by well-vascularized soft tissue. Many severe complications are avoided if this step is completed early. In some patients, the use of local and distant tissue flaps after severe high-energy injury to limbs is restricted due to the unavailability of viable local soft tissue or poor local healing potential due to a compromised vascular supply (i.e., single-vessel limb, conditions after revascularization procedures). Revision flap coverage may not be an option after previous flap necrosis, and amputation remains the standard option for such patients, especially for the lower limb. Extensive bone and tissue loss must be treated with bone grafting (often massive) and early wound coverage using major complex soft tissue reconstructive procedures. Free microsurgical muscle-skin flaps to cover the bone with living vascular tissue are often necessary (Sherman et al. 2006; Mack et al. 2008).

Urgent repair of major blood vessels in patients suffering from open fractures with vascular injuries (Gustilo type 3C fractures) usually requires vascular grafting because the debrided ends cannot be brought together and sutured end to end without tension (Lerner et al. 2009). The autologous graft is preferred to vascular prosthesis when there is significant wound contamination. The graft material must be covered by healthy soft tissue. Similarly, loss of major nerve continuity will call for further complex secondary nerve grafting. Often this protocol is fraught with the likelihood of major complications, particularly infection and grafting failures and donor area morbidity, requiring repeated, highly skilled specialist interventions. In severely traumatized patients, this multi-surgery approach cannot be reconciled with the basic principle of "damage control" and avoidance of the "second hit" (Lerner et al. 2009).

Previous studies on mangled extremities recommend wound closure within the first 72 h in order to reduce complications and shorten hospitalization time (Sherman et al. 2006). Recent reports demonstrate successful wound coverage after more than a month (Mack et al. 2008). Emerging new technologies such as negative-pressure wound therapy (NPWT) have enabled delayed wound coverage (Bernstein and Chung 2007; Ullmann et al. 2006). The easiest soft tissue method of reconstruction is not always the best. Initial soft tissue reconstruction starts with *primum non nocere.* When definitive closure is not achieved during primary wound management, any skin tension should be avoided. Exposed bones, tendons, nerves, or vessels should be covered as soon as possible to avoid drying these structures and further complications. NPWT is a good temporary alternative to flaps and helps in decreasing the local edema.

Many flaps have been described with great success for limb soft tissue coverage. Of the hundreds of flaps described, the most frequently used are the fasciocutaneous and muscle flaps.

Complex combined soft tissue and bone defects are managed with regional, distant, or free flaps (Ullmann et al. 2006). The goal is to restore the missing segments and avoid shortening. Among the most commonly used fasciocutaneous flaps for severe limb injuries are the anterolateral thigh (ALT), scapula, parascapula, radial forearm, and lateral arm. The muscle flaps that are frequently used in these circumstances are the latissimus dorsi, serratus anterior, and rectus abdominis flaps. The omentum flap has the advantage of being thin and large but has a short pedicle. The ALT and radial forearm have longer pedicles with possibility of more proximal anastomosis outside of the zone of injury. Often the vessels around the zone of injury were crushed and could have intimal detachment, which is hard to identify without transection of the vessel. Venous grafts can be used to connect the pedicle to a more proximal area.

6.3 Bone Defect Management Using Acute Shortening and Angulation

When a bone segment is missing, the alternative to shortening is a bone graft or flap. For defects less than 6 cm, bone grafts can successfully be

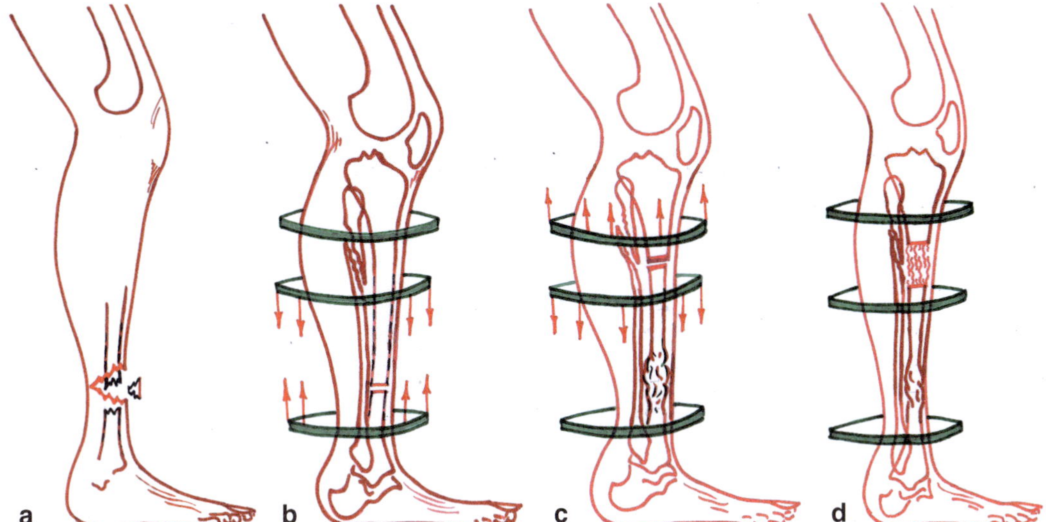

Fig. 6.1 Schematic representation of the temporary acute shortening technique. (**a**) Presentation of the limb on admission – open fracture with bone and soft tissue loss. (**b**) Debridement with acute shortening and stabilization in the external circular frame. (**c**) Proximal elongation tibial osteotomy is performed. (**d**) Limb length is restored by bone regeneration at the osteotomy site

used. Among the bone flaps that are most common for the lower and upper limb are free fibula, iliac crest, and vascularized rib. When the bone defect is more than 6 cm, it is recommended to use a vascularized bone instead of a graft. There are reports demonstrating that the bone quality after fibula flap is lower than the callus obtained by distraction (Bernstein and Chung 2007; Yokoyama et al. 2001). The use of a bone graft or flap requires minimum or no local contamination in order to enhance their survival.

Sometimes soft tissue coverage procedure is a complicated task, especially in patients with single-vessel patency. Bone shortening followed by graduated distraction is a good option when flaps are too risky (Fig. 6.1).

Acute shortening with or without angulation enables good bone molding and quality while avoiding complicated reconstructive soft tissue procedures. The temporary gross deformity thus created offers ample soft tissue necessary to cover the bones which are placed in contact. This maneuver reduces the need for any grafting procedure that would otherwise be used to decrease wound size and bring the wound edges together completely without tension (Ullmann et al. 2006; Simpson et al. 2001). A multiplicity of surgical repeat debridements is avoided using this method, since the initial debridements can be as radical as necessary in the knowledge that the wound can be closed and the need for bone and soft tissue grafting is much reduced. Furthermore, primary vascular and nerve end-to-end repair is facilitated without the need for grafting (Lerner and Soudry 2011). It is also a preferable procedure for heavily contaminated wounds where, after debridement, suspicion remains regarding wound contamination and potential postoperative complications.

The peripheral pulses, color, and capillary refilling must be checked during acute malposition procedures, to make sure that the angulation does not cause any vascular compromise. The extent of the acute shortening must be within safe limits which allow a good distal blood flow. The acute shortening and angulation must be abandoned if signs of vascular compromise appear. For this reason, this procedure should be performed without draping the distal part of the injured limb during the operative procedure, to allow continuous checking of the peripheral pulse, capillary refilling, and Doppler examination.

If the distal blood flow is compromised, compression between proximal and distal bone fragments must be immediately released. When the bone defect is greater than the safe limit for acute shortening, the limb can be shortened during the operative procedure only to the safe limit. Then, the remaining gap between bone fragments can be gradually closed using an external fixation frame during the early postoperative period.

Performing an acute shortening or shortening-angulation procedure can achieve primary closure of the soft tissue defect without tension on the edges of the wound. For a transversely oriented soft tissue defect, acute shortening produces adequate area for contact of the wound edges. In contrast, limb shortening for a longitudinally oriented wound can result in divergence of the wound edges, thereby creating a dilemma with regard to closing the soft tissue defect. An S-shaped extension of the wound solves this problem. This simple maneuver permits the closure of the wound by the counter transfer of the conforming skin-fascia flaps (Lerner and Soudry 2011).

Once skin and soft tissue healing at the wound region is well established, the temporary artificial deformity is gradually corrected, and limb axis and length are gradually restored (usually after 3–4 weeks). The axis, shape, and length of the injured limb segment are reconstructed secondarily once the wound is healed, using techniques of gradual realignment and lengthening at the site of an additional metaphyseal corticotomy or osteotomy in the Ilizarov or Taylor external fixation frames. This is performed without the need for additional complex bone grafting procedures. Distraction forces applied to the bone also create tension in the surrounding soft tissues, specifically the skeletal muscles, and initiate the sequence of adaptive changes known as distraction histiogenesis (Ilizarov 1989a, b; Lindsey et al. 2002; Meffert et al. 2000). Double- or multiple-level elongation corticotomies should be used for dealing with large bone defects, significantly shortening total time of elongation and skeletal external fixation.

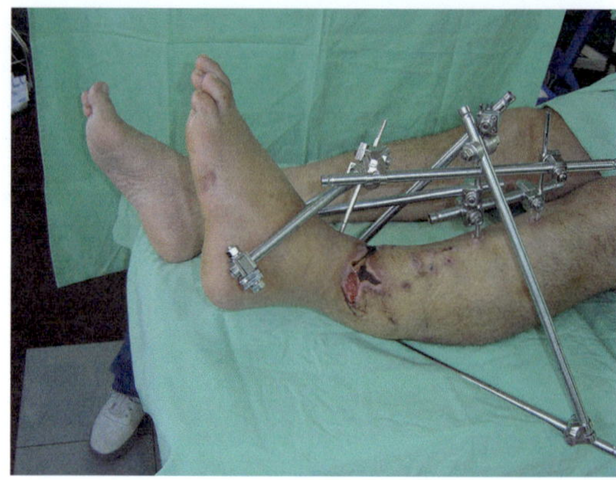

Fig. 6.2 Clinical image showing external fixation of the open tibial fracture after performing an acute temporary shortening and anteromedial angulation

The distraction technique allows restoration of relatively large bone defects without the need for bone grafts and complicated flaps, avoiding morbidity of donor sites and other serious complications. Additionally, the mechanical quality of the distracted bone is superior to cancellous bone and structural bone grafts.

In patients who suffer from a one-side-located extensive soft tissue defect (especially wounds located on the anterior aspect of leg), the fracture site bone remains uncovered, even after performing the acute shortening procedure. In addition, further bone resection is often unacceptable. On the other hand, residual bone exposure indicates the need for soft tissue reconstruction by flaps as the only remaining alternative. However, acute shortening combined with angulation directed to the side of the main soft tissue loss to cover the exposed bone is the treatment of choice. The angulated bone fragments are fixed using a tubular external fixator or hinged Ilizarov external fixation frame (Fig. 6.2).

The hinges of the Ilizarov device, located above the angulation site, must be locked. Subsequent, gradual progressive correction of the angulation can be initiated only when the soft tissue wound is completely closed (usually 3–4 weeks after the malpositioning procedure). The Ilizarov external fixator induces soft tissue lengthening by stretching the skin and the scars,

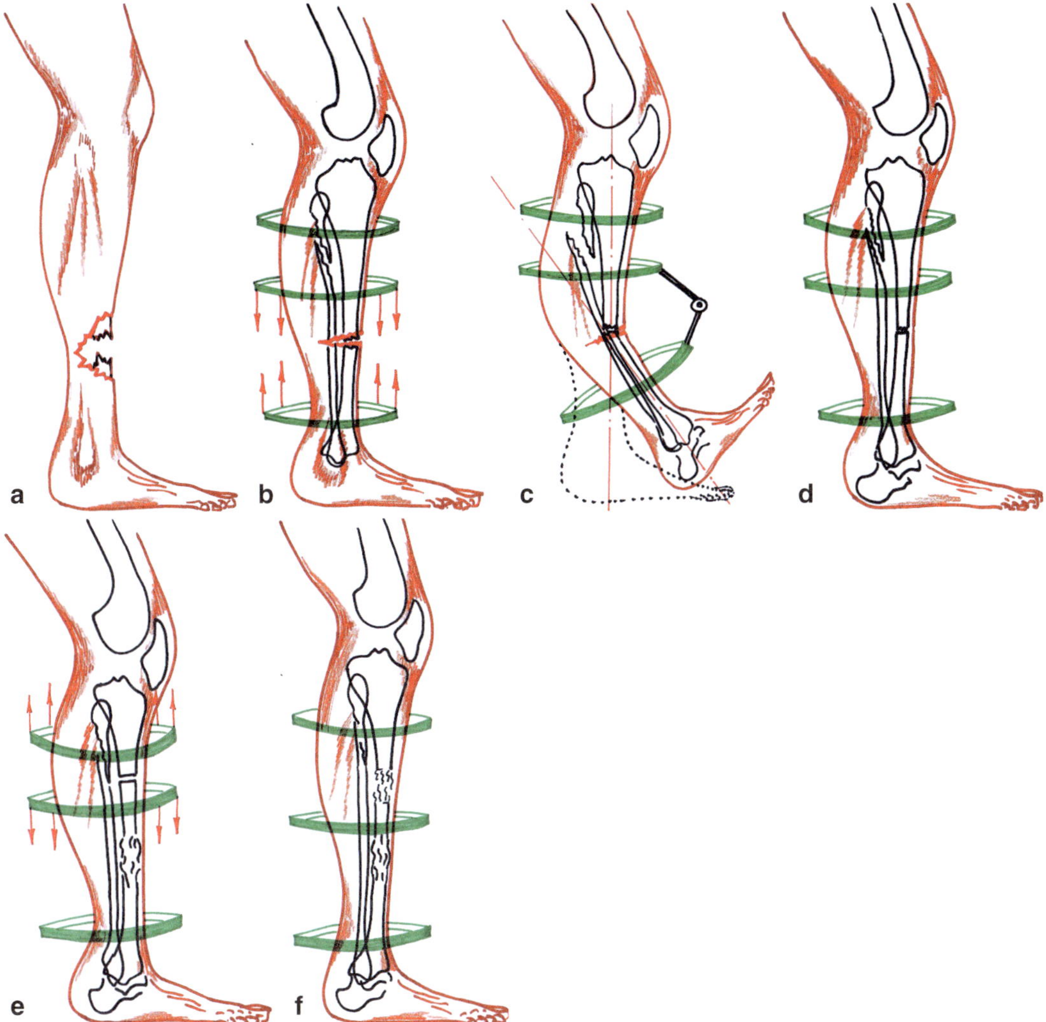

Fig. 6.3 Schematic representation of the temporary acute shortening and angulation technique. (**a**) Presentation of the limb on admission – open fracture with bone and soft tissue loss. (**b**) Debridement with acute shortening and stabilization in the external circular frame. Note uncovered fracture site after performing shortening procedure. (**c**) Acute angulation is performed to diminish the soft tissue wound and coverage of the fracture site. (**d**) The leg is gradually realigned using the Ilizarov frame. (**e**) Proximal elongation tibial osteotomy is performed. (**f**) Limb length is restorated by bone regeneration at the osteotomy site

resulting in a good soft tissue envelope at the end of bone distraction. When realignment of the limb's segment is achieved, an elongation corticotomy can be performed (Fig. 6.3).

In some patients with combined bone and soft tissue loss, the bone fragments remain exposed and deprived of soft tissue coverage, even after performing acute shortening and angulation.

Supplementary rotational displacement of the ends of the injured segment can bring about a decrease of the wound size and approximate the skin edges (temporary acute shortening-angulation-malrotation procedure) (Lerner et al. 2009) (Fig. 6.4). Gradual derotation of the limb in the external fixation frame should be performed later, together with distraction of the bone and

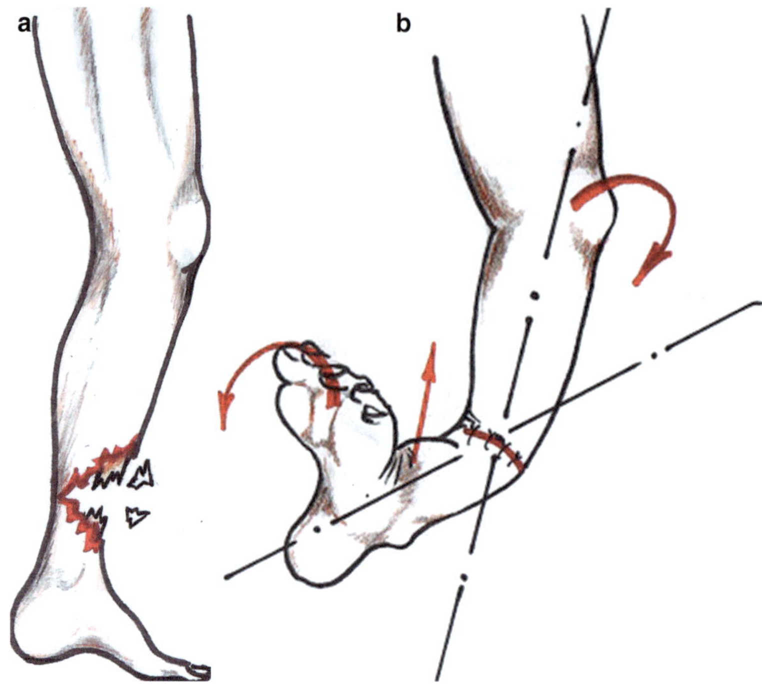

Fig. 6.4 Schematic representation of the temporary acute shortening, angulation, and malrotation technique. (**a**) Presentation of the limb on admission – open tibial fracture with extensive bone and soft tissue loss. (**b**) Debridement with acute temporary "shrinkage" (shortening, angulation, and malrotation) is performed to diminish the soft tissue wound and cover the fracture site and bone ends

limb length restoration. Similar maneuvers can be performed in a Taylor spatial frame (Rozbruch et al. 2006a, b).

Conclusion

Acute temporary malalignment by shortening and malangulation ("shrinkage") of the severely injured limb segment allows immediate soft tissue coverage using remaining vital soft tissues to cover the fracture site and exposed bone ends in extensive limb injuries. Large wounds with exposed bone heal rapidly by the apposition of healthy soft tissues. Acute shortening with subsequent progressive lengthening of the bone is also an accepted alternative for patients with an absolute or relative contraindication for free and local flaps.

Limb axis correction and tissue induction or reconstructions are then achieved by gradual realignment and distraction through one or more corticotomies using the Ilizarov callotasis bone induction technique. This is controlled by circular or hybrid frame external fixation constructs. Lack of donor site morbidity, decreased operating time (important for patients with multiple organ trauma), good handling of both soft tissue and bone defects, and low complication rates are the main advantages of acute shortening for complex limb injuries (Lerner and Soudry 2011; Meffert et al. 2000; Rozbruch et al. 2006a; Simpson et al. 2001). The gradual distraction rate provides acceptable cosmetic results, and the bone and soft tissue losses are handled simultaneously.

References

Bernstein ML, Chung KC (2007) Early management of the mangled upper extremity. Injury 38 Suppl 5:S3–S7. doi:10.1016/j.injury.2007.10.038, S0020-1383(07) 00436-6

Ilizarov GA (1989a) The tension-stress effect on the genesis and growth of tissues. Part I. The influence of stability of fixation and soft-tissue preservation. Clin Orthop Relat Res 238:249–281

Ilizarov GA (1989b) The tension-stress effect on the genesis and growth of tissues: part II. The influence of the rate and frequency of distraction. Clin Orthop Relat Res 239:263–285

Lerner A, Fodor L, Soudry M (2006) Is staged external fixation a valuable strategy for war injuries to the limbs? Clin Orthop Relat Res 448:217–224. doi:10.1097/01.blo.0000214411.60722.f8, 00003086-200607000-00032

Lerner A, Reis ND, Soudry M (2009) Primary limb shortening, angulation and rotation for closure of massive limb wounds without complex grafting procedures combined with secondary corticotomy for limb reconstruction. Curr Orthop Pract 20(2):191

Lerner A, Soudry M (2011) Armed conflict injuries to the extremities: a treatment manual. Springer, New York

Lindsey CA, Makarov MR, Shoemaker S, Birch JG, Buschang PH, Cherkashin AM, Welch RD, Samchukov ML (2002) The effect of the amount of limb lengthening on skeletal muscle. Clin Orthop Relat Res 402:278–287

Mack AW, Helgeson MD, Tis JE (2008) Contralateral structural femoral autograft use in treatment of an open periarticular knee fracture to perform knee arthrodesis. J Orthop Trauma 22(8):576–580. doi:10.1097/BOT.0b013e318180f10b, 00005131-200809000-00013

Meffert RH, Inoue N, Tis JE, Brug E, Chao EY (2000) Distraction osteogenesis after acute limb-shortening for segmental tibial defects. Comparison of a monofocal and a bifocal technique in rabbits. J Bone Joint Surg Am 82(6):799–808

Rozbruch S, Weitzman AM, Tracey Watson J, Freudigman P, Katz HV, Ilizarov S (2006a) Simultaneous treatment of tibial bone and soft-tissue defects with the Ilizarov method. J Orthop Trauma 20(3):197–205, 00005131-200603000-00006

Rozbruch SR, Fragomen AT, Ilizarov S (2006b) Correction of tibial deformity with use of the Ilizarov-Taylor spatial frame. J Bone Joint Surg Am 88 Suppl 4:156–174. doi:10.2106/JBJS.F.00745, 88/suppl_4/156

Sherman R, Rahban S, Pollak AN (2006) Timing of wound coverage in extremity war injuries. J Am Acad Orthop Surg 14(10 Spec No):S57–S61, 14/10/S57

Simpson AH, Andrews C, Giele H (2001) Skin closure after acute shortening. J Bone Joint Surg Br 83(5):668–671

Ullmann Y, Fodor L, Ramon Y, Soudry M, Lerner A (2006) The revised "reconstructive ladder" and its applications for high-energy injuries to the extremities. Ann Plast Surg 56(4):401–405. doi:10.1097/01.sap.0000201552.81612.68, 00000637-200604000-00014

Yokoyama K, Itoman M, Nakamura K, Tsukamoto T, Saita Y, Aoki S (2001) Free vascularized fibular graft vs. Ilizarov method for post-traumatic tibial bone defect. J Reconstr Microsurg 17(1):17–25

Salvage of Infected Periarticular Fractures

Stuart A. Green

Contents

7.1 Introduction

7.1.1 Causation

Infected periarticular fractures constitute one of the most challenging problems in orthopedic surgery. In some cases, the injuries result from open fractures, as a result of either blunt trauma (e.g., motor vehicle collisions) or penetrating trauma (such as gunshot wounds, war injuries, and so forth). Often, however, the initial injury was closed, but the displacement of the fragments following the injury led to open reduction and internal fixation. What often starts out as a triumphant reconstruction by the surgeon ends up as a tragedy as wound breakdown over hardware introduces microorganisms into areas of vulnerable tissue with marginal circulation at best.

Whether the initial injury is open or closed, communication of the infection within the joint space results in a chronic low-grade pyarthrosis that gradually erodes articular cartilage. More significantly, however, the infection cannot be eradicated by antibiotics no matter how long administered or how heavy the dosage. In this situation, microorganisms are protected from the antibiotics as long as the microbes continue to occupy the space.

7.1.2 Surgical Strategy

The only viable method of eliminating such an infection is to resect the joint along with its articular cartilage down to, and through, the

S.A. Green, MD
Department of Orthopaedic Surgery, School of
Medicine, University of California, Irvine, CA, USA
e-mail: sgreen@uci.edu

M. Kocaoğlu et al. (eds.), *Advanced Techniques in Limb Reconstruction Surgery*,
DOI 10.1007/978-3-642-55026-3_7, © Springer Berlin Heidelberg 2015

subchondral bone. Indeed, one must continue to remove osseous tissue if there is any question of viability. Fortunately, removing subchondral bone results in exposure of cancellous bone, tissue that has, in its normal state, good circulation and therefore a capacity to deliver antibiotics locally that have been administered parenterally.

7.1.2.1 Primary Arthrodesis

In some locations, resecting the bone on both sides of the joint leaves sufficient osseous tissue to permit arthrodesis in fairly good alignment. In the past, it was necessary to accept a short limb as a natural consequence of debridement of an infected joint. With the introduction of limb elongation using distraction osteogenesis, it is possible to restore limb length and alignment to a degree never before thought possible.

7.1.2.2 Knee

The knee joint is a typical in this regard. Virtually any amount of bone can be resected from the periarticular region down to healthy bleeding osseous tissue on both sides. Compression of the properly prepared bone surfaces, typically using external skeletal fixation usually leads to union, but with a short limb. Restoring limb length in such a situation is relatively easy and can be done to either the tibia and fibula or via the femur. The patient in this situation, however, is left with a stiff knee gait pattern that is often preferable to an above-knee prosthesis. However, the stiff knee constitutes a social handicap, particularly in various forms of conveyance where an individual who has had a knee fused surgically must take an aisle seat in an airplane or bus with the fused knee projecting into the aisle.

7.1.2.3 Hip

Fortunately, resection arthrodesis of the knee is rare. Even rarer still is resection arthrodesis of the hip. The problem usually follows multiply failed total hip replacement and is therefore covered in published materials dealing with such implants.

7.1.2.4 Ankle

Resection arthrodesis of the ankle, however, is far and away the most likely scenario when one considers this therapeutic approach in the face of a periarticular infection following fracture.

With the above thought in mind, this chapter will focus on the options available to deal with an infection, particularly a recalcitrant one, of the distal tibia that extends into the ankle joint. This is, after all, the most common situation an orthopedic surgeon will likely encounter in civilian practice that would require extensive resection and reconstruction by arthrodesis in an effort to prevent amputation of the limb above the infected region.

7.2 Autogenous Bone Grafting

7.2.1 Implant Issues

Salvage of an infected fracture of the distal tibia—whether initially open or closed—requires a strategy individualized to the presenting problem. If hardware is present, it may be left in place if it securely stabilizes a fracture site associated with viable bone. Most cases, however, require removal of hardware, debridement of dead bone, and application of external fixation for control of sepsis. Autogenous bone grafting is usually needed to reconstruct any residual osseous defect. At times one observes a case in which an unsuspected, chronic ankle joint infection caused persistent sepsis. The infection seems to track into the ankle through open fracture lines after wound breakdown. In such situations, the chronic ankle joint infection must be eradicated (by arthrodesis) to control sepsis (Fig. 7.1a, b).

An infection occurring in a surgically treated fracture of the distal tibial plafond may prove impossible to eradicate (Bourne et al. 1983; Childress 1965; Coonrad 1970; Cox 1965; Gay and Evrard 1963; Green et al. 1996; Green and Roesler 1987; Ruedi and Ailgower 1979; Ruedi and Allgower 1969; Scheck 1965). The presence of nonviable bone fragments and hardware within the septic focus, combined with a thin or deficient soft tissue envelope, makes reconstructive surgery extremely challenging (Leach 1984; Ovadia and Beals 1986; Pierce and Heinrich 1979).

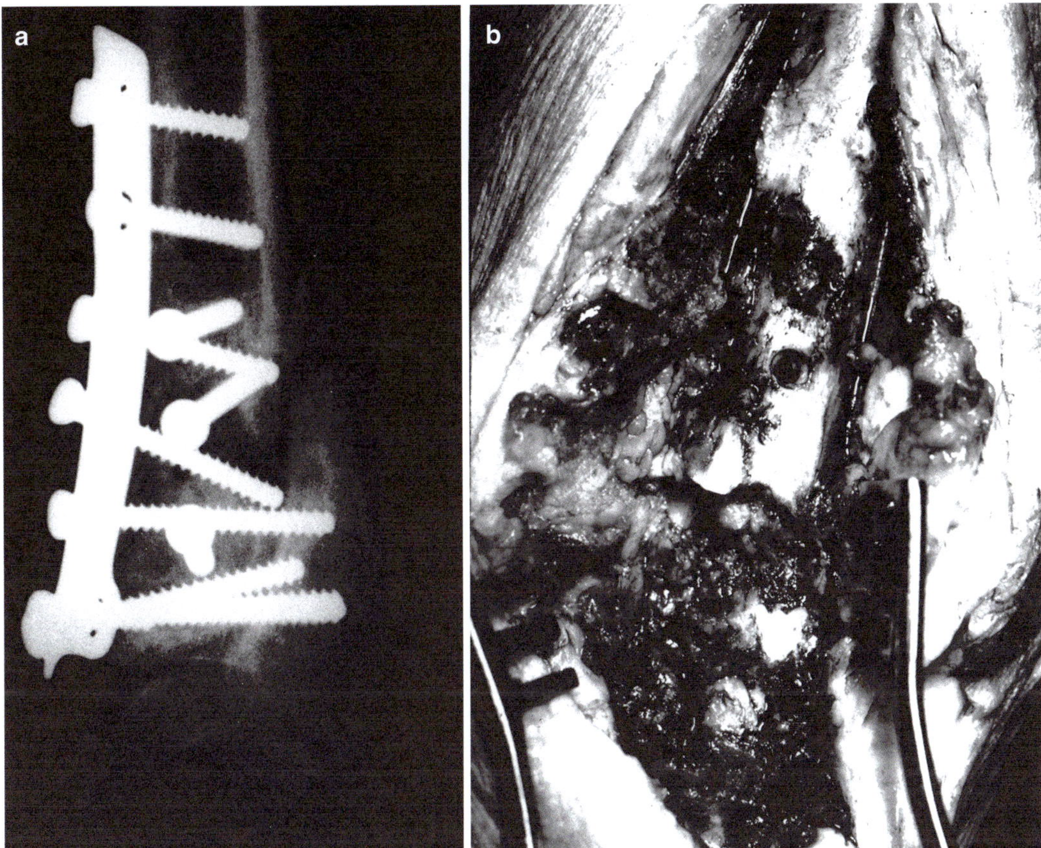

Fig. 7.1 Typical appearance of infected, surgically repaired distal tibia. (**a**) Exposed hardware, screws backing out. (**b**) Removal of hardware reveals nonviable bone requiring debridement

Rarely, the treating physician may elect to leave the initial internal fixation in place, even though the hardware is exposed in an open wound. In our series, we selected this option for two patients; both had excellent stable internal fixation with only exposed screw heads and radiographic evidence of progressive osseous healing. Generally, the infection in such cases starts out as localized skin slough over a screw head or other prominent piece of hardware several weeks or months after the original injury. Inflammatory changes must be limited to the skin immediately surrounding the slough. By leaving the hardware in place, the surgeon may aid fracture healing, but only if fixation is secure (Burwell and Charnley 1985).

When considering whether to "wait out" the local skin slough (leaving the hardware in place),

the physician should avoid wishful thinking, hoping that the infection does not involve deeper osseous tissues. The compression-type pilon fracture often creates nonviable bone fragments that can become the focus of persistent sepsis if microorganisms enter through an area of skin breakdown. Serial radiographs should show disuse osteopenia of all bone fragments; nonviable bone will remain relatively dense on X-ray films as time passes.

In some cases, early healing of a fibular fracture, combined with evidence of progressive healing of the tibial fracture, may suggest that a septic medial (or anterior) tibial buttress plate (if present) can be removed to eliminate the infection. (Fractures originally requiring such a plate, however, have the potential for angulating, especially if there is substantial supramalleolar comminution. In general, these fractures will collapse into varus or apex posterior angulation if not united. Furthermore, motion at such a nonunion site helps perpetuate the infection, leading to an unstable, infected nonunion at the level of the leg where there is only limited soft tissue cover. For this reason, removal of hardware before union of the distal tibial fracture should be accompanied by a strategy (either external skeletal fixation or a non-weight-bearing cast) to prevent fracture angulation.

7.2.2 Classification System

Kallem and Waddell's classification of distal tibial fractures(Kallem and Waddell 1979) recognizes two basic categories based on the mechanism of injury: rotation fractures and compression-type fractures. With rotation fractures, the distal tibial fractures into two or more large fragments (with minimal or no anterior tibial comminution), combined with a transverse or short oblique fracture of the distal fibula. The compression-type fracture has marked anterior tibial comminution, multiple distal tibial fragments, and superior migration of the talus. (The distal fibula may or may not be fractured in the compression-type injury.)

7.2.3 Series Report

At the Problem Fracture Service at Rancho Los Amigos Medical Center, the author treated 13 infected fractures involving the distal tibial metaphysis and plafond.

7.2.3.1 Demographics
The demographic details of this series of patients is of interest. The average age of the patients was 43 years. Ten patients had no associated injuries, while three patients suffered a variety of injuries, including a peroneal palsy, a severe head trauma, and polytrauma with multiple long-bone fractures.

Ten of the patients in this series had compression-type fractures, and three had rotation fractures. Eight patients had open injuries, and five sustained closed fractures.

7.2.3.2 Mechanism
The mechanism of injury was a fall in seven patients, a motorcycle accident in three patients, a twisting injury in one, an assault in one, and unknown in one patient. Seven of the 13 patients were initially treated with open reduction and internal fixation. Interestingly, all but one of the seven patients with internally stabilized fractures experienced a loss of fixation that would have required hardware removal and reoperation even if an infection had not developed.

7.2.3.3 Cultures
All patients had culture-positive drainage at the time of the initial evaluation at our clinic. *Staphylococcus aureus* was the most common organism encountered, followed by Enterobacteriaceae species and *Pseudomonas aeruginosa*. Ten patients had positive cultures for more than one organism. Since these injuries became infected from without inward, polymicrobial contamination is not surprising.

7.2.3.4 Pre-Ilizarov Protocol
Our protocol for managing the infected pilon fracture employs the basic principles of septic fracture care (Cave 1965; Green 1982, 1983; Leach 1984; Muller 1982). Debridement of all nonviable bone is essential, along with removal of all hardware that may serve as a nidus of infection. Following debridement, the distal tibia must be stabilized to prevent angulation and shortening (Weller 1982). Of the 13 patients in our series, 11 were placed in an external fixator following hardware removal. Since the fixator must span the ankle joint, full pins are needed distally, almost always into the calcaneus (Fig. 7.2).

Rigid external fixation may have to remain in place 8–12 months during reconstruction. Eventually, the calcaneal transfixion pins may become loose or septic, necessitating their premature removal. Placing one or more pins or wires pin across the midmetatarsal arch or forefoot when the frame is initially applied allows the construction of a triangular frame connecting the single metatarsal full pin to the pin cluster in the calcaneus and another pin cluster in the mid-tibia. Extraordinary stability and fixator longevity can

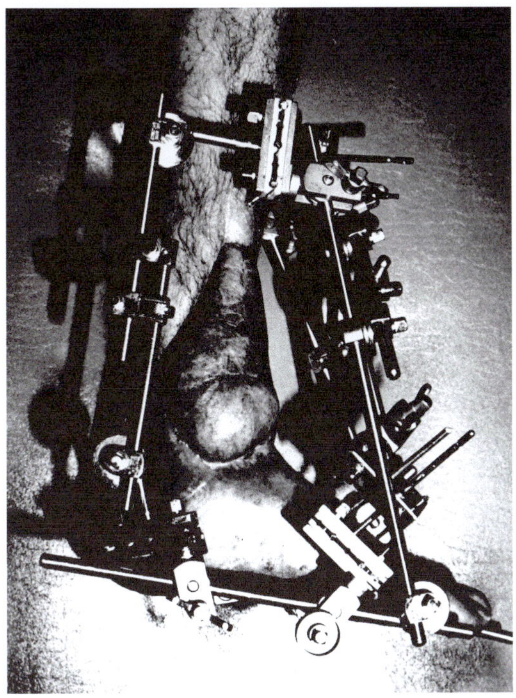

Fig. 7.2 Stable external fixation with Hoffmann apparatus. Note that the frame spans the area of surgery with pins in the calcaneus and forefoot. A microvascular flap covers the area of resection

be achieved in this manner, which creates a triangle between the tibia approximately and the heel and forefoot distally.

7.2.4 Mounting Principles

External skeletal fixation of the calcaneus is technically demanding. Numerous fixator configurations are possible for this type of reconstruction. All of them, however, should, at the very least, completely surround the limb, with either a quadrilateral system or a circular system. In this manner, transfixion implants in the foot are easily secured to the frame.

7.2.4.1 Quadrilateral Configurations

With quadrilateral external fixation, multiple pins within the same pin gripper placed into the tuber of the calcaneus should be in an oblique row, slanting downward and posteriorly, following the angle of the bone. Fluoroscopy aids pin placement with such devices.

7.2.4.2 Monolateral Configurations

Attempting to obtain consolidation after resection of the distal tibia and upper talus with a monolateral fixator is difficult and probably unwise. To do so, one would have to use threaded half pins, most likely inserted from the lateral side of the limb. Unfortunately, the cancellous nature of the calcaneus will not hold half pins for the many months required for the kind of surgery contemplated here. Instead, pin loosening becomes a distressing problem. The calcaneus is a small bone to start with and can quickly turn to Swiss cheese in appearance if implants work loose.

7.2.4.3 Ring Configurations

Certain fixators with ring configurations allow tensioned smooth or beaded wires to crisscross the calcaneus, thereby stabilizing it. The addition of one or more wires in the forefoot completes the distal configuration.

As for the proximal tibial mounting, any stable configuration that uses either wires alone, half pins alone, or combinations of pins and wires (including centrally threaded or fully threaded transfixion pins that attach to the frame on both sides of the limb) will do.

In two of our patients, and several others we have seen in consultation, thorough debridement of the infection, including removal of hardware and excision of nonviable bone from the distal tibia, failed to cure the infection. In these cases, we also observed progressive radiographic narrowing of the ankle joint caused by a subclinical pyarthrosis of the ankle. When wound breakdown over hardware or elsewhere occurs, it is best to assume that the joint infection tracks down a fracture line from the open wound into the ankle joint itself. Once there, the microbes establish a chronic infection that drains to the wound surface via a persistent fracture defect in the tibial plafond (Fig. 7.3a, b). For this reason, the usual clinical signs of joint infection—swelling, fever, and intense pain—may be absent. Instead, there is a slow, progressive bacterial degradation of articular cartilage manifested

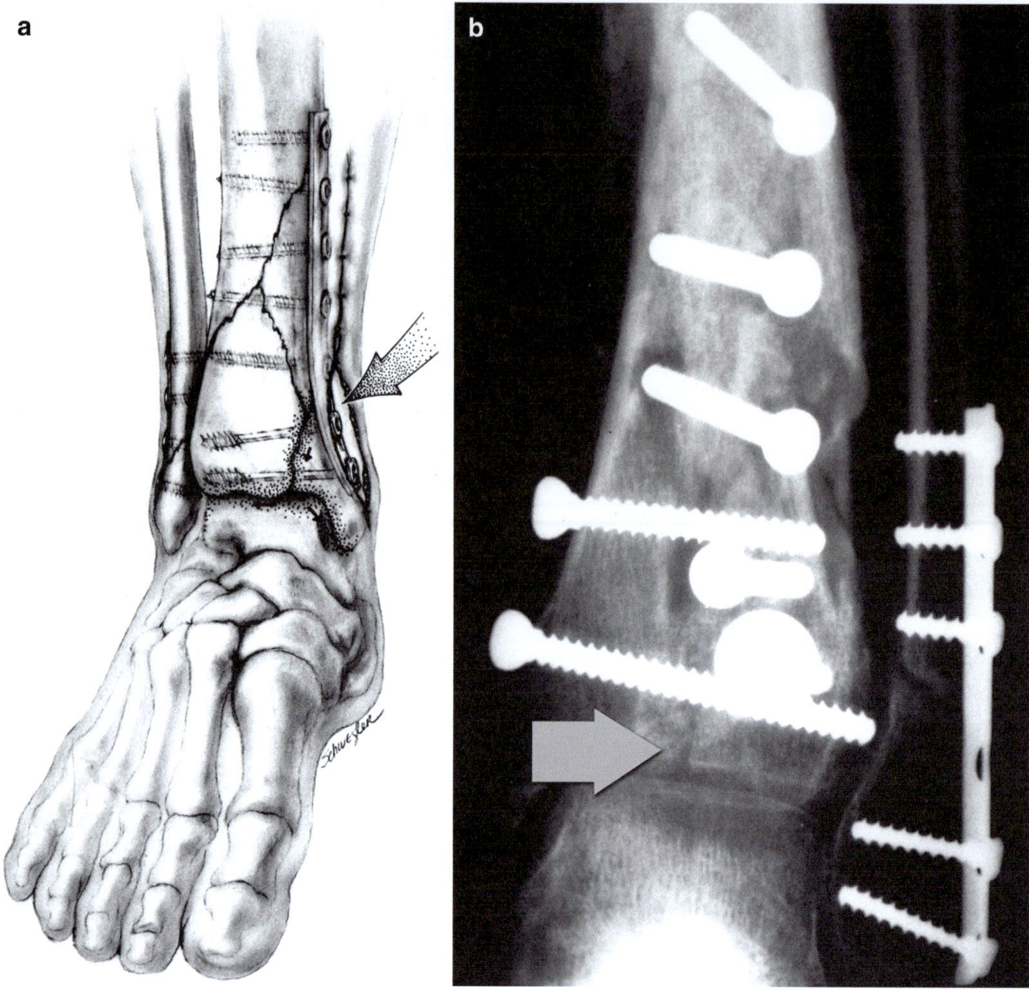

Fig. 7.3 Entry of microbe into the ankle joint space after wound breakdown. (**a**) Diagram showing passageway of bacteria along plate and screws into open fracture lines into the ankle joint. (**b**) *Arrow* points to open fracture line allowing entry of bacteria into the ankle joint from infected exposed hardware

by joint-space narrowing and, possibly, juxta-articular bone erosion.

7.2.5 Resection Principles

A chronic pyarthrosis of any joint is often difficult to eradicate under the best of circumstances and frequently necessitates arthrodesis (Weise and Weller 1982). When a chronic pyarthrosis of the ankle is combined with a chronic osteomyelitis of the distal tibial metaphysis, a classic joint-fusion procedure is impossible because debridement of both the distal tibia [metaphysis and the tibia] plafond leaves a large cavitary bone defect that opens anteriorly or anteromedially. With debridement of the upper talar articular surface as well, the defect extends down into the body of the talus.

7.2.5.1 Papineau Procedure

An open cancellous bone graft—the so-called Papineau procedure(Green 1994; Papineau 1973)—has been proven to be a reliable technique for filling in the defect created by extensive debridement of osseous tissue (Fig. 7.4).

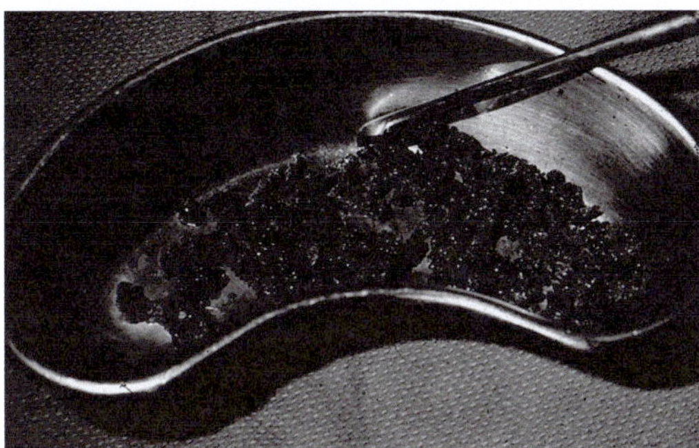

Fig. 7.4 Fresh autogenous bone graft from the iliac crest, the "gold standard" for bone graft material

7.2.5.2 Microvascular Reconstruction

Free, microvascular, composite-tissue transfers—utilizing either the ipsilateral iliac crest or a rib—might also be useful for salvage. Union to the body of the talus, however, would be difficult to achieve. Alternately, coverage can be obtained with a soft tissue free flap, followed by closed bone grafting. (We do not use the contralateral fibula for reconstruction of an infected pilon fracture. In the event the reconstruction fails and the septic limb has to be amputated; we prefer to leave the good leg undamaged.)

7.2.5.3 Structural Considerations

When the reconstructive plan requires extensive bone grafting to fill a cavitary defect across the ankle joint, prolonged immobilization in an external fixator frame is required until the graft matures. Unfortunately, full corticalization of a cancellous bone graft takes 2–5 years, and prolonged bracing is necessary thereafter.

At the ankle, the foot projects forward at a right ankle to the tibia, creating a substantial bending movement in the "ankle" fusion site. A nonunion of the ankle graft mass—actually a motion-induced pseudoarthrosis—occurred in some patients in our series. One way to prevent this problem is to "corticalize" the graft by incorporating the distal fibula. For this reason, we do not remove the distal fibula when performing an arthrodesis of the ankle in infected pilon fractures. (By the time the patient has reached the point where secondary bone grafting of an osseous-articular defect is needed, any fibular

fracture has probably already healed, permitting placement of a graft between the distal fibula and lateral side of the talus.)

The bone graft should be extended proximally between the distal tibia and fibula in the region normally occupied by the interosseous tibiofibular ligament. The goal of surgery is to create a solid mass of bone connecting the lower leg to the talus by whatever means possible.

In several cases, we noted that the infection of the distal tibial metaphysis, while perhaps requiring extensive debridement of the anterior cortex, generally spares the posterior and posterolateral distal tibia. When attempting fusion of the ankle for an infected pilon fracture, the surgeon might be able to abut the posterior cortex of the distal tibia to the posterior edge of the remaining upper talus, thereby enhancing the stability of the construct. This measure alone will do much to speed consolidation in cases managed with a bone graft in the ankle defect..

In spite of our best efforts, we had a substantial number of patients with unfavorable outcomes. Eight of the 13 patients had their fractures unite, but 2 of these 8 had persistent sepsis that we could not eradicate. There were two nonunions, and one patient required a below-knee amputation. Four patients required an ankle fusion to control chronic ankle pyarthrosis. The six patients whose fractures united and were free of infection (less than 50 % of the series) all had stiff ankles and scarred, dystrophic-looking skin around the distal tibia.

7.3 The Masquelet Technique

In virtually all circumstances, it is preferable to insert a bone graft into a closed rather than an open space. Likewise, an ideal situation is to have a cavity receptive to the bone graft already prepared and sterilized. During the last decade or so, the Masquelet technique has become popular among reconstructive surgeons (Donegan et al. 2011; Giannoudis et al. 2011; Karger et al. 2012).

A skeletal defect is filled with antibiotic impregnated bone cement, left in place long enough for a membrane to form around the cement mass. It has been shown that this membrane secretes growth factors, including BMPs, transforming growth factor-beta, and VEGF. When the membrane becomes mature, the cement spacer is carefully removed, leaving the surrounding membrane in place to serve as a bed for the bone graft.

7.4 Reamer Irrigator Aspirator (RIA)

Reports of donor site morbidity associated with the process of obtaining iliac crest bone graft has led surgeons to alternative sources. A popular method of attaining bone involves the use of a device, the Reamer Irrigator Aspirator (RIA), that extracts bone from the marrow cavity of long bones, especially the femur (Cuttica et al. 2010; Stafford and Norris 2010). The user consists of a very sharp intramedullary reamer that withdraws a bone marrow as it advances. A surprising volume of bone can be obtained in this manner. The RIA, like the iliac crest bone graft, is not without its problems. Over-reaming the endosteal surface has resulted in early or delayed fractures of the femur. Nevertheless, the popularity of this product and ease of use suggest it will be around for a long time.

7.5 Distraction Osteogenesis

G. A. Ilizarov provided orthopedic surgeons with an incomparable tool for limb reconstruction when he unlocked from within bone the capacity to produce virtually unlimited quantities of new osseous tissue to fill bone defects (Ilizarov 1952, 1968, 1989a, b; Ilizarov et al. 1972; Ilizarov and Ledioev 1969). This feature of distraction osteogenesis greatly expands the indications for limb salvage surgery in the presence of infected or nonviable bone. Now, as long as the distal part of the limb is worth saving (good sensation and circulation), intercalary reconstruction is usually possible.

Distraction osteogenesis, one of the most remarkable developments in the history of limb reconstruction, plays a particularly significant role in the reconstruction in resection arthrodesis. This is particularly true with respect to the ankle (Green and Roesler 1987). After all, removing the distal part of the tibia and some or all of the talus leaves a gap, which typically exceeds in volume that of a golf ball, and is often much larger. Closing such a gap results in the limb shortening that nowadays can be overcome with distraction osteogenesis.

7.5.1 Bifocal Treatment

Although it may seem desirable to have the new bone formation in the region of the arthrodesis, it is far safer to simply attempt to obtain a joint fusion and eradication of the infection in one location (the ankle) while either simultaneously or sequentially restoring limb length through a different part of the limb segment. Typically, with respect to the ankle, restoration of limb length by distraction osteogenesis should take place in the proximal tibia.

The basic principles of debridement of infected and nonviable tissue remains, as always, the hallmark of restorative orthopedic surgery (Thordarson et al. 1997; Zarutsky et al. 2005). In the ankle, resection of the distal tibia leaves an empty soft tissue sleeve. As long as the remaining tibia has good quality of circulation, the amount of bone removed can be replaced by an osteotomy performed elsewhere in healthy bone, followed by distraction osteogenesis to overcome the defect. Oftentimes, strategies are necessary to prevent the soft tissue sleeve created by resection of nonviable and infected bone from collapsing inward and thereby blocking intercalary transport fragment from reaching its target.

As with the process used to sterilize area for eventual cancellous or RIA bone grafting, the Masquelet technique also helps prepare a proper bed for movement of the intercalary bone segment when using the Ilizarov method. A cylindrical tube of antibiotic impregnated methyl methacrylate can serve as a spacer that functions in a dual capacity in preparation for distraction osteogenesis: first, help sterilize the region where infected bone had been removed and, second, encourage the formation of a membrane through which the transport segment can pass. Since the elution of antibiotics from the surface of a spacer decreases quickly with the passage of time, it may be worthwhile to exchange the spacer more than once as the intercalary segment moves toward its target. In such circumstances, a smaller spacer is used with each exchange.

7.5.1.1 The Intercalary Segment

It has been shown that prolonged transportation of the intercalary moving segment reduces the viability of the and of that segment as it approaches its target (Green 1991a, b, 1994; Green et al. 1992). In all likelihood, this is a consequence of the movement of the intercalary segment, which outstrips its own blood supply (Fig. 7.5).

7.5.1.2 Docking Site

In light of this observation, surgeons experienced in technique of a bone transport reconstructive surgery (known in Ilizarov jargon as "bifocal simultaneous distraction-compression osteosynthesis" since actions are occurring simultaneously at two locations in the limb segment, distraction at the osteotomy site and compression at the docking site) will frequently bone graft docking site. In Kurgan, surgeons routinely enter the docking site percutaneously with curette when there is about 1 cm to go before contact and scrape away the nonviable bone at the end of the intercalary moving segment.

Either approach, bone grafting or curettage of the docking site, is designed to shorten the amount of time it takes to obtain union between the intercalary fragment and the target fragment and to increase the likelihood of successful osteosynthesis, without having to wait too long for union to occur.

Bone grafting the docking site is typically done when the intercalary fragment makes contact with the target fragment. At times, the surfaces are uneven, pointing to the location where the bone graft will do the most good (in the gap between the bone ends). Some surgeons will insert the bone graft when there still exists

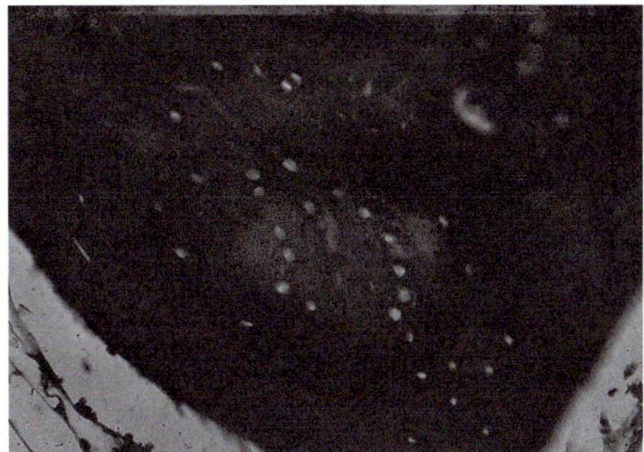

Fig. 7.5 Histology to the tip of a bone transport segment; notice empty osteocyte lacunae, a sign that the end of the fragment is not viable

considerable space between intercalary fragment and the target fragment. The concept employed in such cases is to allow the bone graft to begin to mature while the intercalary fragment is plowing into it. While the idea is appealing, there is no literature that either supports or refutes the wisdom of such a strategy.

7.5.1.3 Oblique Directional Wires

When there is a very long skeletal defect, pulling the intercalary segment through the limb with transverse tension wires connected to a ring is often depicted as the classic method to achieve such a goal (Green 1991a, b, 1994; Green et al. 1992). However, the wires cut through the skin and underlying soft tissues by compression and necrosis of whatever lies in the pathway of the wires as they move in conjunction with their ring. While such a therapeutic approach to large segmental defects—whether occurring as the result of traumatic osseous tissue loss or surgical resection of infected, nonviable, or malignant bone—the experience is often a miserable one for the patient. Necrotic tissue immediately adjacent to the moving wires typically becomes infected, with the surrounding skin and soft tissues reacting with inflammatory features. Ideally, zone of necrosis is small, hardly larger in diameter and the wires themselves. Occasionally, however, the zone of necrosis extends out a few millimeters on either side of the advancing wire, resulting in unsightly scars when the entire process is complete.

With the above consideration in mind, the group in Kurgan, Russia, use oblique directional wires, rather than transverse wires, to pull the intercalary segment through the limb. Such wires traverse the defect in a longitudinal direction after passing through the intercalary segment, often in a crisscross pattern. They typically exit the limb beyond the target fragment. Because such wires cross within the defect region, their crossing angle becomes more and more obtuse as the intercalary fragment approaches the target fragment. In doing so, they not only block the intercalary fragment from reaching the target fragment, but they also can no longer pull intercalary fragment because they have gradually become more transverse (rather than a longitudinal). Hence, it becomes obvious that, as the intercalary fragment approaches the target fragment, longitudinal direction wires must be removed, and the final docking of the intercalary fragment to the target fragment achieved with the use of transverse wires tensioned to a mobile ring within the configuration.

Obviously, considerable advanced planning is necessary to set up a frame that has components capable of achieving a combination of longitudinal traction on the intercalary segment with directional wires followed by conversion of the device to one that can achieve final compression osteosynthesis at the docking site.

Among the considerations necessary to achieve this highly desirable strategy for overcoming a large segmental defect using a combination of techniques that starts out with a longitudinal direction wires and ends with the transverse tensioned wires are the following: placement of an empty ring somewhere toward the middle of the configuration that will be in the proper position to secure transverse tension wires passing through the moving intercalary segment; such a ring must be in the location that allows it to move freely along the longitudinal connecting rods without hitting up against nuts or clickers or sockets during its course of action; the distal ring securing the target fragment must be free of obstructing elements that would block the moving ring from dragging the intercalary fragment to the target fragment with sufficient additional

range to permit into fragmentary compression; and finally, the components used to achieve the initial longitudinal distraction must be placed in a way that will allow easy access to, and not interfere with, the empty transport ring.

7.5.1.4 Conversion from Oblique to Transverse Wires

While it seems desirable to perform any bone grafting procedure at the target site at the same time a conversion from a longitudinal transport system to a transverse transport system is being accomplished, there is a risk with this approach. After all, the longitudinal traction wires, because they exit the skin, must be considered contaminated. Therefore, microbes must, of necessity, inhabit the space between the intercalary fragment and target fragment if the wires have passed through this region. It is also possible to use longitudinal direction wires that do not actually pass through the region of defect but are, instead, parallel to that region in the soft tissues. In such a case, there is probably less risk of contamination of the bone graft by microbes then that might occur if the wires are passing through the defect region.

The safest strategy, therefore, is to perform the conversion from longitudinal traction wires to transverse tensioned traction wires as a step separate from bone grafting the docking site. Usually, the longitudinal direction wires lose their pulling the capacity when the intercalary fragment about 2–4 cm from the target fragment. This is an ideal time to convert the frame from one with longitudinal traction wires to one with transverse tensioned wires. Obviously, such transverse tension wires will cut through the skin creating the problems that are generally avoided by using longitudinal tensioned traction wires. However, the patient will be a lot happier if the surgeon can avoid creating 14 or 15 cm longitudinal scars, rather than 2–4 cm long scars, during the bone transport process.

With distraction osteogenesis, virtually any size bone defect can be overcome, limited only by the patience of the surgeon and patient (Easley et al. 2008; Eralp and Kocaoglu 2008; Green 1994, 2011; Green et al. 1992; Ilizarov et al. 1972;

Ilizarov and Ledioev 1969; Paley et al. 1989; Salem et al. 2006; Santangelo et al. 2008). Thus, the resection of bone on the tibial side of the zone of infection is not an important consideration; generous resection of all questionable bone should be the rule in such cases. The situation on the talar side of the problem, however, is just the opposite.

In almost every case, an infection of the distal tibia extends into the ankle joint space through fracture lines in the tibial plafond. Hence, the articular cartilage of the talus is usually degraded or completely (occasionally partially) digested by microbes inhabiting the joint. Therefore, at the very least, the articular cartilage must be removed for two reasons: First, the advancing end of the moving intercalary tibial fragment cannot unite to the articular cartilage of the talus. Indeed, simply debriding the cartilage by curettage and leaving the subchondral sclerotic bone will usually prove unsuccessful. Instead, it will be necessary to expose the cancellous bone of the talus to the advancing edge of the intercalary fragment if there is any hope to obtain union.

More commonly, the infection extends some distance into the talus making debridement of the infected and nonviable upper portion of the talus an important part of the procedure. Because of the small size of this bone, 10–15 mm of resection is probably the maximum tolerable. At this point, one enters into the portion of the talus that is not thick enough to support bodyweight. For this reason, one should slice off portions of the talus in thin increments, looking for smooth bone uninterrupted by cavitary lesions or other evidence of infection.

7.5.2 Tibiocalcaneal Arthrodesis

There comes a point at which one can no longer take off additional talus material without endangering the outcome. At this point, the decision has to be made to remove the entire talus and attempt arthrodesis to the calcaneus. This requires removing the entire upper surface of that portion of the bone that will become the docking site, thereby exposing the cancellous portion of the calcaneus to the surgical area (Fig. 7.6a–g).

In some cases, it is possible (and, in fact, even desirable) to set the distal portion of the tibia into the surgically created cavity in the calcaneus and surround this portion of the construct with fresh cancellous bone graft, supplemented, perhaps, with BMP and other kinds of biological augmentation.

With this kind of debridement, the entire body of the talus is removed, but typically the neck and head are retained.

7.6 Primary Limb Shortening Versus Bifocal Treatment

One important consideration with such reconstructions is whether to close the skin around the resected skeletal defect by compression at the time of debridement surgery. When possible, immediate compression has numerous advantages. For one thing, a complex bone transport case, involving simultaneous distraction in one part of the limb in conjunction with compression at the site of debridement, is converted into a simple limb lengthening (Sen et al. 2006). Moreover, the limb lengthening part of the surgery can be postponed, if necessary, to a later procedure once consolidation of the ankle fusion is complete. Bear in mind, however, that immediate compression of the distal tibia to either a thinned talus or a scooped-out calcaneus can create redundant skin and subcutaneous soft tissues that prevent safe closure of the operative incisions.

7.6.1 The Charnley Transverse Incision

Even when wound closure is obtained, kinking of the lymphatic vessels causes undue (and perhaps dangerous) swelling of the foot. There are several ways to deal with this problem if anticipated in advance. One option involves transverse, rather than longitudinal, incisions. The extensive debridement and resection required often preclude such an approach, but it might be possible to approach the ankle through the transverse

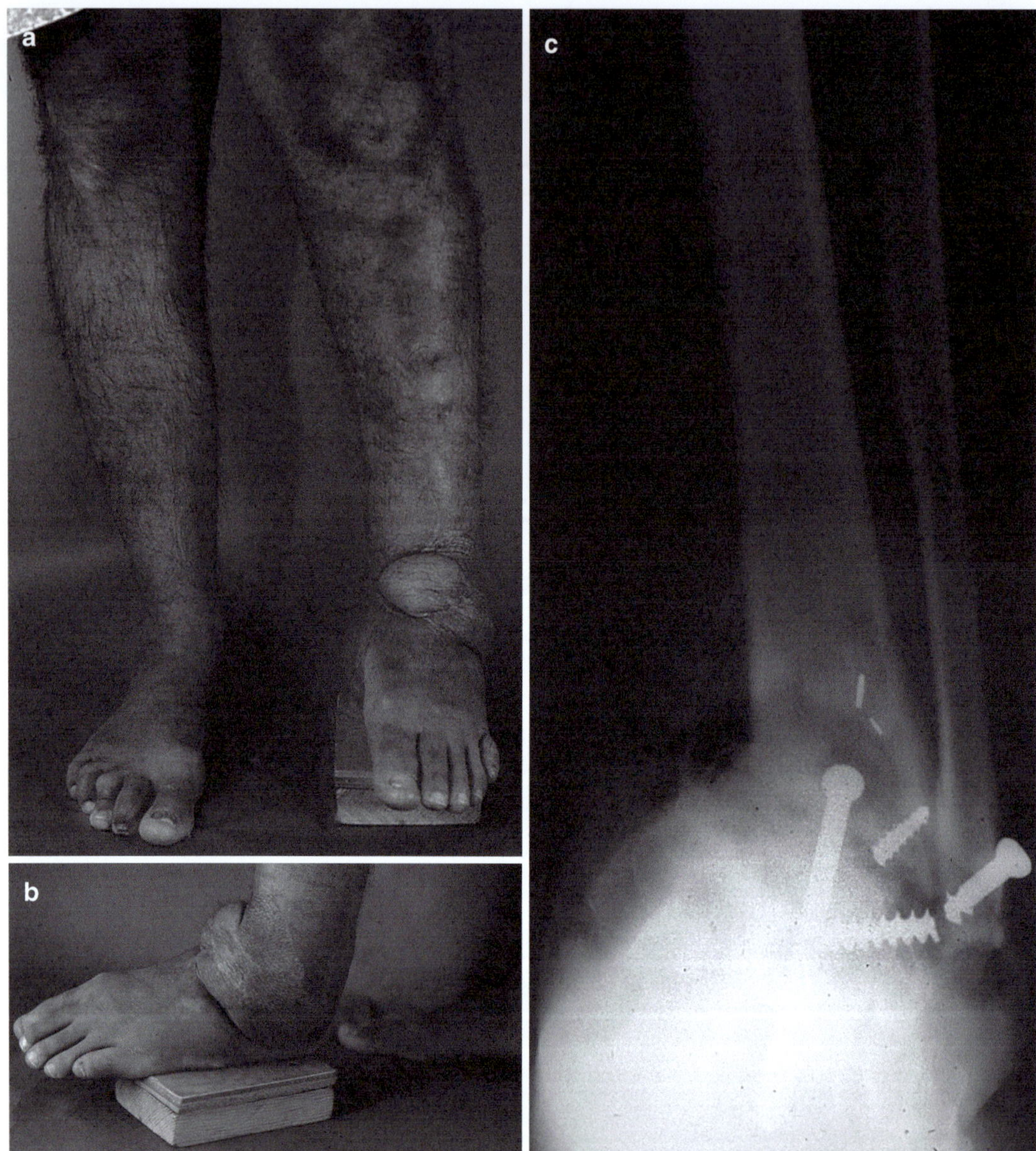

Fig. 7.6 Reconstruction of a limb requiring extensive debridement of distal tibia and entire talus, with tibiocalcaneal arthrodesis. (**a**) Clinical appearance of the limb before reconstructive surgery. (**b**) Side view. (**c**) X-ray appearance of ankle prior to reconstruction. (**d**) Reconstruction with Ilizarov fixator, with tibiocalcaneal arthrodesis. *Arrow* points to proximal corticotomy. (**e**) Final X-ray appearance of the limb after reconstruction. (**f**) Final clinical appearance after reconstruction and revision of skin flap. (**g**) Side view

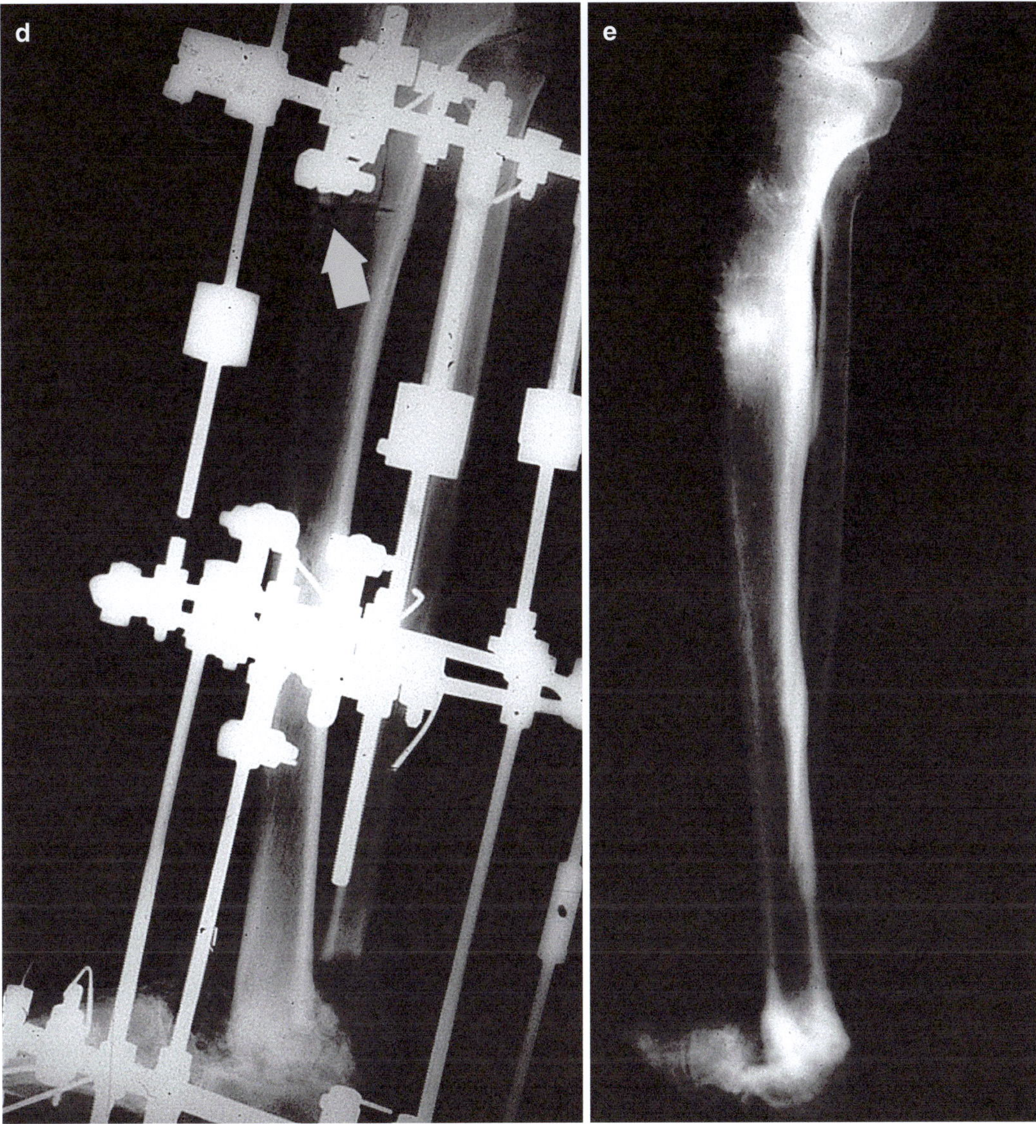

Fig. 7.6 (continued)

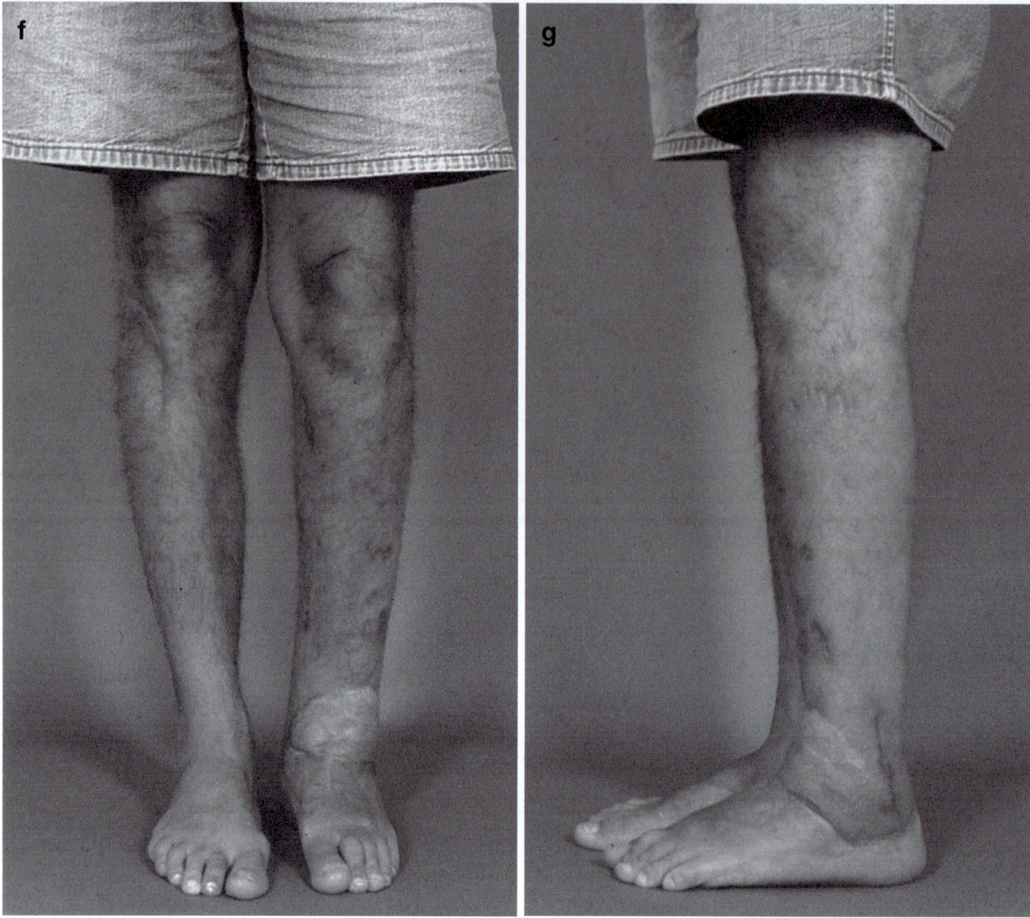

Fig. 7.6 (continued)

anterior approach designed by John Charnley for ankle fusions (Charnley 1953). This approach transects the extensor tendons to the toes, the dorsal nerves to the foot, and the anterior tibial artery as it becomes the dorsalis pedis artery. (The extensor tendons are later repaired prior to closure with the Charnley anterior approach.) Hence, the approach is contraindicated when the posterior tibial artery is compromised.

7.6.1.1 Modified Charnley Incision

It is possible to make a modified anterior Charnley transverse incision by leaving a skin and soft tissue bridge in the region containing the neurovascular and tendon structures and performing the bone. However, this approach makes the bone resection technically difficult, especially when the amount of distal tibial resection exceeds the operative window afforded by the incision.

As a general principle, it is probably unwise to compress the soft tissue sleeve around any resected region of a limb more than 4 cm.

As with the bone graft technique, eliminating joint resection regions with Ilizarov's methods required a stable long-term external fixation frame for the foot. This involves securing both the hindfoot with crossed wires (either with or without supplementary half or full pins) and forefoot fixation, typically with crossed wires or parallel wires, although here too, supplementary half pin fixation (especially in the first metatarsal shaft) adds to stability.

7.7   The Amputation Option

The sometimes unpredictable outcome of a persistent infection following an open or surgically treated comminuted pilon fracture suggests that a patient with a dystrophic leg and neurologic or vascular compromise of the foot considers an amputation at the below-knee level, especially if he or she understands that the reconstruction of the leg might require one or more years in an external fixator—with an uncertain outcome, at best. We do not consider an amputation in this circumstance to be a failure of treatment; instead, the limb ablation is the natural consequence of a severe pilon fracture, whether initially open or closed, since the magnitude of the initial injury precludes a satisfactory outcome under the best of circumstances. We are especially reluctant to recommend reconstructive surgery when the plantar surface of the foot lacks sensibility.

References

Bourne RB, Rorabeck C, Macnab J (1983) Intra-articular fractures of the distal tibia: the pilon fracture. J Trauma 23:591–596

Burwell HN, Charnley AD (1985) The treatment of displaced fractures at the ankle by rigid internal fixation and early joint motion. J Bone Joint Surg 47(B):634–660

Cave EF (1965) Complications of the operative treatment of fractures of the ankle. Clin Orthop Relat Res 42:13–19

Charnley J (1953) Compression arthrodesis. Livingstone, Edinburgh

Childress M (1965) Vertical transarticular pin fixation for unstable ankle fractures. J Bone Joint Surg 47(A): 1323–1334

Coonrad RW (1970) Fracture dislocation of the ankle joint with impaction injury to the lateral weight-bearing surface of the tibia. J Bone Joint Surg 52(A):1337–1344

Cox FJ (1965) Fractures of the ankle involving the articular surface of the tibia. Clin Orthop Relat Res 42:51–55

Cuttica DJ, Devries JG, Hyer CF (2010) Autogenous bone graft harvest using reamer irrigator aspirator (RIA) technique for tibiotalocalcaneal arthrodesis. J Foot Ankle Surg 49:571–574

Donegan DJ, Scolaro J, Matuszewski PE et al (2011) Staged bone grafting following placement of an antibiotic spacer block for the management of segmental long bone defects. Orthopedics 34:730–735

Easley ME, Montijo HE, Wilson JD et al (2008) Revision tibiotalar arthrodesis. J Bone Joint Surg Am 90: 1212–1223

Eralp L, Kocaoglu M (2008) Distal tibial reconstruction with use of a circular external fixator and an intramedullary nail. Surgical technique. J Bone Joint Surg Am 90:181–194

Gay R, Evrard J (1963) Les fractures recentes du pilon tibial chez l'adulte. Rev Chir Orthop Rel Pes 49:397–512

Giannoudis PV, Faour O, Goff T et al (2011) Masquelet technique for the treatment of bone defects: tips-tricks and future directions. Injury 42:591–598

Green SA (1983) Complications of external skeletal fixation. Clin Orthop Relat Res 180:109–116

Green SA (2011) The Ilizarov method of distraction osteogenesis. In: Hamdy RC, McCarthy JJ (eds) Management of limb length discrepancies. American Academy of Orthopaedic Surgeons, Rosemont

Green SA (1991a) The Ilizarov method: Rancho technique. Orthop Clin North Am 22:677–688

Green SA (1991b) Osteomyelitis: the Ilizarov perspective. Orthop Clin North Am 22:515–521

Green SA (1994) Segmental defects: a comparison of bone grafting and bone transport for segmental skeletal defects. Clin Orthop Relat Res 300:111–117

Green SA (1982) Septic non-unions. In: Unthoff H (ed) Current concepts in external fixation. Springer, Berlin

Green SA, Jackson J, Wall DM et al (1992) Management of segmental defects by the Ilizarov intercalary bone transport method. Clin Orthop Relat Res 280:136–142

Green SA, Lewis DA, Marinow H (1996) Pilon fractures treated with circular external fixation. Orthop Trans 20:330

Green SA, Roesler S (1987) The infected pilon fracture. Tech Orthop 2:37–42

Ilizarov GA (1968) General principles of transosteal compression and distraction osteosynthesis. In: Proceeding of the scientific session of institutes of traumatology and orthopedics. USSR, Leningrad, pp 35–39

Ilizarov GA (1952) A method of uniting bones in fractures and an apparatus to implement this method. In:

Ilizarov GA (1989a) The tension-stress effect on the genesis and growth of tissues: part I. The influence of stability of fixation and soft-tissue preservation. Clin Orthop Relat Res 238:249–281

Ilizarov GA (1989b) The tension-stress effect on the genesis and growth of tissues: part II. The influence of the rate and frequency of distraction. Clin Orthop Relat Res 239:263–285

Ilizarov GA, Kaplunov AG, Degtiarev VE et al (1972) Treatment of pseudarthroses and ununited fractures, complicated by purulent infection, by the method of compression- distraction osteosynthesis. Ortop Travmatol Protez 33:10

Ilizarov GA, Ledioev VI (1969) Replacement of defects of long tubular bones by means of one of their fragments. Vestn Khir 102:77

Kallem JF, Waddell JP (1979) Fractures of the distal tibial metaphysis with intraarticular extension—the distal tibial explosion fracture. J Trauma 19:593–601

Karger C, Kishi T, Schneider L et al (2012) Treatment of posttraumatic bone defects by the induced membrane technique. Orthop Traumatol Surg Res 98:97–102

Leach R (1984) Complications. In: Rockwood CA, Green DH (eds) Fractures in adults, 2nd edn. Lippincott, Philadelphia

Muller KU (1982) Therapy of post traumatic osteomyelitis. In: Unthoff H (ed) Current concepts of external fixation of fractures. Springer, New York

Ovadia N, Beals K (1986) Fractures of the tibial plafond. J Bone Joint Surg 68(A):543–551

Paley D, Catagni M, Argnani F, Villa A et al (1989) Ilizarov treatment of tibial nonunions with bone loss. Clin Orthop Relat Res 241:146–166

Papineau L-J (1973) L'excision-greffe avec Fermeture Retardee Deliberee dans l'Osteomyelites Chronique. Nouv Presse Med 2:2753

Pierce RO Jr, Heinrich H (1979) Comminuted intraarticular fractures of the distal tibia. J Trauma 19:828–832

Ruedi T, Ailgower M (1979) The operative treatment of intraarticular fractures of the lower end of the tibia. Clin Orthop Relat Res 138:105–110

Ruedi T, Allgower M (1969) Fractures of the lower end of the tibia into the ankle joint. Injury 1:92–99

Salem KH, Kinzl L, Schmelz A (2006) Ankle arthrodesis using Ilizarov ring fixators: a review of 22 cases. Foot Ankle Int 27:764–770

Santangelo JR, Glisson RR, Garras DN et al (2008) Tibiotalocalcaneal arthrodesis: a biomechanical comparison of multiplanar external fixation with intramedullary fixation. Foot Ankle Int 29:936–941

Scheck M (1965) Treatment of comminuted distal tibia fractures by combined dual-pin fixation and limited open reduction. J Bone Joint Surg 47(A):1537–1553

Sen C, Eralp L, Gunes T et al (2006) An alternative method for the treatment of nonunion of the tibia with bone loss. J Bone Joint Surg Br 88:783–789

Stafford PR, Norris BL (2010) Reamer-irrigator-aspirator bone graft and bi Masquelet technique for segmental bone defect nonunions: a review of 25 cases. Injury 41:S72–S77

Thordarson DB, Patzakis MJ, Holtom P et al (1997) Salvage of the septic ankle with concomitant tibial osteomyelitis. Foot Ankle Int 18:151–156

Weise K, Weller S (1982) Arthrodesis of the ankle joint. In: Unthoff H (ed) Current concepts of external fixation of fractures. Springer, New York

Weller S (1982) The external fixator for the prevention and treatment of infections. In: Unthoff H (ed) Current concepts of external fixation of fractures. Springer, New York

Zarutsky E, Rush SM, Schuberth JM (2005) The use of circular wire external fixation in the treatment of salvage ankle arthrodesis. J Foot Ankle Surg 44:22–31

Reconstruction of Segmentary Defects in Chronic Osteomyelitis Using the Combined Technique

8

Mehmet Kocaoğlu and F. Erkal Bilen

Contents

8.1 Introduction

A greater understanding of distraction osteogenesis and its application has enabled the development of a cure for this complex problem. However, these advancements in surgical methodology are countered by the development of antibiotic resistance in bacterial organisms, especially in certain strains of *Staphylococcus aureus* and *Enterococcus faecalis* (Eralp 2011).

Infected cases of osteomyelitis that result in bone defects and soft tissue problems, including infected nonunions, are generally treated using surgical interventions (Paley et al. 1989). In the past, several techniques, such as the Papineau technique, have been used successfully to overcome these issues (Papineau et al. 1979). The main pathology associated with this condition consists of bone necrosis and damage to adjacent soft tissue resulting from the penetration of microorganisms. The extent of bone necrosis is related to multiple factors, including the severity of the trauma, previous surgical interventions, and the type of primary osteosynthesis. The remodeling of dead bone occurs quite slowly and depends on many factors, such as the virulence of the microorganism and the immune status of the host. The original concept of "burn[ing] infection in the fire of the regenerat[ion] (new bone formation)," which was described by Gavriil Abramovich Ilizarov, has evolved into the current philosophy of "the only cure for chronic osteomyelitis is radical debridement until live, bleeding bone is reached," which was

M. Kocaoğlu, MD (✉) • F.E. Bilen, MD, FEBOT
Orthopedic Surgery Department,
Istanbul Memorial Hospital, Istanbul, Turkey
e-mail: drmehmetkocaoglu@gmail.com;
bilenfe@gmail.com

M. Kocaoğlu et al. (eds.), *Advanced Techniques in Limb Reconstruction Surgery*,
DOI 10.1007/978-3-642-55026-3_8, © Springer Berlin Heidelberg 2015

first described by Tetsworth and Cierny (Ilizarov 1992; Tetsworth and Cierny 1999). The extent of debridement necessary to obtain healthy bone results in bone and soft tissue defects that are difficult to reconstruct (Eralp 2011; Eralp and Kocaoglu 2008; Kocaoglu et al. 2004, 2006; Sen et al. 2004).

Callus distraction over an intramedullary nail is a technique that is rarely used for the reconstruction of intercalary defects created by radical debridement. Compared to classic techniques used for the treatment of infected long-bone nonunions, this technique can significantly reduce the external fixation time and the consolidation index (Kocaoglu et al. 2006; Paley et al. 1997).

8.2 Management of Defects

8.2.1 Indications

- Chronic osteomyelitis following surgical procedures (e.g., total knee arthroplasty)
- Bone defects and/or shortening after debridement in cases of chronic osteomyelitis (Figs. 8.1 and 8.2)
- Bone defects and/or shortening after removal of an infected tumor prosthesis (Figs. 8.3 and 8.4)

8.2.2 Examination

Physical examinations should include the following:
- Bilateral ROM of the hip, knee, and ankle joints.
- Measurement of the actual (distance between the anterior superior iliac spine (ASIS) and the medial malleolus) and the apparent limb-length discrepancy (LLD: distance between the umbilicus and the medial malleolus).
- Determination of the number of 1-cm blocks required under the shortened extremity to provide a level pelvis.
- Photographic documentation of each patient, both initially and at the end of the treatment.

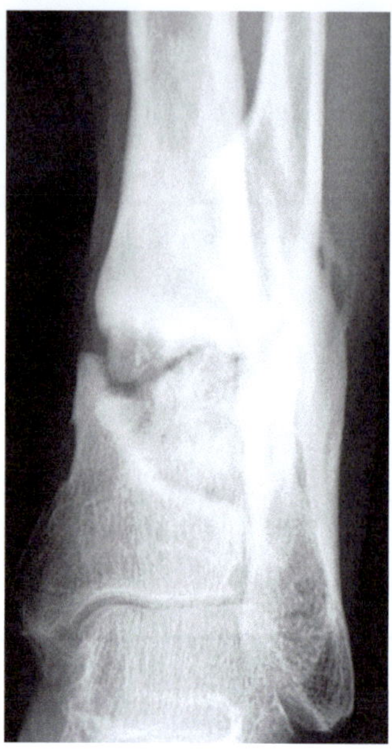

Fig. 8.1 An x-ray of a patient, showing the defect after debridement for osteomyelitis

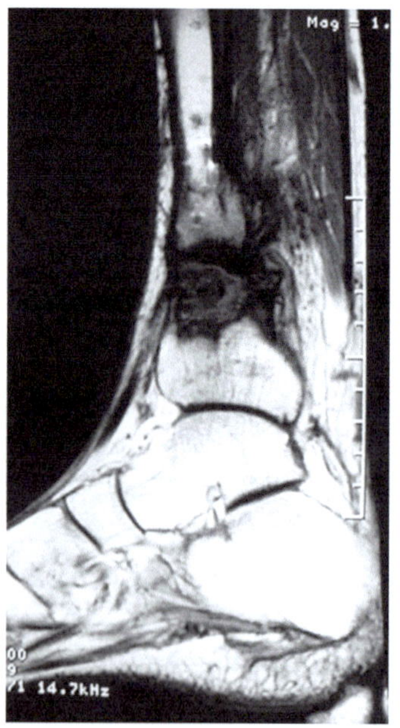

Fig. 8.2 An MRI study of a patient displaying the extent of osteomyelitis

- Assessment of potential joint contractures.
- Careful evaluation and documentation of neurologic and vascular status.

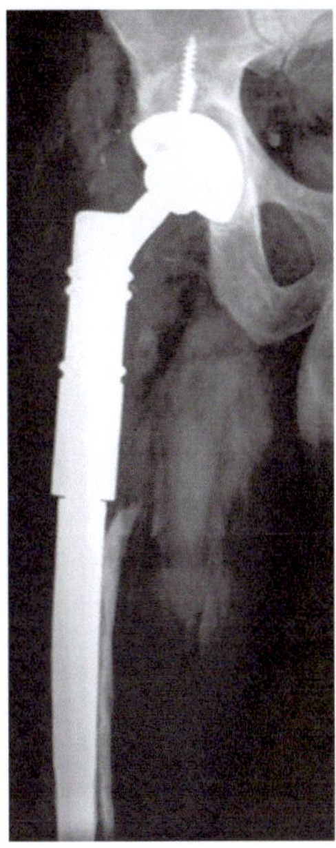

Fig. 8.3 An x-ray of a patient displaying an infected tumor prosthesis, AP view

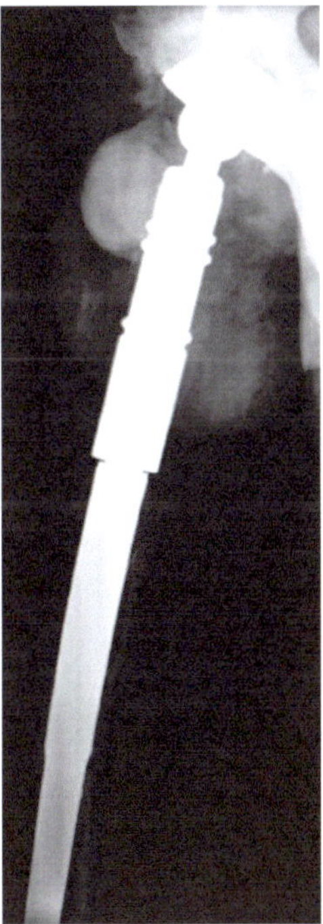

Fig. 8.4 An x-ray of the same patient, lateral view

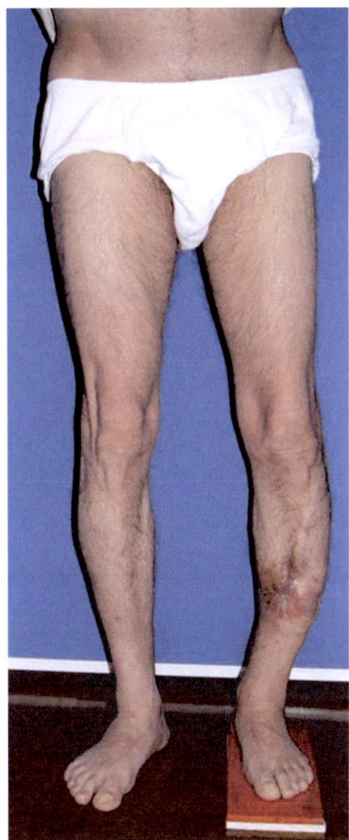

Fig. 8.5 Bone blocks used to determine the extent of shortening

8.2.3   Imaging Studies

- Plain x-rays in both planes (true AP and lateral).
- Orthoroentgenogram in both planes, according to the following guidelines:
  - The knee should be in maximum extension, especially in the lateral view.
  - 1-cm blocks should be used to level the pelvis in the AP view (Fig. 8.5).
- Scaled AP and lateral x-rays of the affected bone segment are necessary to obtain the size and the diameter of the IM nail and to determine the numbers and levels of the osteotomy(ies).
- A computed tomography (CT) scan (to check for sequestra) (Fig. 8.6).
- Magnetic resonance imaging (MRI) to assess the following:
  - The extent of bone infection and abscess formation (MRI may reveal a well-defined

- For cases with a history of thromboembolism, a Doppler ultrasound examination should be performed, and prophylaxis should be initiated.
- Evaluation of nutritional status (albumin, albumin/globulin ratio, and lymphocyte count).

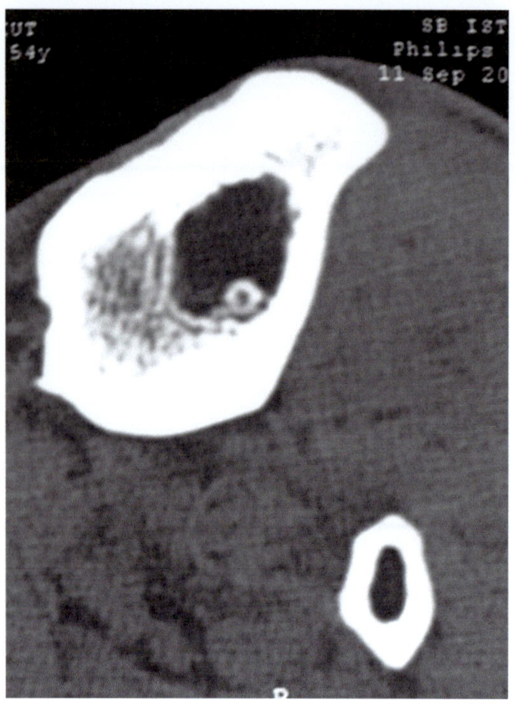

Fig. 8.6 A CT scan of a patient, displaying a sequestrum

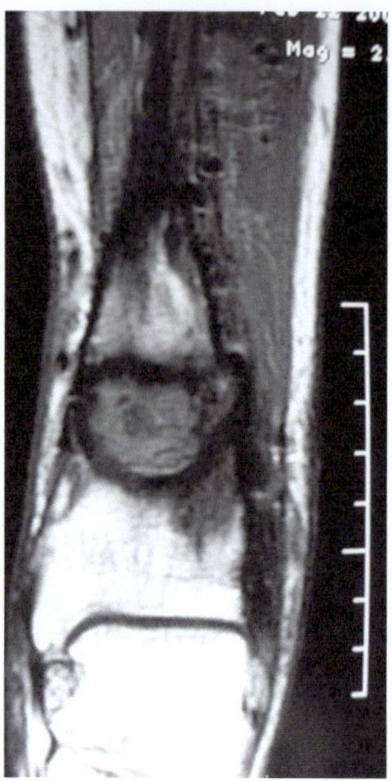

Fig. 8.7 An MRI of a patient showing the extent of the abscess and the active disease

rim with a high signal intensity that surrounds the focus of active disease, which represents the so-called rim sign) (Fig. 8.7) (Dabov 2008)

- The margins of bone resection
- Determination of the vascular status of the affected extremity using Doppler ultrasound (the contralateral side should also be checked if the free flap will be obtained from this side).
- Conventional angiography should be included when there is suspicion following the Doppler examination (Fig. 8.8).
- Tc-99- and indium-111-labeled leukocyte radionuclide scans should be performed to identify any foci of distant infection (or dead bone).
- Fistulography should be applied to track the infection from the inside of the tissue to the surface (Fig. 8.9).

8.2.4 Preoperative Planning

- All data obtained from the clinical examination and imaging studies should be carefully evaluated.

- A deformity analysis should be performed, according to the deformity planning guidelines of Paley and Tetsworth (1992).
- Determination of the level(s) of the osteotomy(ies) and the margins of resection.
- If the defect is at the distal femoral metaphysis, retrograde IM nail insertion should be performed through the intercondylar notch.
- If there is additional shortening, the IM nail should be longer than the femur. The length of the nail outside of the femur should be as long as the planned amount of lengthening (Figs. 8.10a, b).
- If there is only a mid-diaphyseal defect without shortening, an antegrade IM nail may be chosen.
- The diameter and size of the IM nail should be determined based on the scaled AP and lateral x-rays of the affected bone segment(s).
- Paper tracing should be performed to simulate the surgery and to determine the provisional and final position of the bone segment (Fig. 8.11), according to the following factors:
  - The localization of the extra custom-made hole(s) on the IM nail (Fig. 8.12).
  - The location and number of interference screws (poller) should be determined in a

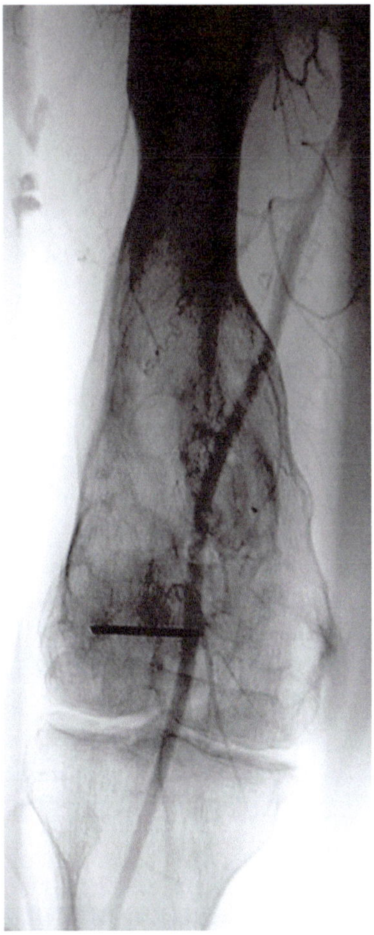

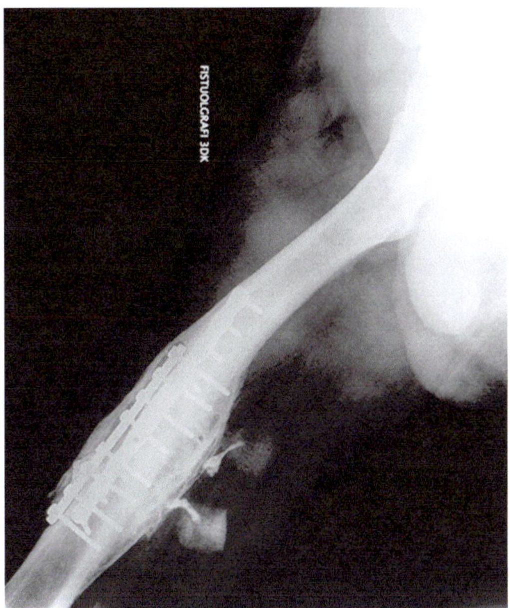

Fig. 8.9 Fistulography of a patient

Fig. 8.8 Conventional angiography from a patient

manner that increases the stability of the reconstruction (Fig. 8.13).

- The incision at the entry point of the IM nail and the osteotomy levels should be mapped out.

8.2.5 Equipment

First Stage
1. Radiolucent table
2. Radiolucent knee support or a rolled, sterile towel
3. Large-field fluoroscopy
4. Flexible intramedullary reaming system
5. Antibiotic-impregnated bone cement or bone cement with appropriate heat-stable antibiotics (gentamicin, tobramycin, teicoplanin, vancomycin, etc.)

6. Steinmann pins of various sizes (for creating antibiotic-impregnated cement rods)

Second Stage
1. Radiolucent table
2. Radiolucent knee support or a rolled, sterile towel
3. Large-field fluoroscopy
4. 6-mm conical hydroxyapatite-coated Schanz screws
5. Unilateral external fixator (EBI Monorail System or Orthofix LRS)
6. Flexible intramedullary reaming system
7. 1.8-mm Kirschner wires (bayonet type)
8. 3.5-mm cannulated drill bits
9. Intramedullary nail (the authors prefer Ortopro 4G Nails from Istanbul, Turkey)

8.2.6 Positioning

- The patient is placed in the supine position on the radiolucent table, and the affected hip should be slightly elevated using a silicone bag under the buttock to provide a lateral view (Fig. 8.14).
- Fluoroscopic images are then acquired from the hip to the ankle joint in both planes prior to the sterile preparation.

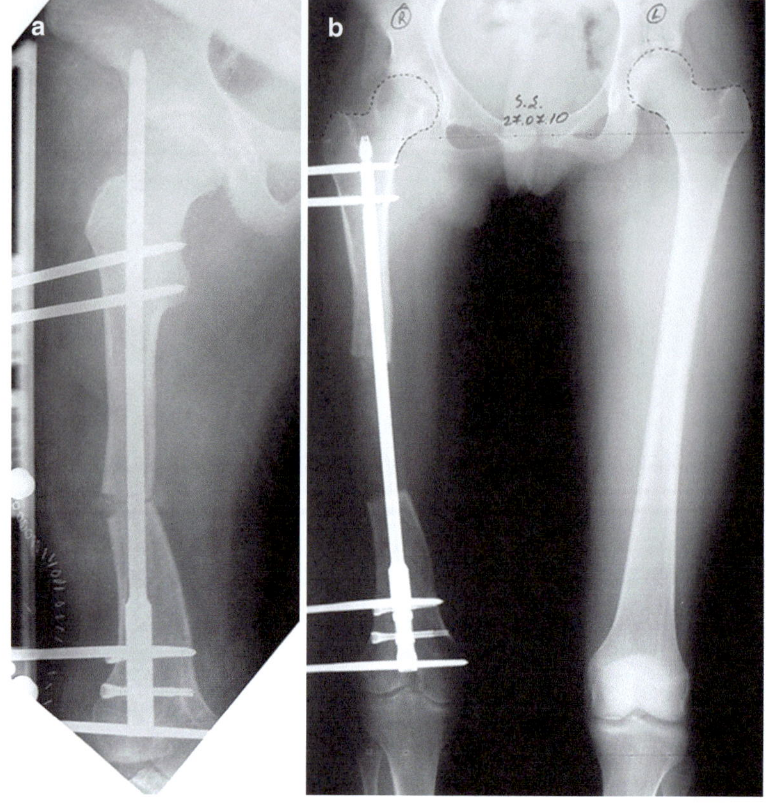

Fig. 8.10 An x-ray of a patient where the IM nail was left in contact with the bone (**a**). The nail length was chosen to fit the original length of the bone, which was determined when the lengthening was complete (**b**)

- Sterile preparation should be used prior to draping the entire lower extremity beginning at the ASIS.

8.2.7 Surgical Technique

First Stage

For the exposure/incision:

- Methylene blue should be injected through the fistula to dye the sinus and its tract.
- The entire sinus tract should be excised with the fistula (fish-mouth incision) (Fig. 8.15).
- If there is no fistula, then a transverse incision is preferred, especially for cases of tibial osteomyelitis. The transverse incision helps to prevent soft tissue buckling due to the extremity shortening induced by the bone excision (Fig. 8.16).
- A wide resection margin is preferred (>7 mm) over marginal excision, as it prevents recurrence.

- Hardware is removed (remove all nails, plate, cerclage wires, screws, etc.) (Fig. 8.17).
- The dead bone can be resected through debridement and the use of multiple drill holes and the osteotomy technique (to prevent heat necrosis, do not use a power saw) (Fig. 8.18).
- If the defect is too large to be closed primarily, then rotational local or free myocutaneous flaps (i.e., latissimus dorsi transfer) may be used (Fig. 8.19).
- All sequestra, purulent material, and scarred necrotic soft tissue should be removed.
- Cortical bleeding, denoted by the Paprika sign, is accepted as an indication that the bone tissue is vital (Fig. 8.20).
- Debridement proceeds until bleeding, living tissue is observed at the resection margins to ensure that all foci of infection are removed (Patzakis and Zalavras 2005; Tetsworth and Cierny 1999).

- It is necessary to ream the medullary canal in 1-mm increments, up to 1–2 mm greater than the previous nail diameter both proximally and distally, after the resection and to check the lengths of both segments.

For the preparation of the custom-made antibiotic-embedded cement spacer:

- The dead space is filled with custom-made antibiotic-impregnated polymethylmethacrylate (PMMA) beads and/or rods (Fig. 8.21).
- Pharmacokinetic studies have shown that the local concentrations of antibiotic achieved are 200 times greater than the levels achieved with systemic antibiotic administration (Dabov 2008).
- The use of an intramedullary rod is preferable, as it provides increased stability and more beads for filling dead space.
- For each 40 g of PMMA, 10 g of cefotaxime, 5 g of vancomycin, 9.6 g of tobramycin, or 2.4 g of teicoplanin should be included (each of these antibiotics is heat stable and bactericidal).
- High-viscosity bone cement powder should be mixed with a form of antibiotic medication in a bowl. A liquid monomer is then added, and the mixture is stirred until the cement is workable.
- Inject the viscous antibiotic-cement mixture with a cement gun into a thorax drainage tube (same outer diameter as the reamer size), and then insert a 5-mm diameter Steinmann pin (as long as the sum of the proximal and distal segments) into the center of the thorax tube (Fig. 8.22).
- The Steinmann pin should be central in position inside of the thorax tube and have a uniform cement mantle (Bhadra and Roberts 2009).
- The thorax tube should be cut to the length of the sum of the proximal and distal segments.
- Before the cement is heated inside of the thorax tube, several beads with cement remnants should be prepared by rolling the remnants into small spheres. Connect the beads using an 18-G wire or No. 5 Ethibond sutures to form a bead chain, and then wait until the cement hardens and cools (this step needs to be performed quickly to allow time for the next step).
- When the cement begins to heat up, cut the thorax tube longitudinally and peal the plastic

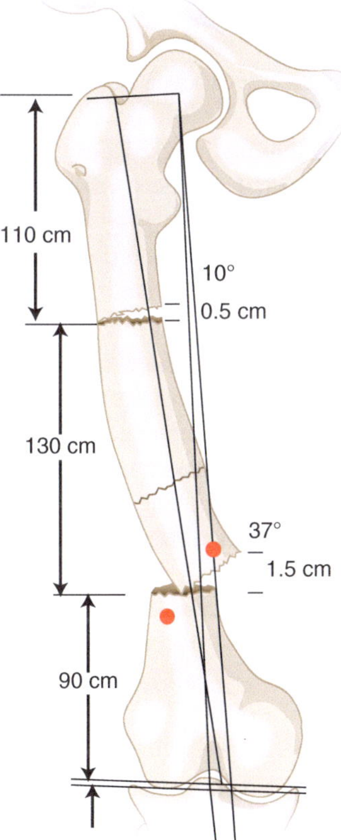

Fig. 8.11 Paper tracing to simulate the surgery

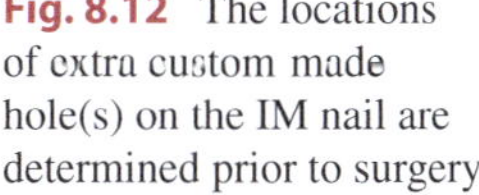

Fig. 8.12 The locations of extra custom made hole(s) on the IM nail are determined prior to surgery

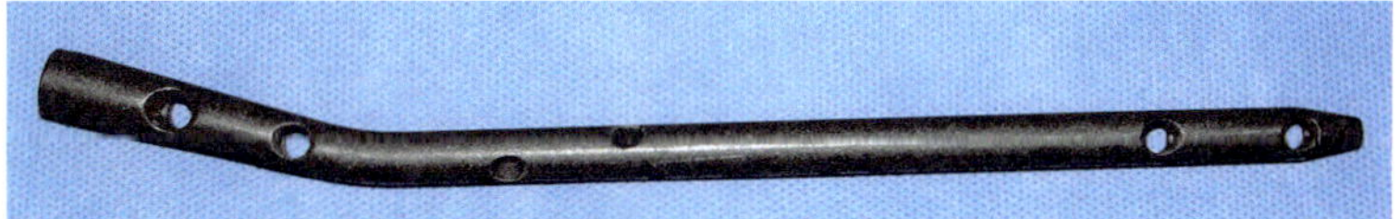

from the hardened cement rod before the plastic begins to melt with the cement (Paley and Herzenberg 2002a).

- The cement rod is placed in the air to cool for a minimum of 10 min. The number of beads on the chain should be recorded to ensure that all beads are accounted for at the time of removal.
- The rod can then be inserted into the medullary canal through the resection area.
- Place the antibiotic beads around the rod and into the dead space (Fig. 8.21).
- Suction drains are not recommended, as the concentration of the antibiotic decreases significantly with use.

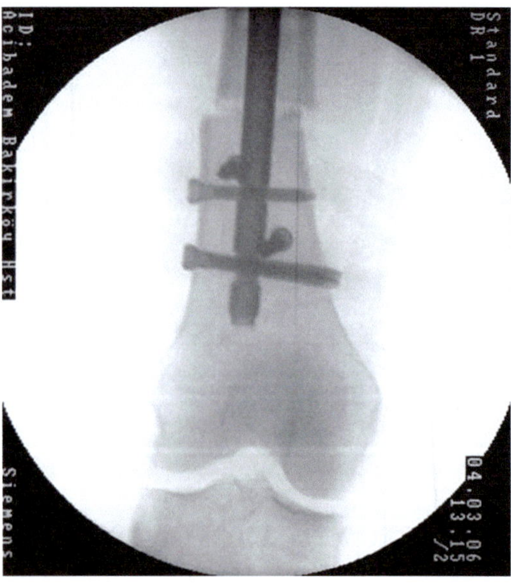

Fig. 8.13 The location and number of poller screws are determined prior to surgery

- The wound should be closed using nonabsorbable, non-braided sutures, such as No. 1 or No. 2 Prolene sutures.
- The limb should be immobilized with a custom-made plastic device or a temporary external fixator (Figs. 8.23 and 8.24).

Second Stage

- The CRP and ESR levels and the clinical status after 6 weeks of antibiotic treatment should be evaluated.
- As a percutaneous procedure, a biopsy specimen should be obtained from a bone gap prior to the second operation and sent for Gram staining and frozen-section analysis. The absence of microorganisms, according to the Gram staining, and the presence of <5 polymorphonuclear leukocytes per high-power field would indicate that the infection has resolved.
- Antegrade nailing is used only for patients with segmental defects and without a limb-length discrepancy (Fig. 8.25).
- Retrograde nailing is preferred for the treatment of a segmental defect in patients with a limb-length discrepancy (Fig. 8.26). The nail is locked distally, and the excess length of the nail is left in the soft tissues and the proximal piriformis fossa as a template for the treatment of LLD (Fig. 8.27). With distraction, the nail glides distally until the correct length is achieved, and the nail is then locked when the lengthening process is complete.
- Paper tracing is necessary to obtain the number and location of the custom-made holes in the intramedullary nail for securing the middle fragment to the nail. This procedure also helps to determine the diameter and length of the nail that should be used (Fig. 8.28).

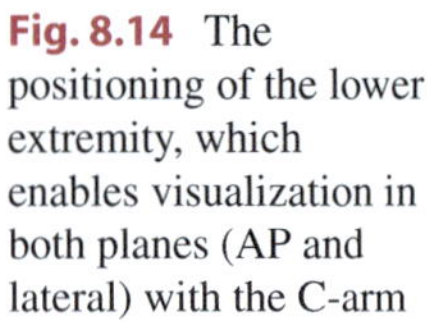

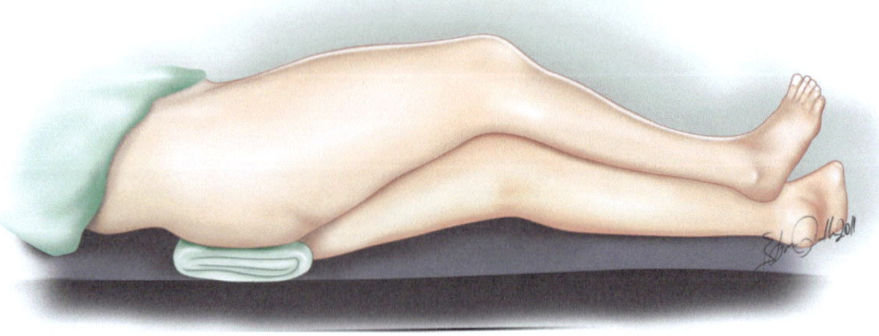

Fig. 8.14 The positioning of the lower extremity, which enables visualization in both planes (AP and lateral) with the C-arm

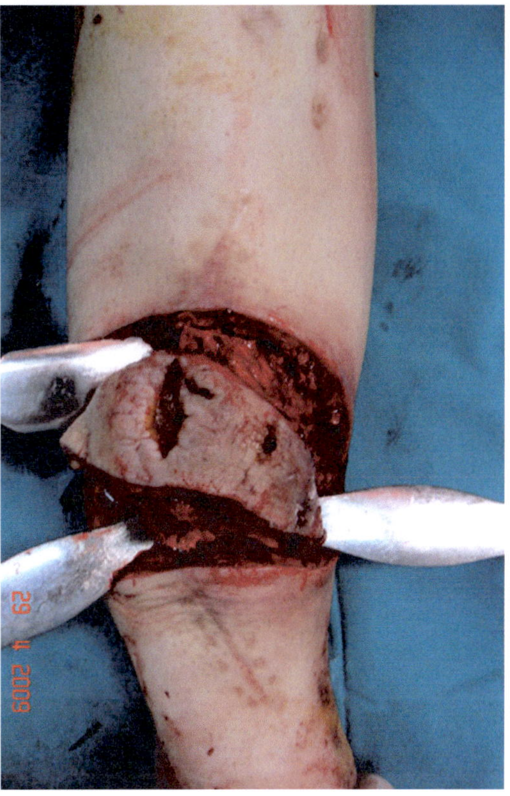

Fig. 8.15 A fish-mouth incision is used to completely remove the sinus tract

Fig. 8.16 A transverse incision is used to avoid buckling after shortening due to bone excision

Treatment of Femoral Defects
- The patient is placed in the supine position on a radiolucent table with his/her limbs in the scissors position and a bolster below the ipsilateral hip.
- Preoperative antibiotics are not administered until the antibiotic rods and beads are removed and the tissue cultures have been obtained.
- The antibiotic-cement rod and beads should be removed through a mini-incision using the previous incision scar from the first stage. The bone tips should be refreshed with the use of a rongeur until the Paprika sign is observed.
- At this time, parenteral intravenous antibiotics should be administered. The administration of first-generation cephalosporins (e.g., 1 g of cefazolin) is recommended, as per routine procedures, because the infection has been eradicated.
- Using a standard approach (through the piriformis for antegrade nailing and through a

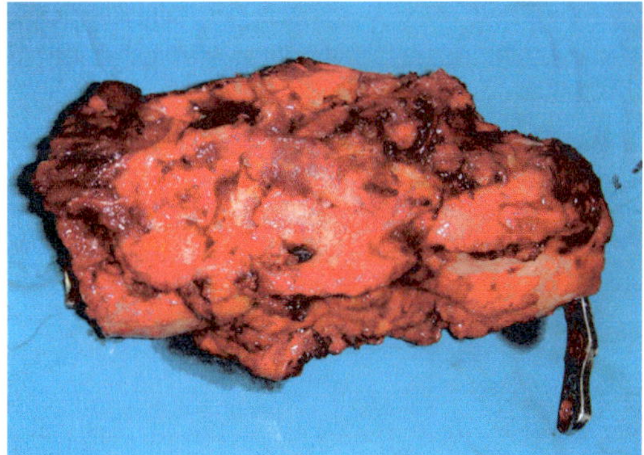

Fig. 8.17 All hardware should be removed

parapatellar incision for retrograde nailing), the medullary canal is reamed over a guidewire to a diameter that is 1.5 mm larger than that of the intramedullary nail that will be used.
- An appropriately placed corticotomy is created percutaneously with an osteotome.

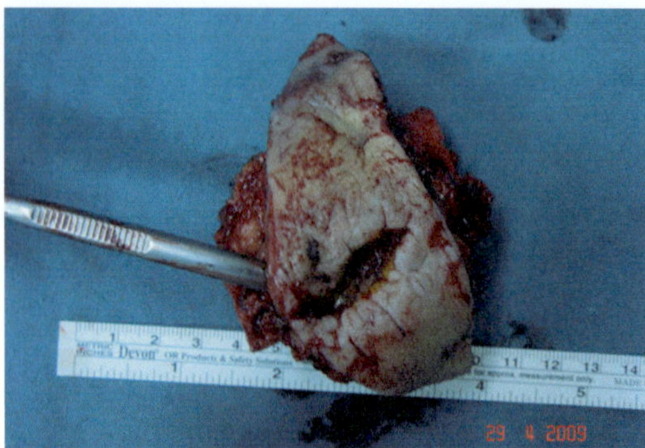

Fig. 8.18 The dead bone is resected via the multiple drill-hole and osteotomy techniques

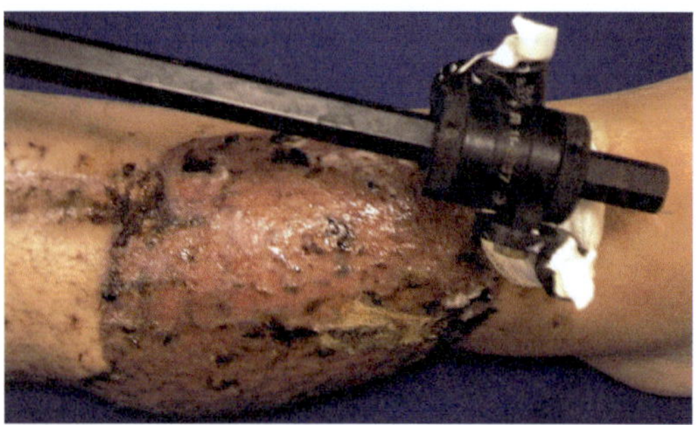

Fig. 8.19 Free flaps are utilized as needed

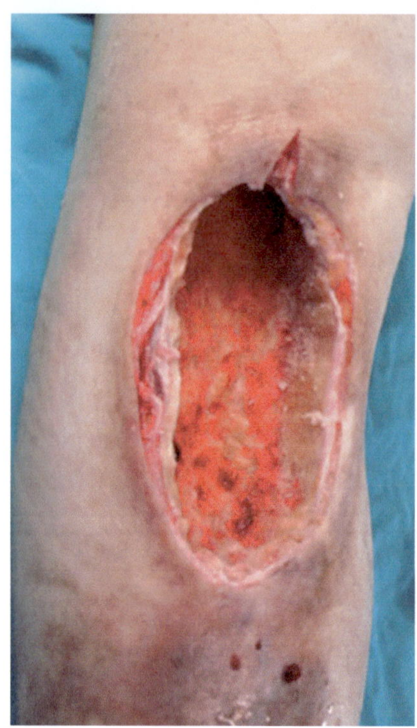

Fig. 8.20 The Paprika sign reveals the existence of vital bone tissue

Osteotomies in the long bones can be executed through the use of limited percutaneous incisions with either the Gigli-saw or the multiple drill-hole technique. (The power saw should not be used, as it may cause heat necrosis of the bone.)

- Finally, an intramedullary nail with custommade holes (Ortopro 4G IM nails are preferred) is inserted through the piriformis fossa or the intercondylar notch for retrograde nailing.
- Regular tibial nails are preferred for retrograde femoral nailing because their curve helps to correct any sagittal deformity that is present (Fig. 8.29).
- Two to three 6-mm conical hydroxyapatitecoated Schanz screws are placed perpendicularly to the anatomic axis of each segment both proximally and distally (as well as at the middle segment when present) using the cannulated-drill technique (Fig. 8.30) (Paley and Herzenberg 2002b).

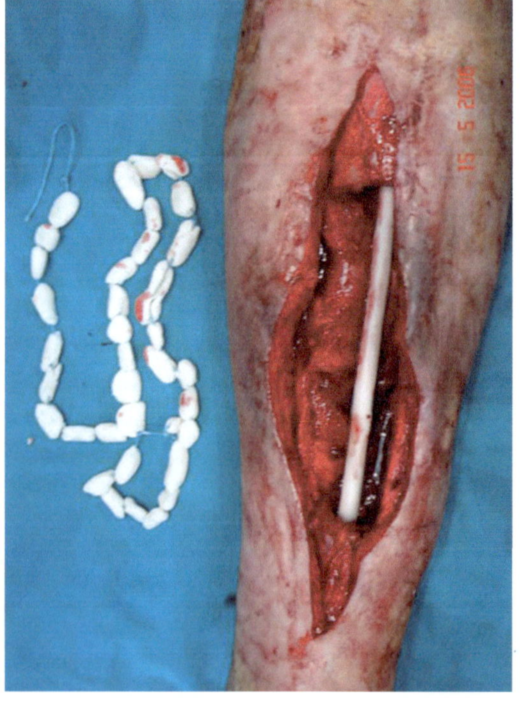

Fig. 8.21 PMMA, which is impregnated with antibiotics, is used to fill the dead space

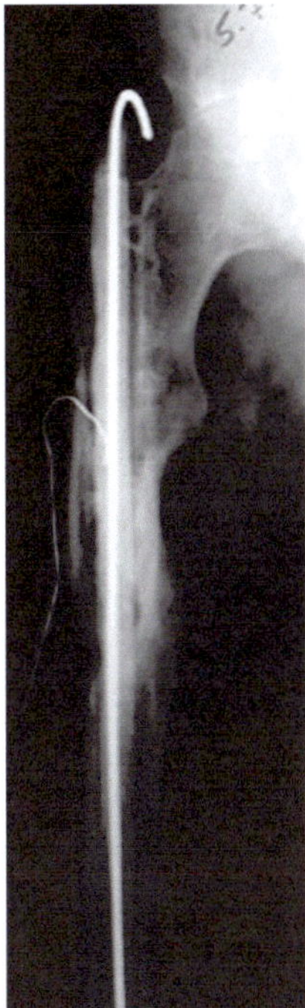

Fig. 8.22 A Steinmann pin is inserted into the thorax tube

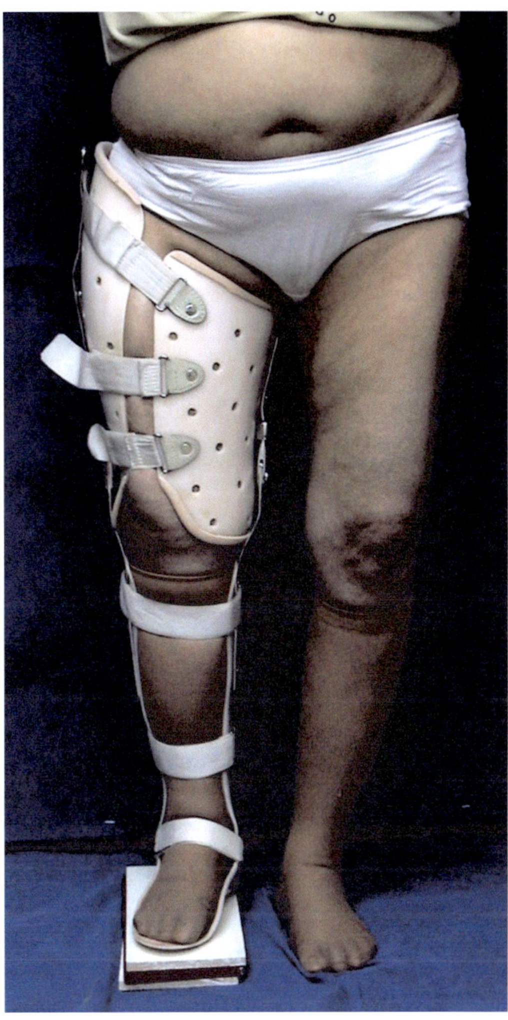

Fig. 8.24 A custom-made device is used to immobilize the limb

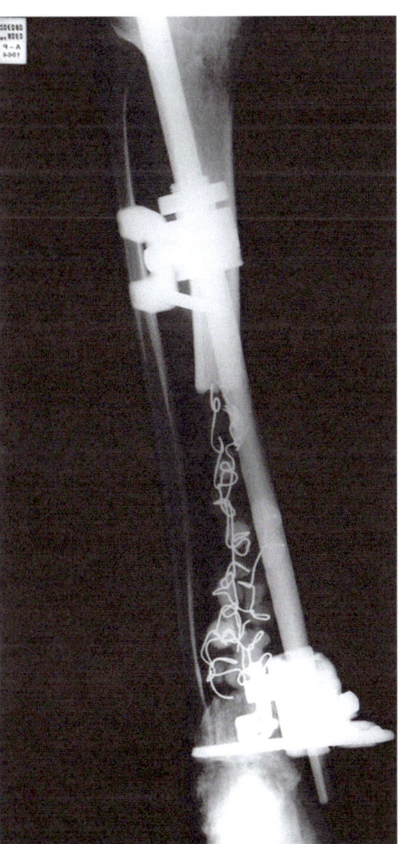

Fig. 8.23 Temporary external fixator application

- The Schanz screws should be placed posteriorly in the following manner, so as not to touch the IM nail (Fig. 8.31):
  - There should be a space of at least 1 mm between the IM nail and the Schanz screws to avoid spreading any pin-track infection into the medullary space (Fig. 8.32).
  - Schanz screws are placed in parallel to the axial plane of each fragment. As a result, once the Schanz screws have been secured to the external fixator after the osteotomy(ies), the rotational deformities will have been corrected (Fig. 8.33).
  - To correct sagittal-plane deformities, the Schanz screws need to be placed in parallel

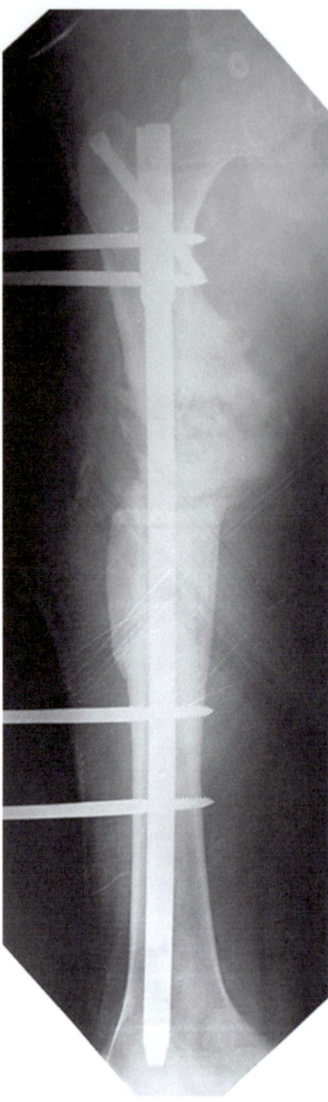

Fig. 8.25 An x-ray of a patient showing antegrade nailing

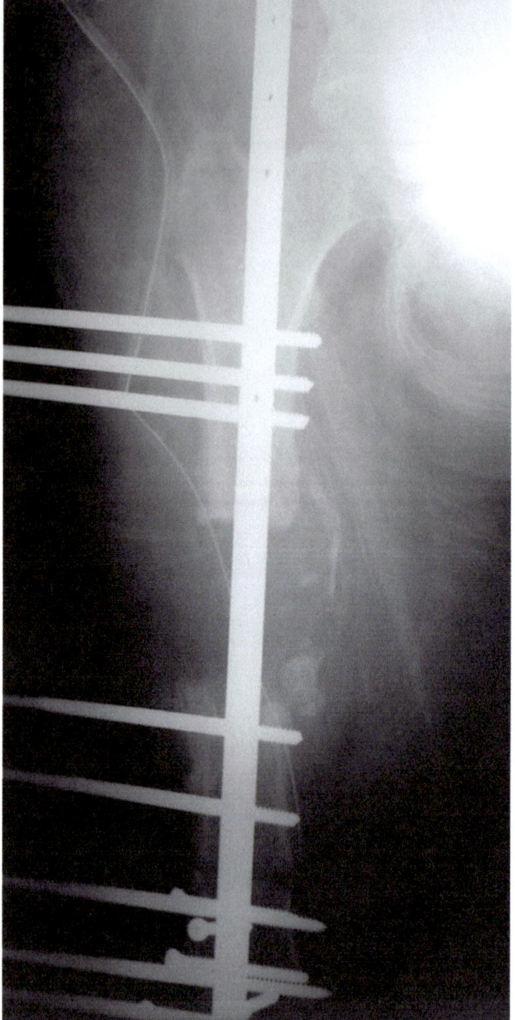

Fig. 8.26 An x-ray of a patient showing retrograde nailing. This patient exhibits LLD in addition to a bone defect

to the sagittal-plane axis of each fragment (Fig. 8.34).

- It is necessary to obtain an intraoperative control x-ray (AP and lateral), according to the following:
  - The x-ray should simulate the preoperative paper tracing.
  - If the desired correction is not achieved, the ex-fix should be readjusted and additional radiographs should be obtained.
- Once a satisfactory correction is achieved, interference screws (poller screws) should be inserted in the frontal plane and/or the sagittal plane to maintain the necessary amount of translation and to narrow the medullary canal, especially in the metaphyseal area (Fig. 8.35) (Krettek et al. 1999a, b; Seligson 2000).
- It is necessary to secure the Schanz screws to a monolateral external fixator (EBI monorail system or Orthofix LRS).
- The distraction testing (0.5 cm) is performed with the ex-fix as follows, to confirm that the distraction is occurring at the level required to lengthen the osteotomy:
  - After a successful distraction test, the gap should be compressed to the original position.

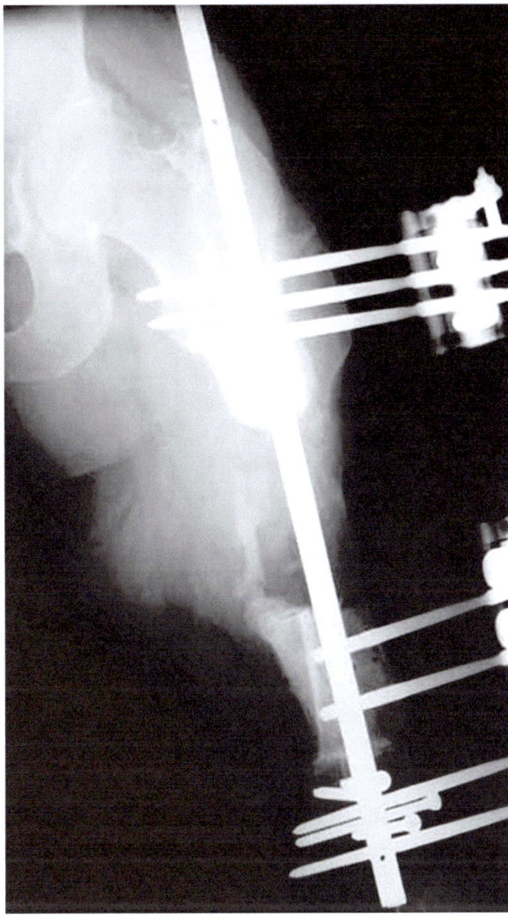

Fig. 8.27 An x-ray of a patient showing an IM nail remaining outside of the proximal end of the bone. This nail will slide into the bone when the lengthening is complete

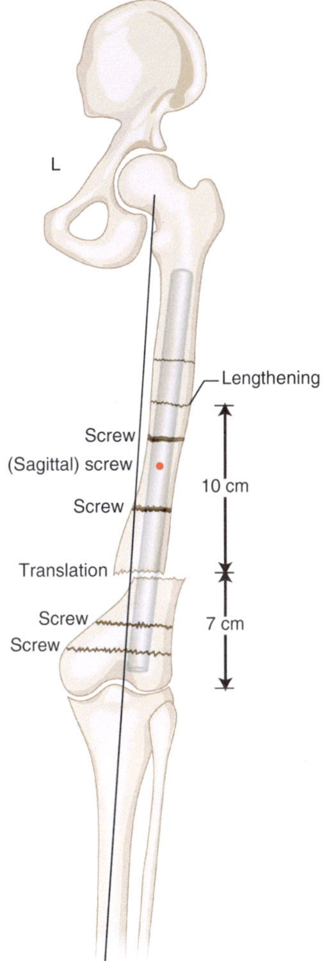

Fig. 8.28 Paper tracing of a patient used to simulate the surgery to determine the number and location of the custom-made hole(s) on the IM nail and to determine the size and length of the IM nail

- If the distraction test is unsuccessful, it is necessary to extract the nail and then overream the canal to a size that is 2 mm larger than the nail. Then, the steps should be repeated.
- Epidural analgesia is preferred, to ensure a comfortable postoperative period in addition to the following:
  - Epidural analgesia decreases the risk of postoperative DVT.
  - However, epidural analgesia may mask the signs of compartment syndrome, although the risk of compartment syndrome in cases of femoral lengthening is quite low (Tornero et al. 2010).
- Treatment of Tibial Defects
- After the removal of the antibiotic beads and rod through the incision that was made during the first stage (Fig. 8.36), it will be necessary to perform a percutaneous fibular osteotomy if there is an associated LLD.
- Each bone segment that is 1.5 mm larger than that of the intramedullary nail should be reamed.
- Insert the IM nail in a standard antegrade fashion.
- Lock the nail proximally and distally using the freehand technique (Fig. 8.37), according to the following guidelines:
  - If there is LLD, the nail should be locked distally and not proximally (Fig. 8.38).
  - For patients with LLD and segmental defects, the intramedullary nail that represents the

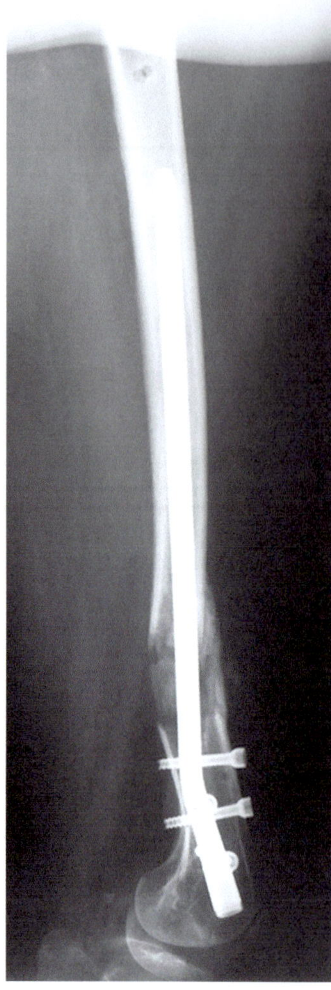

Fig. 8.29 A tibial nail may be preferred for retrograde femoral nailing to correct sagittal-plane deformities

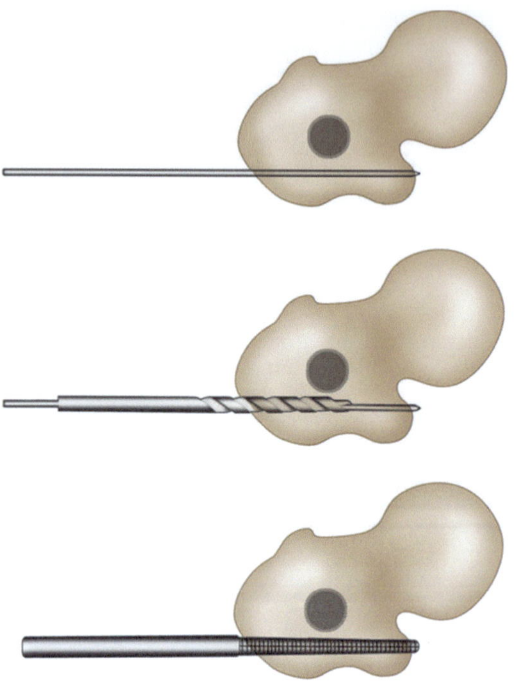

Fig. 8.30 The cannulated-drill technique for Schanz screw placement

eventual desired length of the tibia should be inserted and left in a proximal position, so that it can slide distally during treatment (Fig. 8.39).

- The debridement wound should be closed at this stage, prior to the application of the circular external fixator, as it would be difficult to perform this task at a later time.
- A circular-type external fixator should be applied in the following manner, with one ring for each segment (Fig. 8.40):
  - The long axes of the circular external fixator and the IM nail must be parallel to both the frontal and sagittal planes (Figs. 8.40 and 8.41).
  - Care should be taken so as not to create a rotational malalignment while applying the external fixation.
  - It is always necessary to fix the lateral malleolus with an olive wire to the frame (Fig. 8.42).
  - The fibular head should always be fixed with a Schanz screw through the proximal tibia to the frame (Fig. 8.43).
  - It is essential to ensure that the Schanz screws and K-wires do not touch the IM nail to avoid getting the nail stuck and spreading any pin-track infection into the medullary cavity.
- Perform the percutaneous tibial osteotomy as planned on the paper tracing, according to the following guidelines:
  - The posterior portion (posterior to the IM nail) of the osteotomy should be performed using the Gigli-saw technique (Fig. 8.44), whereas the anterior portion of the osteotomy (anterior to the IM nail) should be completed using the multiple drill-hole technique (Fig. 8.45) (see Chap. 3).

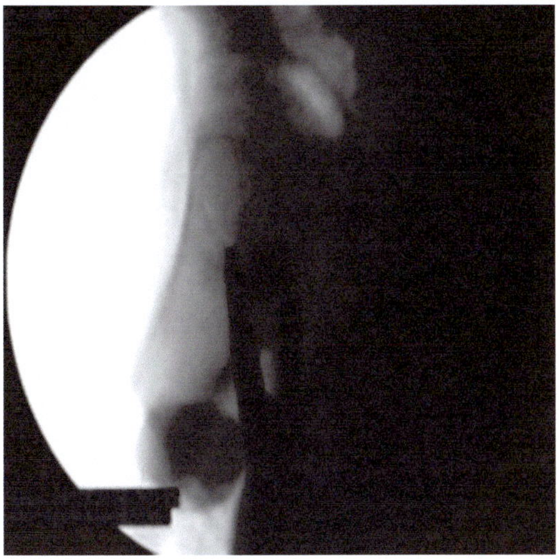

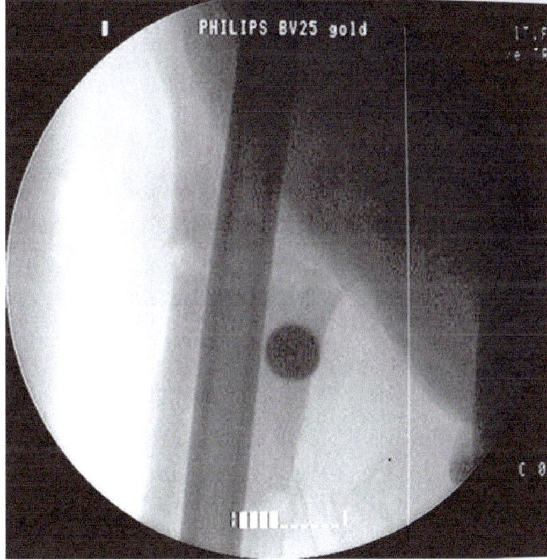

Fig. 8.31 The Schanz screws should be placed posteriorly to leave space for the IM nail

Fig. 8.32 There should be at least 1 mm between the IM nail and the Schanz screws to prevent any pin-track infection from spreading into the medullary cavity

- At this stage, the distraction test is carried out to ensure that the bone segment can slide over the IM nail properly.

8.2.8 Postoperative Period

- Dressing changes begin during the first 48 h, and gentle normal saline cleansing around the pin sites and nonocclusive dressings every 3rd day are preferred.
- On the day of the operation, isometric quadriceps and knee range-of-motion exercises are initiated.
- Ice application, for 3 weeks and four times per day for 20 min, is recommended for the knee joint.
- On the first postoperative day, full-weight bearing with the help of two crutches is allowed.
- The patient is discharged from the hospital on the second or third postoperative day if he/she is able to walk independently with two crutches and exhibits an active, unlimited range of motion at the adjacent joints (hip and knee joints for femoral applications or knee and ankle joints for tibial applications).
- Daily physical therapy is recommended after discharge from the hospital and until the end of the treatment period.
- Distraction begins at the seventh postoperatively day (the so-called latency period) at a rate of 0.25 mm four times per day (i.e., 1 mm per day).
- During the lengthening and/or bone-transport periods, we recommend that radiographs be obtained every 2 weeks to monitor the distraction progress (the amount of lengthening, the quality of the regeneration, the presence of any mechanical failure, and/or osteolysis around the Schanz screws). At each visit, patients should be evaluated for ROM of the adjacent joints, pin-site status, stability of the external fixator, and neurovascular status (clinical status, especially the presence of drop foot) (Figs. 8.46a–c).

8.2.9 Removal of the External Fixator

When the desired amount of lengthening and/or bone transport has been achieved, the patient then undergoes the second stage of surgical treatment, according to the following guidelines:

- The patient should be placed in the supine position on the radiolucent table so that the

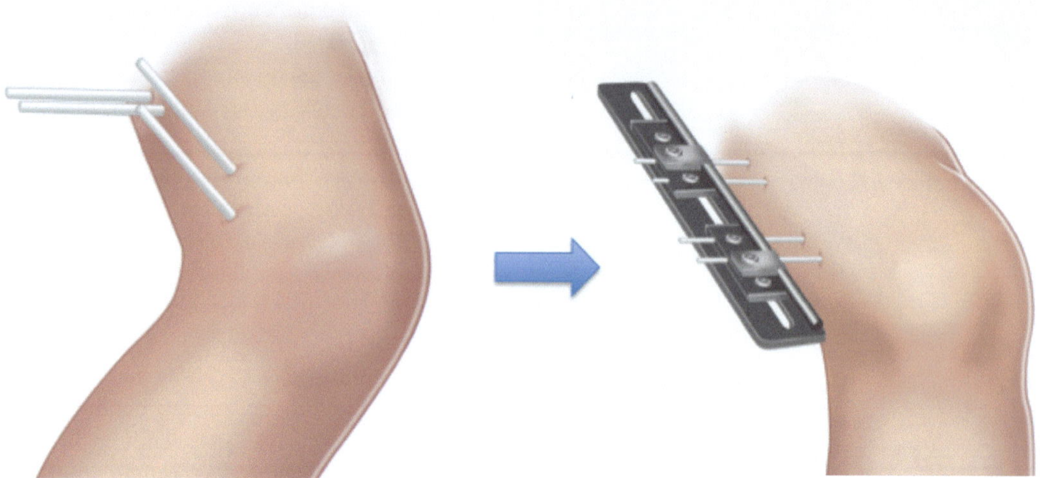

Fig. 8.33 The Schanz screws should be inserted in parallel to the axial plane of each bone fragment to correct any rotational deformity

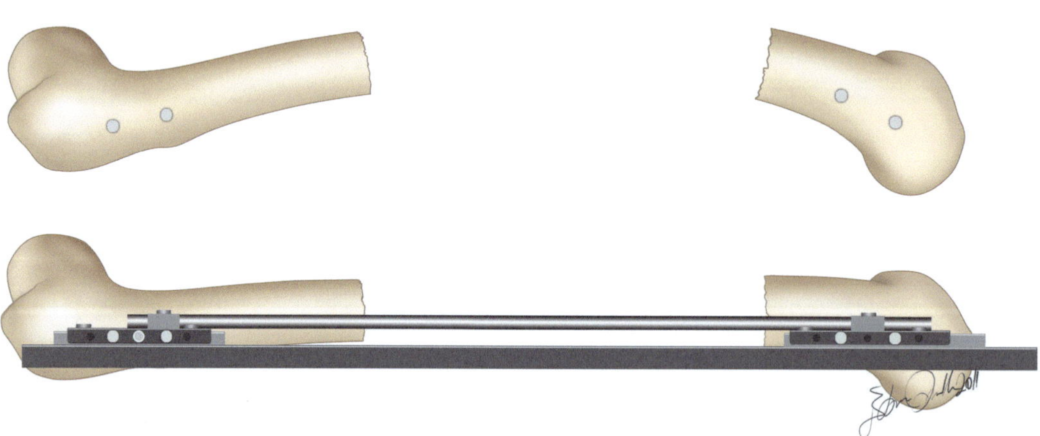

Fig. 8.34 The Schanz screws should be inserted in parallel to the sagittal axis of each fragment to correct any sagittal deformity

physician can check the empty holes made by the IM nail with an image intensifier in both planes prior to the steps required for sterile preparation.

- The patient is then prepared as in the first procedure from the hip to the toes.
- After the entire extremity is prepared, the external fixator is cleansed with Betadine solution and is then wrapped with towels.

- Interlocking the empty holes on the IM nail is performed using the cannulated-drill technique (Figs. 8.47 and 8.48).
- The external fixator is only removed when the IM nail has been locked statically and secured mechanically with interference screws, if necessary.
- The addition of iliac autografting to the docking site is preferred to enhance bone healing.

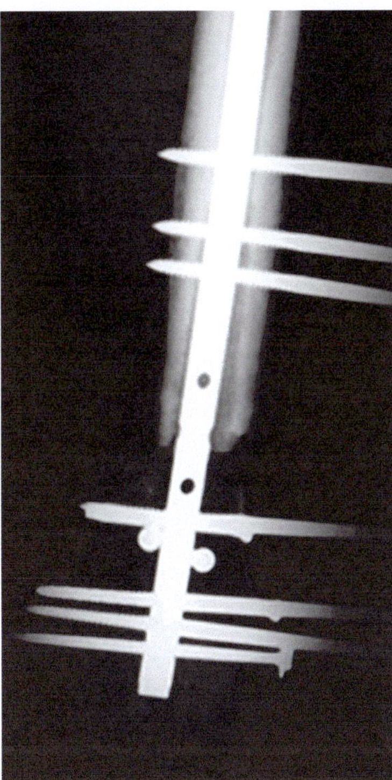

Fig. 8.35 Poller screws are used to narrow the medullary canal and thus increase the stability, especially in the metaphyseal area

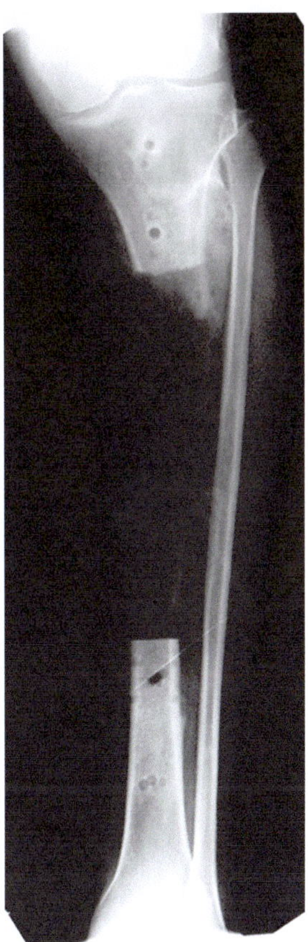

Fig. 8.36 Antibiotic beads and the rod are removed through the incision from the first stage

- This is typically performed as an outpatient procedure.

8.2.10 Follow-Up After the Second Procedure

- At this point, the patient is allowed to bear his/her full weight with the use of two crutches until full consolidation of the regeneration has occurred.

- The first visit after patient discharge from the hospital should occur on the 7th postoperative day. At this visit, the wounds are checked for any problems, but no x-rays are needed at this time.

- Follow-up for the consolidation of the regeneration and the healing of the osteotomy(ies) for deformity correction is checked via AP and the use of lateral x-rays at monthly intervals. During this follow-up visit, the ROM of the adjacent joints and muscle strength are assessed.

Fig. 8.37 For cases with no LLD, the IM nail is locked statically, proximally, and distally

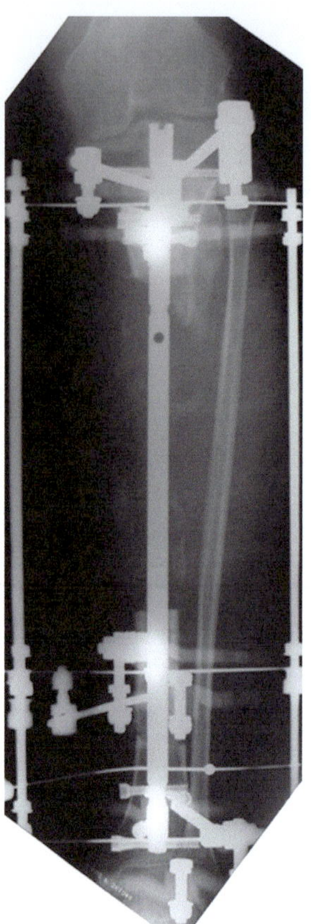

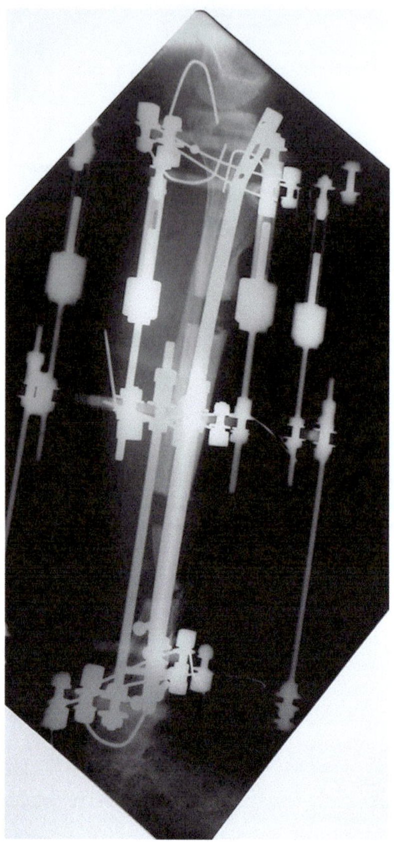

Fig. 8.38 For cases with LLD, only one end of the IM nail is locked

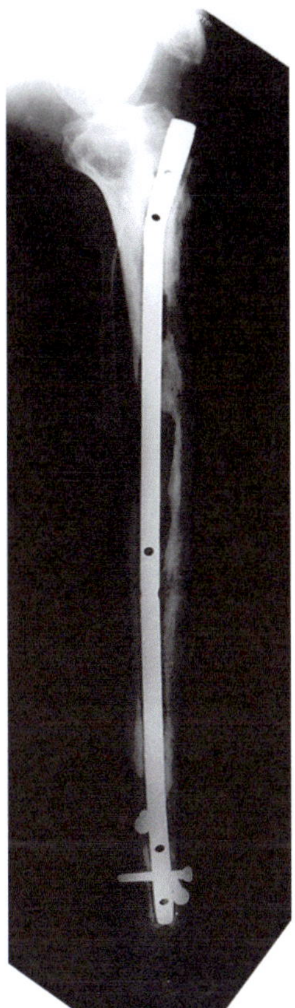

Fig. 8.39 One end of the IM nail can be left outside of the bone prior to lengthening

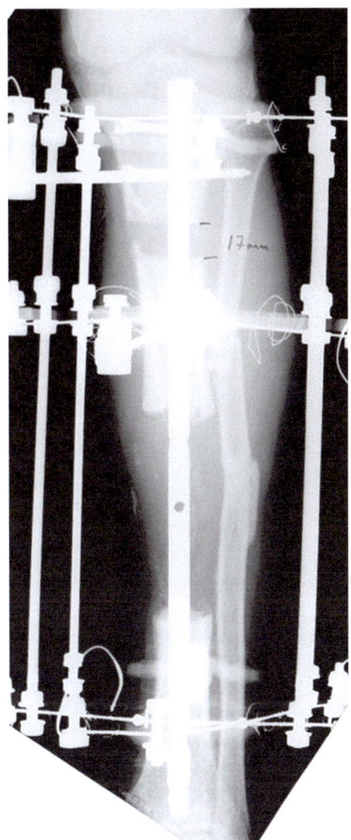

Fig. 8.40 A circular external fixator, which consists of rings in each segment, is applied

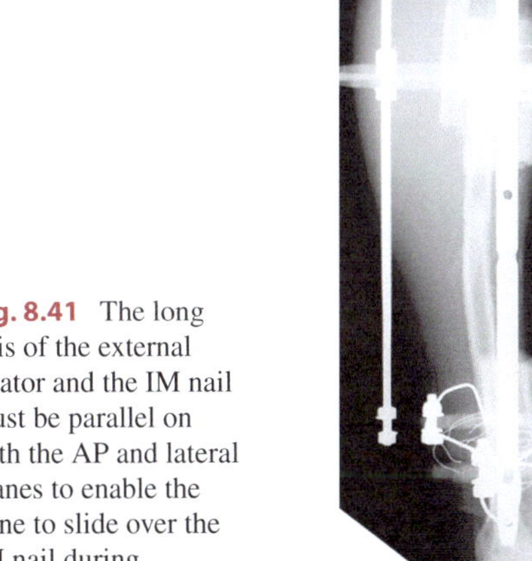

Fig. 8.41 The long axis of the external fixator and the IM nail must be parallel on both the AP and lateral planes to enable the bone to slide over the IM nail during lengthening

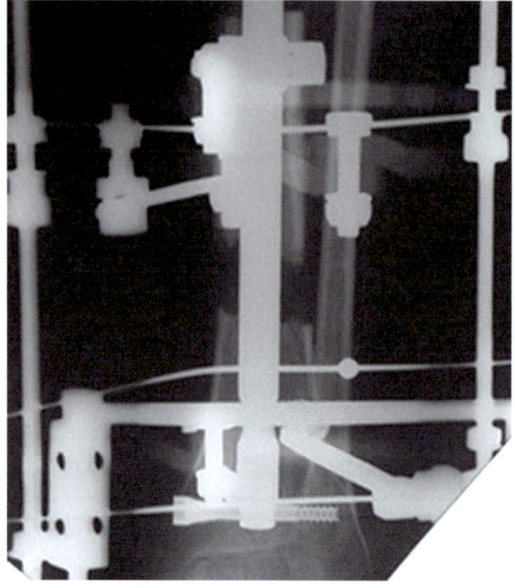

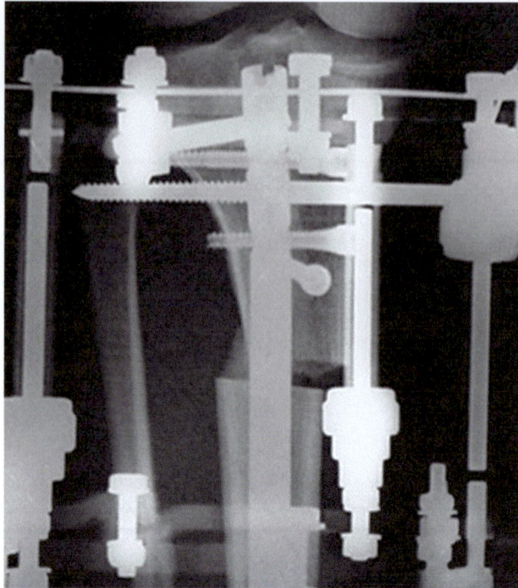

Fig. 8.42 The lateral malleolus is fixed with an olive wire to the frame

Fig. 8.43 The fibular head is fixed to the frame as well

Fig. 8.44 The posterior portion of the osteotomy is performed with the Gigli-saw technique

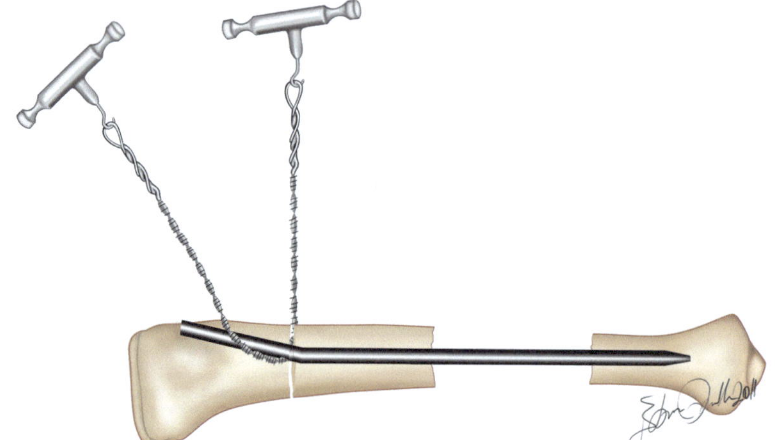

Fig. 8.45 The anterior portion of the osteotomy is performed with the multiple drill-hole technique

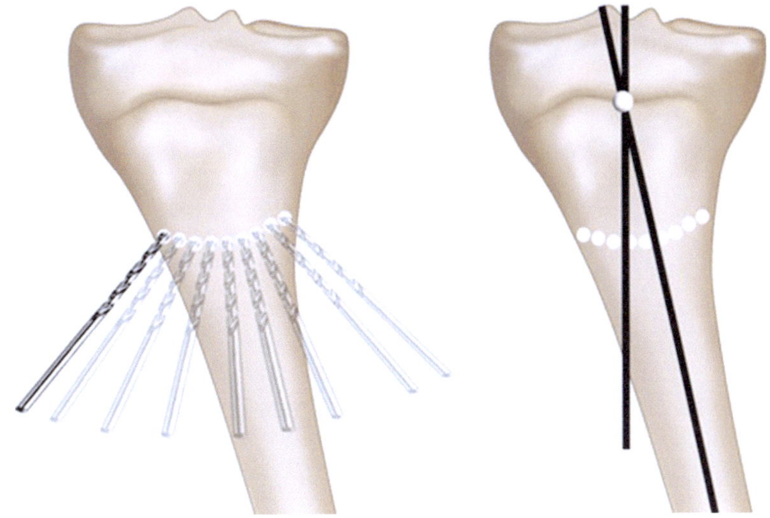

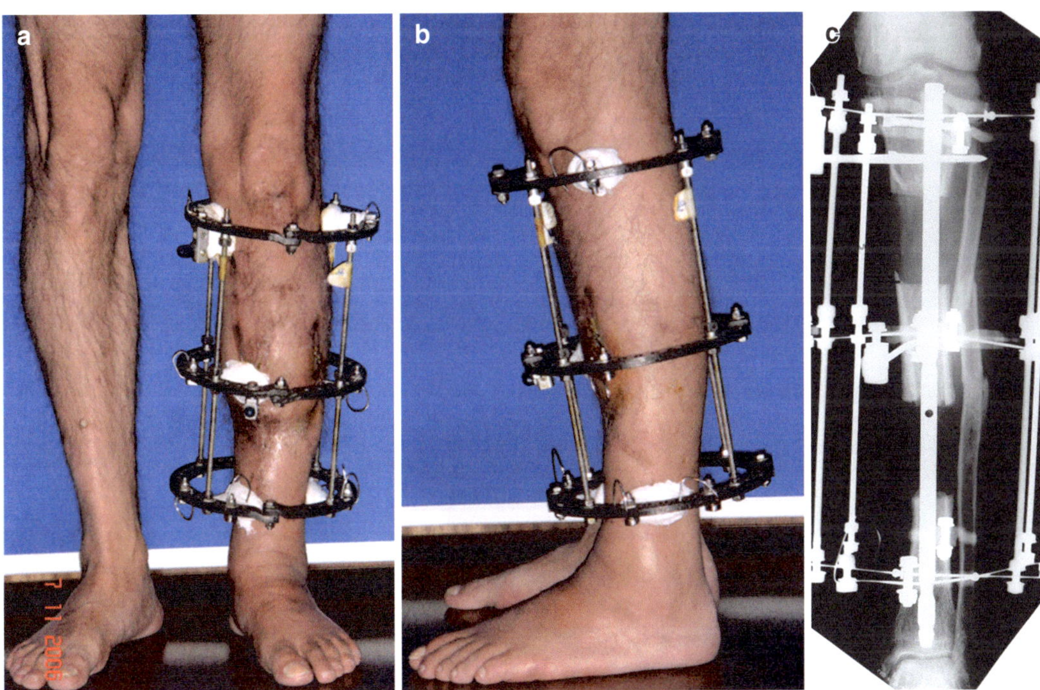

Fig. 8.46 (**a–c**) Different stages in the treatment of a patient with an osteomyelitis defect

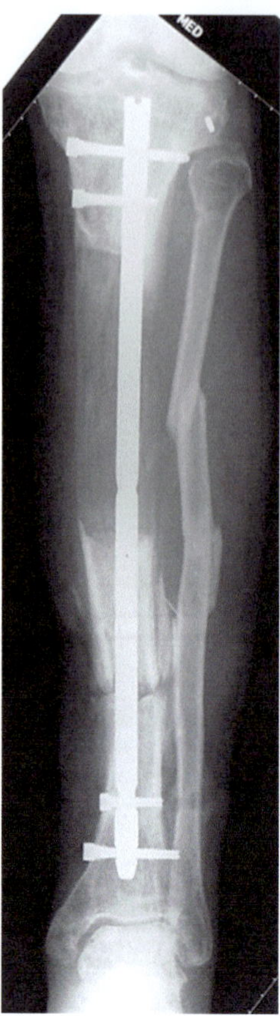

Fig. 8.47 The empty holes of the IM nail are locked using the cannulated-drill technique

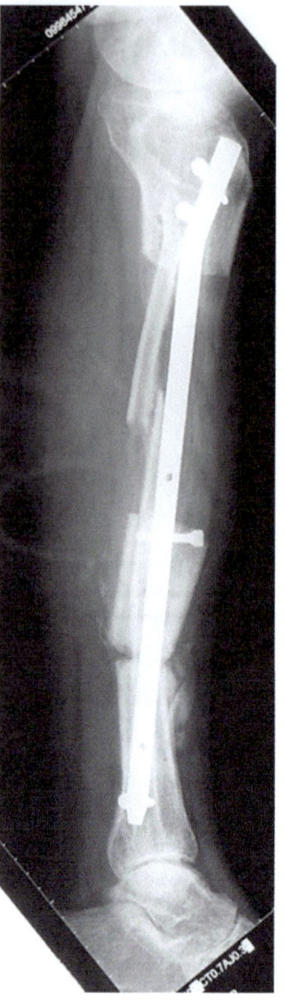

Fig. 8.48 The empty holes of the IM nail are locked using the cannulated-drill technique

References

Bhadra AK, Roberts CS (2009) Indications for antibiotic cement nails. J Orthop Trauma 23:S26–S30

Dabov GD (2008) Osteomyelitis. In: Canale ST, Beaty JH (eds) Campbell's operative orthopaedics. Mosby/Elsevier, Philadelphia

Eralp L (2011) Osteomyelitis. In: Lerner A, Soudry M (eds) Armed conflict injuries to the extremities. Springer, Berlin

Eralp L, Kocaoglu M (2008) Distal tibial reconstruction with use of a circular external fixator and an intramedullary nail. Surgical technique. J Bone Joint Surg Am 90:181–194

Ilizarov GA (1992) The treatment of pseudarthroses complicated by osteomyelitis and elimination of purulent cavities. In: Ilizarov GA (ed) Transosseous osteosynthesis. Springer, Heidelberg

Kocaoglu M, Eralp L, Kılıcoglu O et al (2004) Complications encountered during lengthening over an intramedullary nail. J Bone Joint Surg Am 86: 2406–2411

Kocaoglu M, Eralp L, Rashid HU et al (2006) Reconstruction of segmental bone defects due to chronic osteomyelitis with use of an external fixator and an intramedullary nail. J Bone Joint Surg Am 88:2137–2145

Krettek C, Miclau T, Schandelmaier P et al (1999a) The mechanical effect of blocking screws ("Poller screws") in stabilizing tibia fractures with short proximal or distal fragments after insertion of small-diameter intramedullary nails. J Orthop Trauma 13(8):550–553

Krettek C, Stephan C, Schandelmaier P et al (1999b) The use of Poller screws as blocking screws in stabilising tibial fractures treated with small diameter intramedullary nails. J Bone Joint Surg Br 81(6):963–968

Paley D, Herzenberg JE (2002a) Intramedullary infections treated with antibiotic cement rods: preliminary results in nine cases. J Orthop Trauma 16(10):723–729

Paley D, Herzenberg JE (2002b) Hardware and osteotomy considerations. In: Paley D, Herzenberg JE (eds) Principles of deformity correction. Springer, Berlin

Paley D, Tetsworth K (1992) Mechanical axis deviation of the lower limbs. Preoperative planning of multiapical frontal plane angular and bowing deformities of the femur and tibia. Clin Orthop Relat Res 280:65–71

Paley D, Catagni MA, Argnani F et al (1989) Ilizarov treatment of tibial nonunions with bone loss. Clin Orthop 241:146

Paley D, Herzenberg JE, Paremain G et al (1997) Femoral lengthening over an intramedullary nail. A matched-case comparison with Ilizarov femoral lengthening. J Bone Joint Surg Am 79:1464–1480

Papineau LJ, Alfageme A, Dulcoit JP et al (1979) Chronic osteomyelitis. Open excision and grafting after saucerization. Int Orthop 3:165–176

Patzakis MJ, Zalavras CG (2005) Chronic posttraumatic osteomyelitis and infected nonunion of the tibia: current management concepts. J Am Acad Orthop Surg 13:417–427

Seligson D (2000) Poller screws. J Orthop Trauma 14(6):454

Sen C, Kocaoglu M, Eralp L et al (2004) Bifocal compression-distraction in the acute treatment of grade III open tibia fractures with bone and soft tissue loss: a report of 24 cases. J Orthop Trauma 18(3):150–157

Tetsworth K, Cierny G III (1999) Osteomyelitis debridement techniques. Clin Orthop Relat Res 360:87–96

Tornero EF, Martínez IG, Tonal BG et al (2010) Comparison of hemostatic markers under different techniques for anesthesia-analgesia in total hip or knee replacement. Rev Esp Anestesiol Reanim 57(6):333–340

Reconstruction Techniques for Mega Bone Defects

9

Levent Eralp, Cengiz Şen, and İlker Eren

Contents

Abbreviations

AP	Anteroposterior
CRP	C-reactive protein
CT	Computerized tomography
K-wires	Kirschner wires
MRI	Magnetic resonance imaging
ROC	Receiver operating characteristic

9.1   Indications

Treatment of long bone defects remains a therapeutic challenge. Moreover, the risk of infection as well as vascular and/or neurologic problems is enhanced due to numerous previous surgical treatments. Due to increased difficulties and complication rate, defects above 8 cm are accepted as massive or mega bone defects (Fig. 9.1). Considering the etiology and condition of the patient, treatment of massive defects requires a two-staged approach. The first stage is assessment of the patient's general health and limb's local viability to overcome underlying or initiative pathology. The second stage is reassessment of the condition after the first intervention and deciding on the long-term strategy. This approach can be delineated as "to save what's left

L. Eralp (✉) • C. Şen
Department of Orthopaedics and Traumatology,
Istanbul Universtiy, Istanbul, Turkey
e-mail: drleventeralp@gmail.com;
senc64@gmail.com

İ. Eren
Department of Orthopaedics and Traumatology,
School of Medicine, Koc University, Istanbul, Turkey
e-mail: ilker.eren@gmail.com

M. Kocaoğlu et al. (eds.), *Advanced Techniques in Limb Reconstruction Surgery*,
DOI 10.1007/978-3-642-55026-3_9, © Springer Berlin Heidelberg 2015

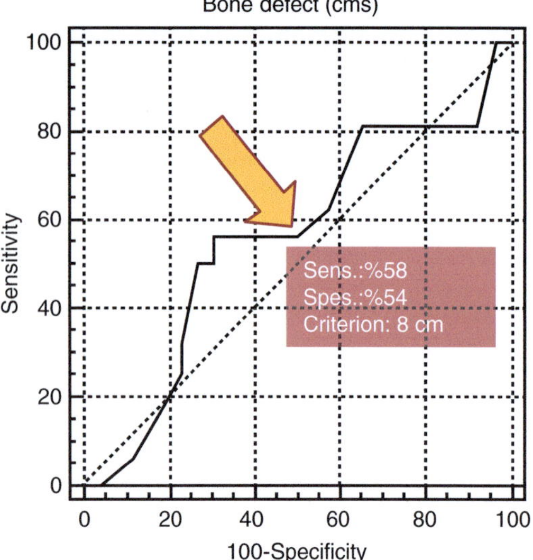

Fig. 9.1 The cutoff point values for the comparison of "amount of bone defect in cm" and "occurrence of complications" have been calculated using receiver operating characteristic (ROC) curve analysis (Istanbul Faculty of Medicine, Orthopaedics and Traumatology Archive)

behind, when the storm is over" for trauma and infections. Indications can be summarized as:

- Tumor resections leading to bone defects
- Bone losses due to trauma or defects following repetitive debridement of open fractures with marked soft tissue defect
- Chronic osteomyelitis requiring segment resection

9.2 Examination/Imaging

9.2.1 Physical Examination

- The skin condition of the limb has an important role in the treatment. Viable skin envelope should be assured before bone reconstruction. When necessary, definitive treatment can be delayed or combined with soft tissue procedures.
- Most of the patients with massive defects have vascular impairment due to previous injury or surgery. Vascular status assessment is vital, as the intervention itself may lead to additional injuries or insufficiency.
- Proximal and distal joint range of motions and any existing deformity should be noted and corrected if necessary.

9.2.2 Imaging

- True size anteroposterior (AP) and lateral radiographs are necessary for planning. In case there is deformity, a meticulous planning should be done before surgery with long-standing AP and lateral X-rays.
- In case vascularized fibula graft is planned, both *fibulae* should be visualized by X-rays.
- For osteomyelitis and tumor, magnetic resonance imaging (MRI) is mandatory. Extent of the resection and remaining bone stock has to be noted using MR, before surgery. MRI is also valuable for diagnosing skip metastasis (or skip abscesses) which will increase resection length and also for grading osteomyelitis.
- If there is known or suspected vascular impairment due to previous surgery, current pathology, or trauma, conventional or computerized tomography, angiography, or Doppler ultrasound can be performed.

9.3 Surgical Anatomy

- One must be familiar with all exposures possible in the limb, as the case may require any due to previous intervention. If it exists, the previous incision should be used to avoid any skin breakdown.
- Any possible described exposure can be used. It should be individualized to the patient, by means of diagnosis, required neurovascular dissection, and preferred treatment method.
- During surgery, the common peroneal nerve and both anterior and posterior tibial arteries are at risk.
- Titanium cages require high amounts of graft, as it is used impacted. Both allografts and autografts can be used. In case autograft is preferred, posterior iliac approach should be preferred.

9.4 Positioning

- Patient is prepared supine, with a sandbag under the ipsilateral buttock to prevent external rotation.
- Prepare graft harvesting site if necessary.

- Even if one fibula is planned for harvesting, both limbs should be prepared.
- Fluoroscopy and radiolucent table are necessary throughout the operation.

9.5   External Fixation

9.5.1   Procedure (Segment Transport)

- A circular external fixator is used for the segment transport technique. The frame consists of three rings applied to the same rods in order to allow sliding of the transported bone (Fig. 9.2).
- *Technique*: The resection area is determined by preoperative planning with X-rays. The frame should consist of three rings connected with the same rods as it allows sliding for segment transport. Following bone resection, the connective parts of the external fixator are assembled, required for either internal or external transport. If internal transport is planned, one of the rings is used as a "dummy" ring (no connection to the bone) for further compression of the docking site. However, we currently prefer doing the external transport technique due to its comfortability and easy facility. The osteotomy site for lengthening is prepared. First, the proximal reference wire is inserted and fixed to the most proximal ring. Then the distal reference wire is inserted and fixed to the most distal ring at the ankle level. Finally, all rings are fixed to the bone with Kirschner wires (K-wires) and Schanz pins (Fig. 9.3).

Pearls
- Use hydroxyapatite screws to decrease pin tract infection.
- Use a kind of spacer to avoid skin invagination.
- Use intramedullary cable technique (Kucukkaya et al. 2009).
- Choose bone transport over intramedullary nail technique (Kocaoglu et al. 2004, 2006).

Pitfalls
- Long waiting time for docking
- Invagination of skin
- Skin irritation and pain due to sliding bone

9.5.2   Procedure: Acute Shortening and Relengthening

- *Preconstructed Frame:* The circular external fixator is used as well for this technique. In this technique, the external fixator consisted of four rays; the rings were connected via different rods as needed. In the cases of distal tibial lengthening and short distal tibial fragments less than 4 cm, the frame is extended to include the foot in order to provide adequate stability (Fig. 9.4).
- *Technique:* The area of resection is determined by preoperative X-rays. A transverse incision is performed over the nonunion or fracture site and the resection is done. The resection of that site is done using an oscillating saw under saline irrigation to prevent heat necrosis. At this moment, the fibula is also resected not to prevent the docking of tibial bone ends. Moreover, the resection is performed until bleeding bone is achieved especially for nonunion cases. Then, acute shortening is done as long as the blood circulation of the foot exists. If the distal arterial circulation is maintained which is confirmed by capillary refilling, pulse oximeter, and Doppler ultrasound, respectively, as needed, the operation could be continued. If the circulation does not allow more shortening, gradual shortening should be reserved at 2 mm/day postoperatively. Following the shortening procedure, the skin is closed and the resected bone ends are temporarily fixed using K-wires or intramedullary Steinman pin. Then proximal and distal reference wires are inserted and fixed to the rings at the most proximal and distal level of the tibial bone. Then the middle two segments are fixed using two K-wires. At this stage, X-rays are taken on both planes. If the alignment of the tibia is well, the procedure goes on; otherwise, a malalignment on any plane should be corrected at this stage. Following this stage, fixation is completed at all levels of frame. Finally, an osteotomy is performed to relengthen the tibia at the healthy site of bone.

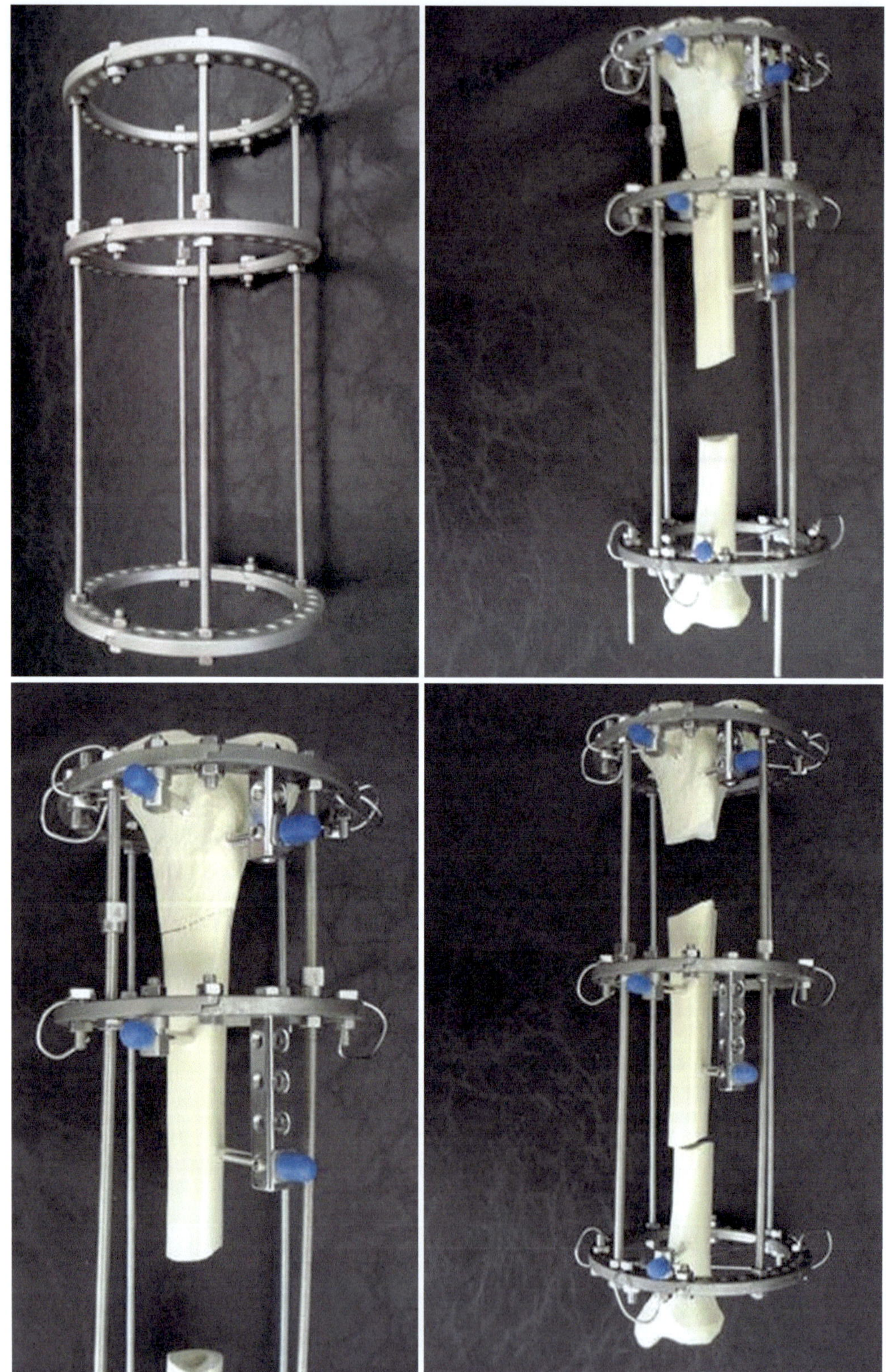

Fig. 9.2 Schematic view of the segment transport method with a saw bone

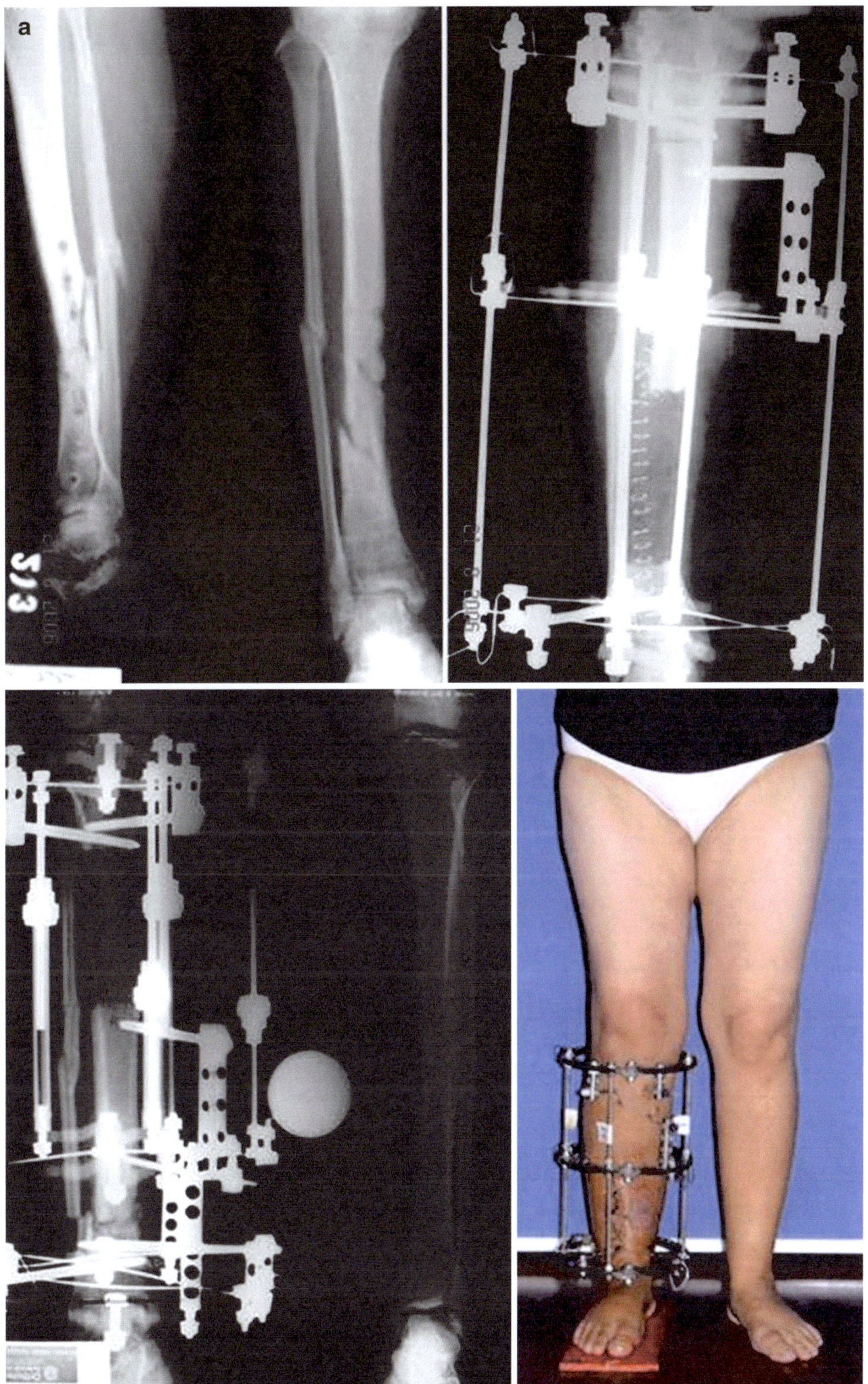

Fig. 9.3 A fifty-one-year-old female patient with chronic osteomyelitis, who underwent a segment transport technique. (**a**) X Rays before surgery, during and after segment transport. (**b**) X Rays and knee flexion after fixator removal

Fig. 9.3 (continued)

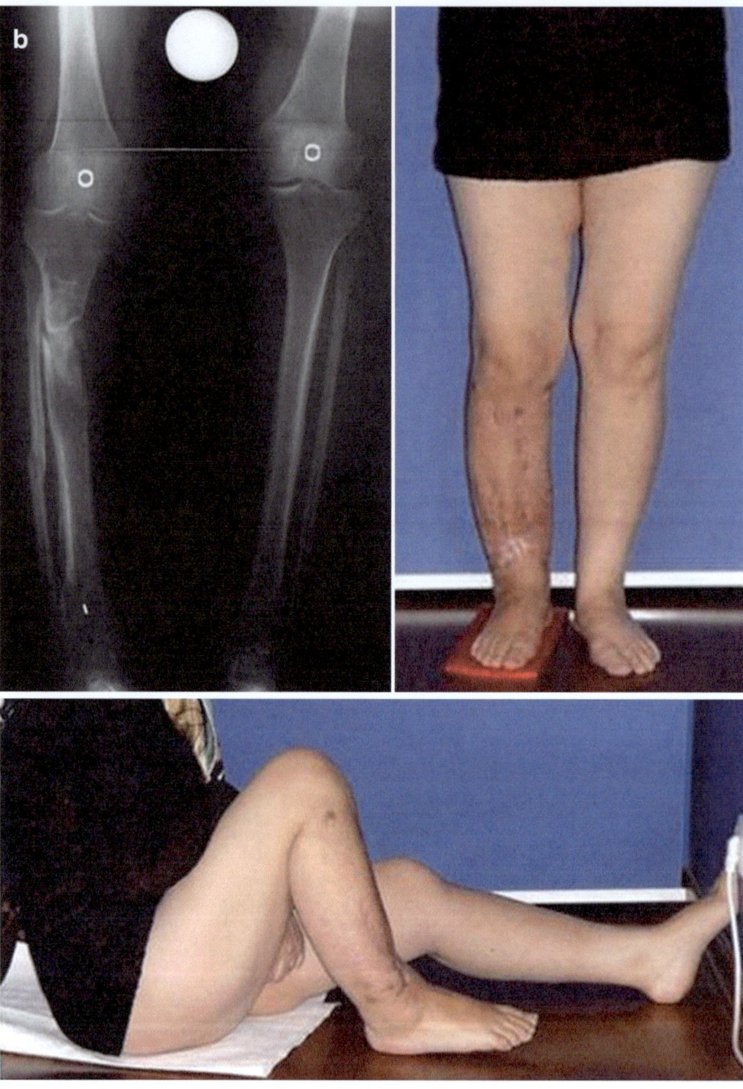

Pearls

- Before assembling the frame, measure the leg size of patients to match with the ring. Choose the size bigger than the leg's size. The room between the leg and ring is getting smaller when you do acute shortening; muscles will become more bulky.
- Check the availability of the radiolucent table before starting the procedure.
- Use transverse incision to close the skin easily.

- Before doing the incision, check the accuracy of the docking area using the image intensifier.
- The docking site should be opened and grafted if progress to union is not observed within 3 months.
- If union is completed, remove the frame and a long-leg brace should be worn for 4–6 weeks.

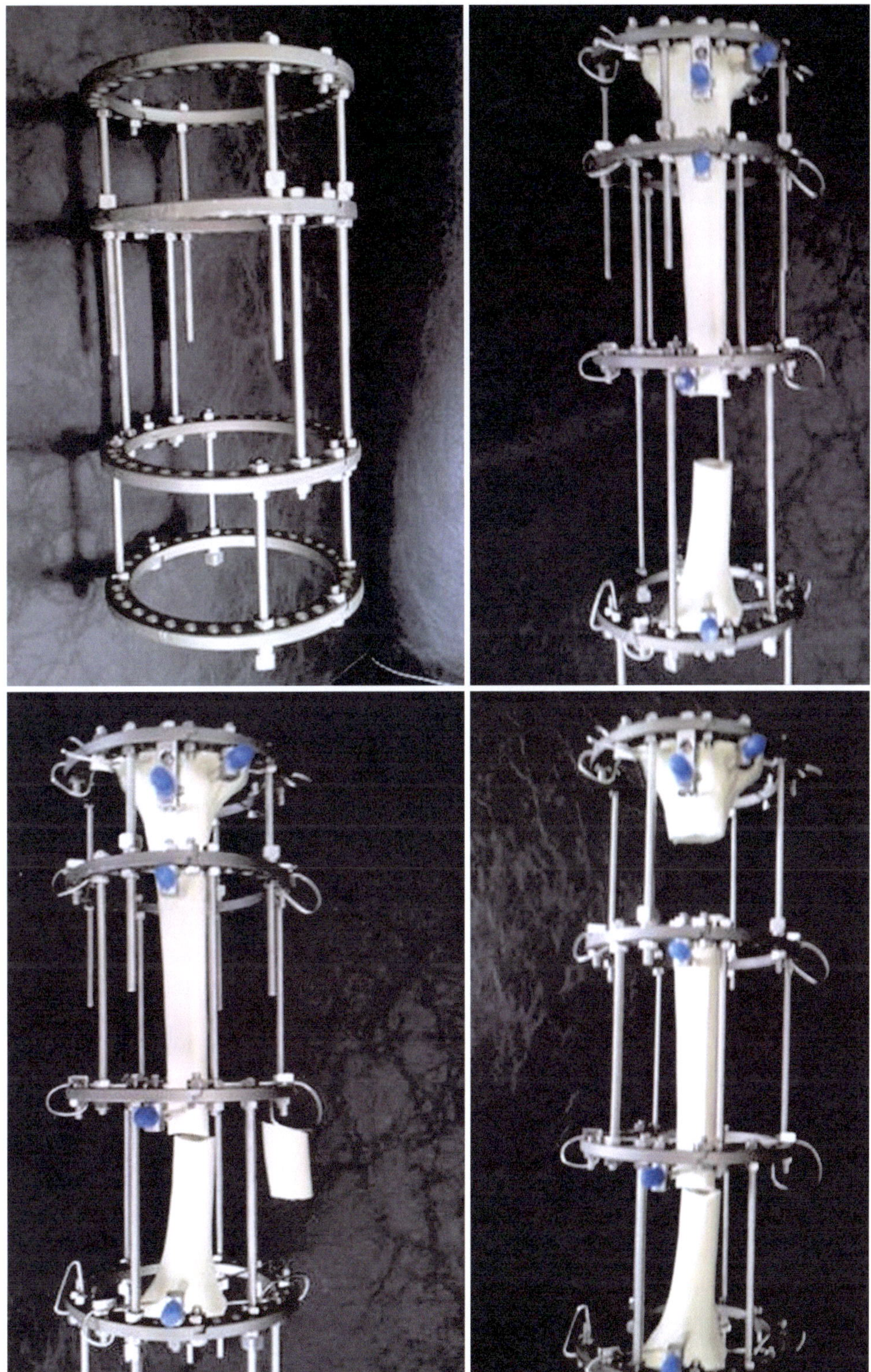

Fig. 9.4 Schematic view of the acute shortening method with a saw bone

Pitfalls

- Fibula resection is mandatory due to shortening of the bone ends acutely. However, this may give rise to instability of the ankle.
- It is absolutely necessary for intensive physiotherapy because muscle relaxation and weakness occur for 4–6 weeks postoperatively.
- You can choose an alternate method for skin cover without resection of the fibula (Gulsen and Özkan 2009).
- Extend the frame to include the foot if you have smaller bone less than 4 cm or plan to lengthen distal bone at the supramalleolar region.
- Check the blood circulation of the foot using Doppler US as well as observe capillary refilling. If you have any doubt of that, distract the docking area until circulation goes completely back to normal.
- Begin daily physiotherapy the day after surgery and wear custom-made shoes with dorsiflexion straps to prevent equinus contractures.
- In infected cases, antibiotic-impregnated beads are implanted following resection. Then, antibiotics specific to the microorganism based on the antibiogram and culture results are used for 6 weeks. At the end of this period, if the levels of C-reactive protein (CRP) and sedimentation returned to normal, reconstruction surgery is then performed as described above (Fig. 9.5).
- *Advantages of the Technique*
  - There is no need for microvascular or plastic surgeon team to close the wound, because acute or gradual shortening at the docking site makes wound closure easier.
  - Acute shortening provides a good opposition at the docking site immediately after resection.
  - Bone ends have maximal viability and potential for union.
  - This exclusive feature of technique gives rise to decreased external fixator time and complication rate.

9.5.3 Controversies

- Segment transport in the management of nonunion with bone loss is a well-known technique. Many studies were reported with successful results. This technique not only solves nonunion problem, but it also addresses leg length discrepancy, correction of deformity, and regain of function of joint motion.
- However, it has some disadvantages such as long external fixation time and docking site problems. Docking site problems include soft tissue invagination, malalignment, reinfection, and nonunion due to an extended time span of bone end opposition.
- Acute shortening and relengthening is less popular compared to segment transport. This technique also provides union and solves some problems such as leg length discrepancy, deformity, and infection.
- Furthermore, it has some advantages such as shorter fixator time and less complication rates because bone ends immediately get into contact either acutely or gradually within a few days postoperatively. Therefore, viable bone ends meet at the docking site in order not to lose stem cells as soon as possible. Besides, it contains a good condition for union. Moreover, it is possible to decrease complication rates because of shorter treatment time.
- However, this technique also has some disadvantages such as loss of resected fibula pieces due to the technical obligation and temporary weakness of muscle power.

9.6 Titanium Cage

- Expected bone defect has to be noted before surgery. Careful planning is the key for success. X-rays and MRI are usually enough for predicting defect. Both the titanium cage and

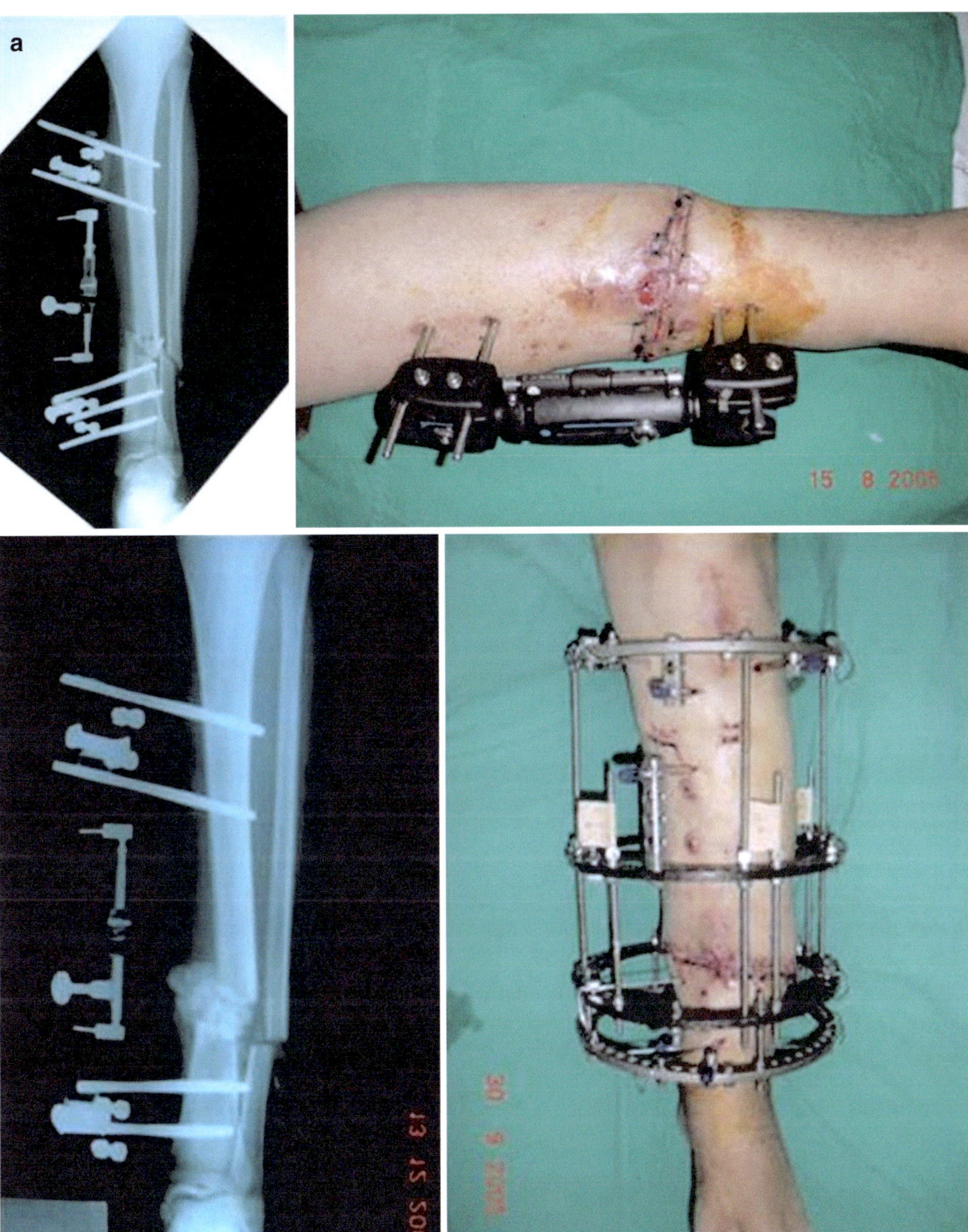

Fig. 9.5 An eighteen-year-old male patient with chronic osteomyelitis, who was treated with acute shortening and relengthening method following radical debridement and antibiotic beads at the first stage. (**a**) X rays with tempo-rary fixator, and clinical photos of the temporary and final fixator setup. (**b**) X rays after segment transport: with and without fixator. Knee flexion is fully achieved

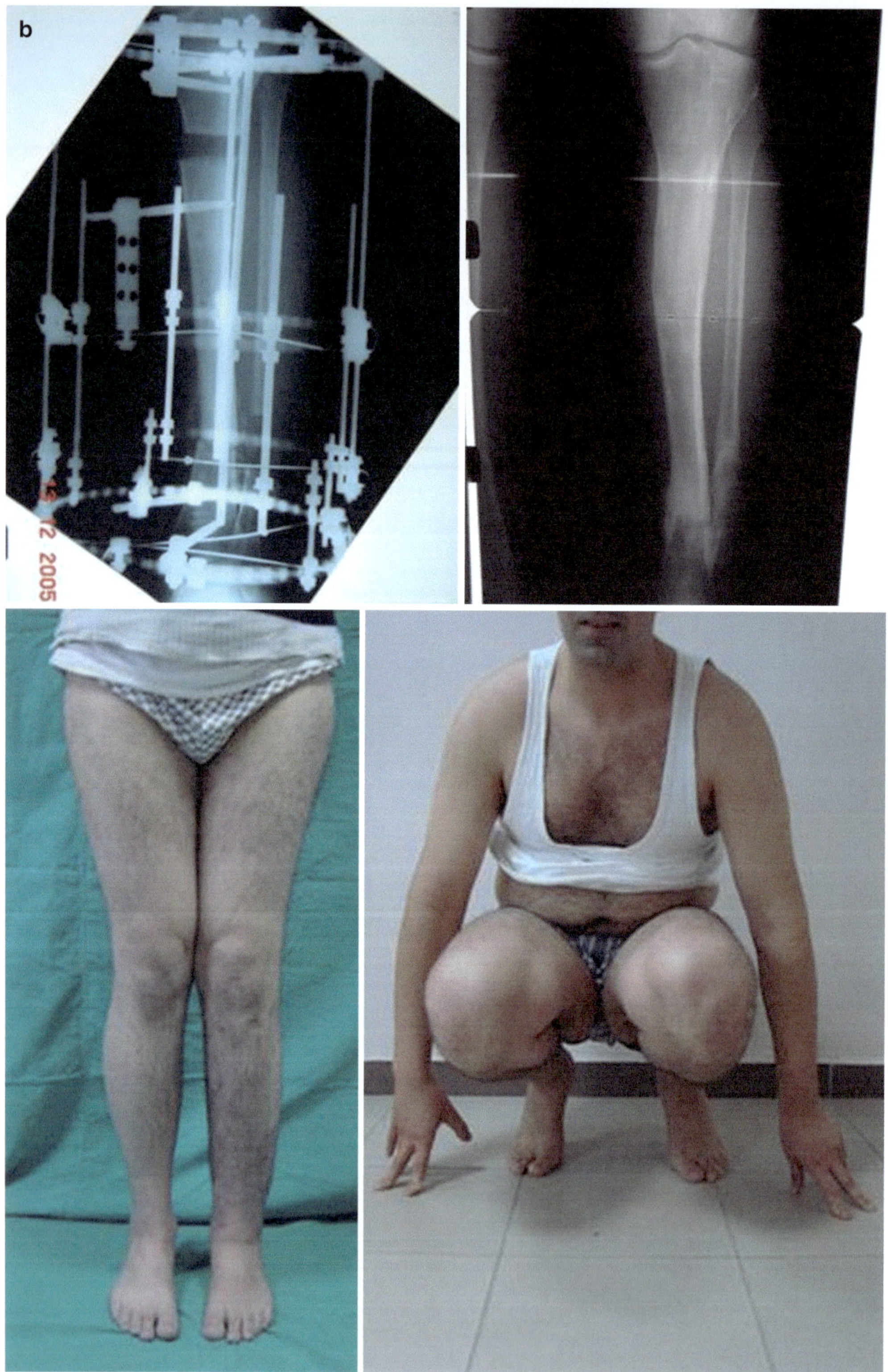

Fig. 9.5 (continued)

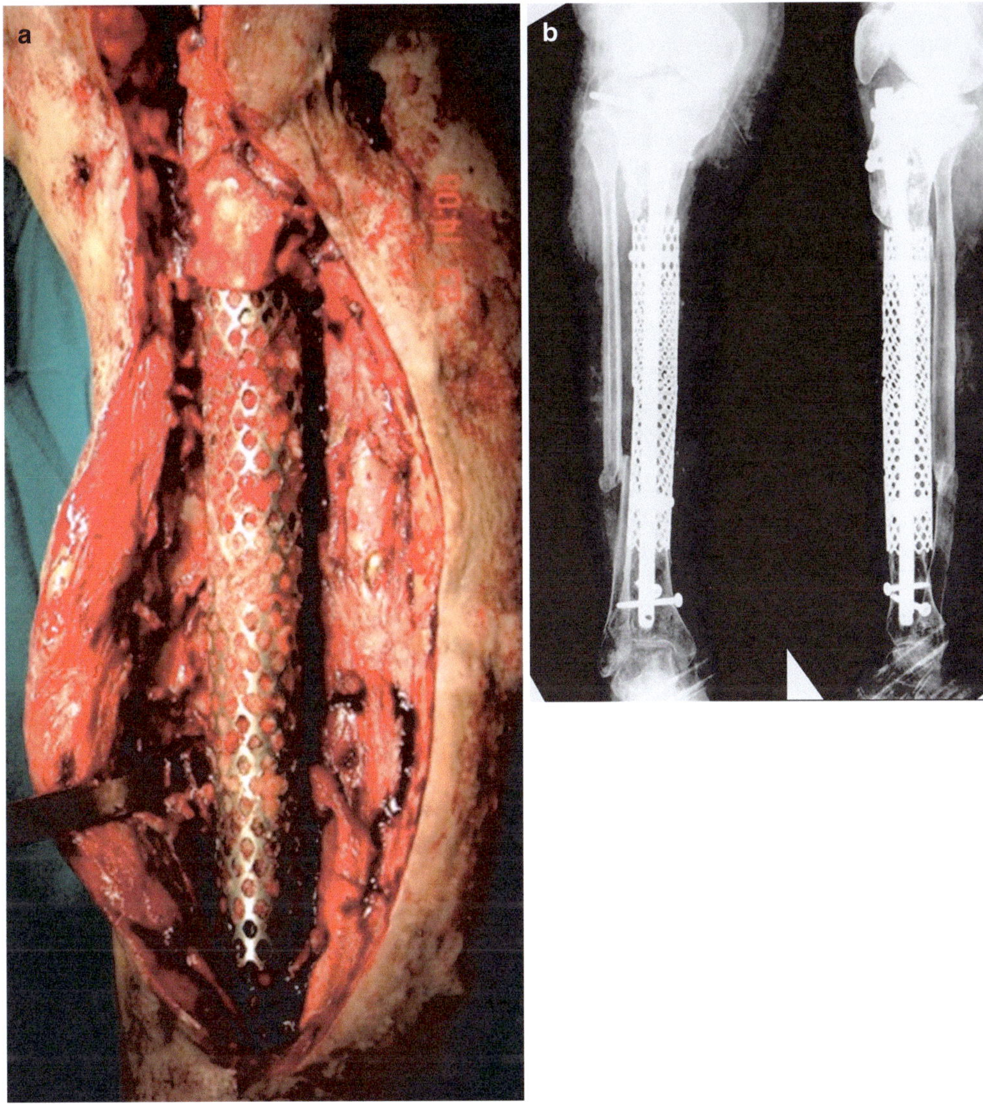

Fig. 9.6 (**a**) Titanium cage is prepared and implanted to the gap. (**b**) After reaming through, it is fixed with an intramedullary nail

the intramedullary nail should be prepared before surgery according to the gap. If necessary, custom-made nails with additional fixation holes can be used.

- After harvesting and morselizing cancellous graft, it is impacted in the cage before implanting. Some cages are prepared in fixed sizes; some are cut during surgery.

- Cage itself will not provide any stabilization. An intramedullary nail is used for that matter. Before positioning the cage, bone is reamed. If necessary, poller screws are used at the metaphyseal region to avoid deformity. Once the nail is advanced until the gap, the cage is placed and the nail is inserted and locked in a standard fashion (Fig. 9.6).

9.7 Free Vascularized Fibula Graft

9.7.1 Exposures

- The fibula is vascularized by the peroneal artery, laying just medial. The artery penetrates the bone at about just distal to the 1/3 proximal segment of the bone. It is harvested from the plane between soleus muscle and peroneal muscles.

9.7.2 Procedure

- *Harvesting Vascularized Fibula:* Once soleus and peroneal muscles are retracted, the septum separating the anterior and peroneal compartments is incised and the interosseous membrane visualized anteriorly. Careful dissection of the membrane is performed protecting anterior tibial vessels and nerve. To expose posterior tibial artery and origin of the peroneal artery, soleus is released posteriorly. Dissection is advanced between peroneal vessels and tibial nerve. The periosteum is incised at the level of osteotomy proximally and distally. A Gigli saw is used for osteotomy. The medial attachment of the fibula and vascular supply is dissected after osteotomy. A small part of tibialis posterior is left over vessels to avoid injury. The artery and vein are ligated and cut proximally and distally.
- Fibula itself has not enough strength to confront physiological forces alone. Thus, combined methods are introduced to overcome this problem. It can be used with massive allografts and irradiated or cryopreserved structural autografts. This support will provide nonliving but structural endurance until the living but weak fibula is remodeled under physiological forces.

- *Technique for Vascularized Fibula Composites (Combination with Cryopreserved Bone Sarcoma)*
  - This technique can only be used for osteoblastic tumors, as the bone has to preserve mechanical integrity for sufficient strength (Fig. 9.7).
  - Before exposure to liquid nitrogen, the surrounding soft tissues have to be removed and medullary canal is reamed (Fig. 9.8).
  - Intramedullary canal of the massive allograft or autograft is prepared by reaming over fibular diameter. It is vital to leave vascular supply enough room in the canal (Fig. 9.9).
  - Before advancing the fibula inside, a window for the vascular supply has to be created on the massive graft. The location of this window has to be on the side of recipient artery and vein of the limb. For this reason, the exact placement of the massive graft has to be carefully adjusted before implanting. If the preserved bone width is not enough for safely advancing fibula through, up to 1/3 of the bone can be removed lengthwise (Fig. 9.10).
  - Prepared massive autograft has to be exposed to liquid nitrogen for 20 min, followed by thawing for 15 min at room temperature (20°), and finally handled in warmed isotonic solution (30°) for 10 min (Fig. 9.11).
  - Definitive fixation is secured by plating with two plates at both sides or one plate bridging through the gap. The surgeon must be aware of the route of the peroneal vessels inside the canal, so that the screws will not penetrate them.
  - The preferred anastomosis and fixation method varies up to the transferred segment and vascular condition of the limb (Fig. 9.12).
  - Grafting osteotomy sites after fixation will facilitate union.

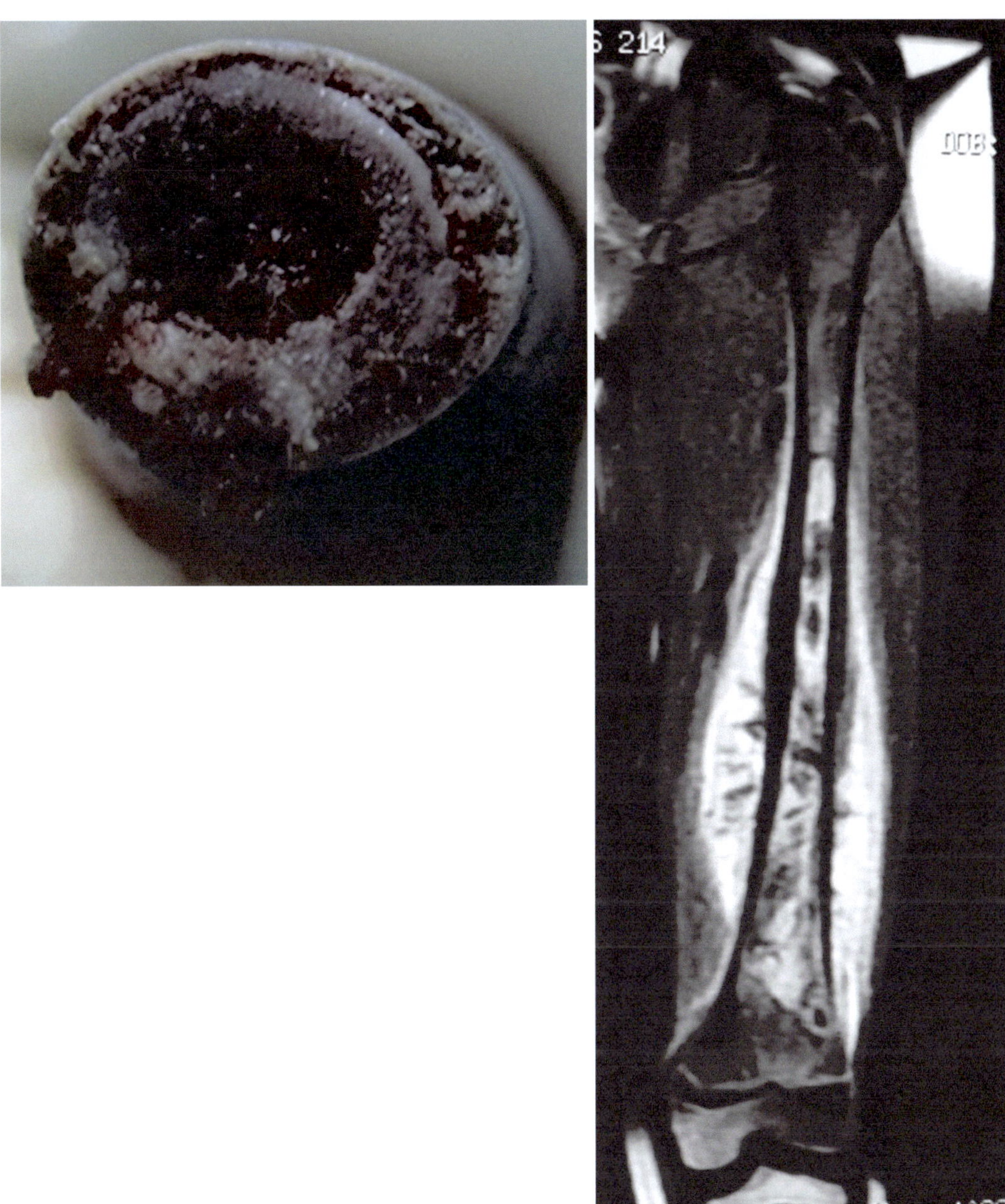

Fig. 9.7 Osteoblastic tumor, located at the distal femur

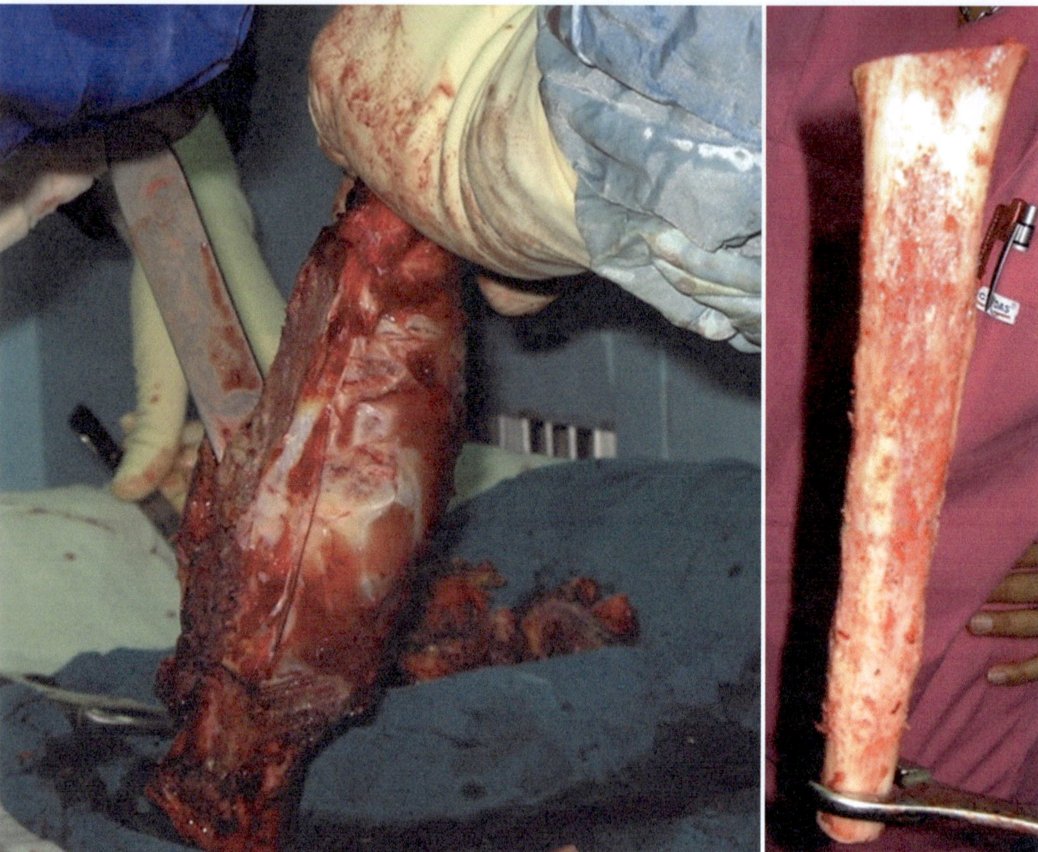

Fig. 9.8 Before exposure to liquid nitrogen, the soft tissues have to be removed

- For tibial diaphyseal defects, transposing the fibula with its vascular supply preserved is also a viable method.

Pearls

- In order to protect peroneal vascular supply, a small ruff of flexor hallucis muscle posteriorly and tibialis posterior muscle medially can be left attached to the fibular graft while harvesting.
- The ends of the fibula may also contribute fixation strength by advancing it through the medullary canal of the patient's remaining bone proximally and distally.
- When it is necessary to bridge defects where the fibula's length is insufficient, double fibula autograft, combined with structural grafts, is an advanced method for bridging such defects. This method is mostly used for extensive tumoral resections, especially for femur.

9.8 Postoperative Care and Expected Outcomes

- Knee and ankle range of motion exercises are encouraged immediately after surgery.

9.8.1 External Fixation

- The ankle joint is positioned in neutral dorsiflexion by using a splint during resting. Weight bearing is permitted with two crutches as tolerated. In acute or gradual shortening cases, more strength exercises are needed because of relaxed and shortened muscles for 4–6 weeks.

- Gradual shortening is continued 2 mm/day as required by starting on the first postoperative day. Lengthening through the osteotomy site is started at 4×0.25 mm per day on the 7th day postoperatively.
- If bony union is not achieved at the end of 3 months postoperatively, autogenous bone grafting is performed. Once union is obtained, the fixator is removed, and a brace is worn for at least 4–6 weeks. During this period, weight bearing is allowed as tolerated.

9.8.2   Free Vascularized Fibula and Titanium Cage

- Patients with cage-nail combination or free vascularized fibula transfer cannot bear full weight until radiological union is evident. This may take months according to the viability of the bone and surrounding soft tissues.
- Radiological assessment is performed monthly.
- Ossification in the cage and at the bone attachments is assessed at 6th month with 3D computerized tomography (CT) scan (Fig. 9.13).
- Failure usually occurs due to infection recurrence or nonunion.

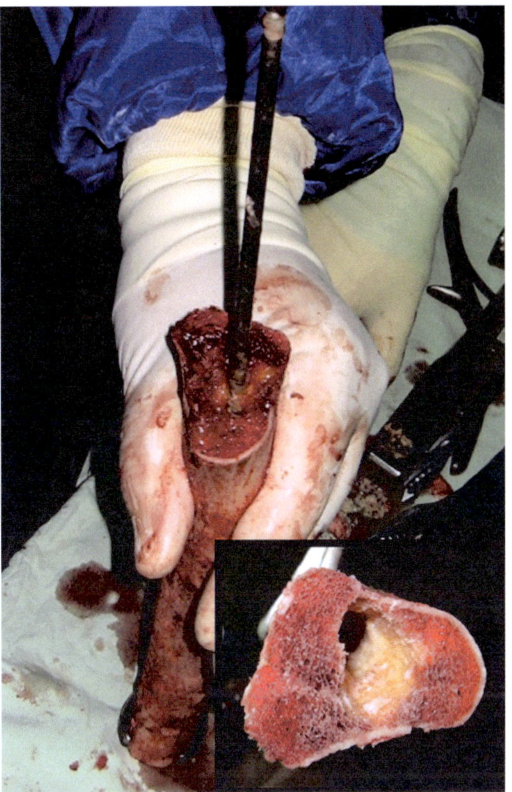

Fig. 9.9 Intramedullary canal is reamed

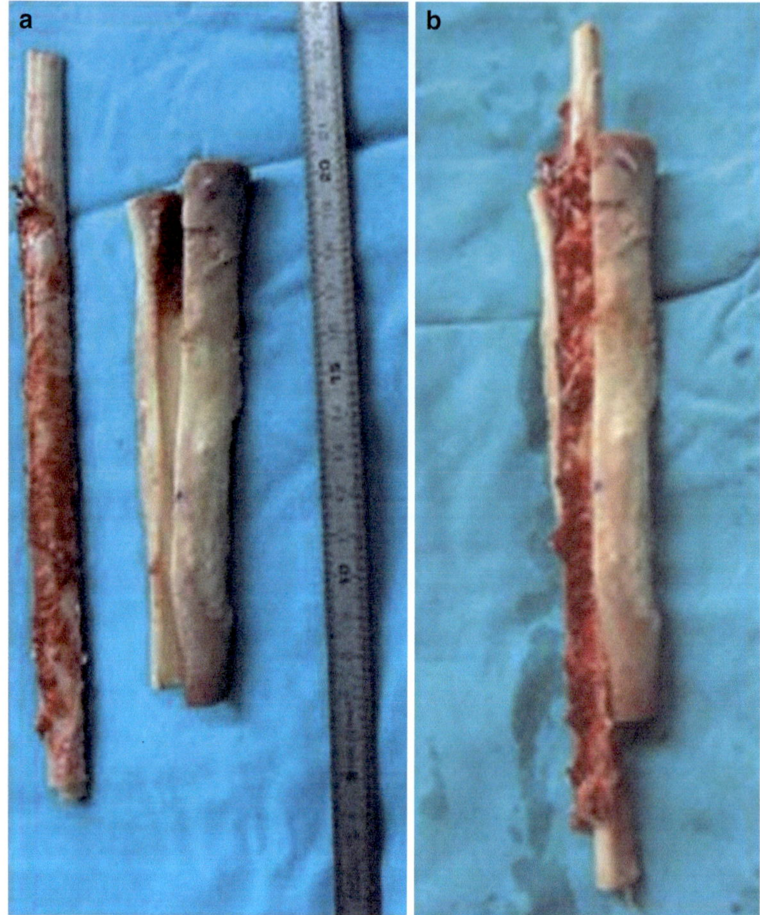

Fig. 9.10 (**a**) Fibula graft and prepared canal, (**b**) Fibula graft placed in prepared canal, preserving vascular supply

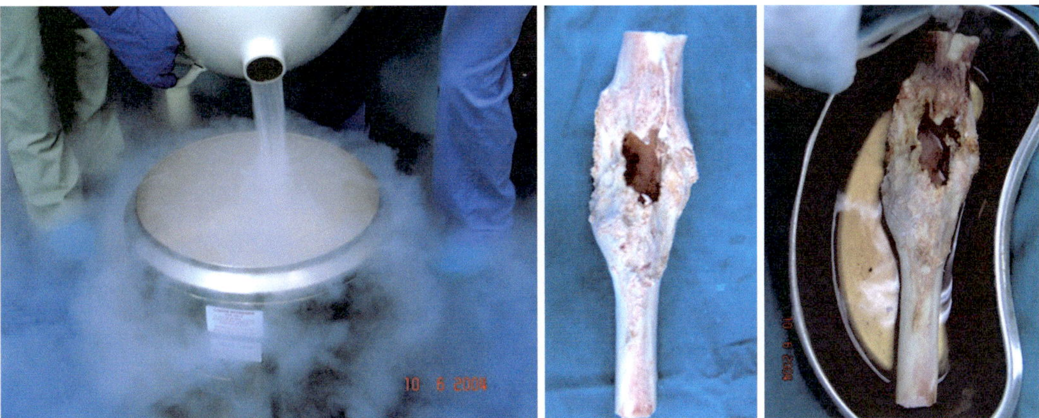

Fig. 9.11 Preparing the bone

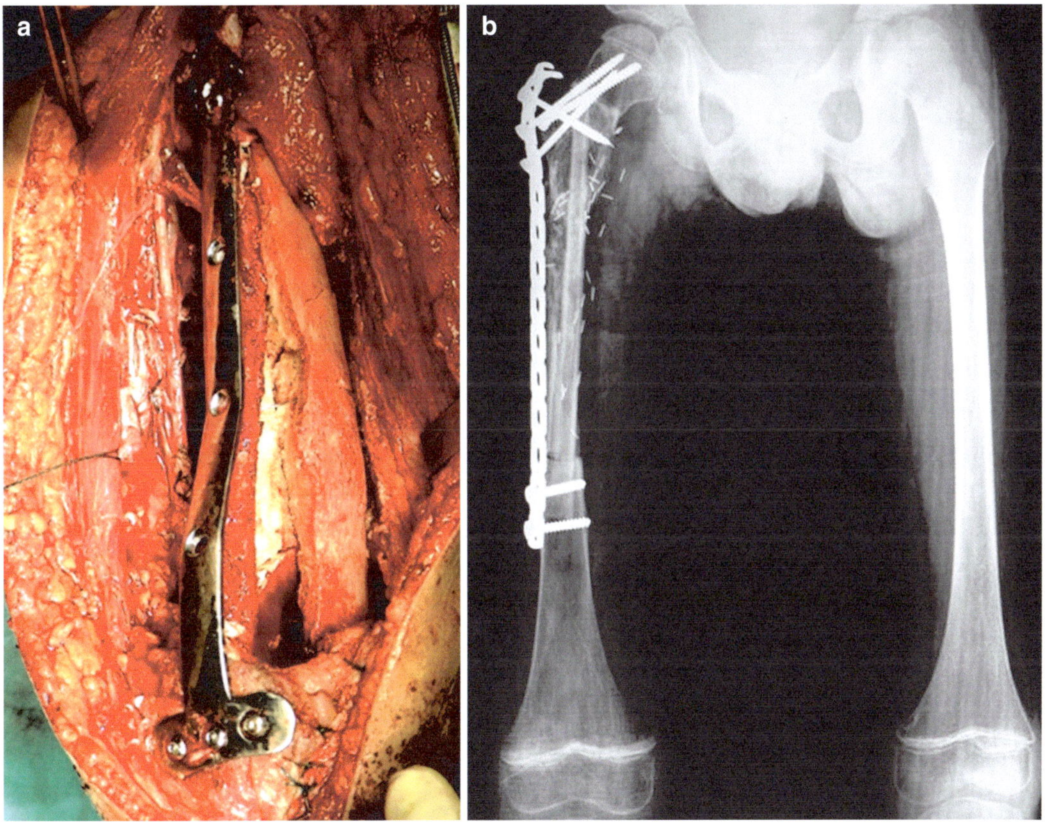

Fig. 9.12 Vascularized fibula with cryopreserved bone implanted and fixed with plate. (**a**) Clinical photos and (**b**) Xray

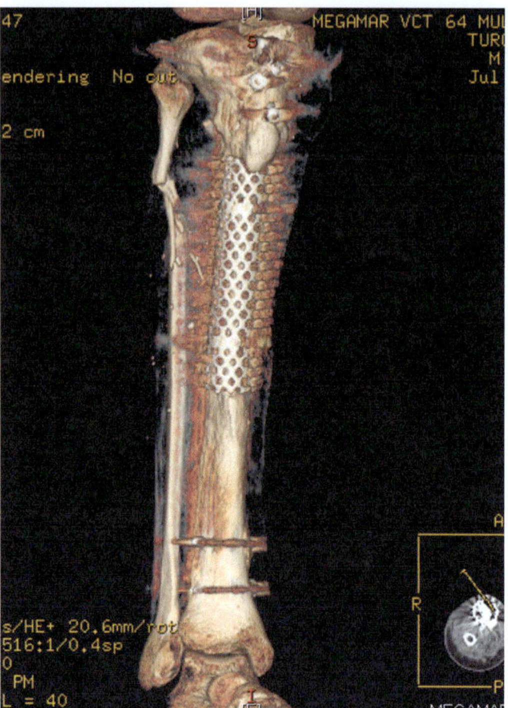

Fig. 9.13 3D computerized tomography scan of the bone at 6th month postoperatively

Conclusions

- Bone segment transfer is the first choice in resections because of chronic infections and traumatic bone loss.
- The current trend is the combined method (external fixator and intramedullary nail) to reduce the external fixator period.
- Acute shortening and relengthening technique should be preferred for the patients with bone loss of less than 7 cm and with good blood circulation of the foot.
- Segment transport methods should be reserved for patients with bone loss of more than 7 cm and with muscle weakness of the foot and ankle, as well as for patients who do not cooperate with the postoperative protocol. Furthermore, in patients with bone defect more than 10 cm, trifocal (two segment transport simultaneously) treatment should be preferred to shorten treatment time.

- Prolonged external fixators may lead to morbidities in patients receiving chemotherapy.
- Other methods are referred in case an adjuvant chemo- or radiotherapy is required, or the patient will not tolerate external fixator for other reasons.
- Vascularized bone grafts preferred after tumor resections to build immediate bone bridging.
- Titanium mesh, allograft, and intramedullary nail combination preserved for patients without any healthy vessel to anastomose vascularized bone/soft tissue flaps and/or insufficient bone stock for segment transfer.
- The idea for the vascularized fibula transfer and titanium cage procedures is based on "close and wrap up the "box" (surgical site) when the operation is finished."
- Lack of planning or encountered complications may end with union with deformity or limb length discrepancy.
- Mega bone defects are one of the most challenging issues of orthopedics. Even with absence of major complications, the majority of the cases take over a year to heal. Patients should be informed about the long-lasting treatment.

References

Gulsen M, Özkan C (2009) Angular shortening and delayed gradual distraction for the treatment of asymmetrical bone and soft tissue defects of tibia: a case series. J Trauma 66(5):E61

Kocaoglu M, Eralp L, Kilicoglu O, Burc H, Cakmak M (2004) Complications encountered during lengthening over an intramedullary nail. J Bone Joint Surg Am 86(11):2406–2411

Kocaoglu M, Eralp L, Rashid HU, Sen C, Bilsel K (2006) Reconstruction of segmental bone defects due to chronic osteomyelitis with use of an external fixator and an intramedullary nail. J Bone Joint Surg Am 88(10):2137–2145. doi:10.2106/jbjs.e.01152

Kucukkaya M, Armagan R, Kuzgun U (2009) The new intramedullary cable bone transport technique. J Trauma 23(7):531

Hiroyuki Tsuchiya and Norio Yamamoto

Contents

10.1 Introduction

Recently, distraction osteogenesis with an Ilizarov ring fixator or a Taylor spatial frame and callotasis with a unilateral fixator developed by de Bastiani have been widely adopted for the treatment of several orthopedic problems such as leg length discrepancy, deformity, nonunion, osteomyelitis, and congenital or acquired skeletal defects (De Bastiani et al. 1987; Ilizarov 1989a, b; Ilizarov and Green 1992). However, bone defects related to trauma, infection, or bone tumor have been treated with autografts, allografts, artificial bone substitutes, spacers, or prostheses. In cases of skeletal reconstruction, bone defects should ideally be repaired with living bone. Living bone that is provided by the distraction osteogenesis technique has the same strength and width as that of native bone. Moreover, the peripheral nerves, vessels, muscles, tendons, ligaments, and skin are also gradually lengthened in proportion with the lengthening of the bone.

In this chapter, the authors introduce applications of external fixators to bone tumor surgery.

10.2 Treatment of Benign Bone Tumors

For the treatment of deformity correction and limb length discrepancy caused by benign tumors, external fixators are extremely useful. For leg length discrepancy, distraction osteogenesis, as

H. Tsuchiya (✉) • N. Yamamoto
Department of Orthopedic Surgery, Graduate School
of Medical Science, Kanazawa University,
13-1 Takara-machi, Kanazawa 920-8641, Japan
e-mail: tsuchi@med.kanazawa-u.ac.jp

M. Kocaoğlu et al. (eds.), *Advanced Techniques in Limb Reconstruction Surgery*,
DOI 10.1007/978-3-642-55026-3_10, © Springer Berlin Heidelberg 2015

opposed to a contralateral shortening procedure, enables the preservation of body height and normalization of body proportions. Moreover, distraction osteogenesis avoids surgery on the unaffected limb and enables simultaneous correction of any associated deformity of the short limb. Closed osteotomy, acute correction, and internal fixation are conventionally used for deformity correction. However, acute correction is limited to the tolerance of both soft tissues and neurovascular elements. Conversely, in gradual distraction using a dynamic external fixator, the magnitude and complexity of the correctable deformity are almost unlimited.

For bone defects after tumor resection, many methods of reconstruction are possible. Bone grafts have limitations in length and strength, especially in children. Autografts require the sacrifice of a healthy organ even in children. Thus, we have used distraction osteogenesis to reconstruct defects. Bone regenerated by distraction osteogenesis provides biomechanical strength, stability, and resistance to infection.

We stress that external fixation is an effective technique for treating deformities and limb length discrepancies resulting from benign bone tumors. In this section, we introduce the treatment of deformity correction and limb length discrepancy caused by Ollier's disease, fibrous dysplasia, osteofibrous dysplasia, nonossifying fibroma, and multiple or solitary exostosis because these diseases are relatively common.

10.2.1 Ollier's Disease

Ollier's disease is a unilateral enchondromatosis of long bones. Disability results from leg length discrepancy and deformity. Angular deformities in the frontal plane lead to mechanical axis deviation of the lower limb and malposition of the joints. A normalized mechanical axis could prevent pathological fracture.

The conventional treatment for the enchondroma itself is curettage and bone grafting, which may result in severe deformities. Osteotomies are performed as often as necessary to correct these deformities. However, bone stabilization is difficult to obtain using internal devices. Accurate correction of the malposition and joint orientation are critical for normal function and to prevent joint degeneration.

To correct limb length discrepancy and deformities by distraction osteogenesis, an Ilizarov ring fixator or a Taylor spatial frame are extremely beneficial (D'angelo et al. 1996). Surgeons need to put wires or pins through the enchondroma because it usually spreads throughout the whole medullary cavity of bones. The authors recommend using extra wires or pins for sufficient stability.

It is still controversial whether distraction osteogenesis at the site of enchondroma causes malignant transformation. However, distraction osteogenesis has the possibility of treating the disease. With the use of distraction, abnormal cartilage is converted successfully into normal mature bone without curettage of the lesion (Jesus-Garcia et al. 2001). In our series, normalized area is reconverted into enchondroma with time. Even if distraction osteogenesis is performed at the enchondroma site, external fixation index is almost the same as distraction osteogenesis of normal bone (Figs. 10.1 and 10.2).

10.2.2 Fibrous Dysplasia

Fibrous dysplasia is an anomaly characterized by widening of the affected bone with cortical thinning and the presence of fibro-osseous tissue in the interior of the bone. Polyostotic fibrous dysplasia that is associated with autonomous endocrine hyperfunction and café au lait spots is known as the McCune-Albright syndrome.

Pathological fractures and deformities are common. Shepherd's crook deformity is a well-known progressive varus deformity with shortening of the femur. Valgus osteotomy, plating, and hip nailing are common surgical procedures for femoral lesions.

However, conventional treatment is curettage of the lesions and bone grafting, but the authors do not recommend this treatment. Curettage of fibro-osseous lesions causes massive bleeding and grafted bone is gradually absorbed. Curettage

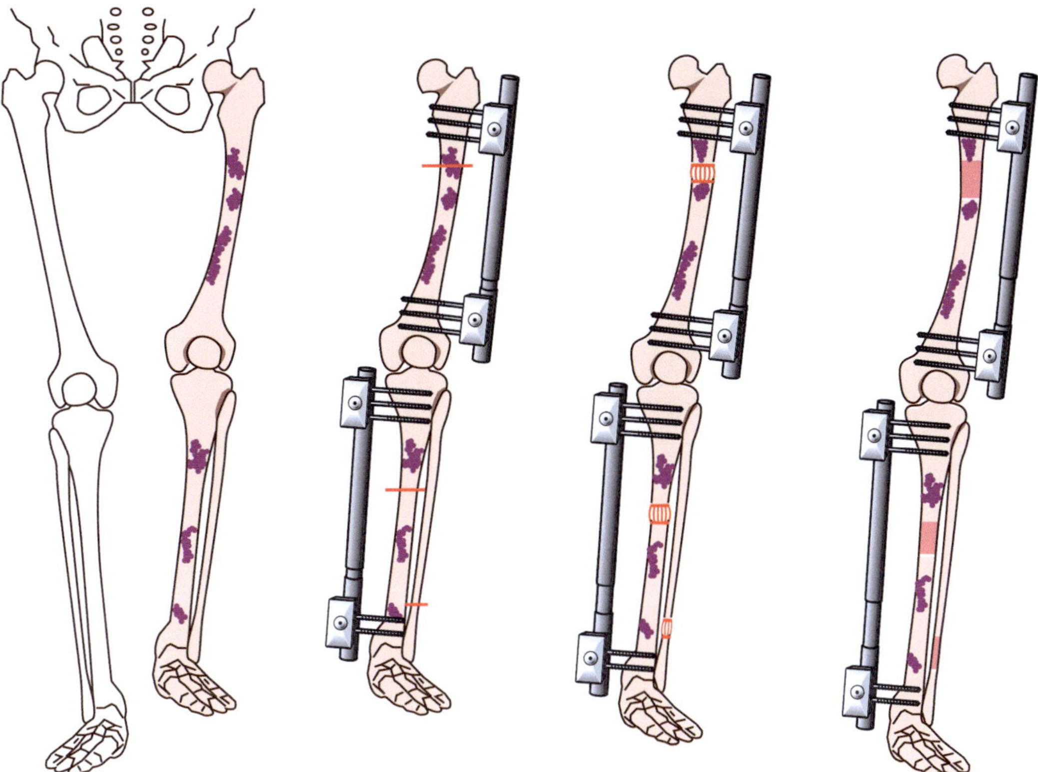

Fig. 10.1 A case of enchondromatosis with a simple leg length discrepancy. Ipsilateral femoral and tibial shortening were present. We performed simultaneous ipsilateral femoral and tibial lengthening using unilateral external fixators

of the lesions and bone grafting might lead to frequent recurrence of dysplastic bone.

Surgeons who treat patients with fibrous dysplasia need to consider the importance of the deformity correction but not of the fibrous dysplasia region itself. It is important to correct the deformity and to obtain a normal mechanical axis to prevent pathological fracture and deformity progression. Extension of fibrous dysplasia into the interior of the bone becomes quiescent with the cessation of growth.

Our recommended treatment consists of osteotomy and gradual deformity correction using an Ilizarov ring fixator or a Taylor spatial frame and mechanical axis realignment of the proximal part of the femur without internal fixation. Even at the site of fibrous dysplasia, bone formation is similar to normal bone.

For severe deformities at the femoral neck, curettage and cortical fibula bone grafts should be performed to prevent further deformity (Fig. 10.3).

10.2.3 Osteofibrous Dysplasia (Ossifying Fibroma)

Osteofibrous dysplasia is either the benign counterpart of a neoplastic process that produces an adamantinoma or the result of spontaneous regression of an adamantinoma. The lesion is most often found in the shaft of the tibia. This tumor actively grows during childhood and adolescence and then becomes quiescent with the cessation of growth.

Conventional treatment involves curettage and bone graft, but local recurrence is frequent, and

Fig. 10.2 A case of severe left lower limb deformity due to Ollier's disease. Radiograph of anteroposterior view of lower limbs before surgery (**a**); operative planning for the first surgery (**b**); in the first step, osteotomy and gradual deformity correction were performed on the femur with Taylor spatial frame (**c**); after removal of the Taylor spatial frame (**d**); in the second step, lengthening of the tibia and ankle mobilization were performed with Taylor spatial frame (**e**); after completion of the treatment (**f**)

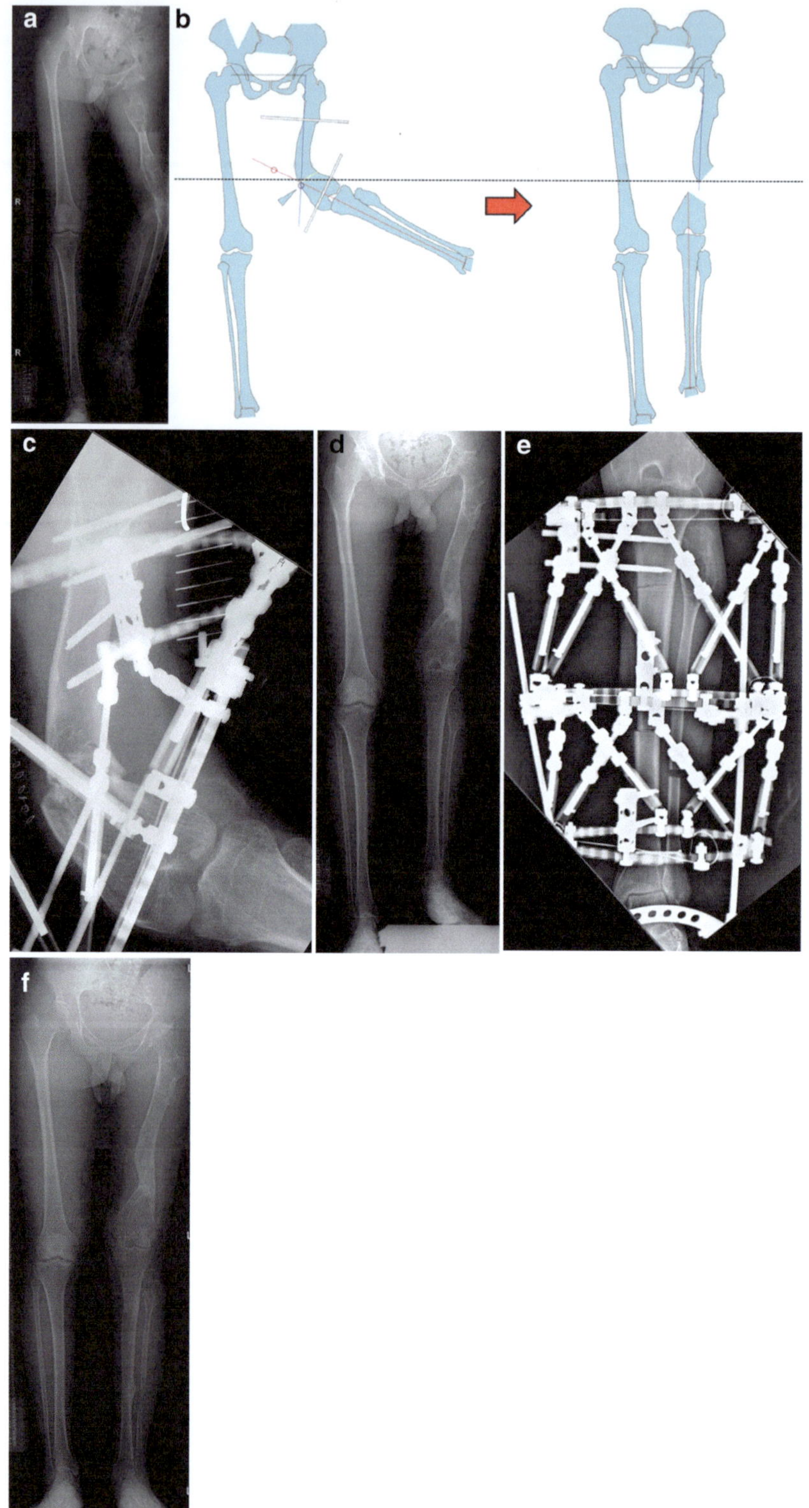

the cortex thins and expands with the bowing deformity. Curettage and bone grafting are likely to induce severe deformity and leg length discrepancy, especially in children under the age of 5 years, in addition to a high incidence of recurrence.

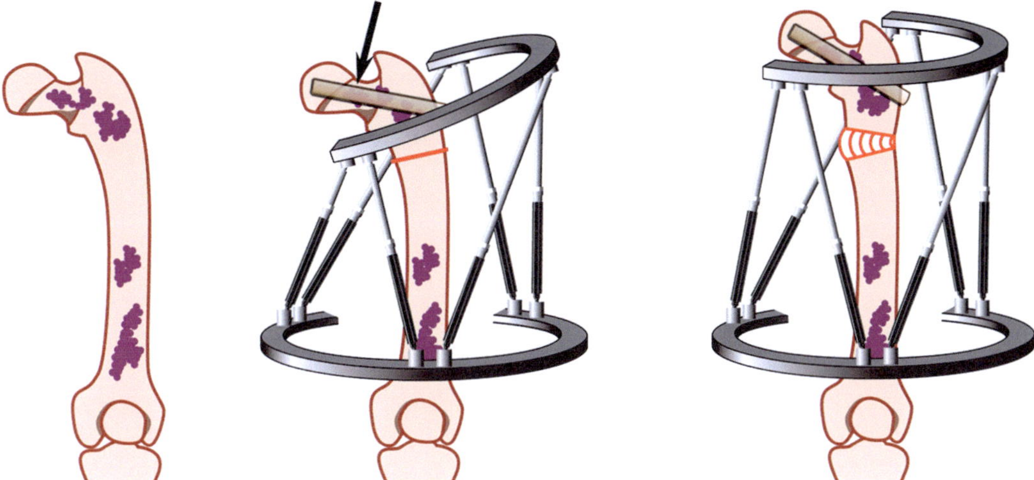

Fig. 10.3 A case of fibrous dysplasia with a cystic bone tumor lesion, pathological fracture, and varus deformity of the proximal femur (Shepherd's crook deformity). We performed tumor curettage, fibula bone graft, and deformity correction. *Black arrow* indicates grafted fibula

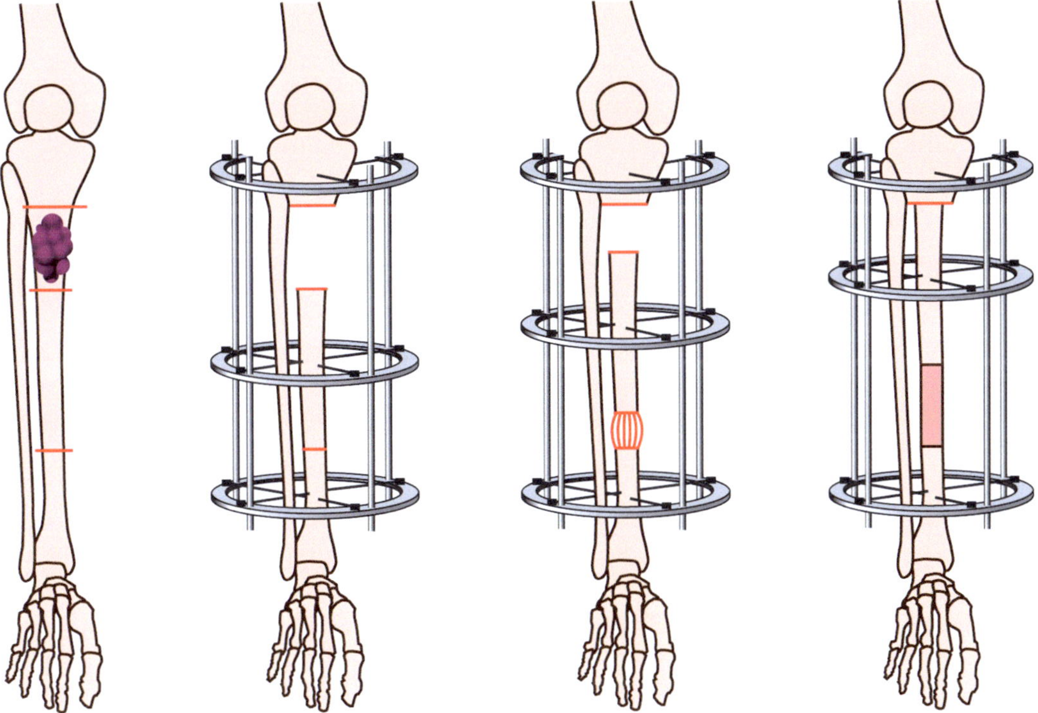

Fig. 10.4 A case of osteofibrous dysplasia with thinned and expanded tibial cortex with a bowing deformity. We performed bone transport after en bloc tumor resection to reconstruct the defect

With sufficient informed consent from the patient or persons in parental authority, we recommend en bloc tumor resection and reconstruction with bone transport because this treatment avoids complications and recurrence (Fig. 10.4) (Karita et al. 2004; Tsuchiya et al. 2004).

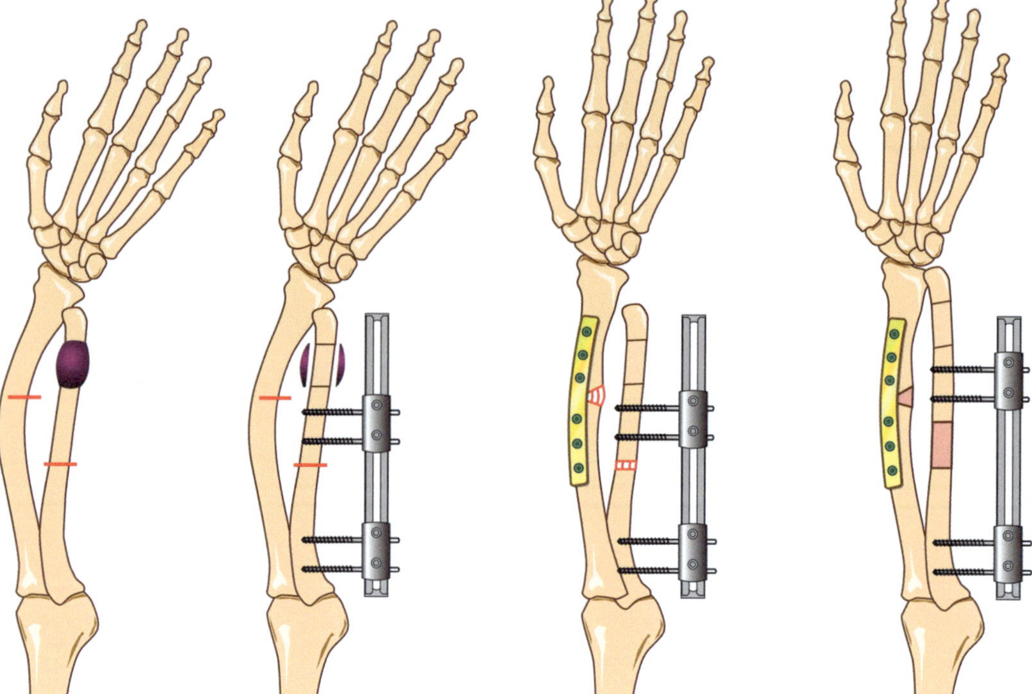

Fig. 10.5 A case of exostosis with shortening of the ulna, ulnar tilt of the distal epiphysis of the radius, and ulnar deviation of the hand. Radial head is dislocated. We performed ulnar tumor resection, radial deformity correction and internal fixation, and ulnar lengthening using a unilateral fixator. In proportion to ulnar lengthening, dislocation of the radial head was completely reduced. The ulna is overlengthened several millimeters to prevent recurrence of the deformity

10.2.4 Exostosis (Osteochondroma)

Multiple exostoses are a hereditary disorder of enchondral bone growth and result in asymmetrical retardation of longitudinal bone growth. The most common deformity of the forearm is a combination of relative shortening of the ulna, bowing of either or both forearm bones, increased ulnar tilt of the distal epiphysis of the radius, ulnar deviation of the hand, progressive ulnarward translocation of the carpus, and dislocation of the proximal radial head. Our treatment involves three steps: Step 1 is tumor resection, step 2 is osteotomy of the radius and ulna followed by a radial correction using internal fixation or an unilateral fixator, and step 3 is ulnar lengthening (Fig. 10.5).

10.3 Treatment of Malignant Bone Tumors

Tumor surgery for malignant bone tumors has evolved from amputation to limb-saving and joint-saving surgery (Tsuchiya et al. 1999b). Reconstruction can result in some difficulties such as an extensive defect, loss of healthy soft tissue, and the need for chemotherapy in some cases.

Biological reconstruction after tumor resection is extremely beneficial for the patients. Once the resected area is completely reconstructed from natural tissue, the patients do not need to worry about infection or breakage for their entire lifetime, unlike with a mega-prosthesis. The distraction osteogenesis technique for biological reconstruction is safe and provides the best qualified living bone. However, the main disadvantage of this technique is the mental burden and complications resulting from long-term external fixation.

Epiphyseal preservation and reconstruction using the distraction osteogenesis technique can provide excellent outcomes in selected cases resulting in sturdy reconstruction and reproduction of the native limb. The Ilizarov fixator or the Taylor spatial frame is used mainly for juxta-articular reconstruction, and a unilateral fixator is used for diaphyseal reconstruction or arthrodesis.

Limb lengthening is beneficial for growing children who suffer from leg shortening as a result of tumor excision or irradiation of the epiphyseal plate. Arthrodesis using distraction osteogenesis is also effective for the treatment of infected tumor prostheses. Furthermore, distraction osteogenesis for late limb length discrepancy and failure after limb-saving surgery appears to be similar to that of benign conditions because there is little influence of chemotherapy or irradiation and soft tissue is also repaired.

It is easier to manage benign and low-grade tumors because expertise and experience are needed for the treatment of high-grade tumors. In the latter case, accurate timing of antibiotic administration, change of dressing, and adjustment of lengthening rate are essential to achieve successful reconstruction.

10.4 Reconstruction After Excision of Malignant Tumor

10.4.1 Selection of Patients

The most important consideration for the use of this procedure is the indication. Patients with a low-grade tumor can be safely treated by distraction osteogenesis because they have no risk induced by chemotherapy and healthy soft tissues are well preserved, which leads to good bone regeneration. Both diaphyseal and metaphyseal defects are the most suitable to be reconstructed by distraction osteogenesis. Distraction osteogenesis enables joint preservation and provides excellent limb function. Patients with less than a 15 cm defect are good candidates for this procedure. However, patients with $a > 15$ cm defect can be treated in combination with an intramedullary nailing. The intramedullary nailing shortens the treatment period.

On the contrary, distraction osteogenesis in patients with a high-grade tumor requires expertise and experience. In such cases, accurate timing of antibiotic administration, change of dressing, and adjustment of lengthening rate are essential to achieve successful reconstruction during chemotherapy. However, once a physician obtains the necessary means, skill, or know-how, patients with a favorable chemotherapy response are also good candidates for this treatment because a good prognosis is expected.

10.4.2 Technique of Distraction Osteogenesis

Distraction osteogenesis is performed with an Ilizarov ring fixator, a Taylor spatial frame, or a unilateral fixator. In each case, the surgeons need to properly use these fixators, taking into consideration the location, deformity, and duration. We prefer to use four basic methods: simple lengthening, bone transport, shortening-distraction, and lengthening combined with intramedullary nailing. Intramedullary nailing is extremely helpful to reduce external fixation time. When primary intramedullary nailing is feasible before distraction, lengthening is performed over an intramedullary nail with either proximal or distal locking screws (primary nailing) (Fig. 10.6). Screws are placed on the unlocked side after distraction is complete as the external fixator maintains the length of the distraction. In some cases, intramedullary nailing is performed after the completion of distraction (delayed nailing) when primary nailing is difficult to apply (Tsuchiya et al. 1997, 1999a).

10.4.3 Principles of Reconstruction

Limb-saving surgery has become common in malignant tumor surgery. Preservation or restoration of the affected limb without endangering

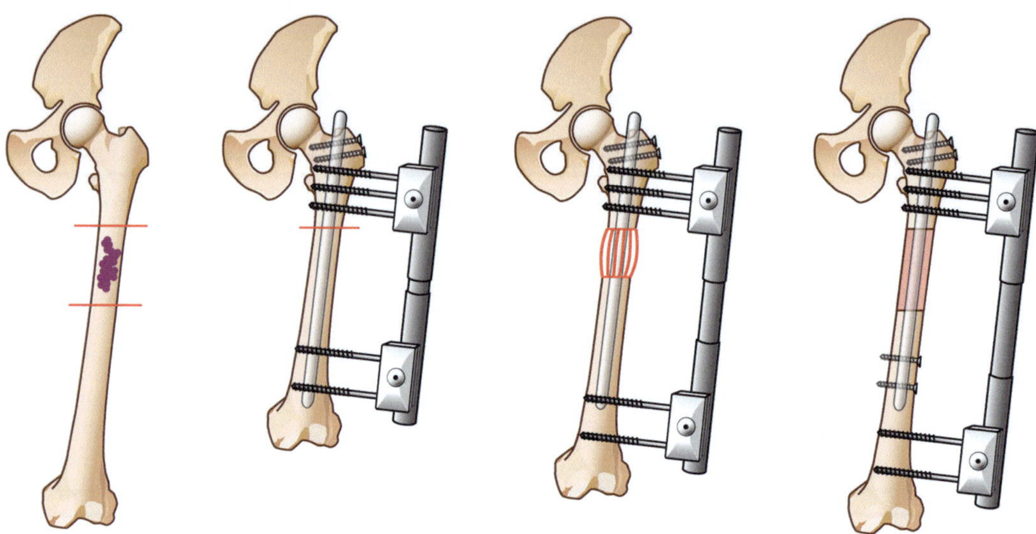

Fig. 10.6 A case of central low-grade osteosarcoma in the mid-femur. Marginal excision was performed and the defect was shortened. Shortening-distraction combined with intramedullary nailing (type 1 diaphyseal reconstruction) was performed. Transfixation screws in the distal femur are initially inserted. After completion of the distraction, the unilateral fixator was removed and transfixation screws were inserted

patients' lives is a recent subject of interest (Tsuchiya et al. 1999b).

Several modalities are available for the treatment of bone loss such as autografts, allografts, heat-treated recycling bones, biomaterials, prostheses, and distraction osteogenesis. Ideal bone reconstruction should combine resistance to infection, durability, long-lasting stability and biological affinity, and eventually good limb function (Tsuchiya et al. 1997). A characteristic of distraction osteogenesis is the regeneration of living bone together with surrounding soft tissues like the muscles, tendons, nerves, and skin. In 1989, to refine limb-saving surgery and provide natural limb, the linkage between distraction osteogenesis and primary reconstruction after massive tumor resection was established in our institute. Recently, several investigators reported the advantages (Tsuchiya et al. 1996, 1997, 1999a; Cara et al. 1993; Gonzalez-Herranz et al. 1995; Kapukaya et al. 2000; Millett et al. 2000; Ozaki et al. 1998; Said and el-Sherif 1995; Stoffelen et al. 1993; Tsuchiya and Tomita 2003) or disadvantages (Ozaki et al. 1998) of distraction osteogenesis for tumor surgery. The authors published a classification of reconstruction techniques comprising five types based on the location of the bone defect. Type 1 is diaphyseal reconstruction, type 2 is metaphyseal reconstruction, type 3 is epiphyseal reconstruction, type 4 is subarticular reconstruction, and type 5 is arthrodesis (Fig. 10.7) (Tsuchiya et al. 1997).

Tumor reconstruction by means of distraction osteogenesis consists of several steps: preconstruction of a frame, adequate tumor excision to prevent local recurrence, and osteotomy and distraction with or without chemotherapy. The distraction procedure is the same as that used for trauma or congenital cases. After adequate tumor excision, distraction osteogenesis can be applied safely and successfully with an Ilizarov fixator, a Taylor spatial frame or a unilateral fixator. Diaphyseal defects are simply treated by bone transport or a shortening-distraction procedure with or without an intramedullary nail. We usually use the shortening-distraction procedure when the defect is less than 10 cm in the femur or 5 cm in the tibia. Careful attention should be paid for nerve injury and circulatory disturbance. Difficulty of wound closure and invagination of soft tissues are also limiting factors to perform shortening of the defect.

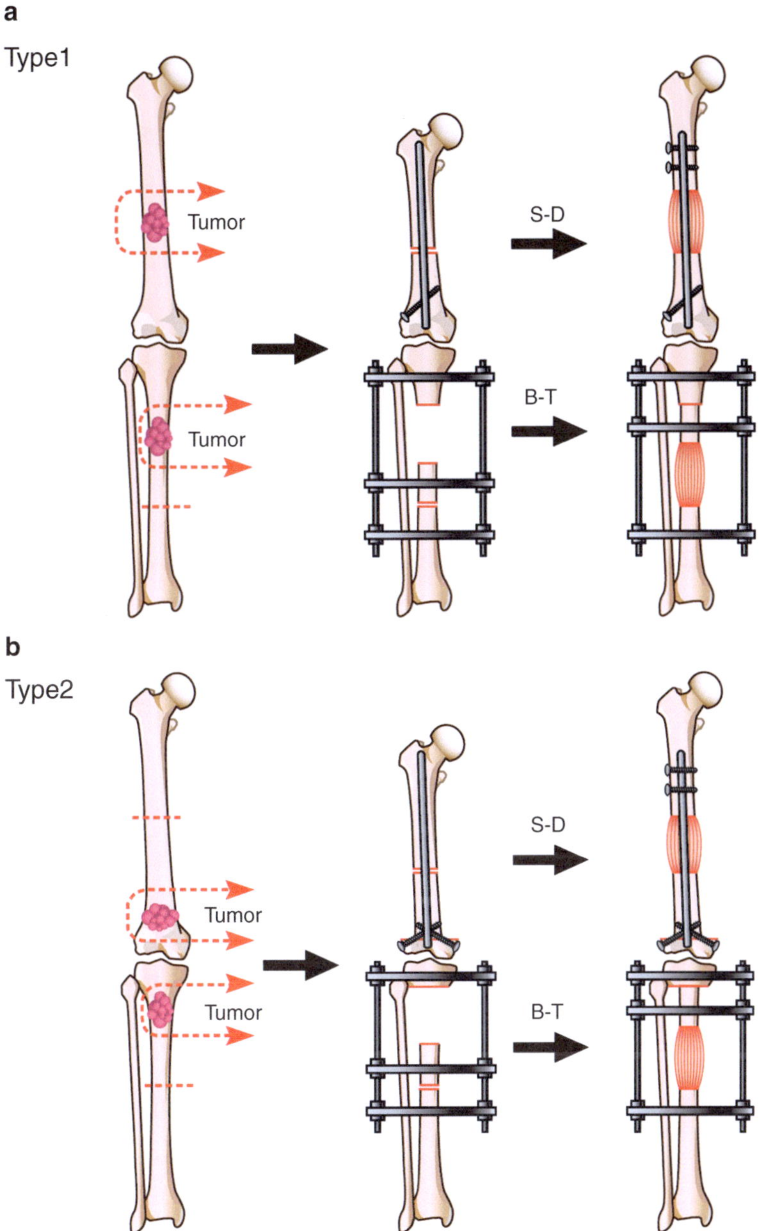

Fig. 10.7 The classification of reconstruction by distraction osteogenesis using bone transport or shortening-distraction: type 1, diaphyseal reconstruction (**a**); type 2, metaphyseal reconstruction (**b**); type 3, epiphyseal reconstruction (**c**); type 4, subarticular reconstruction (**d**); and type 5, arthrodesis (**e**)

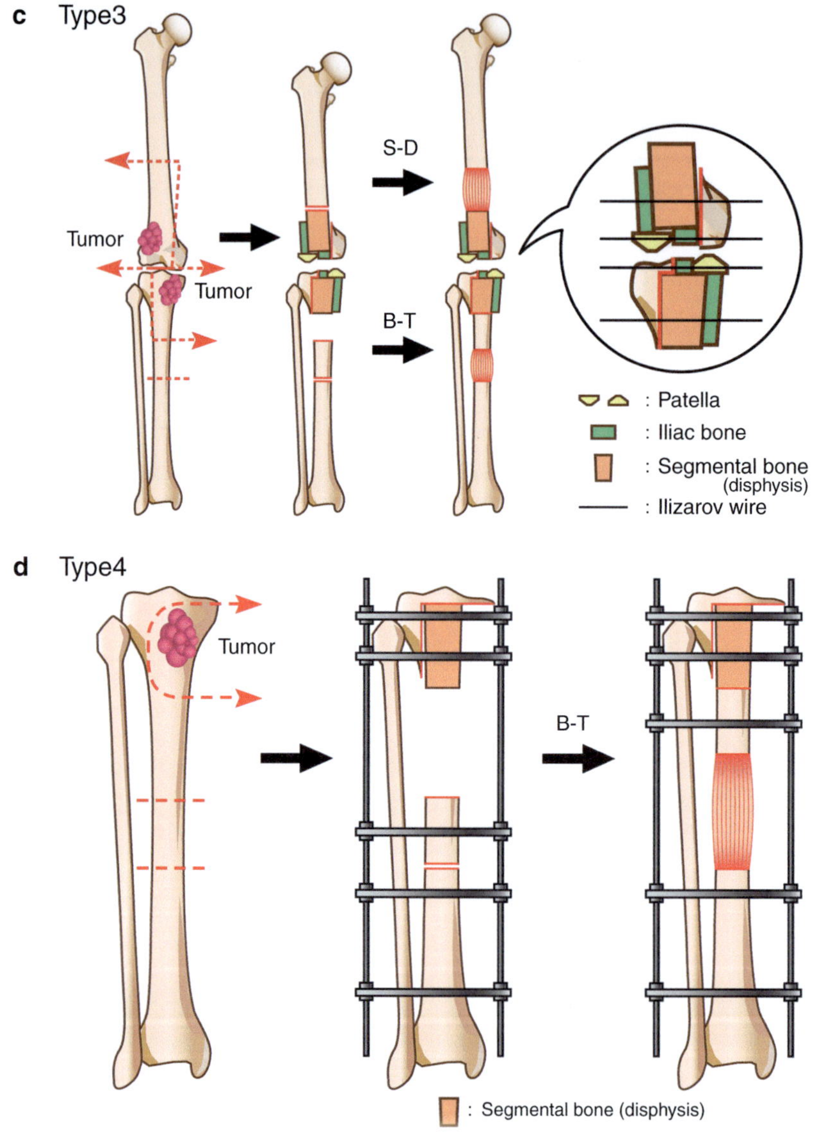

Fig. 10.7 (continued)

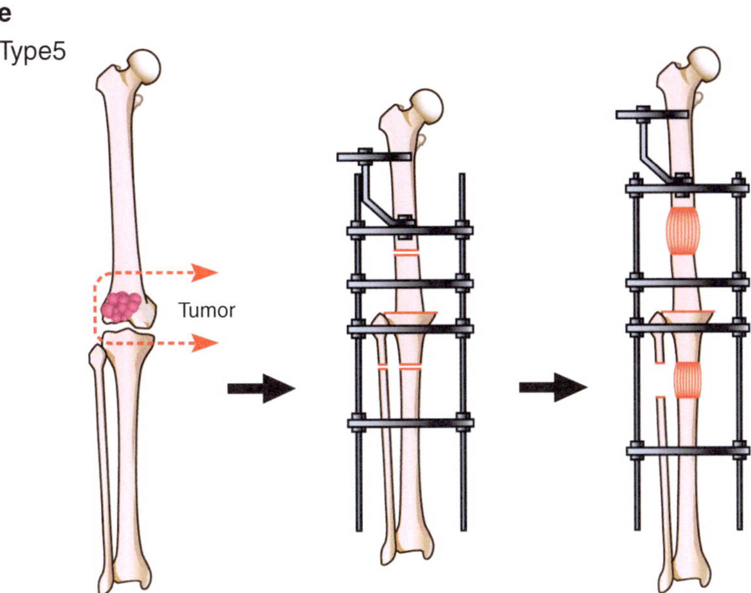

Fig. 10.7 (continued)

For postoperative rehabilitation, weight bearing while using crutches and motion exercises of the joint are initiated after subsidence of bleeding and wound pain. In knee joints when the patella tendon is reattached to its original place with a spike washer, the authors give a 3-week interval between surgery and joint motion exercise.

Low-grade malignant tumors such as adamantinoma, chondrosarcoma, parosteal osteosarcoma, or low-grade central osteosarcoma are usually treated with a wide or marginal excision. However, chemotherapy is not performed for low-grade malignant tumors. Sometimes a healthy soft tissue has to be sacrificed during tumor excision and such a loss may lead to poor blood supply for regeneration.

High-grade malignant tumors such as osteosarcoma, Ewing's sarcoma, and MFH are usually treated with a wide or radical resection accompanied by loss of healthy soft tissue. In most cases, chemotherapy is performed pre- and postoperatively, sometimes in conjunction with radiotherapy. The clinical effects of chemotherapy and radiation on bone formation are still unclear, but may be negative (Tsuchiya 2003; Tsuchiya and Tomita 2003).

With the support of caffeine-assisted chemotherapy, a maximum amount of healthy soft tissue can be preserved. In our series, good bone formation is achieved by means of an intentional marginal procedure that allows a maximum of residual healthy soft tissue to remain, which surrounds the resected area. In addition, important structures such as epiphysis and ligaments for joint stability can be preserved (Tsuchiya et al. 1999b). Epiphyseal sparing is the key to providing natural limbs because epiphyseal sparing and reconstruction with distraction osteogenesis is the only chance for patients to restore the affected limb to almost normal.

The indication of epiphyseal preservation is decided by tumor extension on MRI and response to preoperative chemotherapy. Epiphysis can be preserved when there is no or little involvement of the tumor on MRI and a remarkable response of preoperative chemotherapy is observed. The effectiveness of chemotherapy is evaluated using plain x-ray, angiography, MRI, and thallium scintigraphy. If the results of two or more imaging examinations showed effectiveness of the treatment, the patient is considered to have a remarkable response.

10.4.4 Postoperative Care

Distraction osteogenesis involved several steps: stable fixation of the fragments; bone division; treatment consisting of latency, distraction, and consolidation; assessment of regeneration; and removal of the frame. Distraction is started 7–14 days after osteotomy at 0.5 mm twice daily or 0.25 mm four times daily. This is later reduced to zero when the callus formation is delayed or impaired, or increased to 1.5 mm per day when the callus formation is likely to consolidate prematurely. In cases with significantly poor callus formation, compression and distraction of a moving segment (accordion maneuver) is performed. In rare cases, iliac bone graft to the lengthened site is applied after the failure of these procedures.

The external fixator is removed when consolidation is considered to be sufficient. Usually, consolidation takes one and a half to two times as long as distraction. After removal of the external fixator, a cast or an orthosis is applied for approximately 4 weeks.

10.5 Pitfalls and Common Errors

With regard to complications, delayed consolidation, fracture, deep infection, skin invagination, nerve palsy, skin necrosis, deformity, premature consolidation, and joint subluxation or dislocation might be encountered during or after treatment. At present, it is not possible to avoid all complications in limb-saving tumor surgery regardless of what type of reconstructive method is used. However, the authors believe that distraction osteogenesis is most likely to be successful for complications that are caused by surgical treatment because living bone is easier to handle than dead bone or prostheses. These complications are successfully overcome by surgical interventions or conservative treatment.

In conclusion, the authors would like to emphasize that biological reconstruction is always preferable for massive bone loss after tumor excision. Joint preservation and bone regeneration by means of distraction osteogenesis constitute a highly conservative limb-saving surgery.

References

Cara J, Forriol F, Canadell J (1993) Bone lengthening after conservative oncologic surgery. J Pediatr Orthop B 2(1):57

D'angelo G, Petas N, Donzelli O (1996) Lengthening of the lower limbs in Ollier's disease: problems related to surgery. Chir Organi Mov 81(3):279

De Bastiani G, Aldegheri R, Renzi-Brivio L, Trivella G (1987) Limb lengthening by callus distraction (callotasis). J Pediatr Orthop 7(2):129–134

Gonzalez-Herranz P, Burgos-Flores J, Ocete-Guzman JG, Lopez-Mondejar JA, Amaya S (1995) The management of limb-length discrepancies in children after treatment of osteosarcoma and Ewing's sarcoma. J Pediatr Orthop 15(5):561–565

Ilizarov GA (1989a) The tension-stress effect on the genesis and growth of tissues. Part I. The influence of stability of fixation and soft-tissue preservation. Clin Orthop Relat Res 238:249–281

Ilizarov GA (1989b) The tension-stress effect on the genesis and growth of tissues: Part II. The influence of the rate and frequency of distraction. Clin Orthop Relat Res 239:263–285

Ilizarov GA, Green SA (1992) The transosseous osteosynthesis: theoretical and clinical aspects of the regeneration and growth of tissue. Springer, Berlin

Jesus-Garcia R, Bongiovanni JC, Korukian M, Boatto H, Seixas MT, Laredo J (2001) Use of the Ilizarov external fixator in the treatment of patients with Ollier's disease. Clin Orthop Relat Res 382:82–86

Kapukaya A, Subasi M, Kandiya E, Ozates M, Yilmaz F (2000) Limb reconstruction with the callus distraction method after bone tumor resection. Arch Orthop Trauma Surg 120(3–4):215–218

Karita M, Tsuchiya H, Sakurakichi K, Tomita K (2004) Osteofibrous dysplasia treated with distraction osteogenesis: a report of two cases. J Orthop Sci 9(5):516–520. doi:10.1007/s00776-004-0812-5

Millett PJ, Lane JM, Paletta GA Jr (2000) Limb salvage using distraction osteogenesis. Am J Orthop (Belle Mead NJ) 29(8):628–632

Ozaki T, Nakatsuka Y, Kunisada T, Kawai A, Dan'ura T, Naito N, Inoue H (1998) High complication rate of reconstruction using Ilizarov bone transport method in patients with bone sarcomas. Arch Orthop Trauma Surg 118(3):136–139

Said GZ, el-Sherif EK (1995) Resection-shortening-distraction for malignant bone tumours. A report of two cases. J Bone Joint Surg Br 77(2):185–188

Stoffelen D, Lammens J, Fabry G (1993) Resection of a periosteal osteosarcoma and reconstruction using the Ilizarov technique of segmental transport. J Hand Surg Br 18(2):144–146

Tsuchiya H (2003) Distraction osteogenesis for treatment of bone loss in the lower extremity (Letter to the editor). J Orthop Sci 8(6):882–884. doi:10.1007/s00776-003-0728-5

Tsuchiya H, Tomita K (2003) Distraction osteogenesis for treatment of bone loss in the lower extremity. J Orthop Sci 8(1):116–124. doi:10.1007/s007760300020

Tsuchiya H, Tomita K, Shinokawa Y, Minematsu K, Katsuo S, Taki J (1996) The Ilizarov method in the management of giant-cell tumours of the proximal tibia. J Bone Joint Surg Br 78(2):264–269

Tsuchiya H, Tomita K, Minematsu K, Mori Y, Asada N, Kitano S (1997) Limb salvage using distraction osteogenesis. A classification of the technique. J Bone Joint Surg Br 79(3):403–411

Tsuchiya H, Kitano S, Tomita K (1999a) Periarticular reconstruction using distraction osteogenesis after en bloc tumor resection. Arch Am Acad Orthop Surg 2:68–75

Tsuchiya H, Tomita K, Mori Y, Asada N, Yamamoto N (1999b) Marginal excision for osteosarcoma with caffeine assisted chemotherapy. Clin Orthop Relat Res 358:27–35

Tsuchiya H, Sakurakichi K, Yamashiro T, Watanabe K, Inoue Y, Yamamoto N, Tomita K (2004) Bone transport with frozen devitalized bone: an experimental study using rabbits and a clinical application. J Orthop Sci 9(6):619–624. doi:10.1007/s00776-004-0836-x

Joint Contracture Management with External Fixators

İbrahim Tuncay and Leonid Solomin

Contents

İ. Tuncay (✉)
Department of Orthopaedic Surgery and
Traumatology, Bezmialem Vakif University, Istabul,
Turkey
e-mail: ituncay@gmail.com

L. Solomin, MD, PhD
Department of Orthopaedic Surgery and
Traumatology, R.R.Vreden Russian Research
Institute of Traumatology and Orthopedics,
St.Petersburg, Russia

11.1   Knee Flexion Contractures

Knee contractures could be disabling and can result in increased energy expenditure during the gait cycle. Most contractures are because of the congenital syndromes; they may also occur with disorders such as arthrogryposis, sacral agenesis, tibial dysplasias, and hemimelias. These are rare conditions, often associated with permanent muscle atrophy, joint fibrosis, and impaired distal function (Devalia et al. 2007). When evaluating sagittal knee deformity, it is important to differentiate between dynamic contracture, due to tight hamstrings, and fixed flexion deformity, which may or may not include tight hamstrings, depending upon the etiology.

Many surgical procedures have been described to treat fixed flexion knee deformity: lengthening of the hamstrings, posterior capsulotomy, epiphysiodesis of the distal femoral growth plate, femoral and tibial osteotomies, femoral shortening, or arthrodesis (Phillips and Audet 1990; Abraham et al. 1977; Zimmerman et al. 1982). Soft tissue release may be complicated by peroneal palsy, knee subluxation, hyperextension, skin necrosis, and recurrence (Herzenberg et al. 1994). Treatment depends on the deformity severity (Hosny and Fadel 2008).

It is important to recognize that treatment of knee joint stiffness is quite a complicated problem and it is not always possible to solve it by

M. Kocaoğlu et al. (eds.), *Advanced Techniques in Limb Reconstruction Surgery*,
DOI 10.1007/978-3-642-55026-3_11, © Springer Berlin Heidelberg 2015

Table 11.1 Groups of patients with knee joint stiffness and its treatment

Groups	Reason for stiffness	Clinical/laboratory data	Treatment
I	(a) Aftermath of plaster immobilization of fractures of the femur; less frequently, fixing of the knee by bandaging the fractures of the lower leg (b) Complication of lengthening of the femur (extension stiffness) or lower leg (flexion stiffness)	The stiffness is not associated with a cicatricial process in the knee joint; there are no rough unions or malunions between muscle and bone (myofasciodeses) Conservative treatment, including redressment attempts over 2–3 months, have failed	Passive–active development of movement using an external fixation device
II	Aftermath of inflammatory process in the knee joint or intra-articular fracture	The femur muscles are intact or have no marked secondary fibrous changes or atrophy. The points of pathological fixation of the muscles to the femur are not available or not marked. A cicatricial process occurs in the knee joint cavity and para-articular tissues	Arthroscopic release of the knee joint with subsequent passive–active development of movement using an external fixation device
III	United fractures of the distal third and distal part of the femur	The stiffness is not associated with a cicatricial process in the knee joint or it is not marked and is secondary in character. Marked signs of myofasciodesis: cicatricial union of muscles and tendons with bone, union of tissues	"Semiclosed" with a local process or open myolysis with reconstruction of the muscles sliding. If required, release of the knee joint. Subsequent development of movement in the knee joint using an external fixation device
IV	United open fracture, after extensive injury of the soft tissues of the distal femoral muscle; osteomyelitis in remission	The stiffness is associated with a cicatricial process in the para-articular tissues; polylocal myofasciodeses	Open arthrolysis, myolysis with reconstruction of the muscles sliding with subsequent passive–active development of movement using an external fixation device
V	Malunions and nonunions of the distal third and distal part of the femur	The stiffness is associated with a cicatricial process in the para-articular tissues; polylocal myofasciodeses	One-stage operative treatment: Open arthrolysis, myolysis with reconstruction of the muscles sliding; rigid bone fragments fixation with subsequent passive–active development of movement using an external fixation device Two-stage treatment (is more preferable): The first step is bone union with restoration of an anatomical axis of a segment (even at shortening kept). The second stage is open arthrolysis, myolysis with reconstruction of the muscles sliding with subsequent passive–active development of movement using an external fixation device

external fixation only (Ilizarov et al. 1979). Preoperative examination includes electromyography, ultrasonography, computed tomography, magnetic resonance imaging, and particularly contrast roentgenography of the muscles (Ilizarov 1999). Five groups of patients are identified according to clinical situation (Table 11.1).

11.1.1 Soft Tissue Correction with External Fixators

Severe flexion contractures of the knee are a major obstacle to functional ambulation and weight bearing. Such contractures are particularly common in pediatric patients especially in arthrogryposis, congenital pterygium contractures, and multiple other congenital and acquired problems. Management of these deformities are quite challenging (Hosny and Fadel 2008; DelBello and Watts 1996; Heydarian et al. 1984). Gradual correction of the deformity has been reported previously using various external fixators (Herzenberg et al. 1994; Gillen et al. 1996; Ilizarov 1990; Damsin and Ghanem 1996; Saleh et al. 1989). Several authors have used an Ilizarov circular fixator (Damsin and Ghanem 1996), a monolateral fixator (Herzenberg et al. 1994), hinged distraction apparatus (Saleh et al. 1989), or computer software-based fixators.

"Reconstruction of the muscles sliding" involves various variants and modifications of operations to mobilize and reconstruct the quadriceps (Ebraheim et al. 1993; Paley 2002). Lengthening of the distal tendon of the quadriceps in adults is undesirable as it will result in restricted active extension of the lower leg. Besides, external fixation allows a gradual increase in flexion of the lower leg to the necessary angle in the postoperative period (Window 11.1).

Window 11.1

Apart from the indicators given in Table 11.1, it is necessary to take into account:
1. The degree and duration of the stiffness and the patient's age.
2. The patient's attitude to treatment and his/her desire to restore the amplitude of the knee joint movement. Some patients insist on the maximum possible restoration of joint movement, for others restoration of 30–45 % of movement amplitude is sufficient for their social rehabilitation. However, 90° of flexion is usually accepted functional level.
3. The intensity of changes to the articulating surface of the femur. For example, in exten-

sion stiffness, a 40 % shortening of the belly of the rectus and median muscles due to their atrophy and fibrous changes prejudices the possibility of restoration of full active extension of the lower leg.
4. The presence and characteristics of a chronic inflammatory process of the femur or knee joint.
5. The presence of another orthopedic pathology: nonunions or deformities, including shortening of the femur or lower leg.

If extension stiffness occurs during femur lengthening, especially during formation of a regenerate in the distal third of the segment and the closed manipulation failed, external fixation can be used. For this purpose, a transosseous Ilizarov module is mounted on the lower leg (Fig. 11.1a) or the module is based on two half-pins and a wire (Fig. 11.1b). The module is connected by a hinge subsystem to the basic support. This approach should be used if extension stiffness forms during treatment of femoral fractures, specially open injuries to the distal third of the segment. This approach ensures that the emergence of rough cicatricial unions of tendons and muscles with the bone in the place of the fracture is avoided (Trick 11.1).

Trick 11.1

In most cases, all supports of the device fixing the femur are located perpendicular to the anatomical (mid-diaphyseal) axis of the femoral bone. Accordingly, the distal basic ring (as well as all supports) is not parallel to the knee joint plane. Therefore, to install axial hinges, an additional support fixed at the necessary angle to the distal basic support of the femur must be introduced into the assembly. Another possibility is to use complex hinges, one part serving for fixation to the distal basic support of the femur device and the other the axial hinge itself.

11.1.1.1 Surgical Technique with Ilizarov Circular Fixator

For closed reduction of lower leg dislocations, the first stage involves mounting a transosseous module based on wires or a hybrid module (Fig. 11.1) on the femur. A second module that

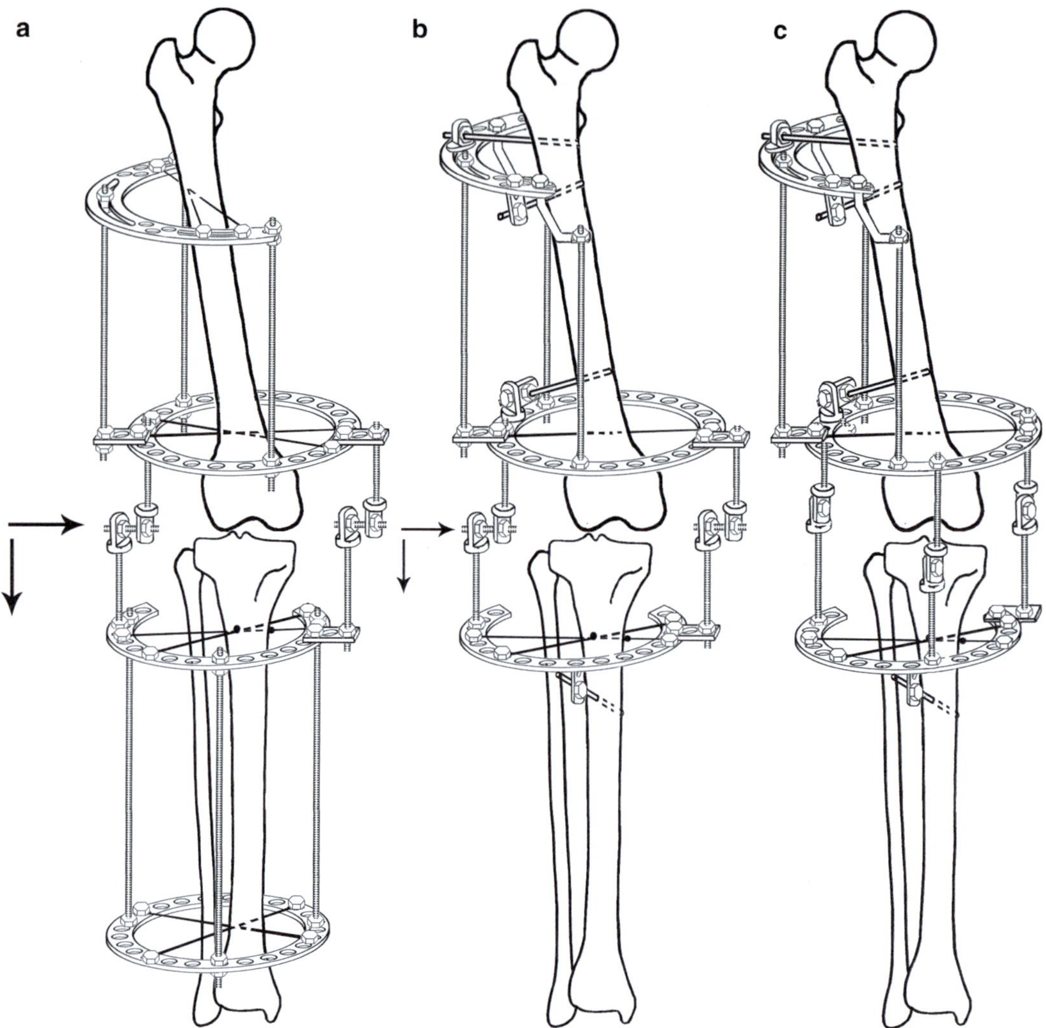

Fig. 11.1 (**a–c**) Schemes for an Ilizarov device (**a**) and a combined (hybrid) device (**b**) for reduction of the lower leg. The external supports of the module fixed to the femur are located parallel to the axis of the femoral condyles. Distraction starts on the 3rd to the 5th day at a rate of 0.25 mm six to eight times a day. The distraction rate is decreased if pain or signs of hyperextension of the great vessels and nerves occur. In lateral (external, internal) dislocations and subluxations, the distraction first must be uniform on all three hinges. After radiographic confirmation of the presence of the necessary diastasis for unhindered movement of the lower leg in the horizontal plane, the subsystem connecting the modules is remounted. The remounting depends on the type of dislocation: anterior, posterior, medial, or lateral. After reduction of the dislocation, the knee joint is fixed in the mid-physiological position for 2–3 weeks. After that the device can be used to develop movements in the knee joint (**c**)

can also be based on wires or a hybrid module is mounted on the lower leg. A hinge-distraction system is installed between the modules. If the dislocation of the shin is a complication of femur lengthening, an additional transosseous module is mounted on the lower leg and connected by a hinge subsystem to the basic frame.

One of the conditions for successful external fixation for knee joint stiffness is to use the reference positions described in the atlas for insertion of transosseous elements.

The second mandatory condition of configuration of the device for increasing knee joint ROM is installation of axial hinges strictly according to an axis of rotation of a knee joint (Fig. 11.2).

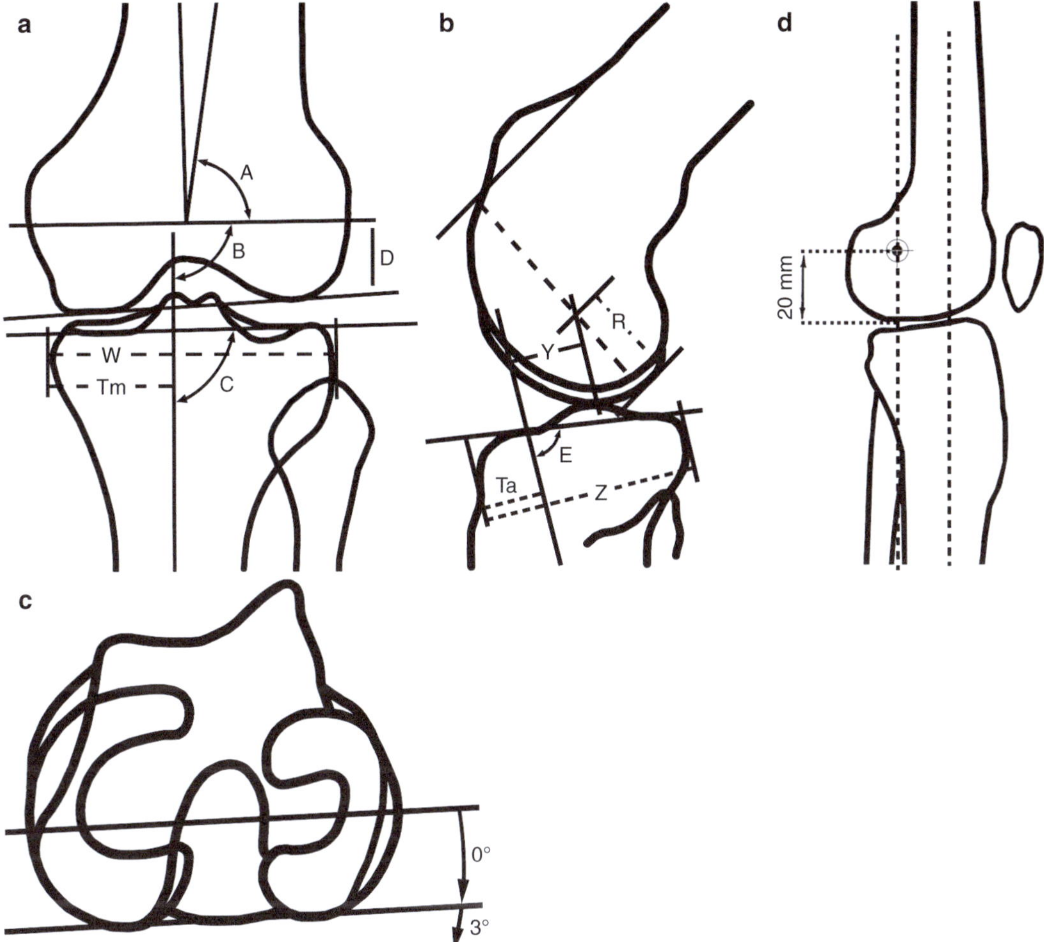

Fig. 11.2 (**a–d**) Orientation of the axis of knee flexion–extension in frontal (**a**), sagittal (**b**), and transverse (**c**) planes. Axial hinges are installed between the transosse-ous modules fixing the femur and the lower leg 2 cm from the joint surface and at the junction of the middle and posterior thirds of the femoral condyle (**d**)

Along with it there is a widely accepted opinion that movements in a knee joint have more complex trajectory than it can be provided by the one-axial hinges. The trajectory of movements in a knee joint can be presented as superposition of points on certain segments of arches of a circle of femoral bone condyles and segments on condyles of a tibial bone. Due to a difference of radiuses, lengths of arches of condyles of femoral bone and segments of tibial condyle movement in a knee joint are carried out on several trajectories with change of the centers of rotation. Thus, the trajectory of movement in a knee joint represents a complex curve, which is differ-ent for external and internal condyles. This provides a rotational component of moving (Iwaki et al. 2000) (Fig. 11.3). Therefore, the use of the devices having the virtual hinge, for example, hexapods, is perspective for knee joint stiffness treatment.

The formation of persistent flexion stiffness of the knee joint that does not respond to conservative treatment can be a complication of lengthening of the lower leg. The lack of loading on the extremity can negatively affect the distraction regenerate; thus, the stiffness needs to be eliminated as soon as possible. For this purpose, a transosseous module is mounted on the femur as

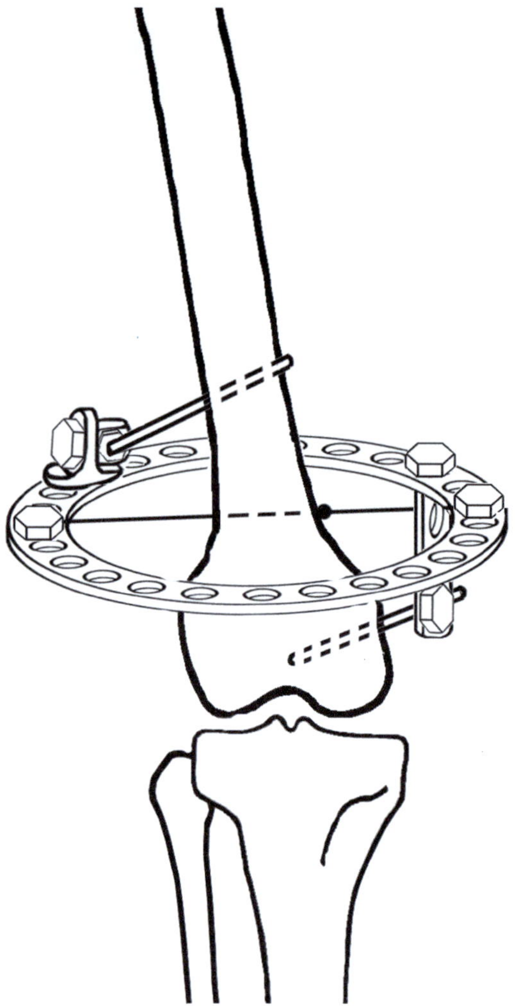

Fig. 11.3 Additional supports for the femur at lower leg lengthening

shown in Fig. 11.1a, or a ring support based on a wire and two half-pins is used (Fig. 11.3).

If patellofemoral synostosis or fibrous union of the patella with the femoral bone has occurred, open or arthroscopic mobilization is required. Extension stiffness of the knee joint is frequently present together with a nonunion, deformity, defect, or shortening of the femur in clinical practice. Simultaneous restoration of the anatomy and function of the injured extremity is the priority in planning the rehabilitation of the patient. At the same time, the operation for single-stage restoration of the knee joint function must be performed with the participation of a sur-

geon with experience of such interventions. Otherwise, the treatment should be divided into stages.

A single-stage operation to treat a traumatic injury simultaneously with mobilization of the knee joint involves the following:

1. In angular and rotational deformity exceeding 15–20°, a shortening of 20–40 mm, osteotomy is recommended with subsequent gradual correction of the deformity.
2. In hypertrophic defect, pseudoarthroses and anatomical shortening of the femur by 2–3 cm, microdistraction is performed to eliminate the inequality in the lengths of the extremities and to restore the anatomy of the bone simultaneously with restoration of the knee joint movement.
3. If external fixation of a nonunion of the femur involves an intervention with an open stage (removal of a metal structure, osteoplasty), it is combined with an operation to mobilize the knee joint.
4. In atrophic nonunions of the femur and shortening of the segment by 40 mm, the bone fragments are openly reduced using, according to the indications, osteoplasty, and corticotomy is performed with osteoclasia of the femoral bone to eliminate inequality in the lengths of the extremities (Kornilov et al. 1992).
5. The operation to treat shortening of a lower extremity that is accompanied by severe stiffness of the knee joint after malunion of intra-articular fractures not more than 1.5 years after trauma starts with surgery to the knee joint. The congruity of the joint surfaces is restored and the joint is mobilized. The second stage involves lengthening of the segment (Reutov et al. 2000).

In replacement of a segmental defect of the femur by the Ilizarov method, operative approaches to improve the function of the knee joint must be postponed at least until adaptation of the transposed fragment to the basic fragment and their stabilization. Arthrolysis and myolysis can be performed in a single step with open adaptation of the transposed and basic bone fragments. Multiple solid myofasciodeses, filling the knee joint cavity with healing tissue, and osteomyelitis favor a two-stage treatment for restoration of the weight-bearing ability of the extremity and then improve knee joint function.

After closed operations the knee joint is stabilized in the position achieved by maximum elimination of the stiffness. However, to reduce pain, we have to reduce the position in the joint achieved by the end of the operation by 30–50 %. It often happens that after open arthrolysis and myolysis, to avoid excessive skin stretching, the skin is taken in with the knee joint flexed less than what was achieved during the operation. To reduce the risk of soft tissue necrosis after surgery, the knee joint is stabilized in a position that ensures good blood supply to the wound edges. If there is a marked cicatricial process occurring in the area of the knee joint, the knee is stabilized in a position close to full extension.

A diastasis of 5–6 mm is created between the joint surfaces in two or three stages. It is important to note that due to the flexure of the transosseous elements, the amount of separation on hinges will not correspond to the joint space. Therefore, the effectiveness of the distraction should be monitored radiographically. Radiographic monitoring of the installation of the axial hinges is also necessary.

On the second or third day after closed osteosynthesis and after arthroscopic release, gradually increasing flexion (extension in the presence of extension stiffness) of the lower leg starts by means of a swivel hinge at an average rate of 2–6° per day in four to six stages. The rate is reduced if pain occurs or if there are signs of irritation of the great vessels and nerves. The manipulations must not cause any pain. The evaluation as to whether the amount of movement of the swivel hinge causes no pain must be made in the morning.

After flexion of the lower leg to an angle of 120° has been achieved (or less if planned preoperatively), extension starts at the same rate. The same is done for flexion stiffness. When the full cycle of flexion extension is completed, it is repeated. The repeat cycle usually takes less time. After 10–15 cycles of passive flexion and extension, the time for a full cycle is reduced to

several minutes. Passive movements are then supplemented by the development of active movements. For this, the arms of the swivel hinge are disconnected. Over 3–7 days a gradual transition is made to the priority development of active movements. The device for the development of movements can be removed after the patient can achieve flexion–extension of the knee joint in 10–20 min.

11.1.1.2 Surgical Technique with Monolateral Fixator

The monolateral fixators for knee contractures consist of laterally based rails fixed to the femur and tibia and connected to each other by a hinge which is centered over the center of rotation of the knee (Fig. 11.4). A minimum of two pins are necessary in both the femur and tibia. The femoral pins may be put on multiple pin clamps so as to cover the whole segment of the femur, but the tibial pins are placed within one clamp in the distal tibia. A distractor is placed posteriorly between the rails, as well as a separate distractor is attached anteriorly between the hinge and tibial pin clamp. The anterior distractor is opened at the end of the procedure to a subjective sensation of increased soft tissue tension as felt by the operative surgeon (Mooney and Koman 2001).

Once full extension is achieved clinically and radiographically, the fixator is left in place for approximately 4 weeks. The device is then removed under anesthesia, and the extremity is placed in a long leg cast in full extension for approximately 4 weeks. Long leg braces are used full time. These are locked in extension except for knee range of motion and strengthening exercises during therapy sessions. Standing and walking are allowed as tolerated.

Historically, initial surgical management has included releases and lengthenings of the hamstrings and posterior capsule if necessary (Mooney and Koman 2001). However, such management is often difficult, since simple soft tissue releases are often insufficient to obtain adequate extension. Serial extension casting, with and without simultaneous soft tissue release, may be effective in mild situations. Complications including fracture, physeal injury, and posterior

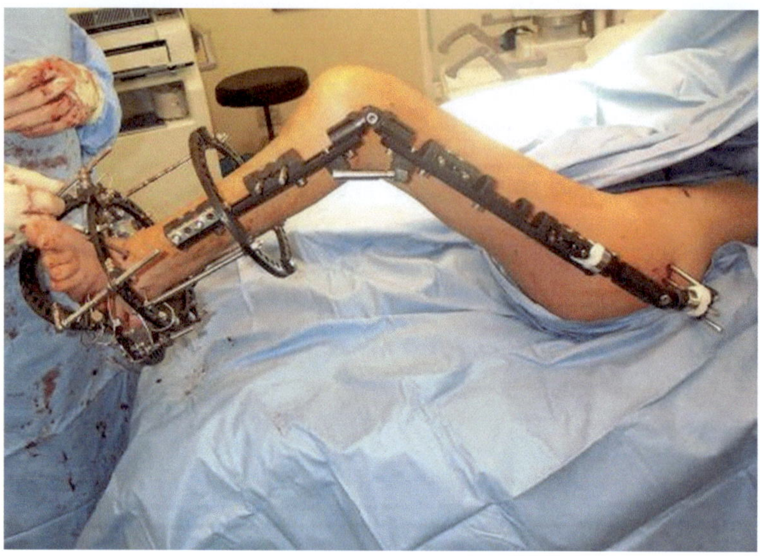

Fig. 11.4 Correction of the contracture with a monolateral fixator

knee subluxation, as well as peroneal nerve injury, have been reported (Heydarian et al. 1984, Mooney and Koman 2001). One study suggests there is no correlation between neurovascular complications and the degree of preoperative contracture or patient age (Asirvatham et al. 1991). It seems the development of complications after acute correction is unpredictable. Ilizarov's law of tension stress (Ilizarov 1990) has been advocated using the circular external fixator to treat these sorts of deformities, as gradual controlled traction on living tissues creates stresses that stimulate regrowth of these tissues.

External fixation has been used for gradual correction, both with and without simultaneous soft tissue release (Herzenberg et al. 1994; Gillen et al. 1996).

Herzenberg et al. described the use of an early monolateral device in two patients in a review of their experience with correction of knee contractures using circular external fixation (Herzenberg et al. 1994). Theoretically, correction with external fixation is more controlled and efficient than acute correction of these deformities. In vivo canine studies have shown that slow gradual correction appears to elongate and stimulate histogenesis within tendons during bone lengthening (Heydarian et al. 1984). Blood vessels and neural structures have been shown to proliferate and elongate during lengthening (Asirvatham et al.

1991). Similar changes should occur in soft tissue structures during correction of joint deformities.

Some recurrence may be noted in follow-up period. It appears that in most patients, similar results were reported by Herzenberg et al., the overall joint motion was essentially unchanged at the end of follow-up but was in a more functional arc at the end of treatment (Herzenberg et al. 1994).

Major knee flexion deformity is disabling, and acute correction of flexion knee contracture with soft tissue release, osteotomy, or both may lead to serious complications (Asirvatham et al. 1991). Soft tissue release may be complicated by peroneal palsy, knee subluxation, hyperextension, skin necrosis, and recurrence (Herzenberg et al. 1994).

11.1.1.3 Surgical Technique with Software-Based Ortho-SUV Frame

The applying of Ortho-SUV Frame technique is in a manner different from the Ilizarov. The virtual hinge is determined by the software of which design is preferred. The software of computer-assisted frame enables to calculate any movement trajectory of one fixator support referring to the other, and the fixator construction allows providing the exact movement of these supports (Solomin et al. 2010, 26).

Based on experimental data, it was revealed that to improve the motion range in the knee joint till 120°/0°/0° and more oval supports should be used. The angulation of the proximal support to the bone should be 90–120°, of distal – 60°. The proximal support should be placed at the distance of 200–210 mm from the knee joint space, and the distal support should be placed at the distance of 120 mm. The use of ring supports and their approximation by 150–120 mm to the joint line enable to reach ROM of 70–90°/0°/0° (Figs. 11.5 and 11.6).

In clinical practice, treatment of false unions, deformity correction, and the femoral bone lengthening can often result in extension contracture of the knee joint or aggravating of the present extension contracture. In such cases, it is also advisable to use a software-based frame instead of a standard hinge assembly. The frame will provide a wider range of movements if the distal ring of the frame on the tibia is at an angle of 60° to the bone. The distal support of the frame should be at a distance of 110–150 mm from the knee joint. If angulated by 60°, it gives additional motion range for the knee joint: 110°/110°/0° (Fig. 11.7).

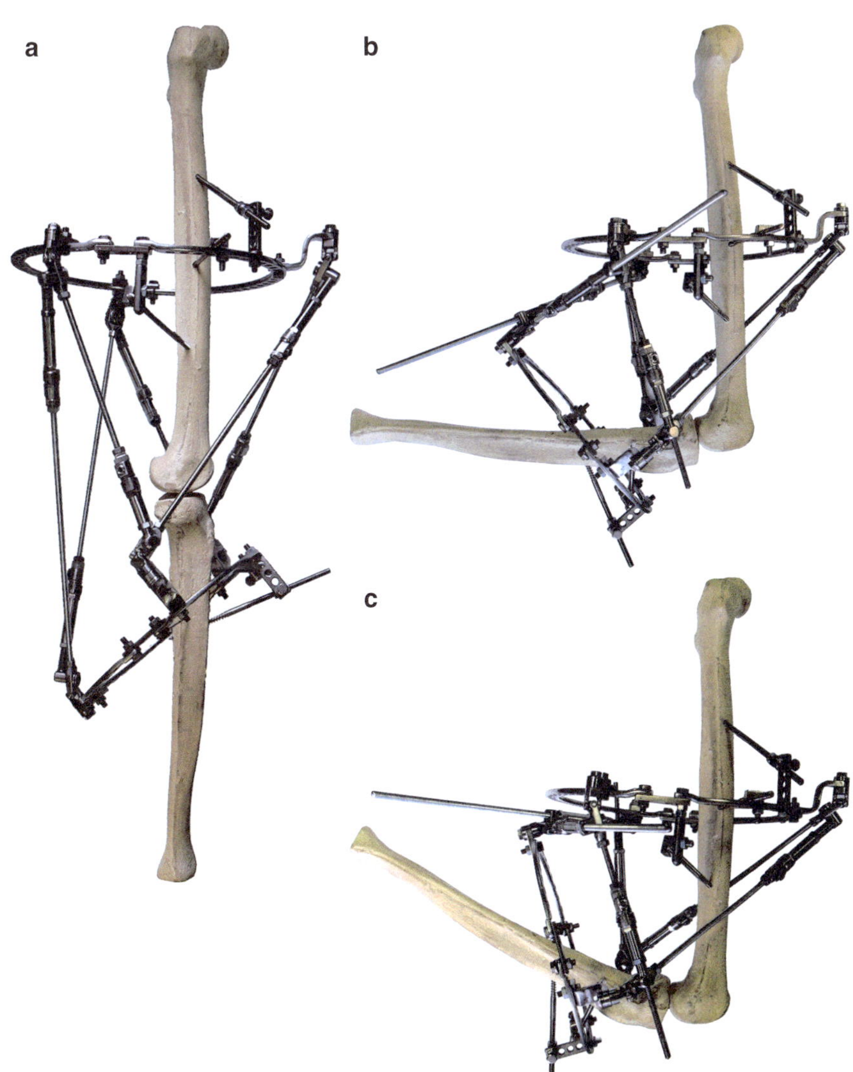

Fig. 11.5 (**a–e**) An Ortho-SUV Frame to work out the motions in the knee joint. (**a–c**) Pattern for various flexion positions in the knee joint. (**d, e**) The software windows

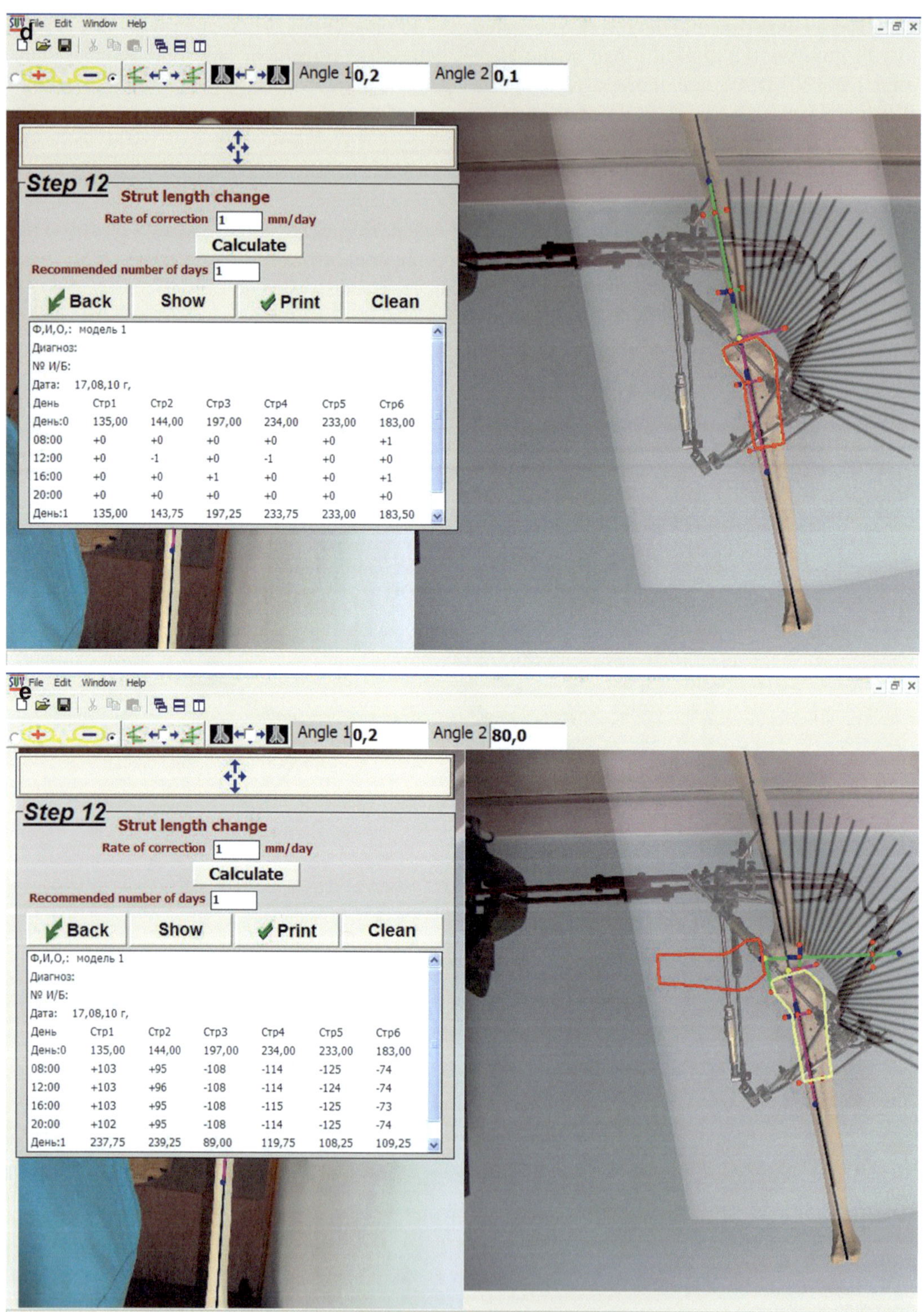

Fig. 11.5 (continued)

Fig. 11.6 (**a–f**) Use of the Ortho-SUV Frame to treat a female patient with persistent extension contracture of the knee joint. (**a**) Before the treatment. (**b**) After arthrolysis, quadricepsplasty, and Ortho-SUV Frame application. (**c**) X-rays during the treatment. Note the correct interrelations in the knee joint. (**d**) Passive workout of movements. (**e**) The result 40 days after assembling the external fixator. (**f**) The result 1 year after the surgery

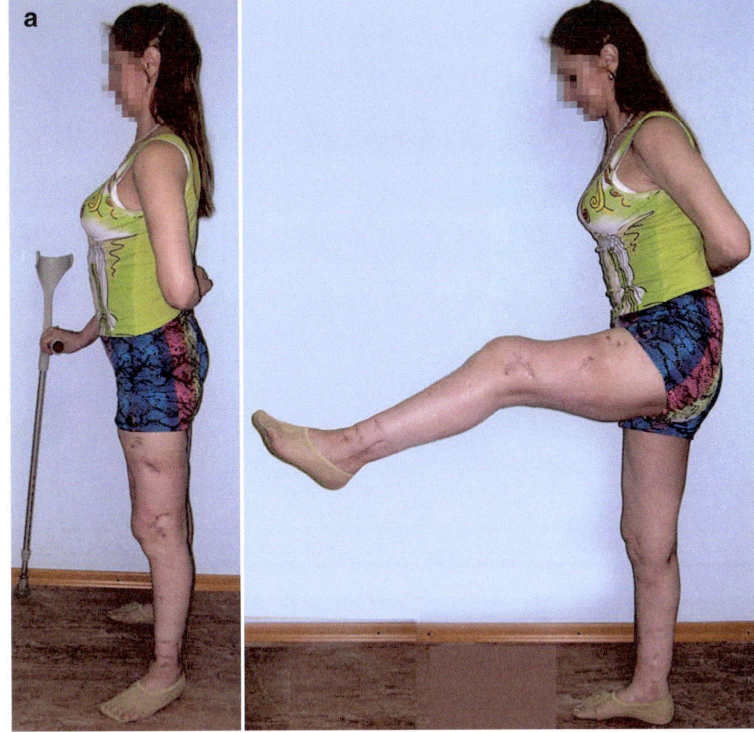

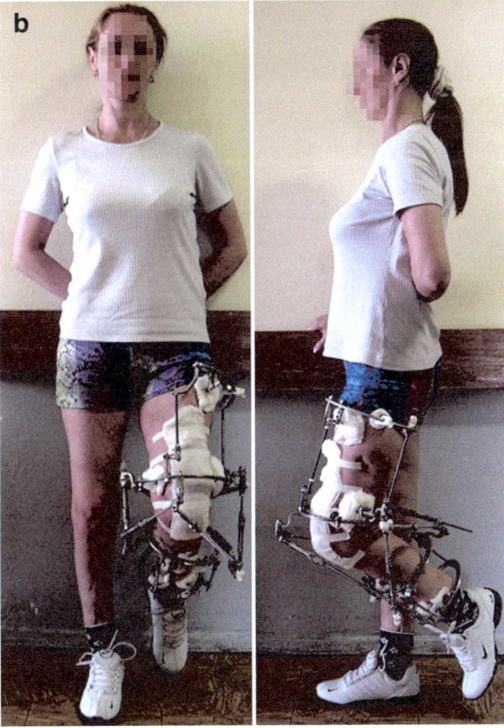

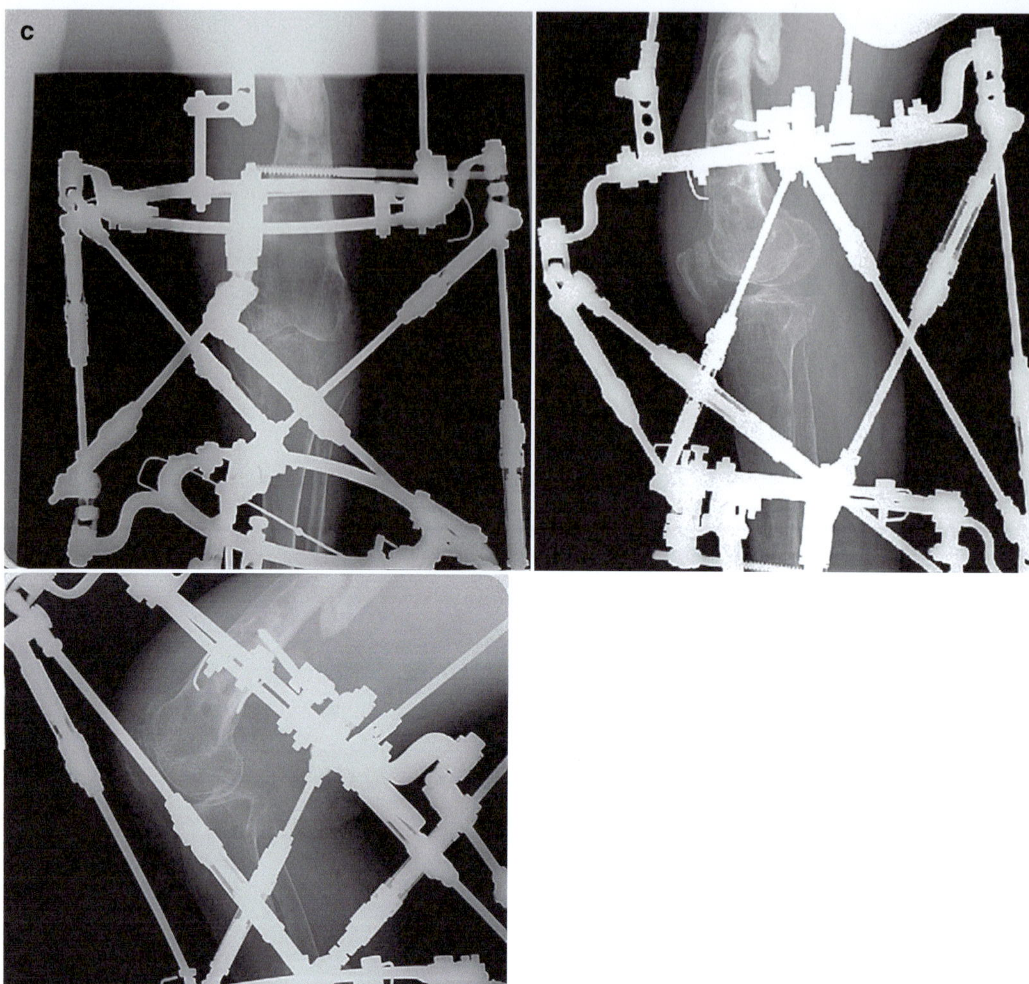

Fig. 11.6 (continued)

Fig. 11.6 (continued)

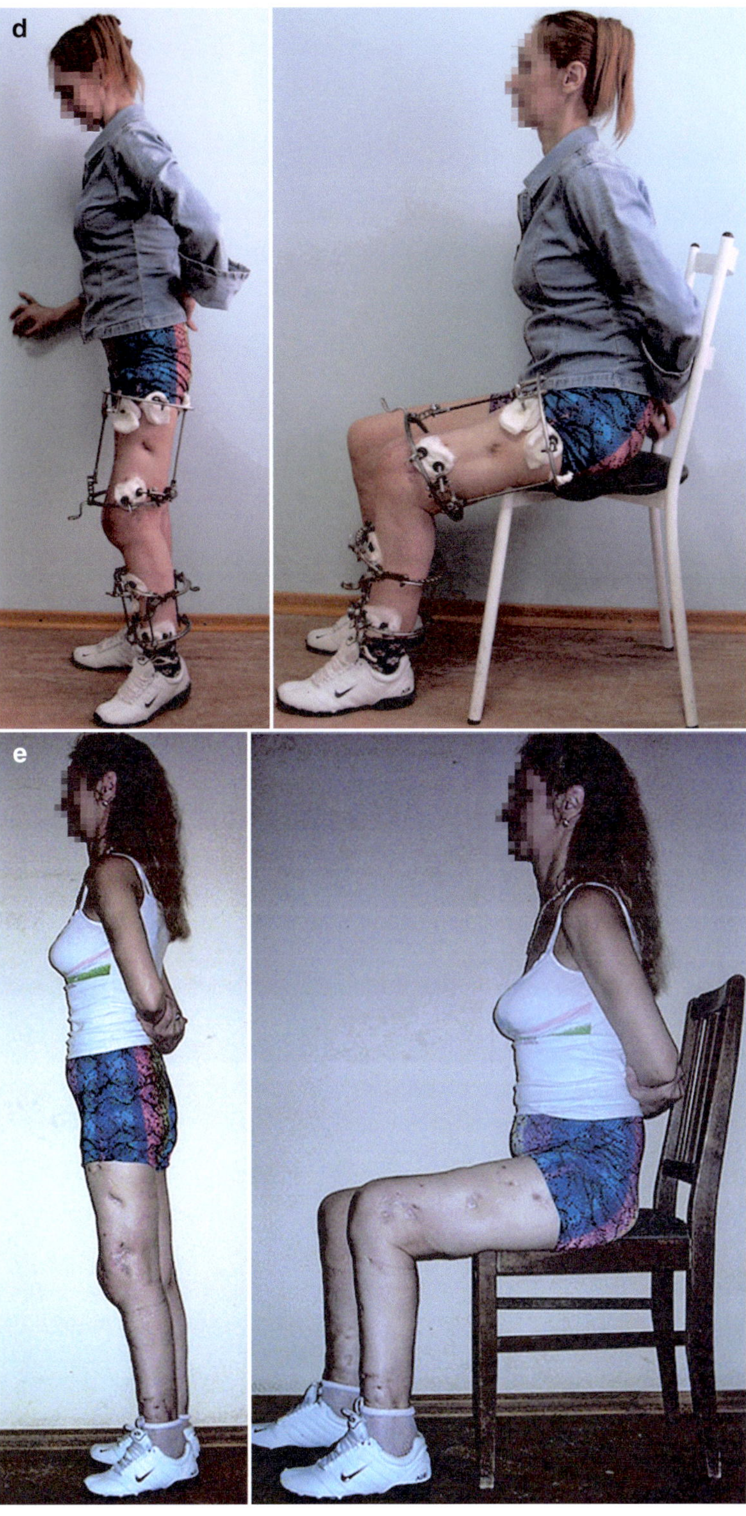

Fig. 11.6 (continued)

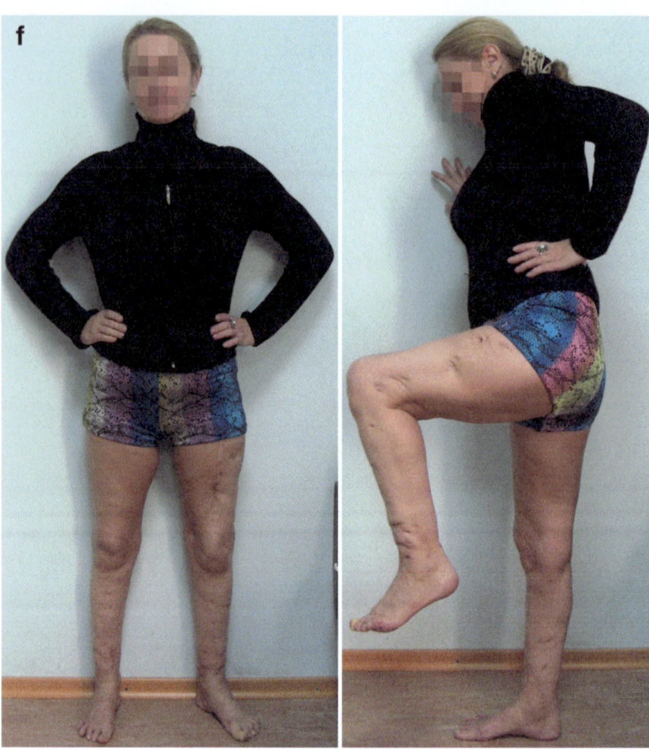

11.2 Ankle Flexion Contractures

The device is assembled from two transosseous modules fixing the lower leg and foot. The modules are connected by a hinge subsystem.

Flexion stiffness of the ankle resulting in talipes equinus is frequent in clinical practice. The most frequent reasons for persistent flexion stiffness are the consequence of breaking the rules concerning plaster immobilization and lower leg lengthening. These complications are grounds for using external fixation by "closed" methods. In stiffness resulting from the diseases that caused persistent relative shortening and changes of the gastrocnemius muscle (like poliomyelitis sequela) or marked osteoporosis, the external fixation operation is performed simultaneously with lengthening of the Achilles tendon. In stiffness emerging after intra-articular fractures of the ankle joint, after a previous infectious process (provided there are no contraindications), arthroscopic release can be performed in one stage at the same time as installation of the external fixation device.

The procedure starts with mounting the transosseous module on the lower leg. If the lengthening of the lower leg is complicated by the presence of pes equinus, the basic device is used. In other cases, two pairs of wires are inserted and are fixed after tensioning to two ring supports. The supports are connected by three rods: V,2-8; V,4-10 – (VII,**8**-2)VII,8-2; VII,4-10.

The lower leg module can be a combined single-support module: VI,12,120; (VII,**8**-2) VII,8-2; VII,4-10 (Fig. 11.8a) or VI,12,120; (VII,**8**-2)VII,8-2; VIII,1,90 (Fig. 11.8c, d). A module based on a lengthened closed half ring ("horseshoe" support) is mounted on the foot. The imaginary biomechanical axis of the ankle joint (rotational axis) passes under the medial malleolus, through the center of the trochlea of the talus, and comes out under the top of the lateral malleolus (Oganesyan et al. 2003).

By means of swivel hinges, gradual extension of the foot is started at an average of 2–6° per day in four to six stages on the second or third day. The rate is reduced if pain occurs or if there are signs of irritation of the great vessels and nerves. The manipulations must not cause any pain. Systematic prescription of analgesics for the development of movements "at any cost" is impermissible. After extension to an angle of 15–20° has been achieved, the foot is stabilized for 3–5 days. After that flexion is started, its rate is limited only by the occurrence of pain or a neurotrophic disorder. After a full cycle of flexion–extension is completed, it is repeated. The repeat cycle usually takes less time. After 10–15 passive flexion and extension cycles, the time for a full cycle is reduced to several minutes. Passive movements can be developed using a special automatic pneumatic attachment (Shevtsov et al. 1995). Passive movements are then supplemented by the development of active movements. For this purpose, the arms of the swivel hinges are disconnected. Over 3–7 days a gradual transition is made to the priority development of active movements.

The device for the development of movements can be removed after the patient has achieved confident movements in the ankle joint.

External fixation is used when dorsal flexion of the foot by 25–30° was not achieved after lengthening of the Achilles tendon. The foot is fixed by the device for 1–2 weeks, after which the hinge subsystem is used in accordance with the above descriptions.

In case of forefoot equinus, a hindfoot should be fixed to the base frame. In this case, the support fixing the forefoot is mobile support (Fig. 11.9).

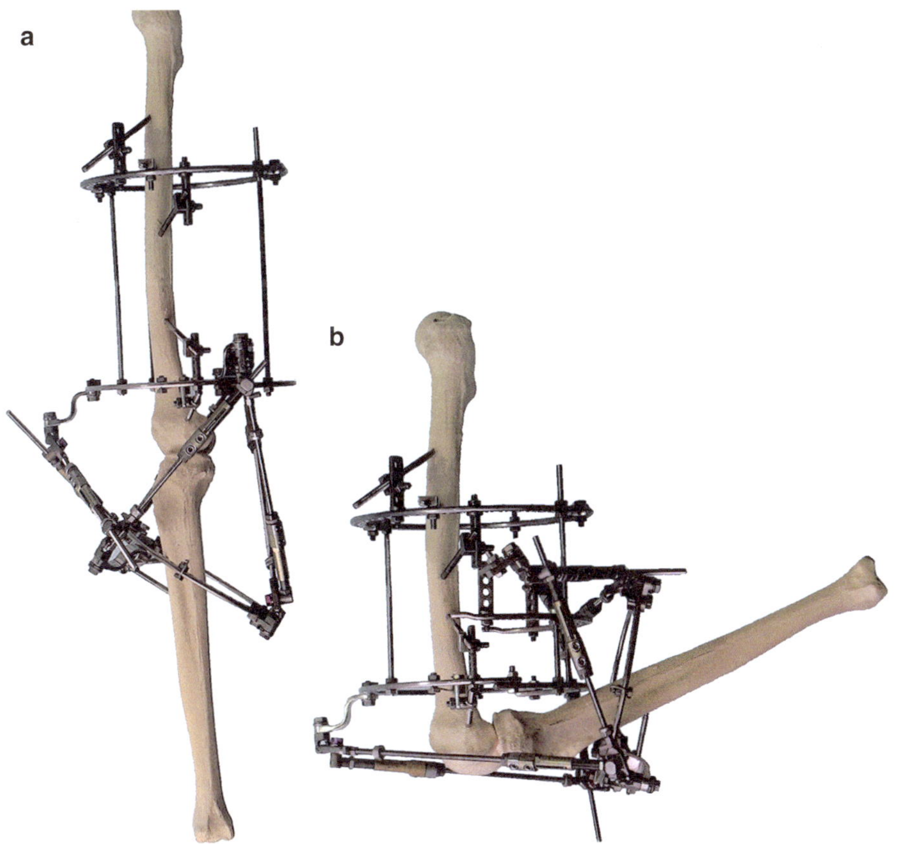

Fig. 11.7 (**a–h**) Ortho-SUV Frame to work out the knee joint movements in the deformity corrections and (or) the thigh lengthening. (**a, b**) Ortho-SUV Frame assembly to work out the knee joint movements in the thigh lengthening. (**c, d**) The female patient during the treatment. (**e–f**) The software window in different flexion positions of the knee joint. (**g–h**) X-rays during the motion workout. Note the correct interrelations in the knee joint

İ. Tuncay and L. Solomin

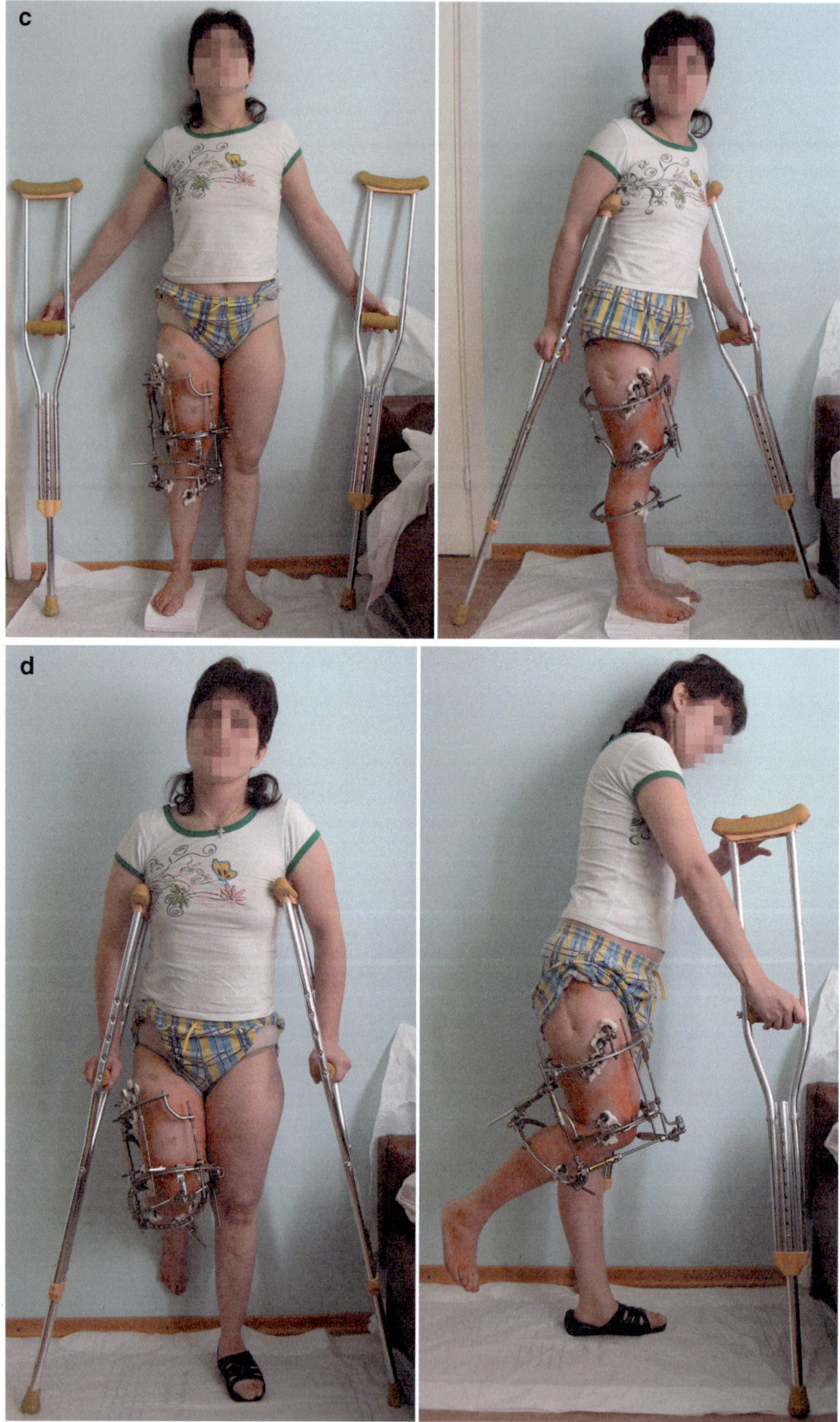

Fig. 11.7 (continued)

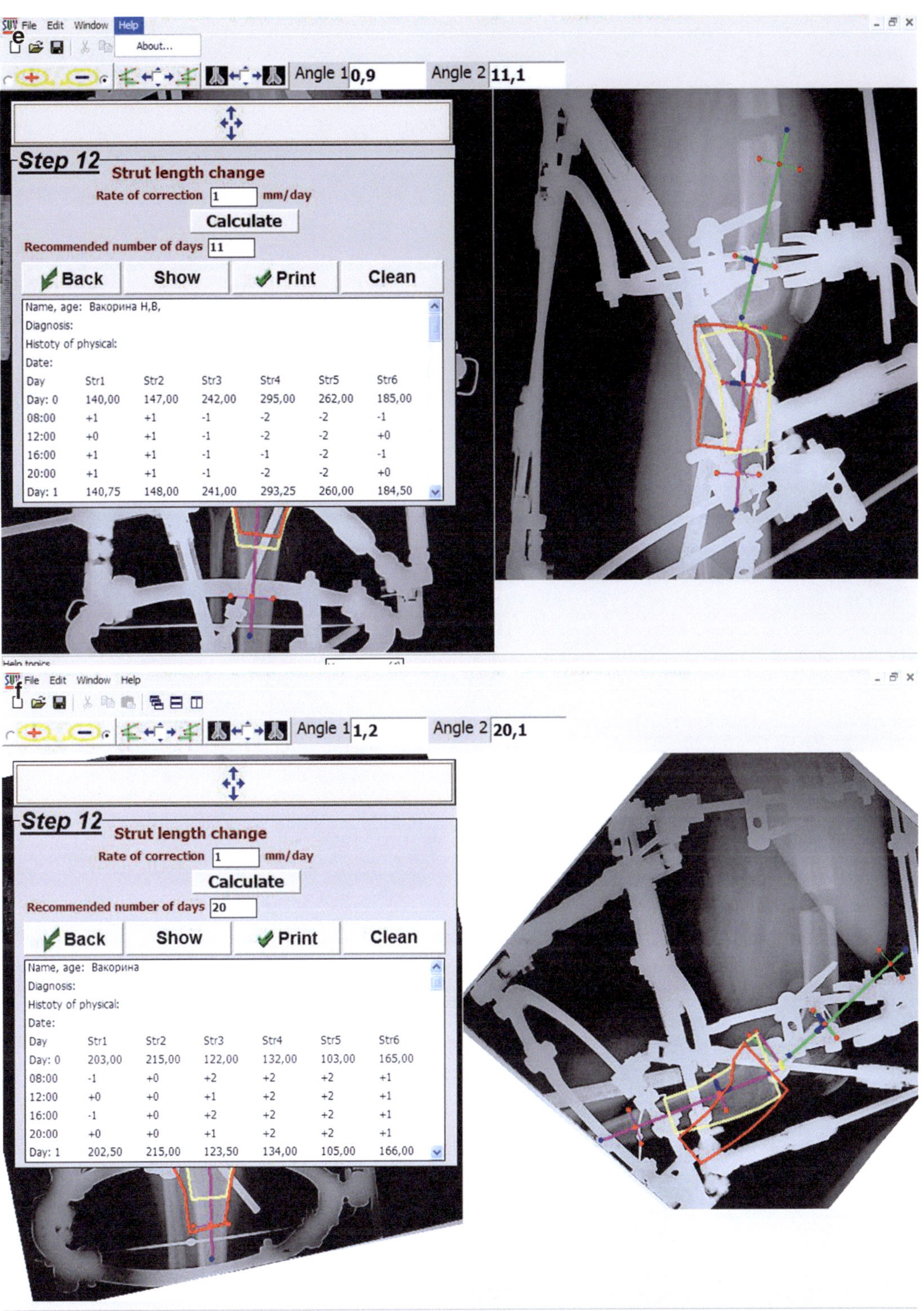

Fig. 11.7 (continued)

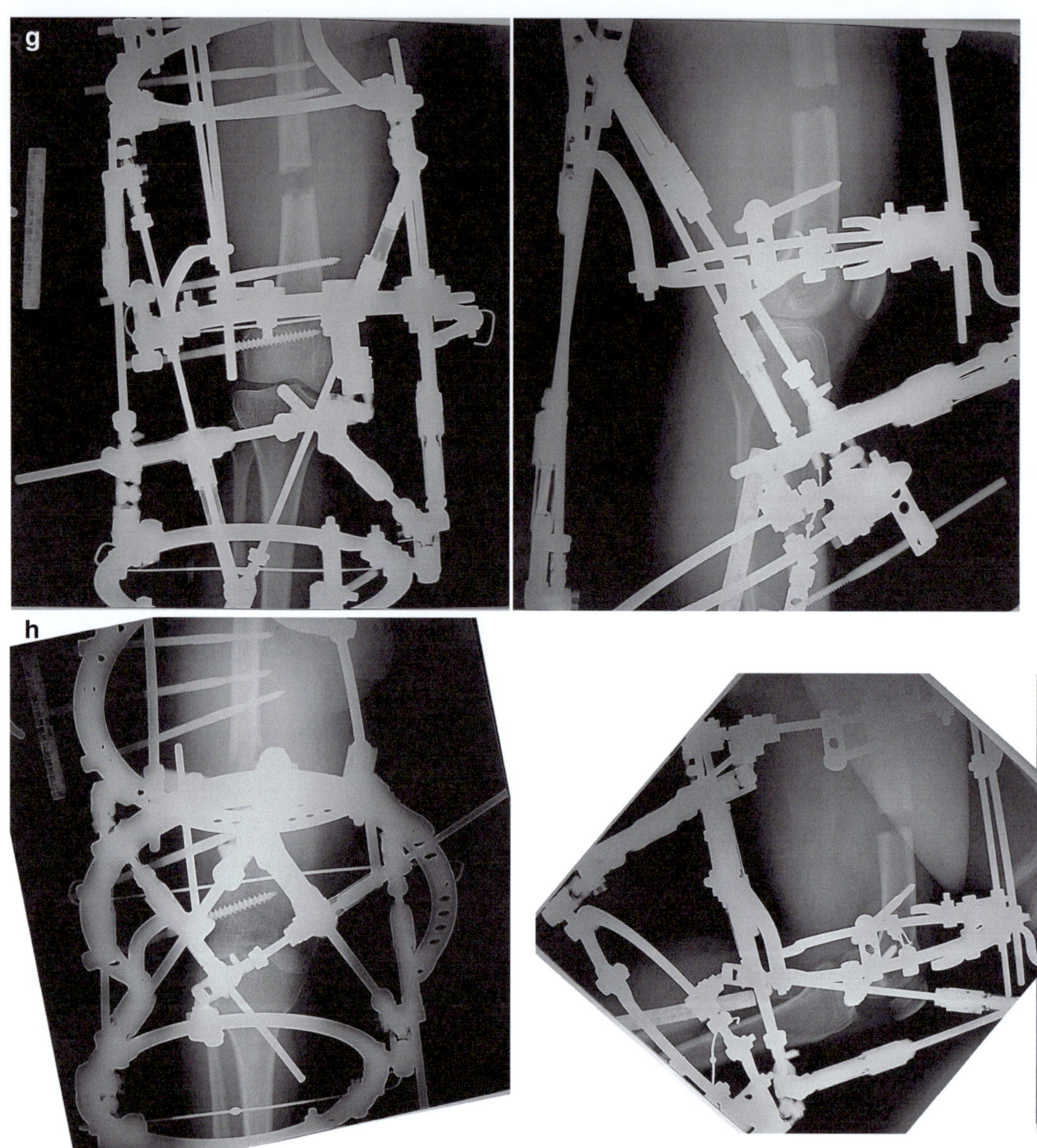

Fig. 11.7 (continued)

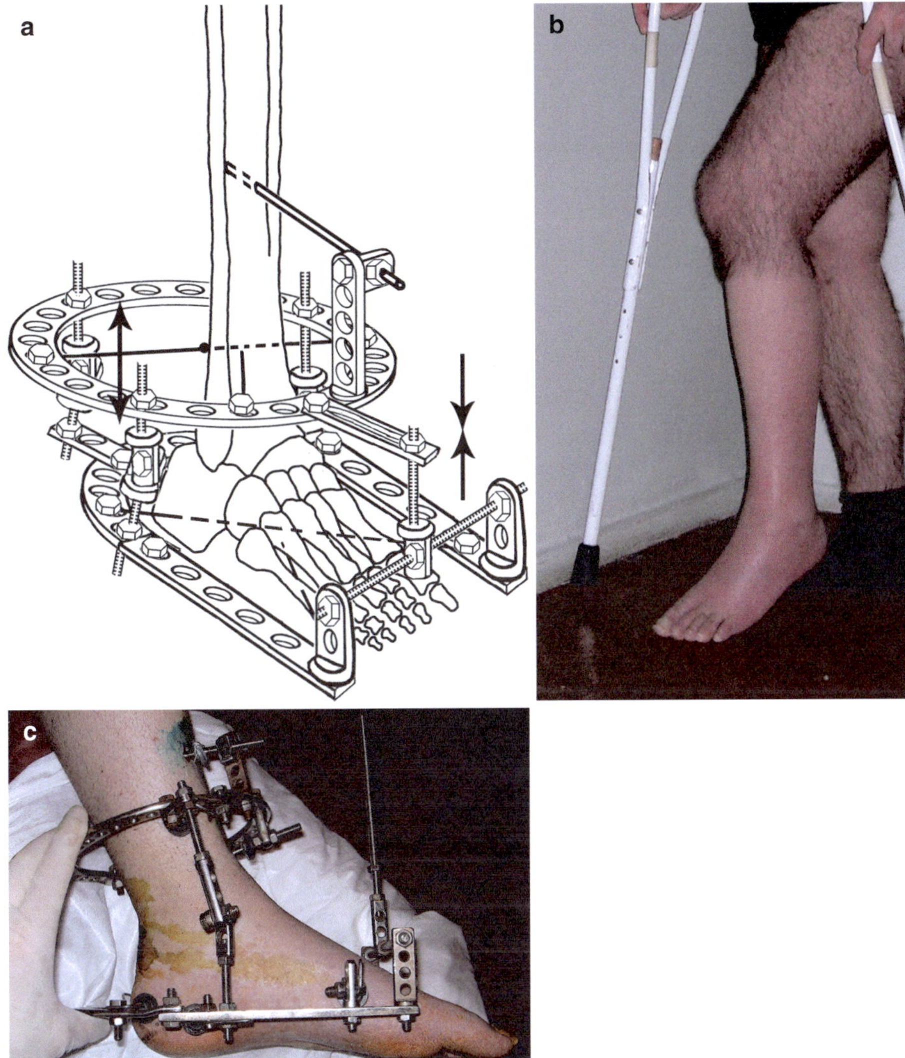

Fig. 11.8 (**a–d**) Technique: a hinge system is installed between the transosseous modules fixing the lower leg and foot. The center of rotation of the axial hinges on the external and internal surfaces of the foot must be located at the level of the center of the head of the talus. One swivel hinge is installed on the posterior aspect of the foot and one on the anterior aspect. The hinge must be at the level of bimalleolar plane. A diastasis of 3–4 mm is cre-ated between the joint surfaces. It is important to note that due to flexure of the transosseous elements, the value of the distraction force on the hinges will not correspond to the value of the distraction force at the joint space. Therefore, the effectiveness of the distraction should be monitored radiographically. Radiography is also neces-sary to make sure that the axial hinges have been properly installed

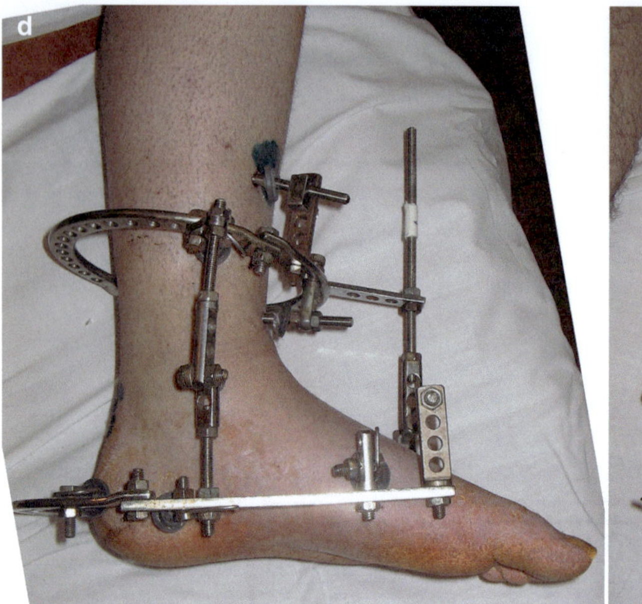
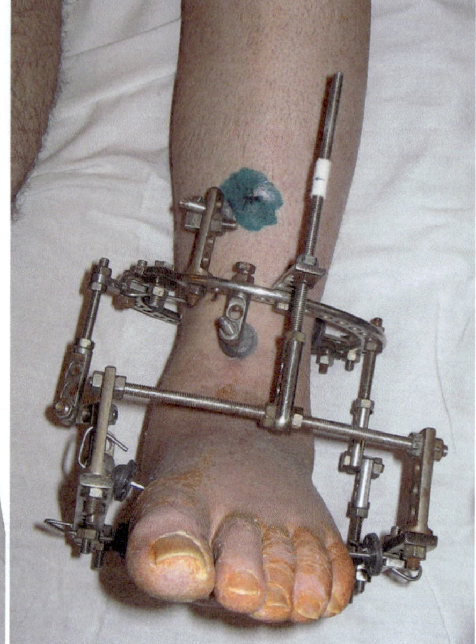

Fig. 11.8 (continued)

11.2.1 Elbow Flexion Contractures[1]

The first stage of the closed reduction of *chronic dislocations of the forearm* involves installation of a double-support module based on a ring and two thirds ring on the shoulder. The support is based on wires (Fig. 11.10a) or may be a hybrid device (Fig. 11.9b). The second module fixing the forearm can also be a wire or hybrid wire/half-pin device: II,6,90; III,**9**-3; IV,6,90 (as shown in the figure) or III,**9**-3; IV,6,70. A hinge-distraction subsystem is mounted between the modules. After reduction of the dislocation, the elbow joint is fixed in the mid-physiological position for 2–3 weeks, after which the device can be used for the development of movement in the elbow joint.

One of the conditions for successful external fixation for *stiffness in the elbow joint* is to use the reference positions shown in the atlas for insertion of transosseous elements (Solomin et al. 2010).

The second indispensable condition of the frame assembly for elbow joint stiffness elimina-tion is installation of axial hinges (one-axial hinge using monolateral devices) strictly accord-ing to an axis of rotation of an elbow joint (Fig. 11.11).

Figure 11.12 shows the assembly developed at the Russian Ilizarov Research Center (Soldatov 2004; Shevtsov et al. 2001). Monolateral config-uration of the device is shown in Fig. 11.13.

A diastasis of 2–3 mm is created between the joint surfaces. Introducing water in the joint under pressure (using the arthroscopic technique) is beneficial.

Using a swivel hinge gradually increasing flexion of the elbow joint starts at an average 2–6° per day in four to six stages. The flexion rate must be reduced if pain occurs or if there are signs of irritation of the great vessels and nerves. The manipulations must not cause any pain. The evaluation as to whether the amount of movement of the swivel hinge causes no pain must be made in the morning. Only after a night without analgesia should an increase in the rate of joint movement be recommended. Systematic prescription of analgesics for the development of movement "at any cost" is impermissible.

---

[1] *With the contribution of J. P. Soldatov.*

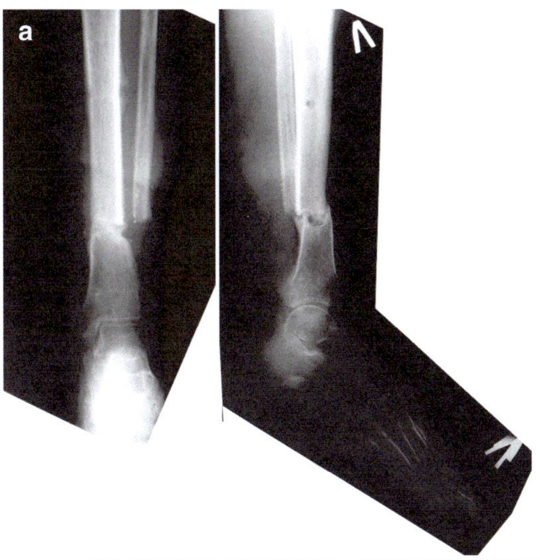

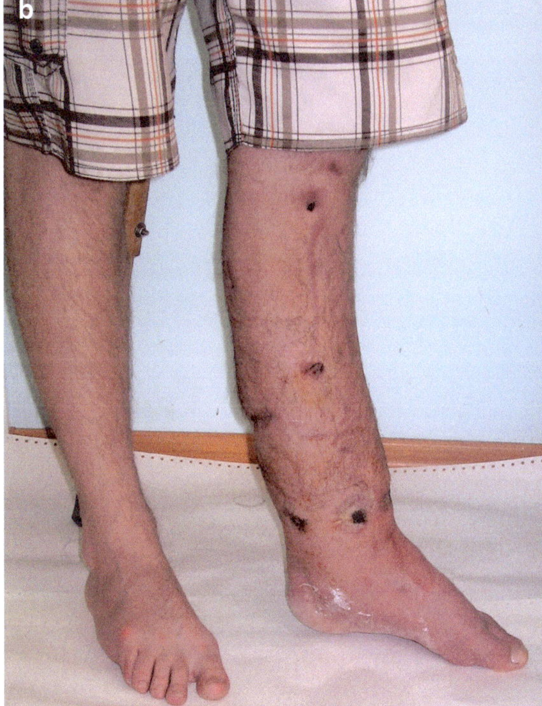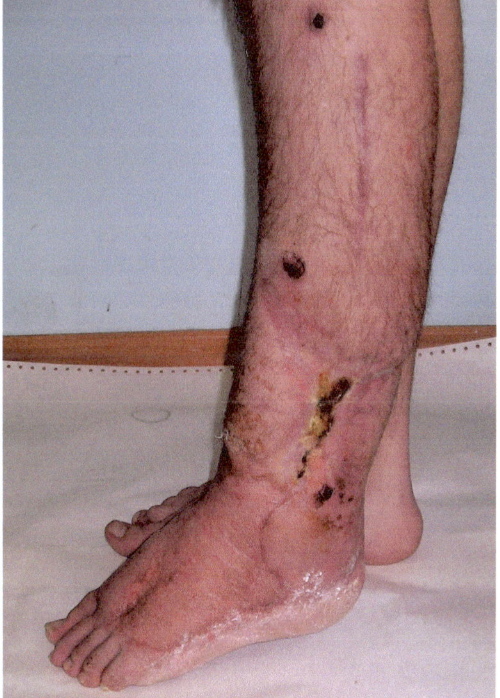

Fig. 11.9 (**a–h**) Elimination of forefoot equinus; external fixation of tibial nonunion. (**a, b**) Before treatment. (**c, d**) After applying software-based Ortho-SUV Frame. (**e, f**) Deformation is eliminated; struts are changed with hinges. (**g, h**) Result of healing

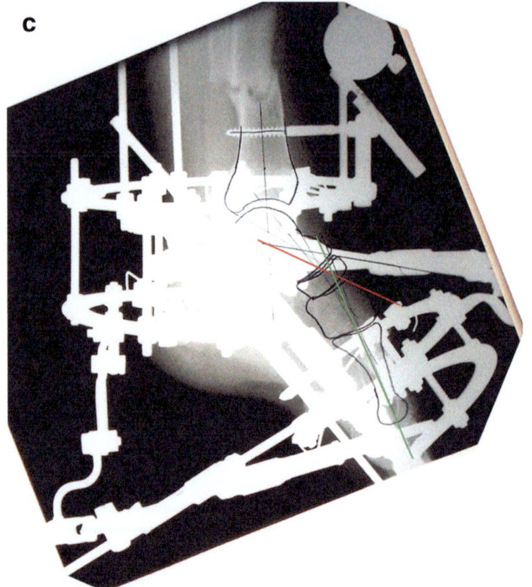

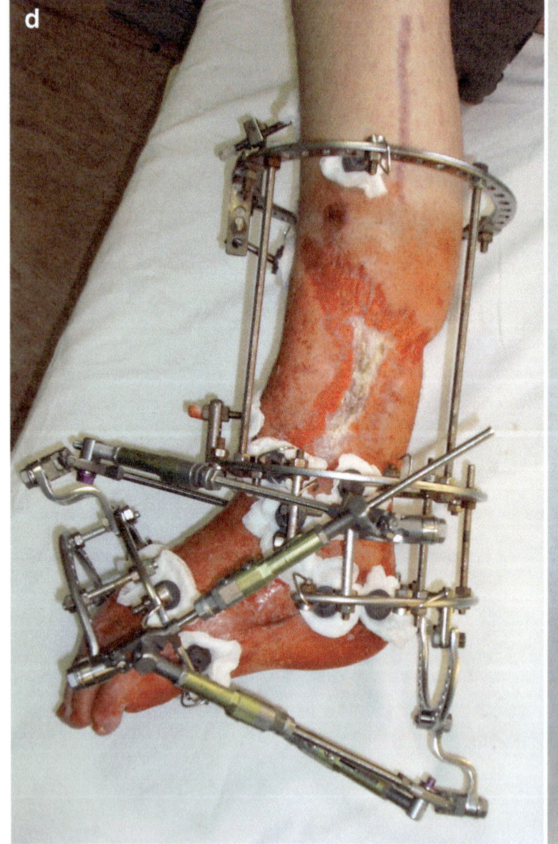

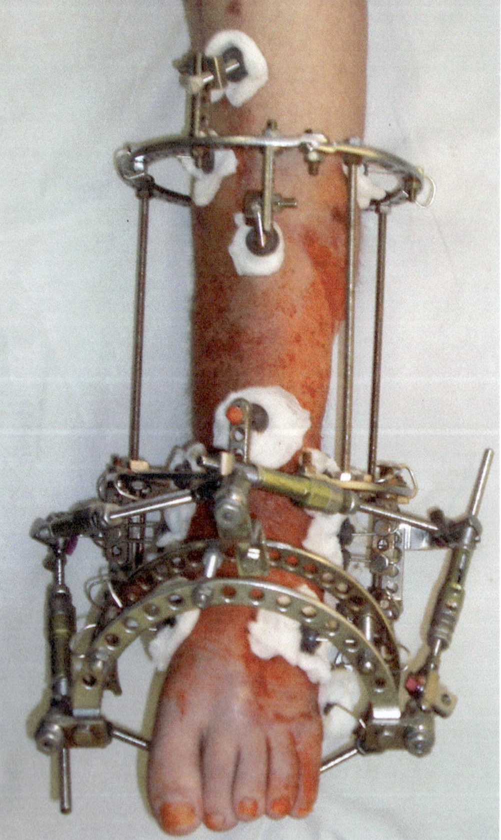

Fig. 11.9 (continued)

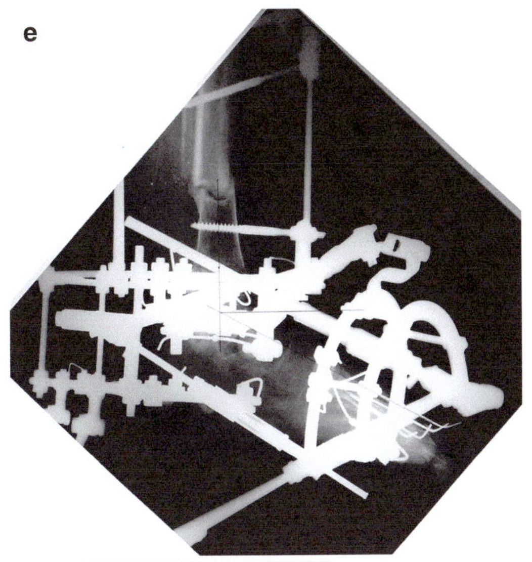

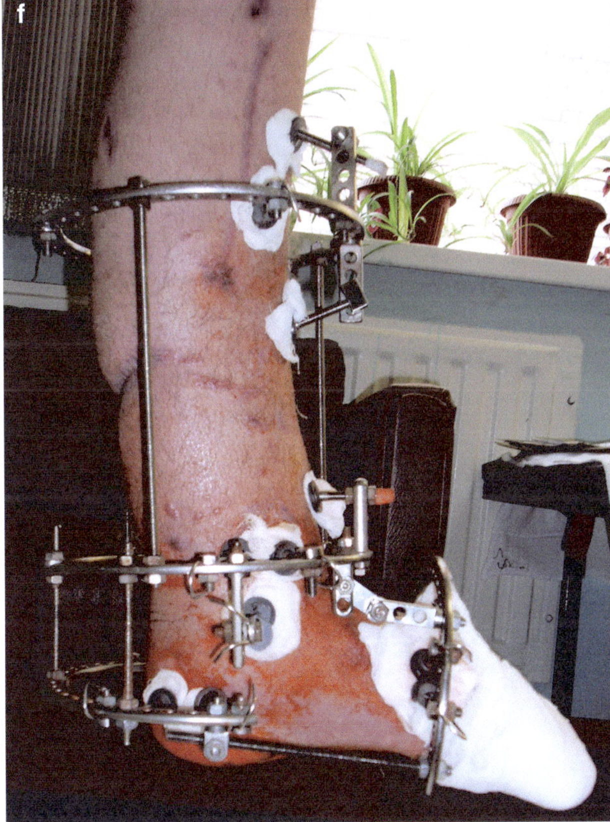

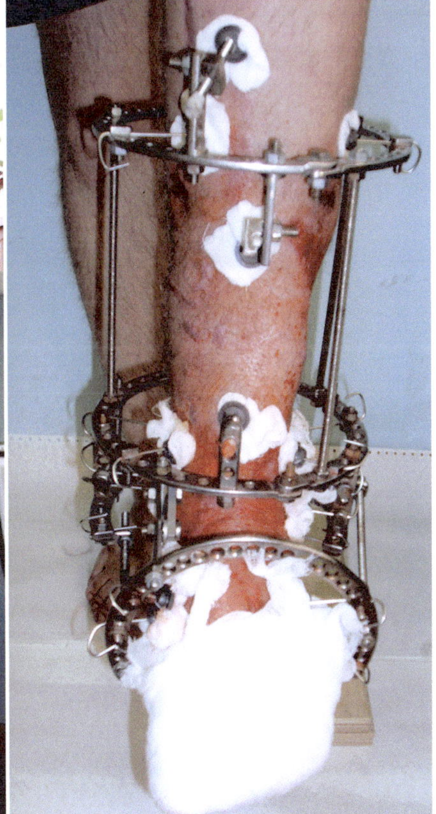

Fig. 11.9 (continued)

Fig. 11.9 (continued)

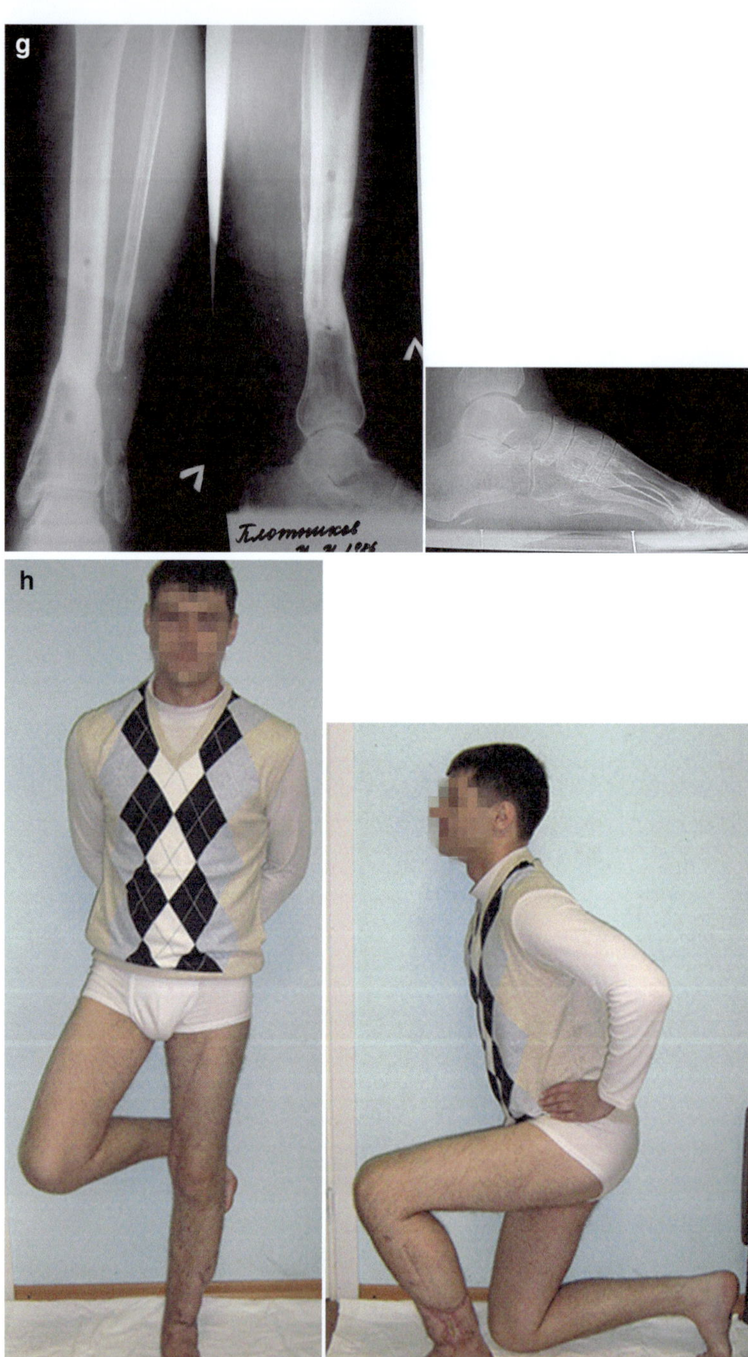

Fig. 11.10 (**a, b**) Schemes for an Ilizarov device (**a**) and combined (hybrid) device (**b**) for reduction of chronic dislocations of the forearm. Distraction starts on the 3rd to the 5th day at a rate of 0.25 mm six to eight times a day. The rate of distraction is decreased if pain or signs of hyperextension of the great vessels and nerves occur. After lateral radiographs confirm the presence of the necessary diastasis for unhindered horizontal movement of the ulnar epiphysis, the subsystem connecting the modules is remounted. Its construction depends on the type of dislocation: anterior, posterior, medial, or lateral. After that the fixator can be used for working out of movements in an elbow joint

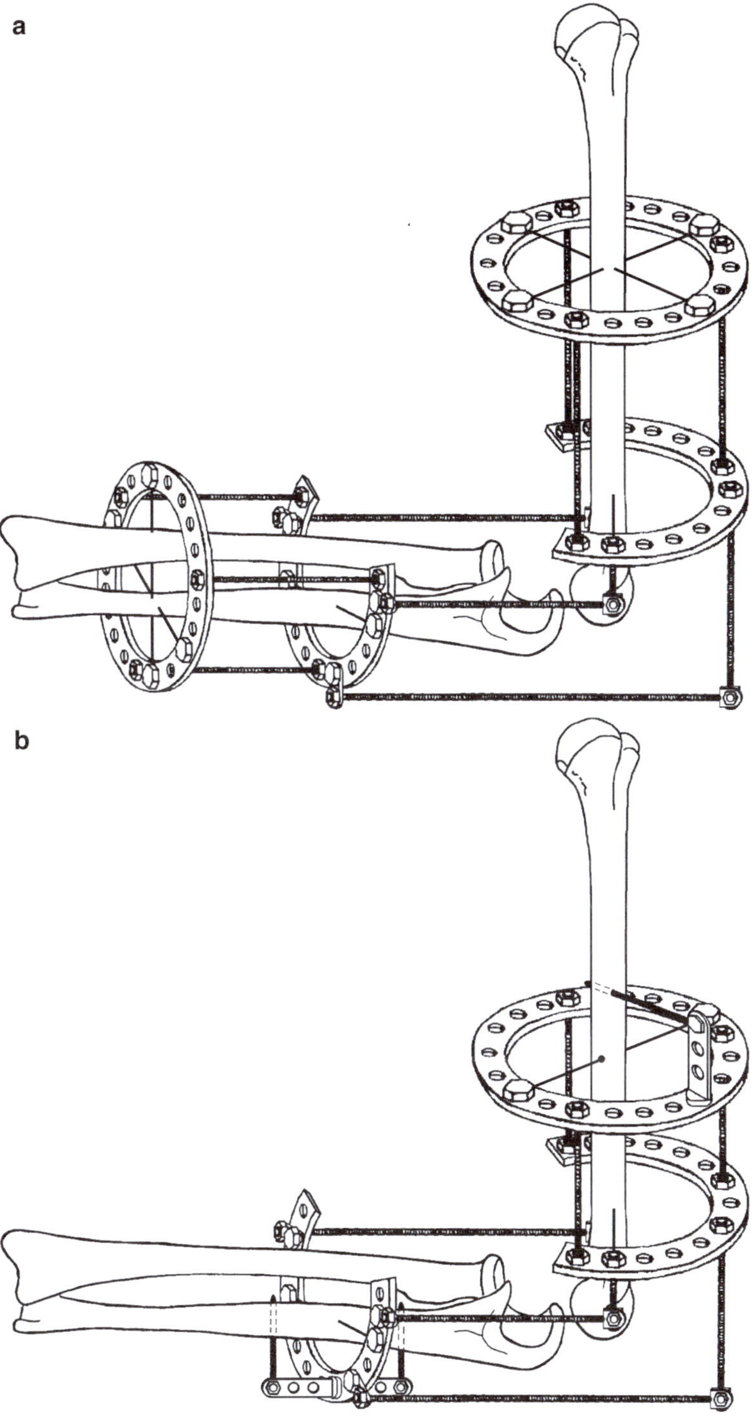

After forearm flexion to an angle of 130–140° has been achieved, its extension starts at the same rate. After the full cycle of "flexion–extension" is completed, it is repeated. The repeat cycle usually takes less time. After 10–15 passive flexion and extension cycles, the time for a full cycle is reduced to several minutes. Passive movements are then supplemented by the development of

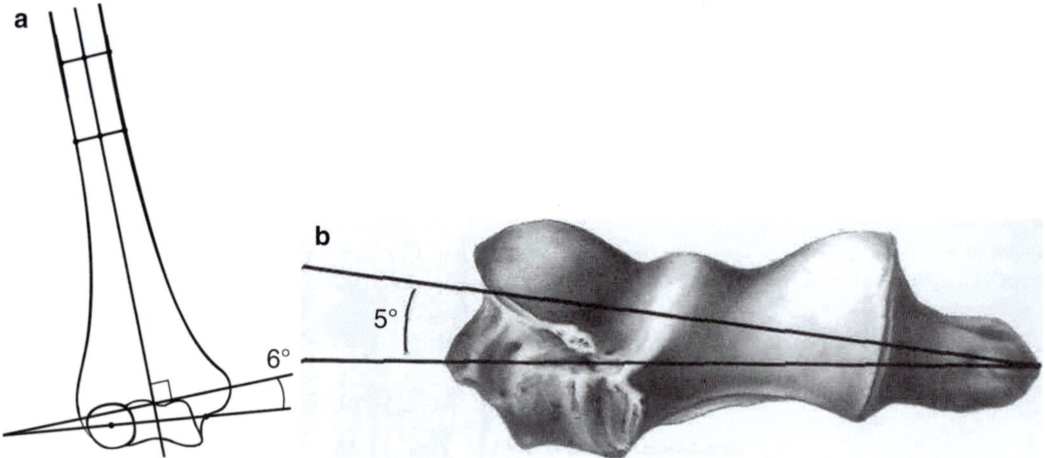

Fig. 11.11 (**a**, **b**) An axis of rotation of an elbow joint in frontal (**a**) and horizontal (**b**) planes

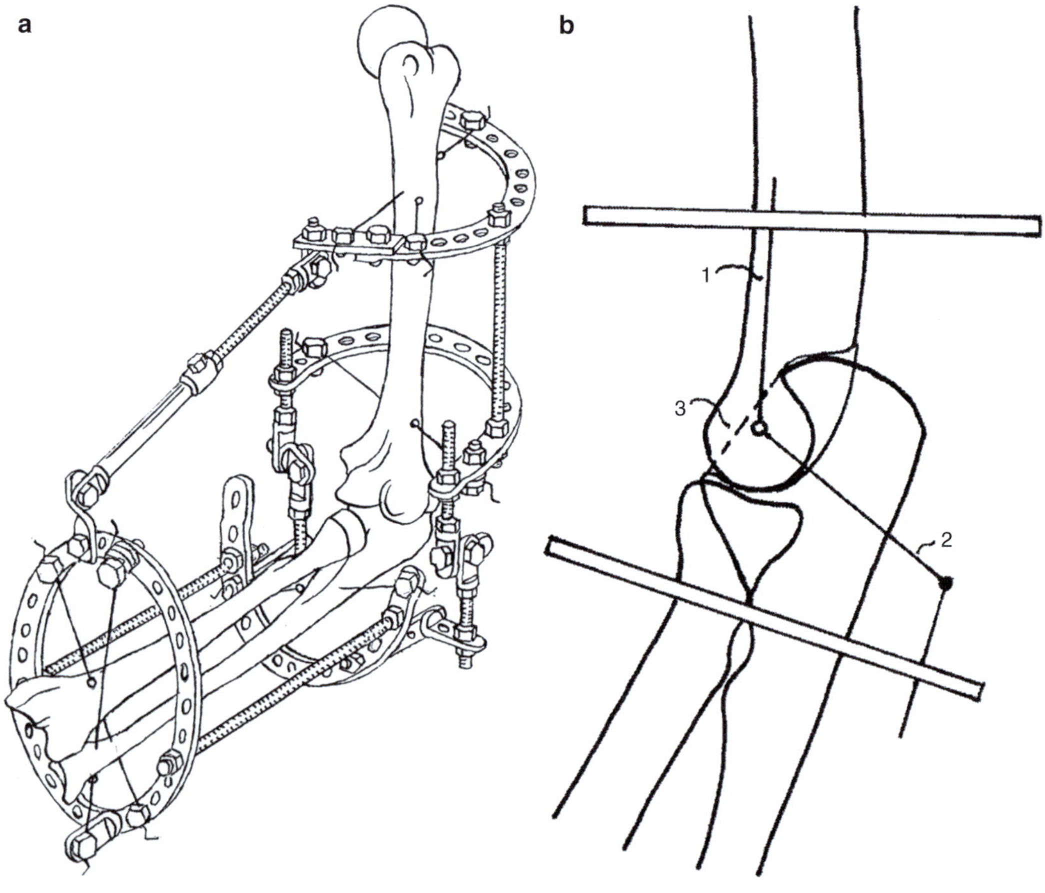

Fig. 11.12 (**a**, **b**) ROM hinged frames. (**a**) Frame assembly of Ilizarov Russian Research Center (Soldatov 2004). (**b**) Two-plane hinge (*1* proximal part, *2* distal part, *3* line between processes of the ulnar bone). (**c**) Alternative "wire – half-pin" assembly

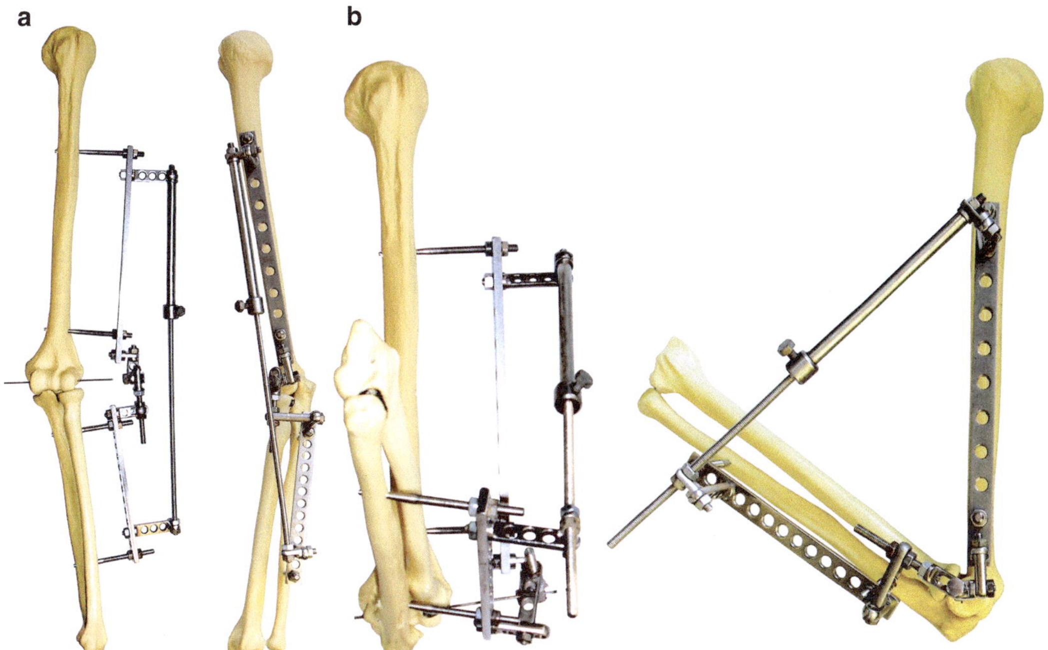

Fig. 11.13 (**a**, **b**) Monolateral configuration of the device for increasing of ROM in elbow joint. The wire is inserted in a projection of an axis of rotation in elbow joint

active movements, for which the arms of the swivel hinge are disconnected. Over 3–7 days a gradual transition is made to the priority development of active movements. Then the device is dismantled and restorative treatment continues.

The procedure for using external fixation devices presented is intended for patients with stiffness with no bone component. If the joint surfaces are congruent, installation of the device is preceded by arthroplasty which may include, according to the indications, partial removal of the ulnar processes, excavation of the olecranon fossa, and removal of ossified material (Figs. 11.14 and 11.15).

In patients with posttraumatic intra-articulate elbow joint fusion, who suffer from the disease over 1 year, the following method is used. At the beginning cup-and-ball (hinged) osteotomy of area of joint fusion using medial and lateral approaches is performed. The ends of humeral and elbow bones should be processed by mills. At this procedure the humeral condyles turn into semicylindrical form and incisura trochlearis ulna gets elliptic (Fig. 11.16). Thus a resection of the ends

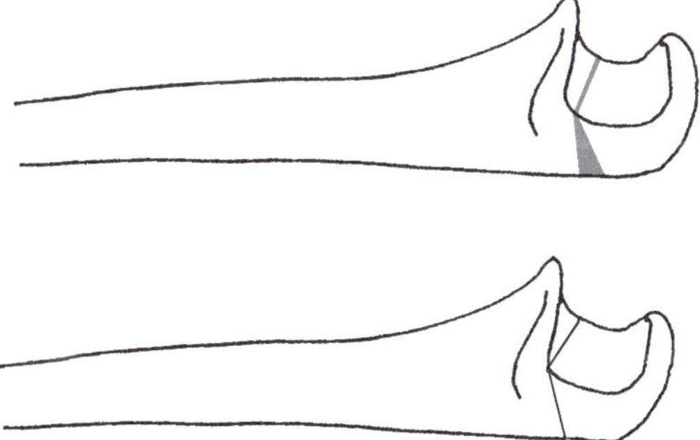

Fig. 11.14 Restriction of extension of the elbow joint because of lack of conformity between the ulnar process and its fossa, decentralization, or hypertrophy of the top of the ulnar process can be corrected by modifying the curvature of the trochlear notch. For this purpose, in accordance with the results of specific calculations, a wedge of bone at the base of the ulnar process is removed. Osteosynthesis of the ulnar process is then performed as for fractures. The supports for tensioning the compression wires are used as the module of the device for the subsequent development of movements in the elbow joint

of a humeral bone and ulna should be 0.5–1 cm. The development of a new elbow joint movement is carried out by means of a hinged frame.

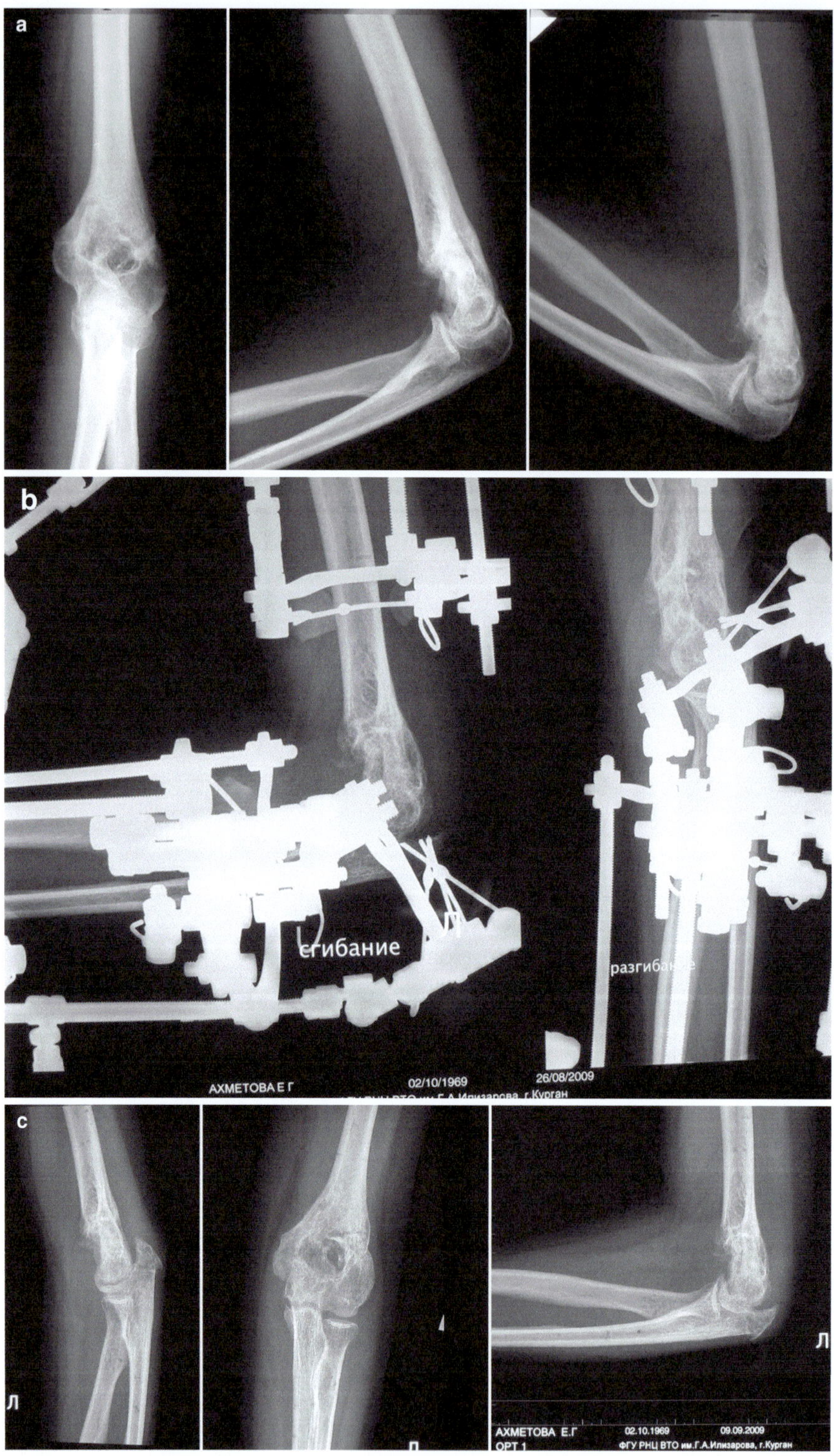

Fig. 11.15 (**a–c**) Roentgenograms of the patient with posttraumatic elbow joint stiffness, caused by deformations of the block of the humeral bone. (**a**) Before treatment with maximum possible extension. (**b**) During treatment. (**c**) After device removal

Fig. 11.16 (**a–d**) Roentgenograms of the patient with elbow joint fusion. (**a**) Before treatment. (**b**) During the cure. (**c**) In 4 months after operation, with the maximum flexion and extension. (**d**) In 9 years after treatment

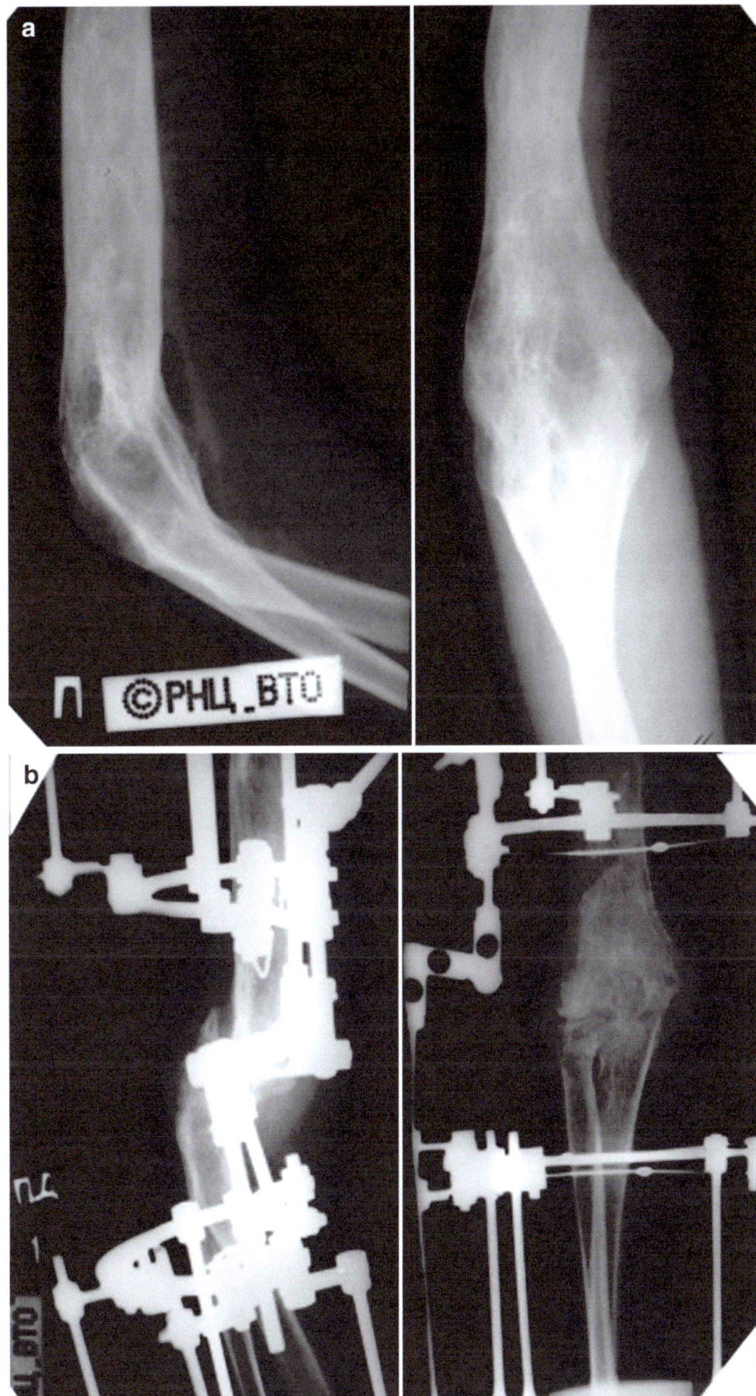

Fig. 11.16 (continued)

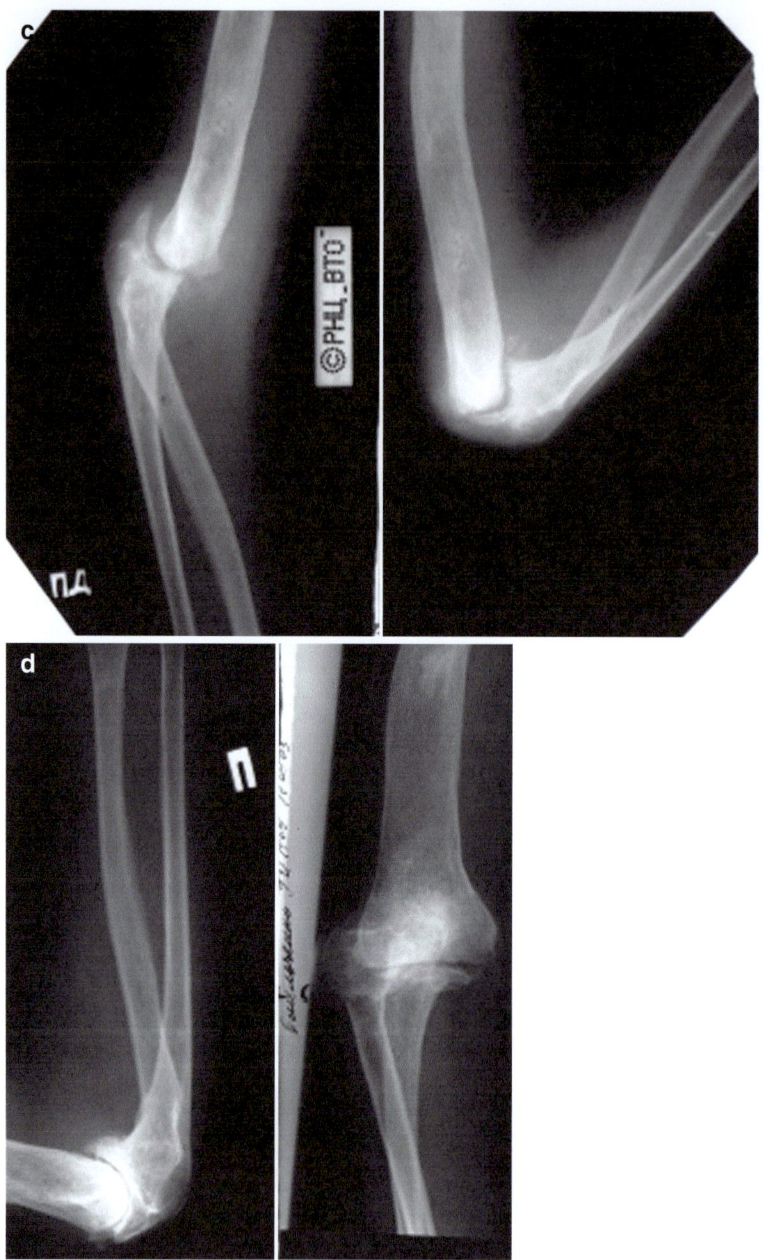

References

Abraham E, Verinder DGR, Sharrard WJW (1977) The treatment of flexion contracture of the knee in myelomeningocele. J Bone Joint Surg Br 59:433–438

Asirvatham R, Rooney RJ, Watts HG (1991) Proximal tibial extension medial rotation osteotomy to correct knee flexion contracture and lateral rotation deformity of tibia after polio. J Pediatr Orthop 11(5):646–651

Damsin JP, Ghanem I (1996) Treatment of severe flexion deformity of the knee in children and adolescent using the Ilizarov technique. J Bone Joint Surg Br 78:140–144

DelBello DA, Watts HG (1996) Distal femoral extension osteotomy for knee flexion contracture in patients with arthrogryposis. J Pediatr Orthop 16:122–126

Devalia KL, Fernandes JA, Moras P, Pagdin J, Jones S, Bell MJ (2007) Joint distraction and reconstruction in complex knee contractures. J Pediatr Orthop 27(4):402–407

Ebraheim NA, Saddemi SR, De Troye RJ (1993) Results of Judet quadricepsplasty. J Orthop Trauma 7:327–330

Gillen JA II, Walker JL, Burgess RC et al (1996) Use of Ilizarov external fixator to treat joint pterygia. J Pediatr Orthop 16:430–437

Herzenberg JE, Davis JR, Paley D et al (1994) Mechanical distraction for treatment of severe knee flexion contractures. Clin Orthop 301:80–88

Heydarian K, Akbarnia BA, Jabalameli M, Tabador K (1984) Posterior capsulotomy for the treatment of severe flexion contractures of the knee. J Pediatr Orthop 4:700–704

Hosny GA, Fadel M (2008) Managing flexion knee deformity using a circular frame. Clin Orthop Relat Res 466:2995–3002

Ilizarov GA (1990) Clinical application of the tension-stress effect for limb lengthening. Clin Orthop Relat Res 250:8–26

Ilizarov GA, Makushin VD, Gerasimov PI, Desjatnik EG (1979) The treatment of stiff joints of the femur and lower leg associated with angular displacement of bone fragments with use of Ilizarov's closed technique (methodological recommendations). RSC "RTO", Kurgan

Iwaki H, Pinskerova V, Freeman MA (2000) Tibiofemoral movement 1: the shapes and relative movements of the femur and tibia in the unloaded cadaver knee. J Bone Joint Surg Br 82-B:1189–1195

Kornilov NV, Karptsov VI, Novoselov KA et al (1992) Comparative analysis of one- and two-stage methods of surgical treatments of femur pseudoarthrosis and malunions associated with knee joint contractures. In: Kornilov NV (ed) Planned surgical interventions (preoperative examination and patient preparation, complications, outcomes). RNIITO, Saint Petersburg

Mooney JF III, Koman LA (2001) Knee flexion contractures: soft tissue correction with monolateral external fixation. J South Orthop Assoc 10(1):32–36

Oganesyan OV, Ivannikov SV, Korshunov AV (2003) The restoration of shape and function of the ankle joint using a caliper traction apparatus. BINOM, Moscow

Paley D (2002) Sagittal plane knee considerations. In: Paley D (ed) Principles of deformity correction, 1st edn. Springer, Berlin/Heidelberg/New York

Phillips WE, Audet M (1990) Use of serial casting in the management of knee joint contractures in an adolescent with cerebral palsy. Phys Ther 70:521–523

Reutov AI, Gyulnazarova SV, Myakotina LI (2000) About functioning of locomotor system of patients with lower extremity shortening associated with permanent limitation in the range of knee motions. Traumatol Ortop Rossii 1:45–49

Saleh M, Gibson MF, Sharrard WJ (1989) Femoral shortening in correction of congenital knee flexion deformity with popliteal webbing. J Pediatr Orthop 9:609–611

Shevtsov VI, Nemkov VA, Sklyar LV (1995) The Ilizarov's apparatus. Biomechanics. Periodika, Kurgan

Shevtsov VI, Makushin VD, Kuftyrev LM (2001) Pseudoarthrosis, long bone defects of the upper extremities and elbow contractures. Zaural'e, Kurgan

Soldatov JuP (2004) Reconstructive treatment of the consequences of damage to the elbow joint with application of the Ilizarov device (dissertation). RSC "RTO", Kurgan

Solomin LN, Korchagin KL, Utekhin AI (2010) Software based "Ortho-SUV Frame" optimal assembly for improvement of knee joint ROM: ICEF&BR. In: 6th meeting of the ASAMI International, Barcelona. http://www.rniito.org/download/ortho-suv-manual-engl.pdf

Zimmerman MH, Smith CF, Oppenheim WL (1982) Supracondylar femoral extension osteotomies in the treatment of fixed flexion deformity of the knee. Clin Orthop Relat Res 171:87–93

12

Joint Distraction for Special Conditions

Dror Paley and Bradley M. Lamm

Contents

D. Paley, MD, FRCSC (✉)
Paley Institute, West Palm Beach, FL, USA
e-mail: drorpaley@gmail.com,
dpaley@lengthening.us

B.M. Lamm, DPM
International Center for Limb Lengthening,
Rubin Institute for Advanced Orthopedics,
Sinai Hospital of Baltimore, Baltimore, MD, USA
e-mail: blamm@lifebridgehealth.org

12.1 Treatment of Perthes Disease of the Hip by Joint Distraction

12.1.1 Introduction

Management of Perthes disease remains controversial despite extensive literature exploring this subject. Obtaining and maintaining hip range of motion are the only principles of treatment that are universally agreed upon. Containment of the femoral head within the acetabulum is thought to have a beneficial role, especially in patients with more than 50 % femoral head involvement (Kamhi and MacEwen 1975). Methods used to achieve containment include abduction bracing (Meehan et al. 1992), femoral (Axer et al. 1980; Lloyd-Roberts et al. 1976) or innominate osteotomies (Salter 1966), and shelf procedures (Willett et al. 1992; Daly et al. 1999). However, these methods are contraindicated when the degree of femoral head collapse and deformation prevent spherical hip motion (Lloyd-Roberts et al. 1976). Unloading of the hip was originally considered important in the treatment of Perthes disease (Eaton 1967). Various methods, such as complete bed rest (Eaton 1967) and use of a Snyder sling (Snyder 1947), have been tried toward this end, but little evidence exists to show that these methods alter the natural history of the disease (Evans 1958; Evans and Lloyd-Roberts 1958). The failure of unloading may be related to the misconception that non-weight bearing is equivalent to

M. Kocaoğlu et al. (eds.), *Advanced Techniques in Limb Reconstruction Surgery*,
DOI 10.1007/978-3-642-55026-3_12, © Springer Berlin Heidelberg 2015

unloading. We now know that muscular forces on the non-weight-bearing hip can apply one to two times the body weight. To truly remove all compressive forces from the hip, the muscular forces must be neutralized. This can be accomplished by hip joint distraction with an external fixator. Distraction of the hip also can reduce subluxation of the femoral head relative to the acetabulum.

Considering that the cartilage of the femoral head epiphysis actively proliferates into the uncovered and presumably unloaded lateral regions of the extruded femoral head (Catterall 1971). We postulated that if the femoral head could be distracted back into the acetabulum, the epiphyseal cartilage might proliferate to fill the gap between the collapsed femoral head and the acetabulum. Furthermore, distraction would stretch out the contracted capsule and muscles around the hip, and improved hip range of motion could be expected. Finally, the repair process and neo-osteogenesis of the femoral head could proceed without risking femoral head collapse. Based on this theoretical rationale, Paley first applied hip joint distraction as a therapeutic approach to Perthes disease in 1989. Although arthrodiastasis of the hip had been used and applied for other pathologies such as chondrolysis (Herring et al. 1992), it had not been used during the resorption phase of Perthes disease prior to this time to the author's knowledge.

12.1.2 Surgical Procedure (Fig. 12.1)

The patient is positioned supine with no bump under the hip. The pelvis should remain level and not tilted toward one side or another. The entire forequarter of the limb, from midline anterior to midline posterior and from ribs to toes, was prepped and draped free.

Step 1: Arthrogram of hip joint.

Anteroposterior and frog leg views are obtained with arthrographic dye in place.

Step 2: Percutaneous adductor tenotomy of adductor longus and gracilis tendons.

Step 3: Psoas tenotomy

Make a 3–4 cm anterior groin line incision. Feel the femoral artery pulse and stay lateral to it. Identify the medial border of the sartorius muscle and dissect deep and medial to it. The femoral nerve is identified and retracted medially. The nerve lies on the medial anterior aspect of the iliopsoas muscle. Dissect down the medial side of this muscle, and on the undersurface of its medial side can be found the psoas tendon. Cut the tendon while leaving a continuous muscle bridge.

Step 4: Insert a flexion-extension axis pin into the femoral head.

A horizontal line of the pelvis is marked on the drapes, guided by the image intensifier (line across the top of both iliac crests or bottom of both ischial tuberosities). The affected lower limb is held with the patella forward, knee in extension, and hip in 15° of abduction relative to the horizontal line of the pelvis. With the image intensifier and a wire, mark a line over the shaft of the femur and a point over the center of the acetabulum. Draw a line from the center of the acetabulum point, perpendicular to the shaft of the femoral line. Place the image intensifier into the lateral view. The dye in the hip joint helps identify the circumference of the femoral head. Draw a line representing the equator of the femoral head in the sagittal plane. Insert a 2.5 mm Steinmann pin into the center of the femoral head from the intersection point of the AP line with the lateral line. These pins should be perpendicular to the shaft of the femur, end in the center of the acetabulum, and be in the midsagittal plane of the femoral head. Because the hip is usually proximally migrated, the center of rotation of the femoral head will be proximal to the center of the acetabulum. The axis pins should be centered on the acetabulum and is therefore more distal to the center of the femoral head.

Step 5: Preconstruct a hinged monolateral external fixator (e.g., Orthofix, EBI, or the SN modular rail system (MRS)) and apply the cannulated hinge over the axis pin.

Step 6: Insert the femoral frontal plane pins.

Adjust the distal clamp to the level desired on the femur. Insert two frontal plane pins with the femur kept in the patella forward position. Leave room for lengthening on the distal fixator.

Step 7: Insert two pins into the anterolateral pelvis.

Roll the operating room table to the opposite side and place the image intensifier over the affect supra-acetabular region. When a triangle is visualized over the acetabulum, the correct plane for the pin is seen. Drill a 1.8 mm wire into this triangle and then tap it in until a hollow sound from hitting a cortex is heard. If the wire is in the correct plane, then level the table and overdrill the wire with a 4.8 mm cannulated drill bit or in smaller children a 3.2 mm cannulated drill bit. Insert a hydroxyapatite-coated half-pin. Repeat the same for a pin either more proximal or more distal to the first.

Step 8: Attach an arch to these first two pins so that the arch is in line with the rest of the fixator based on the constraints of the fixator.

This arch will usually not be perpendicular to the pelvis due to the 15° abduction of the hip joint.

Step 9: Add one transverse and one oblique pin to the pelvic arch for a total of 4 pins in the pelvis. The transverse pin should be in the supra-acetabular region. The oblique pin should be between the transverse and the two anterior pins.

Step 10: Test the hip motion. The hip should move easily in flexion-extension.

Step 11: Perform an acute distraction of the hip joint so that Shenton line is over reduced.

Step 12: Reduce any lateral subluxation of the hip. This is achieved by loosening the fixation of the distal frontal plane pins and pushing the femur medially to reduce the femoral head deeper into the acetabulum.

Step 13: Insert one or two more distal femoral pins in a delta configuration to the frontal plane pins.

Step 14: Add an arch to the distal femur clamp.

Step 15: Add a removable distraction rod anteriorly between the pelvic arch and the distal femoral arch to prevent flexion contracture by keeping the hip extended especially at night.

12.1.3 Postoperative Management of Distraction Treatment for Perthes Disease

Physiotherapy is initiated immediately to work on hip flexion-extension, with emphasis on maintaining hip extension with prone exercises. The therapist must clearly understand that they are not to work on hip abduction, adduction, external rotation, or internal rotation because this would stress the external fixation pin-bone interface. The patient and therapist are taught to measure the true hip motion at the hip hinge rather than doing so clinically (i.e., between the thigh and the spine). The patient is taught how to perform flexion-extension exercises at home, supplementing the hour of daily physical therapy. Patients are allowed 50 % weight bearing while the external fixator is in place.

Flexion contracture of the hip commonly develops. Physiotherapy is important for prevention and treatment of contractures. If a severe degree of flexion contracture occurs, distraction of the hip joint is compromised. Using the removable hip extension bar prevents this complication. The apparatus is left in place for 4 months in patients younger than 12 years and for 5 months in patients 12 years and older. This usually correlates with radiograph re-ossification of the lateral pillar.

Apparatus removal is performed under general anesthesia as an outpatient procedure. Because of the osteoporosis of the femoral head and neck, manipulation of the hip with the patient under anesthesia should not be performed after the removal to avoid fracture of the hip or femur. A bilateral abduction brace (pelvic band with bilateral thigh cuffs and hip hinges) set at 30° of abduction per leg is applied after the removal and was used both day and night for 6 weeks. Resumption of full weight bearing begins on a gradual basis immediately after fixator removal, and full weight bearing is achieved in approximately 4 weeks. After 6 weeks of full-time use, the abduction splint is used only at night for 6 months. Running, jumping, and participation in sports are not allowed for 1 year after treatment. Swimming, cycling, and walking are encouraged. The patient is taught a series of five stretches I call the Perthes exercises. These should be performed twice daily until skeletal maturity.

Perthes Exercises

1. Wide abduction standing
2. Supine hip flexion
3. Prone internal rotation stretches
4. Prone external rotation stretches
5. Prone hyperextension of the hip

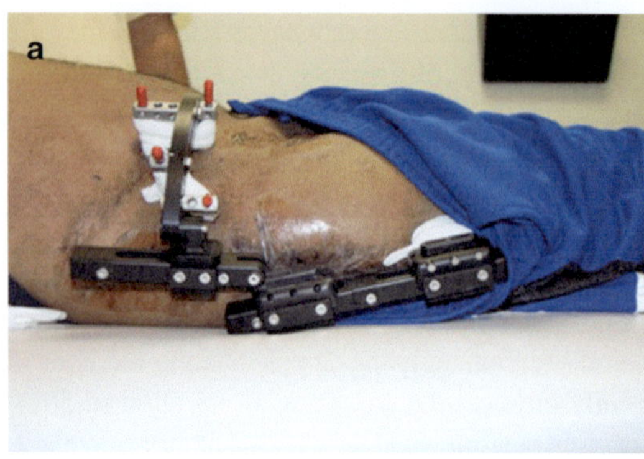
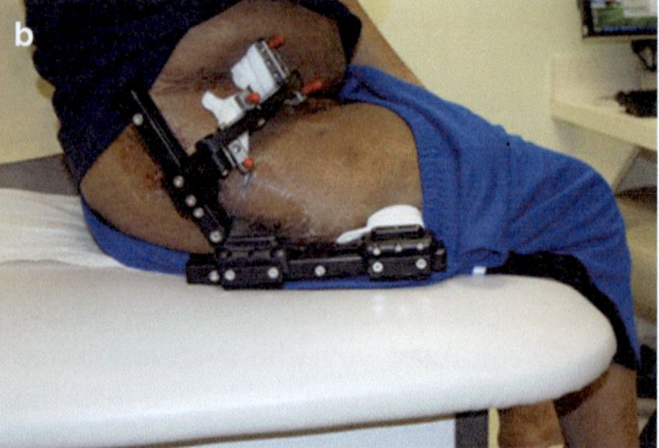

Fig. 12.1 Hip hinge distraction external fixator (Smith and Nephew Modular Rail System) supine (**a**) and sitting (**b**)

12.1.4 Results

Paley and Segev conducted a retrospective study of the first 16 consecutive patients (18 hips) treated by hip joint distraction between July 1989 and July 1999. Fourteen patients had Perthes disease, and two had avascular necrosis of the hip after slipped capital femoral epiphysis. The patient group was comprised of four girls and 12 boys. Two patients had bilateral hip involvement and received the same treatment for both hips. One patient received repeat distraction treatment of the same hip. The mean patient age at the time of disease onset was 9.1 years (range, 6–14 years). The mean patient age at the time of surgery was 10.2 years (range, 6.5–15.6 years). All patients with Perthes disease had whole-head involvement, and the cases were classified as Catterall IV (Catterall 1971; Lloyd-Roberts et al. 1976; Herring et al. 1992; Salter and Thompson 1984) or depending on the date of initial presentation to the senior author. The two patients with slipped capital epiphysis experienced collapse of the femoral head resulting from avascular necrosis.

The treatment protocol used in all these cases was based on previous experience with hip distraction for chondrolysis and hip dislocation and the successful treatment of the first patient in this series in 1989 (Fig. 12.2). Containment surgery by osteotomy was contraindicated for this 11-year-old patient who presented with a very stiff, subluxed, and deformed hip that had previously been treated by bracing for 1 year. Distraction was proposed to reduce the hip,

which had marked proximal migration and subluxation. This patient was considered to have a very poor prognosis before treatment. The striking success of the distraction treatment in this difficult case encouraged us to offer distraction treatment as an alternative therapy for patients who subsequently presented with Perthes disease. Conventional treatment options, such as pelvic and femoral osteotomy and shelf procedures, were discussed with all patients and were offered as surgical management options when patients met the criteria for these procedures. The surgical approach and treatment protocol for all patients treated by distraction was identical to those used for the index patient, and all documentation was conducted in the same way at the same time intervals. Although this study is retrospective in that no formal study was organized or planned in advance, all the data were collected for clinical documentation in a prospective fashion by the treating author. These data were later reviewed for this retrospective study.

The families of all patients who were offered the distraction treatment were first given the phone numbers of one or two previously treated patients so that they could contact them. Families made their decision to proceed with distraction or containment surgical treatment based on their conversations with previous patients and based on information provided by the surgeon regarding conventional treatment. Because of our success in the treatment of Perthes disease, the distraction regimen was additionally applied to all cases of avascular necrosis resulting from

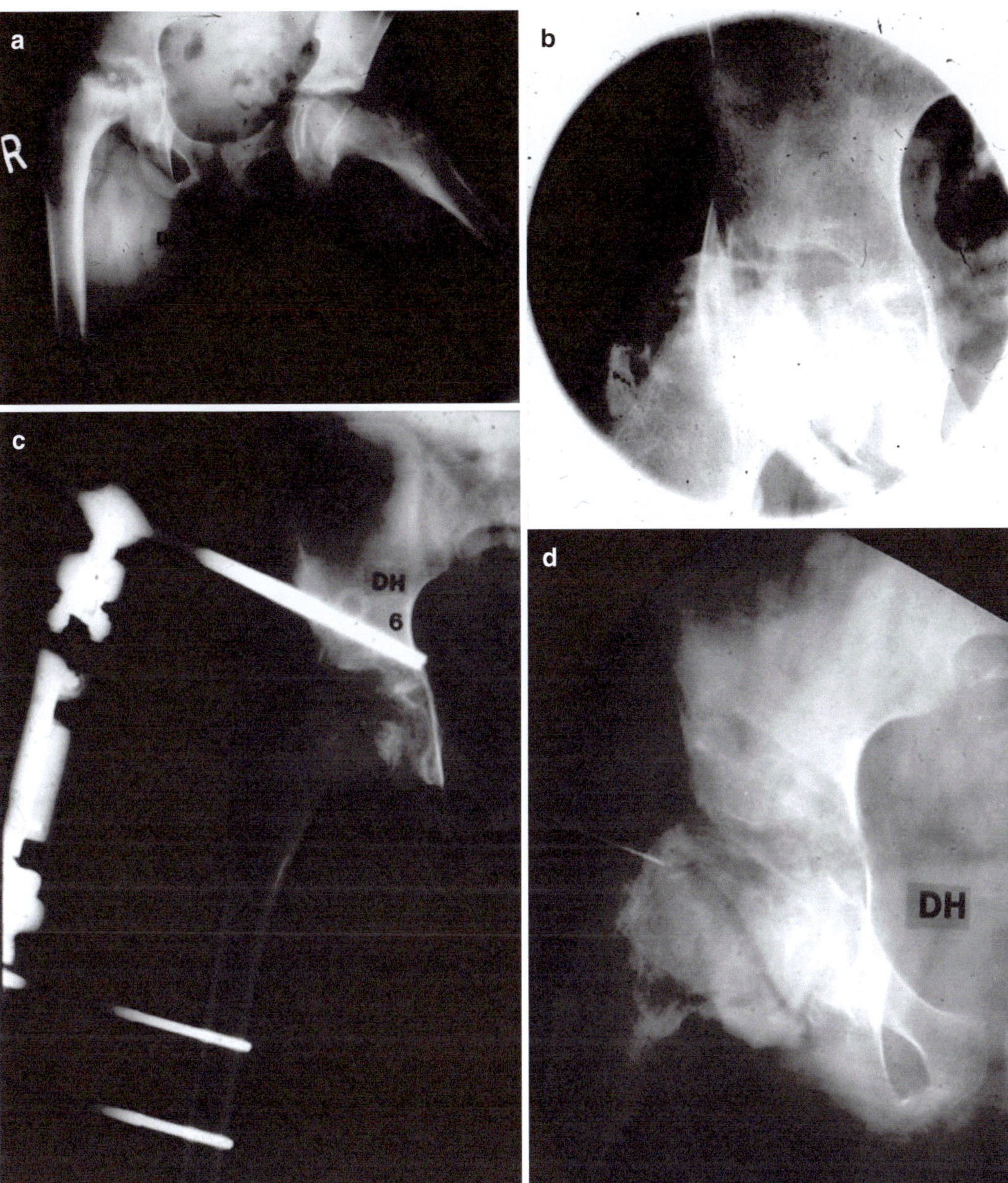

Fig. 12.2 (**a**) An 11-year-old boy with Perthes with fixed flexion-adduction contracture. There is a break in Shenton line with proximal and lateral migration of the femoral head; (**b**) intraoperative arthrogram showing femoral head flattening; (**c**) reduction of the femoral head by application of hinge distraction external fixator with hip in 15° of abduction; (**d**) arthrogram at time of removal of apparatus. The femoral head is rounder; (**e**) follow-up radiograph 22 months after surgery; (**f**) hip abduction 22 months after distraction; hip external (**g**) and internal (**h**) rotation 22 months after distraction; hip abduction 10 years after distraction (**i**, **j**); hip external (**k**) and internal (**l**) rotation 22 months after distraction; AP (**m**) and frog lateral (**n**) pelvis x-rays 10 years after distraction; flexion 10 years after distraction (**o**)

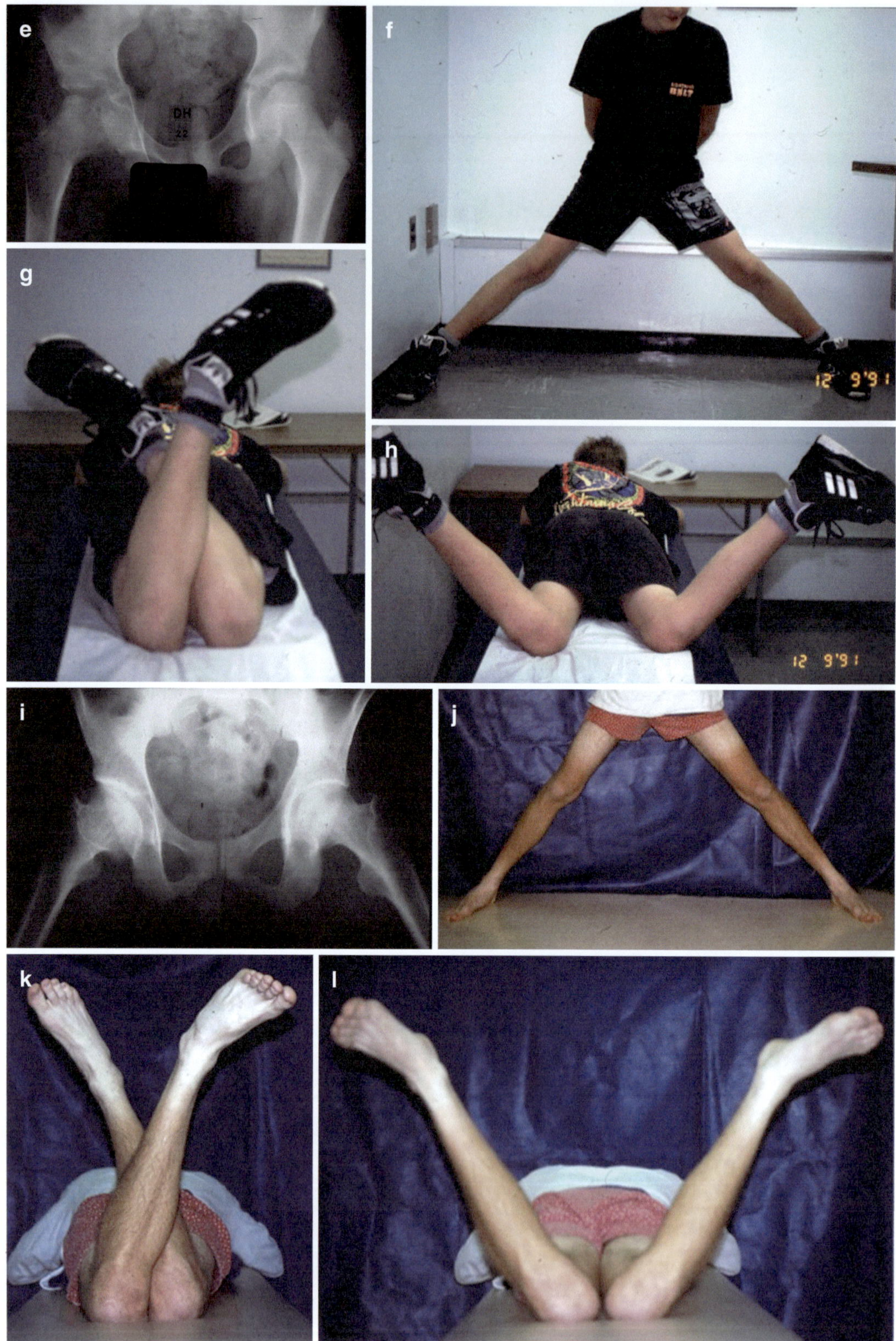

Fig. 12.2 (continued)

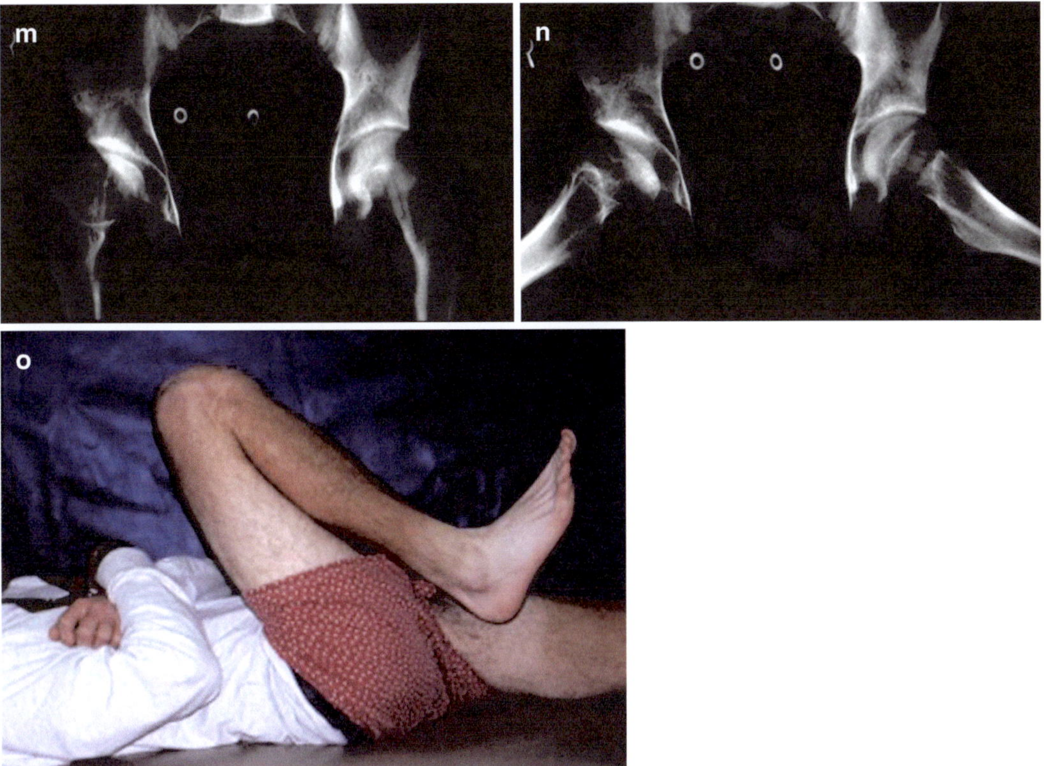

Fig. 12.2 (continued)

slipped capital femoral epiphysis treated during the same time period. To date, all these patients have chosen distraction treatment.

External fixation was in use at our institution for hip joint distraction and distraction of other joints for various indications; the use of the technique to treat Perthes disease was therefore not considered experimental. During the study period, internal review board approval was not required by our institution for the application of hip distraction to cases of Perthes disease or avascular necrosis of the hip. Furthermore, because no formal prospective study was being conducted, this study is considered retrospective. Internal review board approval was obtained to conduct this retrospective study.

All patients, while under general anesthesia, underwent intraoperative arthrography of the hip at the time of external fixator application and post-distraction arthrography of the hip at the time of fixator removal. Patients were examined

every 6 months for the first 2 years and then annually for the remainder of the study period. Clinical observations were evaluated and recorded by the senior author at each follow-up visit and included subjective pain and activity levels, bilateral hip range of motion (flexion, fixed flexion deformity, abduction, adduction, prone internal, and external rotation), knee range of motion, Trendelenburg test, clinical gait assessment, and anteroposterior plus frog leg view pelvic radiographs. The average time from surgery to most recent follow-up visit was 6.7 years (range, 3.5–13.4 years). The clinical evaluations and final follow-up radiographs were tabulated and analyzed.

Based on the total arc of hip range of motion, a clinical sphericity index was calculated to describe how close the hip motion was to being spherical. This index was calculated by dividing the total arc of motion in all three planes of motion (flexion-extension, abduction-adduction, and internal-external rotation) of the diseased hip by 270°, which is the average normal total hip range of motion. The clinical sphericity index is expressed as a percentage of normal total range of motion. The hip was considered to move spherically if the index was greater than two-thirds (67 %) of the normal range.

We also calculated the sphericity of the femoral head using measurements derived from pre- and post-distraction arthrograms. The ratios between the largest diameter of the femoral head divided by the lesser diameter (two times the lesser radius, perpendicular to the largest diameter, and bisecting it in its middle), on the anteroposterior and lateral view arthrograms, were added together and divided by 2 to calculate an index. A normal index for a spherical femoral head is 1.1 (Bennett et al. 2002). The closer the index is to 1.1, the more spherical is the head. The initial and final arthrogram ratios were compared.

The final follow-up radiographs, including those of patients who were not skeletally mature, were graded using the Stulberg et al. (1981) classification system. The following radiographic parameters were measured on the preoperative and final radiographs for the operated and normal hips: sharp acetabular angle, central edge angle, proximal migration of Shenton line, and distance of the medial border of the femoral head from the tear drop. Closure of the proximal femoral physis on the normal side was noted and considered to be evidence of hip skeletal maturity. A premature closure of the diseased hip physis relative to the normal hip also was noted.

Fifteen patients had complained of varying degrees of pain before surgery. At final follow-up, only one patient complained of mild pain that did not require analgesics and did not interfere with daily activities. All patients returned to full school and/or work activities, including sports without limitation. All patients expressed satisfaction with the results and indicated vast improvement in their function compared with their pretreatment abilities. Fifteen patients walked with a limp before the operation, compared with only one patient who walked with mild lurch gait at final follow-up. Fifteen patients had positive Trendelenburg sign before the operation, compared with only one with positive Trendelenburg sign at final follow-up. All patients had full ipsilateral knee range of motion before surgery and at final follow-up.

All our patients experienced marked limitation of motion on the affected side at presentation. At final follow-up, the mean flexion-extension arc of motion was 100° (range, 90–130°). The mean abduction-adduction arc of motion was 54° (range, 25–75°). The mean internal-external rotation arc of motion was 58° (range, 0–90°). The mean total hip arc of motion was 214° (range, 115–285°). The mean arc of motion for the treated hip was 79 % of normal (range, 43–100 %). At final follow-up, 16 of 18 hips that underwent hip joint distraction had their range of motion restored to at least two-thirds normal; two hips had a range of motion below functional range.

During distraction, early, rapid osteoporosis of the femoral head was consistently observed, revealing sclerotic dead bone. This was followed by gradual ossification of the lateral pillar, which usually was completed by 4 months. All patients except two underwent external fixator application after femoral head collapse and during the resorption phase. Two patients underwent application of the external fixator just after the initial subchondral fracture. In both of these cases, the femoral head re-collapsed after fixator removal and subsequently went through a resorption phase. One of these patients underwent a second distraction treatment, and complete success was achieved the second time.

At the most recent follow-up visit, nine patients had reached skeletal maturity as judged by closure of the femoral capital epiphysis in the normal hip. Three hips showed signs of premature physeal closure on the operated side. The mean preoperative Sharp acetabular angle was 45° (range, 40–50°) and at final follow-up was 44° (range, 35–50°). The mean preoperative center-edge angle was 19° (range, 0–30°) and increased to 24° (range, 15–35°) postoperatively. The difference between pre- and postoperative Sharp acetabular angles was not significant ($P=0.094$); the increase in the center-edge angle after treatment was marginally significant ($P=0.051$).

The mean proximal migration measured as a break in Shenton line was 7 mm (range, 0–14 mm) preoperatively and improved to 2 mm (range, 0–12 mm) at the most recent follow-up visit. This difference was statistically significant ($P = 0.002$). The average distance from the medial femoral head to the teardrop was 13 mm preoperatively (range, 8–16 mm) compared with 11 mm (range, 6–18 mm) postoperatively, which was statistically significant ($P = 0.022$). The mean radiographic sphericity index improved from 1.29 (range, 1.1–1.6) at the time of frame application to 1.17 (range, 1.0–1.59) at the time of frame removal, which was statistically significant ($P = 0.001$). The Stulberg classification based on the most recent radiographs was as follows: Class I, one hip; Class II, five hips; Class III, eight hips; and Class IV, four hips (unpublished study).

12.1.5 Complications

Most patients developed minor pin tract infections, which were successfully treated with oral antibiotics. The fixator on one patient had to be removed after only 2 months because of severe pin tract infection. This patient developed recurrent stiffness and subluxation of the hip after the first removal. After the second treatment, the patient was able to maintain a mobile hip with spherical hip motion.

One patient sustained a fractured neck of the femur caused by a fall on the day of fixator removal. The fracture was treated by screw fixation and healed uneventfully.

Two patients each underwent a second application of the fixator for contralateral Perthes disease at 3 years and 3 months and at 1 year and 4 months, respectively, after the index distraction treatment. One patient underwent treatment of Perthes disease shortly after a subchondral fracture of the hip. The course of treatment by distraction was uneventful. However, after fixator removal, the femoral head proceeded to undergo resorption, collapse, and subluxation. Reapplication of the external fixator a year later, during the maximum resorption phase, led to an excellent final result.

As an addendum to this study, I decided to review the radiographs and results of as many patients that could be located in 2009. This represented a 20-year follow-up on the earliest patient. Only 13 of the total hips and 11 of the total patients could be found. All of the Stulberg 4 cases were in the follow-up group. It is interesting to note that all of the Stulberg 4 cases had evidence of degenerative changes, while none of the Stulberg 1, 2, or 3 cases did. Only two of the four Stulberg 4 cases were symptomatic, while the others were not. Femero-acetabular impingement (FAI) was present in all of the Stulberg 3 and 4 cases reviewed. We were unaware of FAI when we first conducted this study. Some of the Stulberg 3 cases are being considered for femoral head reduction osteotomy. The Stulberg grade did not change at final follow-up in 2009. The result grading also did not change since the two painful Stulberg 4 cases were the same symptomatic cases in the original study. It is clear that the four Stulberg 4 cases will all require a hip replacement. It is likely that the Stulberg 3 cases will require some treatment for FAI which could include hip arthroscopy or surgical dislocation of the hip with osteochondroplasty or femoral head reduction osteotomy (Paley 2011).

12.1.6 Discussion

The natural history of Perthes disease and avascular necrosis of the hip joint is directly related to patient age at time of disease onset and amount of femoral head involvement (Gower and Johnston 1971; McAndrew and Weinstein 1984; Yrjonen 1999; Ippolito et al. 1985). Older age and whole femoral head involvement are poor prognostic factors (Ippolito et al. 1987; Norlin et al. 1991; Mazda et al. 1999; Eyre-brook 1936). Treatment by bed rest, non-weight bearing, and abduction orthosis is of limited value and is not well tolerated (Kamhi and MacEwen 1975; Meehan et al. 1992; Eaton 1967; Martinez et al. 1992). Range-of-motion exercises and various forms of surgical containment have constituted the mainstay of treatment for Perthes disease (Lack et al. 1989; Bankes et al. 2000; Klisic 1983) that for children older than 6 years, any method of treatment offers a better prognosis than no treatment. Containment treatment in patients older than 11 years leads to only 40 % satisfactory results (Catterall 1971; Salter and Thompson 1984) compared with an overall age-independent success rate of 70–90 % (Gower and Johnston 1971).

Stiffness, subluxation, and femoral head collapse are considered contraindications to surgical containment treatment. Therefore, the worst cases often are not treatable with containment. Abduction bracing is a nonsurgical containment treatment method. It is fraught with problems of noncompliance, especially in older children, and can lead to hip stiffness unless prescribed in conjunction with aggressive physical therapy (Martinez et al. 1992). Varus femoral osteotomy can achieve the greatest degree of femoral head containment (Lloyd-Roberts et al. 1976). The resulting coxa vara deformity may not remodel and therefore may produce a long-term limp due to abductor muscle dysfunction because the abductor lever arm and muscle tension are altered (Noonan et al. 2001). A pelvic osteotomy alone for containment is more limited in its amount of coverage (Rowe et al. 2006; Lee et al. 2009). All these methods are contraindicated if the hip is stiff, especially if it cannot abduct sufficiently; these hips are suitable for a salvage procedure.

Both varus femoral and pelvic osteotomy methods distort the anatomy and have limited ability to change the shape of an already collapsed femoral head or to reduce subluxation (Lack et al. 1989).

The distraction we describe is not limited by hip stiffness, degree of femoral head deformity, or subluxation. Although distraction is performed with the hip in 15° of abduction, the primary goal is not containment. The epiphyseal cartilage of the femoral head is not primarily damaged from the loss of circulation to the femoral head. Instead, it reacts by proliferating outside the acetabulum, leading to coxa magna and lateral ossification. The cartilage also proliferates medial to the femoral head when the femoral head has migrated laterally and superiorly (Bennett et al. 2002). Proliferation or ossification is not observed superior to the femoral head, where it is in contact with the acetabulum. Because the femoral head cartilage seems to have the potential to grow in the unstressed regions inside and outside the acetabulum, we postulated that if the femoral head were pulled away from the acetabulum and kept there, the epiphyseal cartilage might proliferate into the acetabulum and fill the space created by the previous collapse. The acetabulum would act as a sort of mold for the femoral head. In many ways, this is similar to the theory behind containment. Pulling the femoral head down also would reduce the apparent subluxation of the hip, especially the break in Shenton line. In cases in which collapse has not occurred or has not progressed to maximum, dead bone may be resorbed under the protection of the distractor. If the distractor remains in place long enough, new bone formation can replace removed bone, preventing collapse after fixator removal. Herring (Salter and Thompson 1984) noted that once the lateral pillar has re-ossified, no further collapse is to be expected. Therefore, we chose re-ossification of the lateral pillar as a satisfactory end point for fixator removal.

The radiographic findings obtained during distraction revealed very rapid progression of osteoporosis of the femoral head and neck. The dead bone could readily be distinguished from the live bone by its white sclerotic appearance; the remainder of the femoral head and neck appeared osteoporotic. At approximately 6–8 weeks after surgery, new ossification of the lateral pillar was observed. The lateral pillar was fully reconstituted by 4 months after initiation of the distraction treatment. In children older than 12 years, this took up to 5 months.

Mose (1980) and Stulberg et al. (1981) showed that femoral head sphericity and congruency with the acetabulum are directly related to the long-term prognosis. Distraction leads to improved femoral head radiographic sphericity. Our results documented an average sphericity index improvement from 1.29 before treatment to 1.17 at frame removal, indicating increased roundness of the head and improved joint congruency. These findings were corroborated by the clinical range-of-motion results. All our patients experienced improved hip range of motion with distraction treatment. The clinical sphericity index increased, on average, to 79 % at last follow-up. If we can assume that when something moves like a sphere, it must be shaped like a sphere, it can be said that most of these hips demonstrated spherical three-dimensional motion.

We also observed that distraction did not change the shape of the acetabulum, as evidenced by the lack of change in Sharp angle. The position of the femoral head in the acetabulum, as judged by the center head angle, did change. In 12 of 18 cases, sustained reduction of a previously subluxed femoral head occurred, as revealed by a reduction of Shenton line and a decrease in lateral migration distance. This, too, is consistent with improved hip biomechanics and presumably improved longevity of the hip.

Clinically, the patients were active and had little if any gait abnormality, pain, or weakness after distraction treatment. At the most recent follow-up examinations, all except one of our patients was free from pain, limp, and Trendelenburg sign. All of our patients could walk normally and took part in normal daily activities, including sports, and were happy with their outcomes. Considering that 12 of 16 patients in this study were older than 8 years and that 7 were older than 10 years, the prognosis expected with conventional treatment would not be so favorable. Our overall results with distraction were 95 % satisfactory based on pain and limp. Containment of the hip by femoral osteotomy, when performed in older patients with hip subluxation, may cause an "incongruent incongruency" situation and worsen the condition of the joint (Lloyd-Roberts 1955; Cooperman and Stulberg 1986; Salter 1980).

Distraction treatment of the hip has been termed *arthrodiastasis* and has been used for stiffness of the hip after trauma, chondrolysis, slipped capital femoral epiphysis, avascular necrosis, Perthes disease, and other conditions (Canadell et al. 1993; Aldegheri et al. 1994a). Often combined with capsulectomy and arthrolysis, it has not been used as the primary treatment for Perthes disease (Canadell et al. 1993). One study showed unsatisfactory results of such an application that included use of an Ilizarov external fixator without

a hinge (Kocaoglu et al. 1999). The authors who presented that study have since adopted the hinge distraction method reported herein for the primary treatment of Perthes disease and have achieved vastly improved results. Guarniero (Guarniero 2006) presented the results of a comparative study of two groups of patients diagnosed with Perthes disease, treated by varus femoral osteotomy or hip joint distraction. They reported consistently good results for both groups of patients and noted that the femoral head underwent remodeling faster in the patients treated by hip joint distraction.

Segev who learned this technique from Paley reported on 16 patients with Perthes treated by distraction. The average age was 12 years which is a much older group of patients than most and therefore would have a very poor prognosis. All patients had improved range of motion and improved pain scores. This demonstrated improved prognosis over that expected for such an older group of patients (Segev 2004, 2008; Segev et al. 2004).

Minimal interference with osseous architecture and relative simplicity of hip joint distraction combined with a low complication rate renders this treatment an attractive alternative for more advanced and later-onset cases of Perthes disease. According to Stulberg et al., the most important prognostic factor that affects outcome is residual deformity of the femoral head, coupled with hip joint incongruity. Class I and II spherical hips are compatible with normal longevity of the hip; Class III and IV hips with aspherical congruency usually deteriorate during the sixth decade of life; and Class V hips with incongruity usually degenerate by the fourth decade. This series did not include any cases of incongruity (Class V). Six spherical hips (Class I and II) and 12 aspherical congruity hips (Class III and IV) were included. The long-term prognosis for these patients, therefore, is relatively good, considering that eight of 18 hips were in patients who were older than 9 years at onset of disease.

In this series, we proceeded with treatment once stiffness, subluxation, and collapse were evident in the presence of whole-head involvement in all except two cases in which the treatment was performed immediately after subchondral fracture occurred. The femoral head went on to re-collapse after fixator removal in both patients. One of them (patient 5) underwent reapplication of the fixator and a second distraction treatment without tendon release more than 1 year after the first distraction treatment; a satisfactory result was achieved. Another patient also underwent a second distraction treatment. This patient was a boy who suffered severe deep soft tissue infection of the pelvic pin sites because of poor compliance and poor personal hygiene. For the second distraction treatment, he was treated at a pediatric rehabilitation center; no subsequent difficulty occurred at the pin sites, and an excellent result was achieved after the second treatment. The final results in both of these cases were as good as those achieved by the remainder of the patients after successful one-time treatment. Because distraction does not distort the anatomy, it can be reapplied if it fails the first time. In retrospect, both of the reapplications were avoidable (too early treatment in one case and poor home hygiene in the other). Based on our results, we conclude that immediately after subchondral fracture it is too early to apply treatment. Treatment should not be implemented until femoral head resorption is evident, with or without subluxation and collapse.

Although we did not have a control group at our institution and because most other clinical series would have considered many of the cases in this series to be too severe for conventional containment approaches, we think it is reasonable to conclude that hip joint distraction combined with adductor tenotomy and psoas recession leads to results that are as good as or better than the results of traditional containment treatment methods for patients with Perthes disease and for patients with avascular necrosis after slipped capital femoral epiphysis. In contrast the study previously referred to by Guarniero did have a control group of patients treated by varus osteotomy. The healing of the Perthes head involvement was twice as fast in the distraction group as in the varus osteotomy group. This finding was similar to the results observed in this study. A major advantage of hip joint distraction

is that it is indicated even in cases in which marked stiffness, subluxation, or deformity of the femoral head is present and is not contraindicated for older children. Distraction treatment is particularly indicated for older children with more severe at-risk and poor prognostic signs. In conclusion, distraction treatment offers many theoretical and practical advantages over conventional containment treatment approaches and is a valuable addition to the armamentarium of the orthopedic surgeon who is faced with managing the difficult problem posed by Perthes disease.

12.2 Distraction Arthroplasty of the Ankle

12.2.1 Introduction

A growing number of patients are developing ankle arthritis from various causes. Many patients are seeking alternative treatment options to arthrodesis or total joint replacement. Most patients prefer to preserve their natural ankle joint and ankle motion. Although research into cartilage regeneration and repair is promising, it is too preliminary to offer a viable clinical option for the ankle at this time.

Joint distraction with external fixation has evolved as an alternative to arthrodesis and/or joint replacement. The technique of joint distraction uses the principle of ligamentotaxis to restore the normal joint space, afford less joint loading, and provide an environment in which the joint cartilage can recover. The first reported joint distractions of the knee and elbow were performed in 1975 and of the ankle in 1978 (Volkov and Oganesian 1975; Judet and Judet 1978). Aldegheri et al. (1994), from Verona, Italy, coined the term *arthrodiastasis* in 1979 to describe joint distraction (arthro [joint], dia [through], and tasis [to stretch out]).

Indications for ankle joint distraction are congruent joint surface, pain, joint mobility, and moderate to severe arthritis. The indications may be stretched to include avascular necrosis of the talus. The success of the clinical outcomes varies with respect to the presenting diagnosis.

12.2.2 Existing Method and Results

Van Roermund and colleagues have written extensively about ankle distraction for the treatment of arthritis of the ankle (van Roermund et al. 2002; Marijnissen et al. 2001a, b, 2002, 2003; van Roermund and Lafeber 1999; van Valburg et al. 1995, 1999). Their hypothesis for ankle distraction treatment is that the mechanical stress (weight-bearing forces) on the cartilage is removed to allow for restoration. Weight bearing in the fixator also allows for continued intra-articular intermittent fluid pressure and increased synovial fluid, providing further cartilage restoration. Maintaining the patient within the fixator for 3 months also allows for reduction in the subchondral bone density to increase the resiliency of the joint. These changes will allow the osteoarthritic cartilage to show reparative activity.

The indications cited by van Roermund and colleagues are posttraumatic ankle osteoarthritis with or without equinus contracture in patients who are 20–70 years old and have semi-mobile ankle joints. Their protocol involves application of the Ilizarov device (a two-ring construct) to the tibia with two 1.5-mm Kirschner wires per ring attached via four threaded rods to a U-shaped foot ring (closed distally). A talar wire to prevent distraction of the subtalar joint, two crossing calcaneal olive wires, and one medial olive wire through the metatarsals are fixed to the foot ring. Distraction is performed at a rate of 0.5 mm two times per day for 5 days to achieve a total distraction of 5 mm. This distraction is maintained for 3 months, during which full weight bearing is allowed. The device is not hinged.

The authors (van Roermund et al. 2002; Marijnissen et al. 2001a, b, 2002, 2003; van Roermund and Lafeber 1999; van Valburg et al. 1995, 1999) report that 70 % of their patients showed significant clinical improvement, including decrease in pain and increase in function (results for 50 patients with 2–8 years of follow-up). Joint mobility was sustained with the distraction treatment but was markedly restricted (50 % of normal range). Most notable was the timing of the clinical improvement, with only one-half of the clinical improvement occurring within the first year after the procedure. A slight increase in joint mobility, significant widening of the joint space, and diminished subchondral sclerosis were progressively observed during the 5 years after the procedure. The authors also performed a prospective controlled study which showed that joint distraction led to a statistically significant better clinical outcome than did arthroscopic débridement of the ankle joint alone (Marijnissen et al. 2001a, 2002, 2003). In summary, van Roermund and colleagues (van Roermund et al. 2002; Marijnissen et al. 2003) showed that static ankle distraction alone without range-of-motion exercises yields a positive clinical effect in 70 % of cases.

12.2.3 Paley's Method

Unlike the Dutch group, Paley chose to build the ankle distractor with an anatomically located hinge which allows the patient to perform range-of-motion exercises throughout the entire distraction treatment. In addition, he combined adjunctive procedures to increase range of motion, eliminate impingement, improve stability, and improve joint orientation. This method is referred to as Paley's method and includes hinged ankle joint distraction, allowing joint range-of-motion exercises during treatment; correction of osseous alignment using osteotomy; surgical treatment of muscle/joint contractures by soft tissue releases; and treatment of joint impingement by resection of osteophytes and osteochondroplasty.

12.2.4 Paley Method Technique

12.2.4.1 Adjunctive Procedures
Blocking Osteophyte Resection

If dorsiflexion is limited by anterior distal tibial or talar neck osteophytes, the osteophytes should be resected. An anterior incision is made lateral to the tibialis anterior tendon. The tibialis anterior tendon is retracted medial and the neurovascular bundle lateral. The ankle joint is entered through the posterior sheath of the tibialis anterior tendon. The anterior distal tibia is then resected and the neck of the talus deepened.

The extent of the resection is checked using fluoroscopy. If plantar flexion is limited by posterior ankle osteophytes, they should be resected through a posterolateral incision (i.e., Gallie approach) to gain access to the posterior ankle capsule. To prevent recurrence of these osteophytes, bone wax may be pressed into the cancellous bone. We use nonsteroidal anti-inflammatory drugs (NSAIDs) (e.g., indomethacin, naproxen) postoperatively to inhibit bone formation for 6 weeks. However, NSAIDs are not used if an osteotomy is performed concomitantly (Dahners and Mullis 2004).

Equinus Contracture Release

Equinus contracture can be released by performing either isolated anterior or posterior gastrocnemius recession (i.e., Baumann or Strayer, respectively), gastrocnemius-soleus recession (i.e., modified Vulpius procedure), or Achilles tendon lengthening (Lamm et al. 2005; Paley 2005; Herzenberg et al. 2007). We prefer the isolated gastrocnemius recession or gastrocnemius-soleus recession to maintain triceps surae muscle strength. Operating on the triceps surae structures is not enough to correct the equinus. A posterior capsular release may also be required to restore the ankle joint motion. Acute correction of equinus contractures should be combined with tarsal tunnel decompression to prevent stretch and acute entrapment (Lamm et al. 2007). Both the tarsal tunnel decompression and the posterior ankle capsular release can be accomplished through a posteromedial longitudinal incision. The posterior osteophytes can also be resected through a posteromedial incision. When acute release is not sufficient to reduce the equinus, the residual equinus can be corrected using gradual distraction (Fig. 12.3).

Ankle Joint Realignment

Ankle joint malalignment due to deformities such as valgus and recurvatum may be the cause of ankle joint degeneration (Paley 2005). To increase the longevity of the ankle joint cartilage, reorientation procedures, such as supramalleolar osteotomy, realign the ankle joint plafond. If the tibia-fibula relationship (ankle Shenton line) is incongruent, an isolated tibial lengthening with or without deformity correction or a fibular shortening or lengthening might be necessary to accurately restore the normal ankle anatomy. Fixed subtalar joint compensatory contracture, if present, should be addressed at the time of realignment and distraction. Subtalar contractures can be acutely reduced through a release or gradually corrected with the use of an external fixator. It is important to accurately assess compensatory deformities before surgical intervention (Paley 2005; Lamm and Paley 2004). Correction of ankle alignment is usually done using a supramalleolar osteotomy. This can be carried out acutely and fixed internally while the distraction is performed with external fixation. An alternative is to perform acute or gradual distal tibial realignment and ankle distraction with the same external fixator.

12.2.4.2 Application of Hinged External Fixation for Ankle Joint Distraction (Figs. 12.4 and 12.5)

Step 1—Apply a two-ring fixation block (orthogonal to the tibial axis) to the tibia by using wire(s) and half-pin(s). The tibial external fixation construct should be applied an ample distance proximal to the ankle joint to ensure ease of hinge application. Insert a temporary center-of-rotation wire through the Inman ankle axis of rotation

Fig. 12.3 (**a**) A 45-year-old woman with Ollier's disease status post osteotomies and ankle arthritis. She has equinus deformity of the ankle. (**b**) Lateral radiograph shows anterior ankle osteophytes blocking dorsiflexion. (**c**) After resection of osteophytes and application of a hinged external fixation ankle joint distraction device. (**d**) Lateral radiograph after distraction and correction of ankle joint contracture. (**e**) Anteroposterior and lateral radiographs after removal of the external fixator obtained at 3-year follow-up. (**f**) Lateral view obtained at 3-year follow-up shows recurrence of ankle osteophytes and a plantigrade foot position. The patient has no pain. (**g**) Final clinical photo at 3-year follow-up. The foot is plantigrade

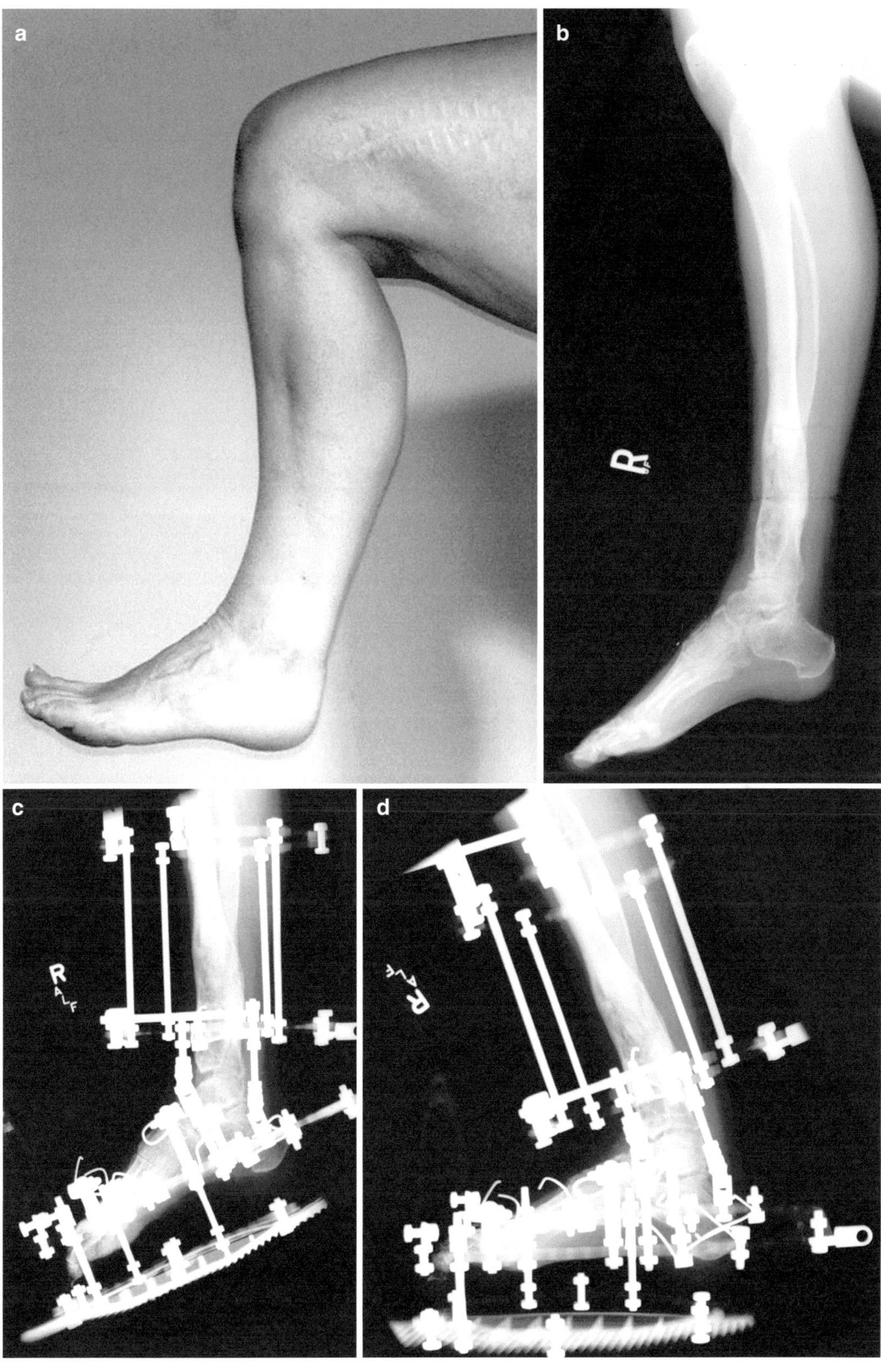

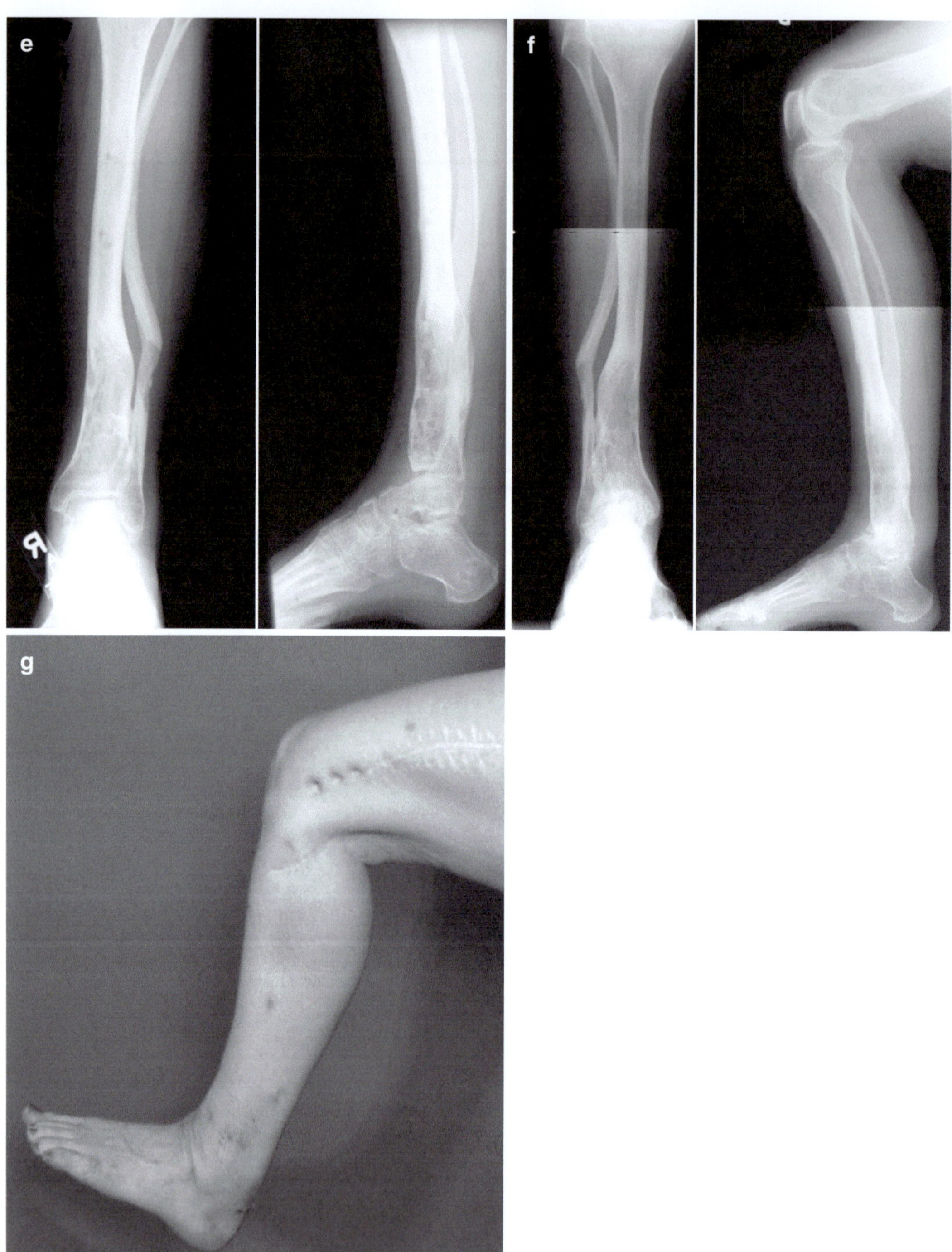

Fig. 12.3 (continued)

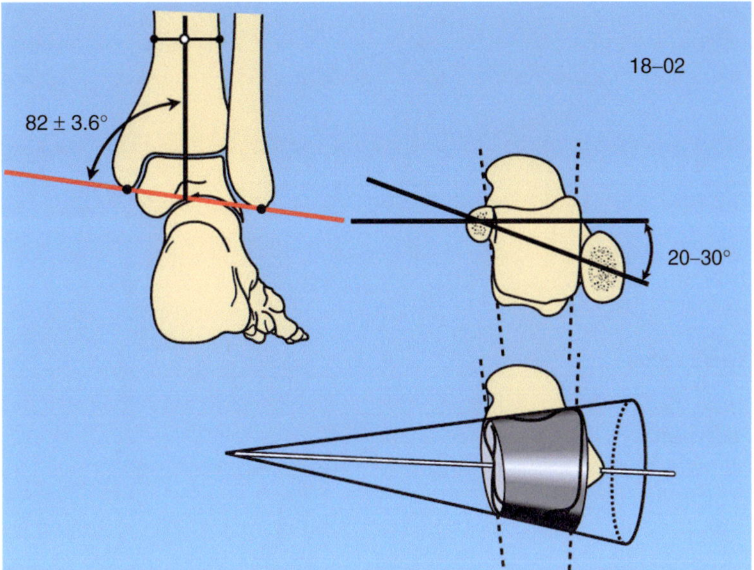

Fig. 12.4 Inman's ankle joint axis illustrated in multiple planes (Reproduced with permission from Paley (2005))

(start from the tip of lateral malleolus to the tip of medial malleolus) (Paley 2005). Then cut this wire short to allow space for hinge adjustment.

Step 2—Mount a closed U-shaped foot ring parallel to the sole of the foot by using two crossed calcaneal wires and two midfoot wires. Then insert two talar smooth wires, one medial to lateral through the talar neck and the other from anteromedial in the neck of the talus to posterolateral to the Achilles tendon. The position of the wires should be monitored with fluoroscopy to make sure they do not enter the subtalar or ankle joints. Mount these two wires to the foot ring and tension them.

Step 3—Attach medial and lateral threaded rods from the tibial to the foot ring making sure the universal hinge align/intersect the ankle axis wire. The universal hinges joint should be centered with the ankle axis wire. The medial hinge is positioned more proximal and anterior than the lateral hinge.

Step 4—Add a posterior distraction rod, which can be removed by the patient for ankle range-of-motion exercises.

I prefer to simultaneously distract both the subtalar and ankle joints acutely. This is accomplished by applying distraction between the tibial and foot fixation before inserting the two talar wires. In addition, after insertion of the two talar wires, 2 mm of acute ankle distraction is performed and checked with the use of fluoroscopy to ensure symmetrical and accurate ankle distraction. The patient starts distraction at a rate of 1 mm per day on postoperative day 1 for a total of 5 days. The goal is to achieve 8–10 mm of symmetrical ankle joint distraction. The external fixation device is maintained for 3 months while allowing weight bearing as tolerated. The patient removes the posterior distraction rod to perform daily ankle range-of-motion exercises and attends physical therapy three times a week.

12.2.5 **Author's Results** (Paley and Lamm 2005; Paley et al. 2008)

Paley and Lamm reported on 32 patients who underwent this ankle joint distraction technique

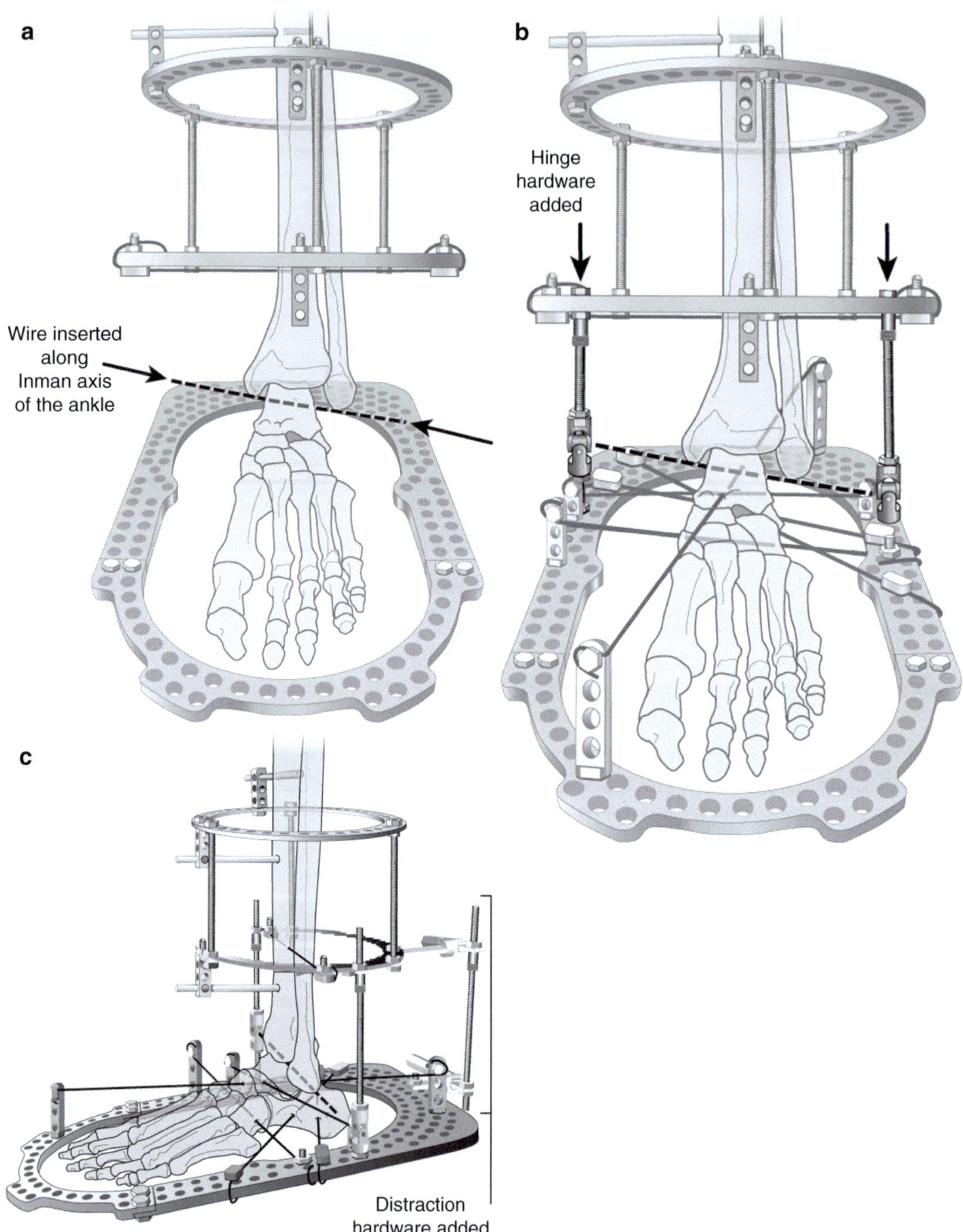

Fig. 12.5 (**a**) Two-ring block of fixation is placed on the tibia by using a wire and three half-pins perpendicular to the tibia bisection in both the transverse and sagittal planes. A center-of-rotation wire is placed through the Inman axis of the ankle (tip of medial malleolus to tip of lateral malleolus). This is a reference wire (*dotted line*) which is cut short and utilized for positioning the medial and lateral ankle hinges. (**b**) The foot ring is mounted parallel to the sole of the foot. Note the foot ring is closed/completed by attaching a half ring to the distal end of the U-shaped foot ring. Fixation of the foot ring is achieved with two crossed wires in the calcaneus, two talar neck wires, and one wire across the midfoot. Universal hinges are placed to intersect the Inman's ankle axis wire. Once aligned the universal hinges are then mounted to the foot ring. Note the medial hinge is more proximal than the lateral hinge. (**c**) A posterior distraction rod is placed and can be removed by the patient for ankle range-of-motion exercises. Note the medial hinge is more anterior than the lateral hinge

and found 78 % of patients had maintained their ankle range of motion and have none to occasional moderate pain that can be managed generally with NSAIDs alone. Only one has required an ankle fusion, and only one has been converted to an ankle joint replacement. The longevity of these results and the higher percent of good or excellent results when compared with other studies suggest that combining adjunctive procedures and articulation with ankle distraction improves the results of this procedure.

12.2.6 Discussion

The reason ankle distraction leads to lasting pain relief when treating ankle joint osteoarthritis is still speculative. It is possible that distraction permits cartilage repair to occur in a protected low-pressure environment. Salter et al. (1980) showed that cartilage repair (fibrocartilage) occurs within a cartilage defect. Fibrocartilage formation is the body's attempt to restore a normal joint surface. Pain from osteoarthritis may be related to the effect of hydrostatic pressure on subchondral bone cyst, whereby the synovial fluid from the joint enters through a cartilage defect (channel) and increases the fluid and thus the pressure within the subchondral bone cyst (van Valburg et al. 1995). Distraction might allow for the formation of fibrocartilage, which adequately seals these channels to the subchondral bone cyst and therefore eliminates the increased fluid (pressure) and the pain. In addition, joint distraction of the hip in cases of Perthes disease has been shown to stimulate epiphyseal cartilage to grow (Paley 2005).

Radiographs obtained after the external fixation is removed show that the joint distraction space of the ankle is not maintained. However, this radiographic finding does not seem to negatively impact the clinical result. Cartilage repair (i.e., fibrocartilage) has occurred although it is not enough to increase the radiographic measured joint space post-distraction but merely seal the cartilage cracks and defects.

Our results showed that the total arc of ankle joint motion was only slightly reduced by the treatment of hinged ankle distraction. This finding is significant in that our technique of hinged distraction did not create any additional ankle joint stiffness. Most notable is that the arch of ankle joint motion was harnessed into a functional range to our goal of 10° of dorsiflexion and at least 15° of plantar flexion. Therefore, if patients have very little ankle motion preoperatively, it is unlikely to become increased by this procedure.

The patients who underwent hinged ankle joint distraction using the protocol detailed above had promising long-term results. Seventy-eight percent (14 of 18 patients) had only occasional moderate to mild pain. Our mean Foot and Ankle Follow-Up Questionnaire ankle distraction score of 71 points is comparable to a recent ankle fusion study in which the score was 74 points (Colman and Pomeroy 2007). Most notably, only one of our patients required conversion to ankle arthroplasty and only one of our patients required an ankle fusion.

As for the longevity of our aforementioned hinged ankle joint distraction treatment protocol, our longest follow-up patient that was tractable was 13 years. That patient is still functioning well with occasional NSAIDs and without further surgery. After 5 years post-distraction treatment, the benefit decreases as shown by our data (Foot and Ankle Follow-Up Questionnaire score was 79 points for the patients with 5 years or less follow-up and 52 points for patients greater than 5 years follow-up). Therefore, the benefit of the distraction treatment decreases after 5 years.

Although 44 % of the patients who underwent treatment at our center could not be located or refused to be included in the study, we think the 56 % who took the questionnaire were representative of the group. Seventy-nine percent have maintained their ankle range of motion and have none to mild pain that can be managed without pain medication or with NSAIDs alone. Only one has required an ankle fusion, and only one has been converted to an ankle joint replacement. The longevity of these results and the higher percent of good or excellent results when compared with other studies (van Roermund et al. 2002; Marijnissen et al. 2003; Marijnissen et al. 2002;

van Valburg et al. 1995, 1999) suggest that combining adjunctive procedures and articulation with ankle distraction improves the results of this procedure.

Conclusions

Ankle joint distraction is a viable alternative to ankle arthrodesis or ankle replacement. A congruent, painful, mobile, and arthritic ankle joint treated with this technique can achieve good results. The à la carte approach (blocking osteophyte resection, muscle/joint contracture release, and osseous ankle realignment procedures) presented in this article is as important for a successful outcome as is the hinged ankle joint distraction technique itself.

References

Aldegheri R, Trivella G, Saleh M (1994) Articulated distraction of the hip. Conservative surgery for arthritis in young patients. Clin Orthop Relat Res 301:94–101

Axer A, Gershuni DH, Hendel D, Mirovski Y (1980) Indications for femoral osteotomy in Legg-Calve-Perthes disease. Clin Orthop Relat Res 150:78–87

Bankes MJ, Catterall A, Hashemi-Nejad A (2000) Valgus extension osteotomy for 'hinge abduction' in Perthes' disease. Results at maturity and factors influencing the radiological outcome. J Bone Joint Surg Br 82(4): 548–554

Bennett JT, Stuecker R, Smith E, Winder C, Rice J (2002) Arthrographic findings in Legg-Calve-Perthes disease. J Pediatr Orthop B 11(2):110–116

Canadell J, Gonzales F, Barrios RH, Amillo S (1993) Arthrodiastasis for stiff hips in young patients. Int Orthop 17(4):254–258

Catterall A (1971) The natural history of Perthes' disease. J Bone Joint Surg Br 53(1):37–53

Colman AB, Pomeroy GC (2007) Transfibular ankle arthrodesis with rigid internal fixation: an assessment of outcome. Foot Ankle Int 28(3):303–307. doi:10.3113/fai.2007.0303

Cooperman DR, Stulberg SD (1986) Ambulatory containment treatment in Perthes' disease. Clin Orthop Relat Res 203:289–300

Dahners LE, Mullis BH (2004) Effects of nonsteroidal anti-inflammatory drugs on bone formation and soft-tissue healing. J Am Acad Orthop Surg 12(3): 139–143

Daly K, Bruce C, Catterall A (1999) Lateral shelf acetabuloplasty in Perthes' disease. A review of the end of growth. J Bone Joint Surg Br 81(3):380–384

Eaton GO (1967) Long-term results of treatment in coxa plana. A follow-up study of eighty-eight patients. J Bone Joint Surg Am 49(6):1031–1042

Evans DL (1958) Legg-Calve-Perthes' disease; a study of late results. J Bone Joint Surg Br 40-B(2):168–181

Evans DL, Lloyd-Roberts GC (1958) Treatment in Legg-Calve-Perthes' disease; a comparison of in-patient and out-patient methods. J Bone Joint Surg Br 40-B(2): 182–189

Eyre-brook A (1936) Osteochondritis deformans coxa juvenilis or Perthes disease: the result of treatment by traction in recumbency. J Bone Joint Surg Br 24: 166–182

Gower WE, Johnston RC (1971) Legg-Perthes disease. Long-term follow-up of thirty-six patients. J Bone Joint Surg Am 53(4):759–768

Guarniero R (2006) Comparative study of two groups of patients diagnosed with Perthes disease, treated by varus femoral osteotomy or hip joint distraction. Perthes Course, Baltimore

Herring JA, Neustadt JB, Williams JJ, Early JS, Browne RH (1992) The lateral pillar classification of Legg-Calve-Perthes disease. J Pediatr Orthop 12(2):143–150

Herzenberg JE, Lamm BM, Corwin C, Sekel J (2007) Isolated recession of the gastrocnemius muscle: the Baumann procedure. Foot Ankle Int 28(11):1154–1159. doi:10.3113/fai.2007.1154

Ippolito E, Tudisco C, Farsetti P (1985) Long-term prognosis of Legg-Calve-Perthes disease developing during adolescence. J Pediatr Orthop 5(6):652–656

Ippolito E, Tudisco C, Farsetti P (1987) The long-term prognosis of unilateral Perthes' disease. J Bone Joint Surg Br 69(2):243–250

Judet R, Judet T (1978) The use of a hinge distraction apparatus after arthrolysis and arthroplasty (author's transl). Rev Chir Orthop Reparatrice Appar Mot 64(5):353–365

Kamhi E, MacEwen GD (1975) Treatment of Legg-Calve-Perthes disease. Prognostic value of Catterall's Classification. J Bone Joint Surg Am 57(5):651–654

Klisic PJ (1983) Treatment of Perthes' disease in older children. J Bone Joint Surg Br 65(4):419–427

Kocaoglu M, Kilicoglu OI, Goksan SB, Cakmak M (1999) Ilizarov fixator for treatment of Legg-Calve-Perthes disease. J Pediatr Orthop B 8(4):276–281

Lack W, Feldner-Busztin H, Ritschl P, Ramach W (1989) The results of surgical treatment for Perthes' disease. J Pediatr Orthop 9(2):197–204

Lamm BM, Paley D (2004) Deformity correction planning for hindfoot, ankle, and lower limb. Clin Podiatr Med Surg 21(3):305–326, v. doi:10.1016/j.cpm.2004.04.004

Lamm BM, Paley D, Herzenberg JE (2005) Gastrocnemius soleus recession: a simpler, more limited approach. J Am Podiatr Med Assoc 95(1):18–25

Lamm BM, Paley D, Testani M, Herzenberg JE (2007) Tarsal tunnel decompression in leg lengthening and deformity correction of the foot and ankle. J Foot Ankle Surg 46(3):201–206. doi:10.1053/j.jfas.2007.01.007

Lee DS, Jung ST, Kim KH, Lee JJ (2009) Prognostic value of modified lateral pillar classification in Legg-Calve-Perthes disease. Clin Orthop Surg 1(4):222–229. doi:10.4055/cios.2009.1.4.222

Lloyd-Roberts GC (1955) Osteoarthritis of the hip; a study of the clinical pathology. J Bone Joint Surg Br 37-B(1):8–47

Lloyd-Roberts GC, Catterall A, Salamon PB (1976) A controlled study of the indications for and the results of femoral osteotomy in Perthes' disease. J Bone Joint Surg Br 58(1):31–36

Marijnissen AC, Vincken KL, Viergever MA, van Roy HL, Van Roermund PM, Lafeber FP, Bijlsma JW (2001a) Ankle images digital analysis (AIDA): digital measurement of joint space width and subchondral sclerosis on standard radiographs. Osteoarthritis Cartilage 9(3):264–272. doi:10.1053/joca.2000.0384

Marijnissen AC, van Roermund PM, Verzijl N, Bijlsma JW, Lafeber FP (2001b) Does joint distraction result in actual repair of cartilage in experimentally induced osteoarthritis? Arthritis Rheum 44:S306

Marijnissen AC, Van Roermund PM, Van Melkebeek J, Schenk W, Verbout AJ, Bijlsma JW, Lafeber FP (2002) Clinical benefit of joint distraction in the treatment of severe osteoarthritis of the ankle: proof of concept in an open prospective study and in a randomized controlled study. Arthritis Rheum 46(11):2893–2902. doi:10.1002/art.10612

Marijnissen AC, van Roermund PM, van Melkebeek J, Lafeber FP (2003) Clinical benefit of joint distraction in the treatment of ankle osteoarthritis. Foot Ankle Clin 8(2):335–346

Martinez AG, Weinstein SL, Dietz FR (1992) The weight-bearing abduction brace for the treatment of Legg-Perthes disease. J Bone Joint Surg Am 74(1):12–21

Mazda K, Pennecot GF, Zeller R, Taussig G (1999) Perthes' disease after the age of twelve years. Role of the remaining growth. J Bone Joint Surg Br 81(4):696–698

McAndrew MP, Weinstein SL (1984) A long-term follow-up of Legg-Calve-Perthes disease. J Bone Joint Surg Am 66(6):860–869

Meehan PL, Angel D, Nelson JM (1992) The Scottish Rite abduction orthosis for the treatment of Legg-Perthes disease. A radiographic analysis. J Bone Joint Surg Am 74(1):2–12

Mose K (1980) Methods of measuring in Legg-Calve-Perthes disease with special regard to the prognosis. Clin Orthop Relat Res 150:103–109

Noonan KJ, Price CT, Kupiszewski SJ, Pyevich M (2001) Results of femoral varus osteotomy in children older than 9 years of age with Perthes disease. J Pediatr Orthop 21(2):198–204

Norlin R, Hammerby S, Tkaczuk H (1991) The natural history of Perthes' disease. Int Orthop 15(1):13–16

Paley D (2005) Principles of deformity correction, 1st edn, Corr 3rd printing. Rev ed. Springer, Berlin

Paley D (2011) The treatment of femoral head deformity and coxa magna by the Ganz femoral head reduction osteotomy. Orthop Clin North Am 42(3):389–399, viii. doi:10.1016/j.ocl.2011.04.006

Paley D, Lamm BM (2005) Ankle joint distraction. Foot Ankle Clin 10(4):685–698, ix. doi:10.1016/j.fcl.2005.06.010

Paley D, Lamm BM, Purohit RM, Specht SC (2008) Distraction arthroplasty of the ankle–how far can you stretch the indications? Foot Ankle Clin 13(3):471–484, ix. doi:10.1016/j.fcl.2008.05.001

Rowe SM, Jung ST, Cheon SY, Choi J, Kang KD, Kim KH (2006) Outcome of cheilectomy in Legg-Calve-Perthes disease: minimum 25-year follow-up of five patients. J Pediatr Orthop 26(2):204–210. doi:10.1097/01.bpo.0000194696.83526.6d

Salter RB (1966) Role of innominate osteotomy in the treatment of congenital dislocation and subluxation of the hip in the older child. J Bone Joint Surg Am 48(7):1413–1439

Salter RB (1980) Legg-Perthes disease: the scientific basis for the methods of treatment and their indications. Clin Orthop Relat Res 150:8–11

Salter RB, Thompson GH (1984) Legg-Calve-Perthes disease. The prognostic significance of the subchondral fracture and a two-group classification of the femoral head involvement. J Bone Joint Surg Am 66(4):479–489

Salter RB, Simmonds DF, Malcolm BW, Rumble EJ, MacMichael D, Clements ND (1980) The biological effect of continuous passive motion on the healing of full-thickness defects in articular cartilage. An experimental investigation in the rabbit. J Bone Joint Surg Am 62(8):1232–1251

Segev E (2004) Treatment of severe late onset Perthes' disease with soft tissue release and articulated hip distraction. J Pediatr Orthop B 13(5):345

Segev E (2008) Correspondence: treatment of severe late onset Perthes disease with soft tissue release and articulated hip distraction (Reply). J Pediatr Orthop B 17(1):55. doi:10.1097/01.bpb.0000210585.97533.0a

Segev E, Ezra E, Wientroub S, Yaniv M (2004) Treatment of severe late onset Perthes' disease with soft tissue release and articulated hip distraction: early results. J Pediatr Orthop B 13(3):158–165

Snyder CH (1947) A sling for use in Legg-Perthes disease. J Bone Joint Surg Am 29(2):524–526

Stulberg SD, Cooperman DR, Wallensten R (1981) The natural history of Legg-Calve-Perthes disease. J Bone Joint Surg Am 63(7):1095–1108

van Roermund PM, Lafeber FP (1999) Joint distraction as treatment for ankle osteoarthritis. Instr Course Lect 48:249–254

van Roermund PM, Marijnissen AC, Lafeber FP (2002) Joint distraction as an alternative for the treatment of osteoarthritis. Foot Ankle Clin 7(3):515–527

van Valburg AA, van Roermund PM, Lammens J, van Melkebeek J, Verbout AJ, Lafeber EP, Bijlsma JW (1995) Can Ilizarov joint distraction delay the need for an arthrodesis of the ankle? A preliminary report. J Bone Joint Surg Br 77(5):720–725 van Valburg AA, van Roermund PM, Marijnissen AC, van Melkebeek J, Lammens J, Verbout AJ, Lafeber FP, Bijlsma JW (1999) Joint distraction in treatment of osteoarthritis: a two-year follow-up of the ankle. Osteoarthritis Cartilage 7(5):474–479. doi:10.1053/joca.1998.0242

Volkov MV, Oganesian OV (1975) Restoration of function in the knee and elbow with a hinge-distractor apparatus. J Bone Joint Surg Am 57(5):591–600

Willett K, Hudson I, Catterall A (1992) Lateral shelf acetabuloplasty: an operation for older children with Perthes' disease. J Pediatr Orthop 12(5): 563–568

Yrjonen T (1999) Long-term prognosis of Legg-Calve-Perthes disease: a meta-analysis. J Pediatr Orthop B 8(3):169–172

Lengthening Reconstruction Surgery for Congenital Femoral Deficiency

13

Dror Paley and Fran Guardo

Contents

D. Paley, MD, FRCSC (✉)
F. Guardo, M.Ed., MPT, DPT
Paley Advanced Limb Lengthening Institute,
Kimmel Building 901 45th St,
West Palm Beach, FL 33407, USA
e-mail: drorpaley@gmail.com,
dpaley@lengthening.us

M. Kocaoğlu et al. (eds.), *Advanced Techniques in Limb Reconstruction Surgery*,
DOI 10.1007/978-3-642-55026-3_13, © Springer Berlin Heidelberg 2015

13.1 Introduction

Congenital femoral deficiency (CFD) is a spectrum of severity of femoral deficiency, deformity, and discrepancy. Deficiency implies a lack of integrity, stability, and mobility of the hip and knee joints. Deformity refers to bony malorientation, malrotation, and soft tissue contractures of the hip and knee. Both deficiencies and deformities are present at birth, nonprogressive, and of variable degree. Discrepancy refers to limb length and is progressive.

13.1.1 Classification

Existing classifications of congenital short femur and proximal femoral focal deficiency are descriptive but are not helpful in prescribing treatment. A longitudinal follow-up of different classification systems (1) showed that they were inaccurate in predicting the final femoral morphology based on the initial radiograph. Furthermore, previous classification systems were designed with prosthetic reconstruction surgery (PRS) (e.g., Syme's amputation or rotationplasty plus prosthetic fitting) rather than lengthening reconstruction surgery (LRS) (equalization of limb length with realignment of the lower limb and preservation of the joints) in mind. The author's (DP) classification system (Fig. 13.1) is based on the factors that influence lengthening reconstruction of the congenital short femur (2).

13.2 Evaluating the Child with Unilateral CFD

13.2.1 History

Most children born with unilateral CFD have no family history of this or other congenital anomalies. Nevertheless, inquiry should be made into family history, exposure to drugs, medications, radiation, or infectious diseases during the first trimester. Many cases are now identified with prenatal ultrasound early in the pregnancy by measuring the lengths of the two femurs.

13.2.2 Physical Exam

There is an obvious leg length discrepancy. Associated fibular hemimelia and ray deficiency may be present. The hip and knee should be examined for flexion contracture greater than the other side. Neonates and young infants normally have such contractures for the first 3–6 months. The range of motion of the hip, knee, and ankle should be recorded.

Characteristic physical examination findings include the following:

Hip: external rotation (ER) deformity or increased ER vs. internal rotation (IR), fixed flexion deformity (FFD) of hip, and limitation of abduction (when coxa vara is present)

Knee: FFD of knee, no limitation of knee flexion, hypoplastic patella, lateral tracking or subluxed or dislocated patella, anteroposterior instability of knee, rotary instability of knee, anterior dislocation of tibia on femur with knee extension followed by reduction of knee with attempted flexion, hypermobile meniscal clunks, and temporary locking of the knee during flexion

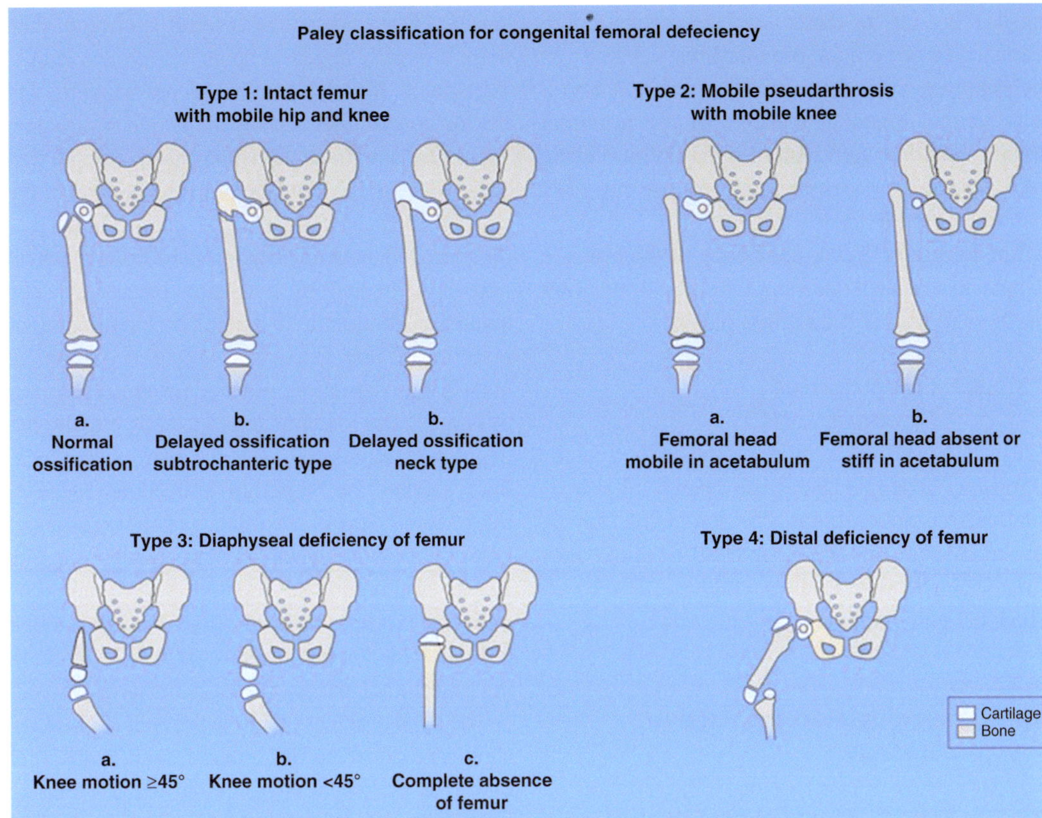

Fig. 13.1 Congenital femur deficiency classification (Conceived by Paley 1998)

Ankle: limitations of ankle dorsiflexion, obligatory eversion with dorsiflexion, hypermobility of ankle to eversion, and lateral malleolus high compared to medial

13.2.3 Radiographic Examination

13.2.3.1 Before Standing Age

Long anteroposterior (AP) pull-down X-ray; this is an AP radiograph of both femurs and tibias with the legs pulled straight and the patellas forward. It allows measurement of length of both femurs and tibia. It does not include foot height. Long lateral radiograph of both lower limbs pull-down with X-ray tube distance the same for both sides; this includes the femur and tibia of each lower limb in maximum extension on the same film. When there is a knee flexion deformity, it also allows accurate measurement of length of femur and tibia on both sides. AP pelvis supine; this allows more accurate measurement of the center-edge (CE) angle of both hips to assess for hip dysplasia. It is also a better-quality X-ray to assess for the ossification of the femoral neck. It is important that the pelvis be level for more accurate measurement.

13.2.3.2 Magnetic Resonance Imaging (MRI)

MRI is useful for assessment of integrity of the proximal femur. It can help determine whether the femoral head is joined to the shaft of the femur via a cartilaginous femoral neck. It can also help determine whether the cartilage of the femoral head is fused to the cartilage of the acetabulum in cases of femoral neck pseudarthrosis. Finally, it helps outline the deformity of the proximal femur. For optimal imaging, the cuts of the proximal femur should be reformatted in an oblique plane to see the entire proximal femur on one cut. MRI can also help outline the intra-articular pathology of the knee identifying deficiency of the cruciate ligament(s) as well outlining the shape of the joint surfaces in frontal and sagittal planes.

13.2.3.3 Computerized Tomography (CT)

CT is only useful at an older age when the acetabulum and proximal femur are nearly fully ossified. Three-dimensional CT reconstruction is useful to compare the normal acetabulum with the dysplastic side. In older children 3D CT can show the pathologic anatomy.

13.3 Surgical Reconstructive Strategy

13.3.1 Step 1: Preparatory Surgery of the Hip and Knee

Prior to lengthening one must determine whether the hip or knee are stable and/or deformed and whether surgical procedures for these joints are required before initiating lengthening. At the hip, if the acetabulum has an acetabular index that has a comparable slope to the opposite normal side, a CE angle is $\geq 20°$, and the neck shaft angle (NSA) is $\geq 110°$, no separate hip surgery is required before the first lengthening. If the acetabulum shows signs of dysplasia, then a pelvic osteotomy should be performed prior to lengthening. Objective evidence of dysplasia is defined by a CE angle of less than 20° (Suzuki et al. 1994) or CE angle greater than 20 degrees with an increased slope of the sourcil (acetabular roof) compared to the other side. Similarly increased acetabular index in young children is equivalent to increased sourcil slope in older children or adults. Coxa vara should be corrected prior to lengthening if the NSA is less than 120°. Similarly external rotation deformity of the hip is a factor to consider for correction at the same time as the acetabular dyspla-

sia. If a Dega type of osteotomy is chosen, then there is usually a gain of about 1 cm in leg length. Associated hip deformities of retroversion, hip flexion contracture, and hip abduction contracture should be simultaneously addressed. The flexion contracture of the hip is treated by recession of the psoas tendon and release of the rectus femoris tendon. Flexion deformity may also be bony in which case it is treated by extension osteotomy. The abduction contracture is treated by lengthening or resection of the fascia lata and if necessary an abductor muscle slide. When all of these deformities are present together and especially with higher degrees of angulation, the reconstructive procedure is called the "superhip" procedure. Many of these more severe cases also have delayed ossification of the femoral neck or subtrochanteric region. Before lengthening the proximal femur should be as ossified as normal for that age. It is not enough to restore the biomechanics to normal by correcting the femoral and acetabular deformities. If there is a delayed ossification of the femoral neck, BMP should be added to the femoral neck to get it to ossify. It is beneficial to femur lengthening to remove the fascia lata. The fascia lata is a thin but very tough limiting membrane which resists lengthening and applies pressure across the knee joint and the distal femoral growth plate. For this reason, it should always be removed or at least cut before lengthening. Rather than throw away the fascia lata, I prefer to use it to reconstruct the absent cruciate ligaments. Although this is not an essential preparatory procedure, I prefer to reconstruct the knee ligaments at the same time as the hip surgery when indicated. Together with the knee ligament surgery a hemi-physiodesis can be added using a plate. The ideal age for the preparatory procedure is between age 2 and 3 years.

13.3.2 Step 2: Serial Lengthenings of the Femur

To determine the number of lengthening surgeries required, a prediction of leg length discrepancy at maturity is carried out. This can be done using the Paley multiplier method (Paley et al. 2000). The first lengthening of the femur can proceed 12 months after the preparatory surgery assuming the femoral neck has ossified. If the preparatory surgery is performed between 24 and 36 months (age 2–3 years), the first lengthening can follow between ages 3 and 4 years, respectively. The exception to this is if the femur is excessively short for an external fixator and it would be beneficial to wait a year or two to allow it to grow or if the femoral neck fails to ossify in the Paley type 1b case. The lengthening goal depends on the total discrepancy at maturity. Since the total discrepancy is large in most cases, we try and achieve as much length as possible safely. The safe range is 5–8 cm if a good physical therapy program is available. In most cases, we achieve 8 cm as long as the patient is able to maintain adequate knee range of motion. As a rule of thumb to make it easy for the parents to remember the age for lengthening, we follow the rule of 4, one lengthening every 4 years (e.g., ages 4, 8, 12). The age for the second lengthening is around 8 years and the final lengthening around 12 years. If each time we can get up to 8 cm, after three lengthenings, the gain is up to 24 cm, and together with the one cm gain from the hip surgery, the total is 25 cm. If more equalization is needed, a physiodesis of the long leg distal femoral growth plate is carried out for an additional 5 cm. In this manner, we can equalize 30 cm of discrepancy with three lengthening surgeries and one physiodesis. If more is required one more lengthening of up to 10 cm can be done, increasing the total to 40 cm. Following the rule of 4, this would be done at age 16 years or older. In some cases, the tibia is also short and contributes to the LLD. During one or more lengthenings of the femur, the tibia would also be lengthened. This will be discussed in more detail later. When the LLD is from both the femur and the tibia, lengthening both at the same time can reduce the total time of external fixation while achieving even more length than is possible with lengthening of only the femur.

13.3.3 Acetabular Dysplasia

It is very common for even mild cases of CFD to have acetabular dysplasia, which predisposes the femoral head to subluxation during lengthening. The acetabulum should be assessed at the age of two by means of a supine AP pelvis radiograph. A CE angle <20° is an indication for pelvic osteotomy. A sourcil angle that is not horizontal ±5° or which is asymmetric from the opposite side is also an indication for pelvic osteotomy even in cases where the CE angle is at 20°. The acetabular dysplasia associated with CFD is not like that associated with developmental dysplasia of the hip. The deficiency is more of a hypoplasia of the entire acetabulum. This is most manifest superolateral and posterior with a hypoplastic posterior lip of the acetabulum. In young children (2–5), the Dega osteotomy is my preferred method to improve coverage (Grudziak and Ward 2001). Although the Dega gives excellent superior and lateral coverage, it is misleading to think that it improves the posterior coverage. Since the posterior lip is an ischial structure located distal to the triradiate, the Dega cannot increase its coverage but rather does not reduce its coverage like a Salter osteotomy does. In older children (6–12 years old) with an open triradiate cartilage, I prefer a periacetabular triple osteotomy, and in adolescents or adults (>13 years old with closed or closing triradiate cartilage), I prefer the Ganz periacetabular osteotomy. In both of these, there is the ability to improve the posterior coverage by internally rotating the periacetabular fragment prior to abducting this fragment for increased lateral coverage. In my early experience I used the Salter or the Millis-Hall modification of the Salter (combining innominate bone lengthening with the Salter) (Salter 1978; Millis and Hall 1979). The problems with this are twofold: (1) the hip becomes more uncovered posteriorly and (2) femoroacetabular impingement tends to develop as they mature since the femoral neck, which is often short and has a poor anterior recess, impinges with the more prominent anterior lip of the acetabulum (which is now retroverted). The Salter osteotomy and its modifications are to be avoided. Similarly, when performing the Dega osteotomy, it is also important to make sure the cut extends posteriorly past the apex of the sciatic notch to end as a T junction with the triradiate as it separates the ischium from the ilium laterally. This will ensure that the Dega osteotomy hinges on the triradiate or medial bone of the ilium rather than rotate the quarter pelvis the way a Salter osteotomy does.

13.3.4 **Proximal Femoral Deformities**
(Fig. 13.2a, b)

There is a wide spectrum of deformity of the proximal femur seen in CFD. This is nicely illustrated in the Pappas classification (Pappas 1983) which is very descriptive but not very useful for directing reconstruction. The mildest cases may have coxa valga (Pappas type 9). The majority of cases however have varying degrees of coxa vara. This coxa vara ranges from mild uniplanar deformity to severe triplanar deformity. Until recently, the pathoanatomy of this deformity was not clear. We now understand that it is a complex combination of bony deformities in the frontal, sagittal, and axial planes, combined with soft tissue contractures affecting all three planes. The severity of these deformities is often but not always milder in type

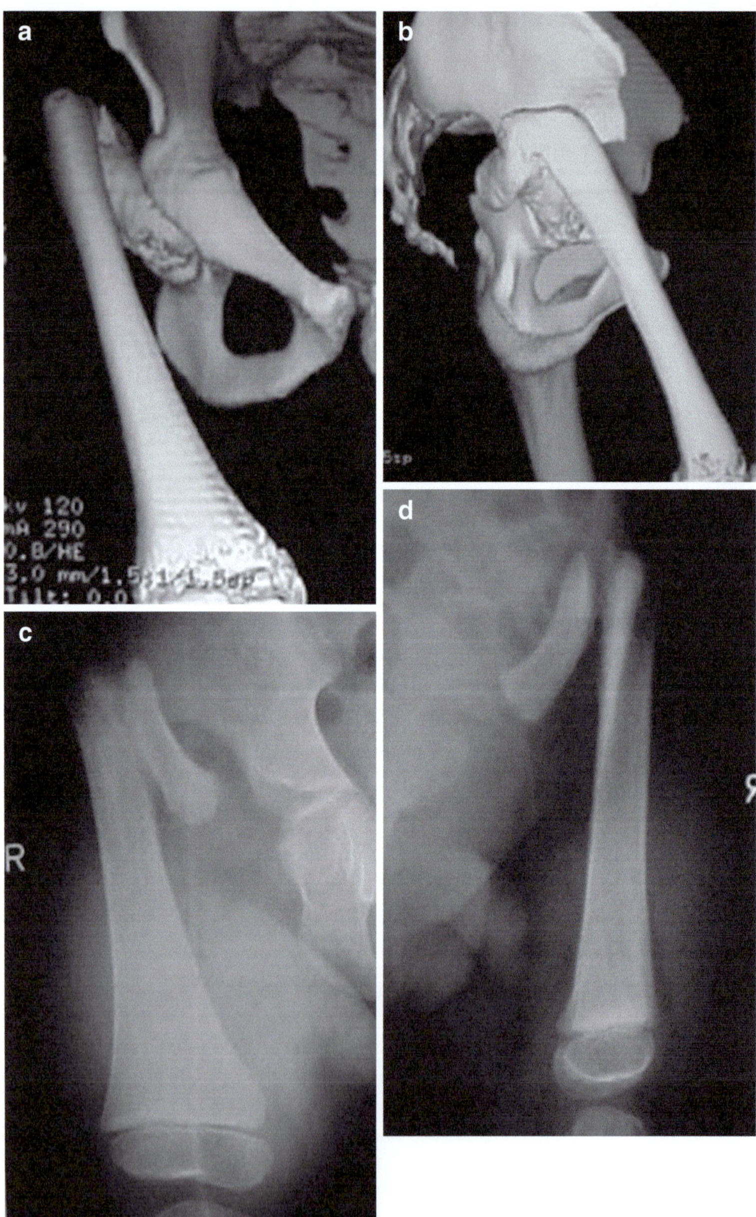

Fig. 13.2 3D CT reconstruction AP (**a**) and lateral views (**b**) showing typical type 1b deformity. Corresponding radiographs AP (**c**) and lateral (**d**)

1a cases and more severe in type 1b cases. Since the natural history of delayed ossification of the proximal femur is to ossify, very severe proximal femoral deformities may be seen in type 1a cases which at one point would have been classified as type 1b (Sanpera and Sparks 1994). Therefore, the difference between type 1b and type 1a may be a matter of the timing of the classification. Had the same 1a case been seen young enough, it might have shown a delay in ossification and been called a 1b and vice versa. In other words, the natural history of all 1b cases is to ossify and become 1a.

The proximal femoral deformity of CFD can occur between the level of the femoral neck to and including the subtrochanteric region of the femur. It is a result of a combination of extra-articular hip joint contractures combined with a bony deformity between the proximal diaphyseal part of the femur and the intertrochanteric or subtrochanteric region of the upper femur segment. Due to combination of frontal plane, sagittal plate, and axial plane angular deformities, the deformity appears differently when observed from a proximal vs. a distal reference perspective. This phenomenon is called "parallactic homologues" (Paley 2005a).

To avoid confusion in the description of the deformity, we need to establish a point of anatomic reference. Since the only deformity of the pelvis is hip dysplasia, I will describe the deformity of each of the two segments of the femur relative to the pelvis with the pelvis in an anatomic position. I will also use the convention of describing the distal relative to the proximal segment with the proximal segment being the anatomic pelvis laying flat on a table.

Proximal femoral deformity relative to the pelvis: The proximal femur consists of the femoral head, neck, and greater and lesser trochanter, including a smaller or larger segment of the femoral diaphysis (neck type vs. subtrochanteric type, respectively). The proximal femur relative to the pelvis is in flexion and internal rotation associated with extra-articular contractures of the hip abductors, hip flexors, and piriformis tendons. In the most severe cases, it is common for the hip flexion deformity to be as much as 90° and the internal rotation deformity to be 45°. Purely flexing the femur 90° places the neck of

the femur horizontal to the pelvis in the frontal projection but at a 45° angle to the sagittal projection of the neck of a femur with a 135° neck shaft angle. The neck would be oriented anteriorly from the head to the trochanter. The flexion therefore makes the neck appear to be retroverted 45° (apparent retroversion deformity) when viewed from distal to proximal. Internally rotating the femur around its mechanical axis, while the hip is in a 90° flexed position, moves the neck from being horizontal to the pelvis (parallel to the line connecting the two ischial tuberosities), to appear 45° abducted to the horizontal of the pelvis (apparent abduction deformity). The neck moves proximally closer to the iliac wing. The greater trochanter faces posterior, medial, and distal towards the sacrum. Since the tip of the greater trochanter is pointing towards the sacrum, the piriformis muscle which originates at the sacrum will be very short and appear contracted. Similarly for the hip abductor muscles, the greater trochanter is so medial and proximal that the hip abductor muscles have never been stretched out to length. Finally the psoas and rectus femoris tendons will also be tight for the same reasons.

13.3.5 Distal Femoral Deformity

The distal femur relative to the pelvis is mostly externally rotated. It may also have some flexion and adduction relative to the pelvis depending on the amount of relative deformities of the proximal and distal segment to each other.

Deformity of the proximal to the distal femur: If we connect the distal femur to the proximal femur, we have a CFD hip deformity. The relationship of the two segments relative to each other is the confusing part. As a reminder, the deformities of the proximal femur to the pelvis include actual flexion and internal rotation deformities, combined with the apparent abduction and retroversion. The deformities of the distal femur to the pelvis include actual neutral to adducted position, neutral to flexed position, and external rotation. In relation to each other, the distal relative to the proximal femur deformities appears very different. The distal femur appears adducted to the proximal segment (coxa vara). I call this apparent since there is no actual abduction of the proximal femur. The proximal femur deformity that appears to be abduction is actually internal rotation of the proximal segment of the femur. There will be a net adduction deformity relative to the pelvis since the adduction of the distal femur relative to the proximal femur is greater than the apparent abduction of the proximal femur relative to the pelvis. Relative to the proximal femur, the distal femur appears to be in extension. I call this apparent extension because the distal femur rotation makes a true flexion deformity of the distal femur appear to be extension. This will become more understandable as we proceed to unravel this complex deformity. Since the apparent extension deformity of the distal femur is smaller than the flexion deformity of the proximal femur, the net is a smaller fixed flexion deformity relative to the pelvis. Relative to the proximal femur, the distal femur appears to be externally rotated. The reason I call this apparent external rotation is because the proximal femur is in apparent retroversion due to its flexion deformity. Because the retroversion is apparent, the relationship between the two is apparent. The smaller apparent retroversion of the proximal segment to the pelvis combined with a larger external rotation deformity of the distal femur leaves a net external rotation deformity relative to the pelvis.

If one could remove all of the soft tissue tethers and place the proximal femur in a normal anatomic position relative to the pelvis but keep the distal femur connected to the proximal femur in its deformed position, what position would the distal femur be in? We start by internally rotating the proximal femur. Because the hip is at 90° of flexion, the internal rotation appears to be abduction. Using the distal femur as a handle, we have to adduct the distal femur until the neck is horizontal. Next we need to extend the proximal femur around the horizontal axis of the pelvis. To rotate around the horizontal axis of the pelvis using the distal femur as a handle, one must consider the apparent adduction deformity of the distal femur (which in extreme cases can make the diaphysis appear parallel to the femoral neck). The maneuver for reduction of the proximal

femur to an anatomic position requires the distal femur to rotate externally and flex. Once the femoral neck is reduced to a normal position, the final position of the distal femur relative to the proximal femur and to the pelvis is adduction, flexion, and external rotation. The adduction and external rotation were anticipated, but the flexion was not. This is due to the principle of parallactic homologues mentioned earlier. The rotation deformity makes the angular deformities appear different when the deformity is moved around and viewed from a different perspective.

Chicken and egg question: which came first: the contractures of the proximal femur or the deformity of the bone of the distal femur relative to the proximal femur? We will never know the answer to this question. The net effect in the frontal plane is that the greater trochanter with its insertion of the abductor muscles (gluteus medius and minimus) is abnormally close to the pelvis. This leads to several problems including impingement of the trochanter with the iliac bone and contracture of the gluteal muscles since the distance between their origin and insertion is short. The fascia lata with its iliotibial band extension to the tibia combined with part of the gluteus maximus is the most lateral of the soft tissue structures. They therefore contribute the greatest to the abduction contracture of the hip. Since adduction of the hip is preserved due to the varus of the femur and since the hip cannot be abducted much because of iliotrochanteric impingement, the abduction contracture is not obvious. It is rather stealth and hidden in plain view. If the bony coxa vara is corrected by osteotomy, without soft tissue releases, the abduction contracture will be uncovered. The abduction contracture will prevent the hip from coming back to a neutral position relative to the pelvis producing a fixed pelvic tilt. An abduction pelvic tilt on the short leg makes the limb length discrepancy (LLD) appear less than before surgery. In the face of an open growth plate or a nonossified neck or subtrochanteric segment, as in Type 1b cases, the abduction contracture leads to recurrence of the coxa vara after osteotomy. The mechanism for this recurrence may be differential growth of the physis, bending at the nonossified tissues, or slipped capital femoral epiphysis.

13.4 Superhip Procedure

Positioning, prepping, and draping for the superhip procedure: The patient should be on a radiolucent operating table, positioned supine close to the edge of the table, bumped up 45°, to roll the pelvis towards the opposite side. The entire side should be prepped and draped free from the nipple to the toes.

Step 1: *Incision* (Fig. 13.3a). A long midlateral incision is made from the iliac wing in a straight line to the tibial tuberosity in the anterior midline of the upper leg. The incision is carried down to the depth of the underlying fascia lata and iliotibial band.

Step 2: *Elevation of flap* (Fig. 13.3b). The subcutaneous tissues are dissected off the fascia of the thigh and pelvic region. The fat is adherent to the fascia and should be dissected preferably with a cautery. It is important not to incise the fascia with the cautery if the fascia is to be used for knee ligament reconstruction. Elevate a large flap of skin and subcutaneous tissues anteriorly allowing it to fold upon itself. Posteriorly a subcutaneous flap is elevated for only 1 or 2 cm. Extend the flap dissection medial to the Smith-Peterson interval (interval between the tensor fascia lata (TFL) and the sartorius) proximally. Distally reflect the flap to the patella if no ligament reconstruction is to be done and all the way to the medial side if ligament reconstruction is to be done. The fascia lata is now fully exposed from the patella to a couple of centimeters posterior to the intermuscular septum distally and from the medial side of the TFL to the mid-gluteus maximus proximally.

Step 3: *Fascia lata release* (Fig. 13.3c). The fascia is incised at the TFL-sartorius interval making sure to stay on the TFL side in order to avoid injury to the lateral femoral cutaneous nerve. The fascial incision is extended distally to the lateral border of the patella ending at the tibia. The posterior incision of the fascia lata starts distally and posterior at the intermuscular septum and extends proximally to overlie the gluteus maximus in line with the incision. The gluteus maximus (GMax) should be separated from the overlying fascia anterior to the poste-

rior fascial incision. The fascia should be retracted anteriorly and away from the underlying muscle, while the GMax should be dissected off of the fascia and the intermuscular septum that separates it from the TFL. The GMax should not be split in line with the fascial incision to avoid denervating the muscle anterior to the split. It can now be reflected posteriorly to allow exposure of the greater trochanter, piriformis muscle, and sciatic nerve. When ligamentous reconstruction using the fascia lata is planned, the fascia lata is cut proximally at the muscle tendon junction anteriorly. The fascial cut should be sloped posteriorly and proximally to include a longer fascia segment posteriorly from the fascia that was dissected off of the GMax. The fascia lata is reflected distally to Gerdy tubercle. The TFL can be left in place without further dissection. It does not have to be separated from the underlying gluteus medius (GMed). The two muscles are often adherent to each other. In fact, it may be confusing at times which fibers are TFL and which are GMed. The distinguishing feature is that the GMed fibers insert on the greater trochanter while the TFL does not. The distal fascia lata also called the iliotibial band (ITB) blends with the underlying lateral knee capsule. It is common to reflect some capsule with the ITB. The fascia should be mobilized all the way until Gerdy tubercle. The fascia can then be divided into two halves using a straight pair of scissors. It should be kept moist while the rest of the surgery proceeds. The two limbs of the fascia are ready for later use in the superknee procedure.

Step 4: *Hip flexion contracture releases*. The dissection is carried beneath the sartorius to find the rectus femoris tendon. The rectus femoris tendon insertion is identified at the anterior inferior iliac spine. The constant ascending branch of the lateral femoral circumflex artery and vein is cauterized prior to cutting the tendon. The conjoint rectus femoris tendon (distal to the split into reflected and direct heads) is cut and allowed to reflect distally. Care should be taken not to go too distal on the rectus femoris to avoid injury to its innervating branch of the femoral nerve. Just medial

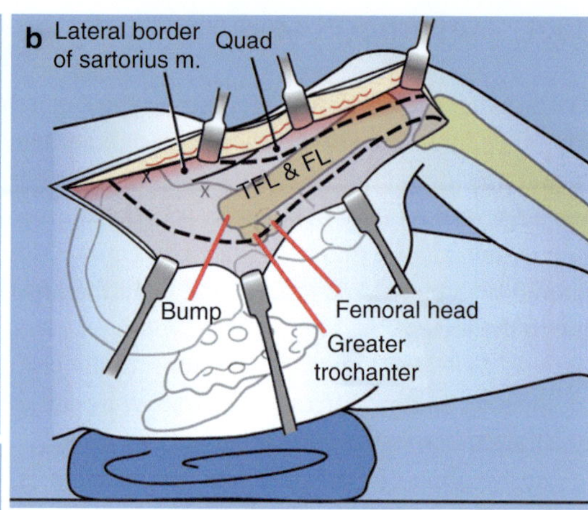

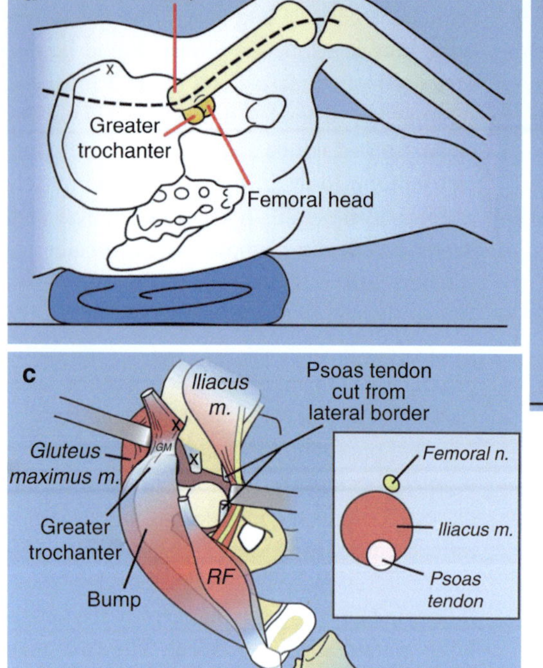

Fig. 13.3 Superhip Procedure (Paley Hip Reconstruction-1). (**a**) The patient is positioned supine with bump under affected hip. A straight midlateral incision is made from the top of the iliac crest to the tibial tuberosity. (**b**) A large anterior flap is raised off of the underlying fascia lata. (**c**) The rectus femoris is released from the anterior inferior iliac spine. The psoas tendon is recessed over the iliacus muscle. The femoral nerve is identified and decompressed. (**d**) The piriformis tendon is released from the greater trochanter. The sciatic nerve is identified and decompressed. (**e**) The remaining flexion deformity of the femur is due to the hip abductor muscles. (**f**) The hip abductor muscles tether the femur and limit its adduction. (**g**) To untether the hip abductors the apophysis is split and the abductor muscles are allowed to slide distally. This is called an abductor slide. It also allows the iliacus muscle to slide distally (flexor slide). (**h**) The abductor and flexor muscles have slid distally allowing the proximal femur to be fully adducted and extended. (**i**) A hip arthrogram outlines the cartilaginous femoral head (**j**) On the lateral view one can visualize concentric circles representing the outside of the femoral head, the perimeter of the femoral neck and the ossification of the ossific nucleus. (**k**) Place a guide wire from the center of the tip of the greater trochanter to the center of the femoral head. (**l**) Insert a second guide wire up the femoral neck at 45° to the first guide wire. (**m**) The red line is the future anatomic axis of the femur. Together with the two guide wires the anatomic axis forms a triangle made up of three angles: 50° (the complement of the NSA = 130°), 85° (MPFA), and therefore the third angle must equal 45°. (**n**) The second guide wire is in the center of the concentric circles and this in the center of the femoral neck and head. (**o**) Use a cannulated chisel to create a path for the blade plate up the femoral neck. (**p**) The chisel should be perpendicular to the posterior edge of the greater trochanter. (**q**) Replace the chisel with a 130° cannulated blade plate. (**r**) The side plate will be parallel to the posterior border of the greater trochanter. This demonstrates the flexion deformity of the upper femur that is present. (**s**) Cut perpendicular and parallel to the side plate and remove a small piece of bone. (**t**) Perform a subtrochanteric osteotomy. (currently I prefer to resect the medial lip to avoid impingement. (**u**) Rotate the femur internally and abduct it out of varus. (**v**) Overlap the bone ends and cut the diaphysis of the distal segment at the level of overlap to shorten the femur. The length is limited by the medial muscles. (**w**) Resect the diaphyseal segment and save it for bone graft for the Dega osteotomy. (**x**) Fix the plate with additional screws in the diaphysis and one up the femoral neck. (**y**) For cases with delayed ossification of the femoral neck, make a drill hole in the superior neck parallel to the blade. (**z**) Insert BMP-2 through this hole into the cartilage of the femoral neck. (**Za**) Perform the Paley modification of the Dega osteotomy. (**Zb**) The Paley modification cuts around the acetabulm all the way to the triradiate cartilage between the ilium and ischium posteriorly and triradiate cartilage medially. Unlike the original Dega no break is made through the medial cortex. (**Zc**) Lever down the roof of the acetabulum using a laminar spreader. (**Zd**) Customize and insert the cortical femoral graft from the bone that was resected from the femur. (**Ze**) Perform an iliac osteotomy to allow closure of the apophysis after the abductor slide. (**Zf**) The iliac bone can be used to graft the acetabulum and the femur osteotomies. (**Zg**) Transfer the recuts femoris tendon to the tensor fascia lata muscle. (**Zh**) Close the apophysis

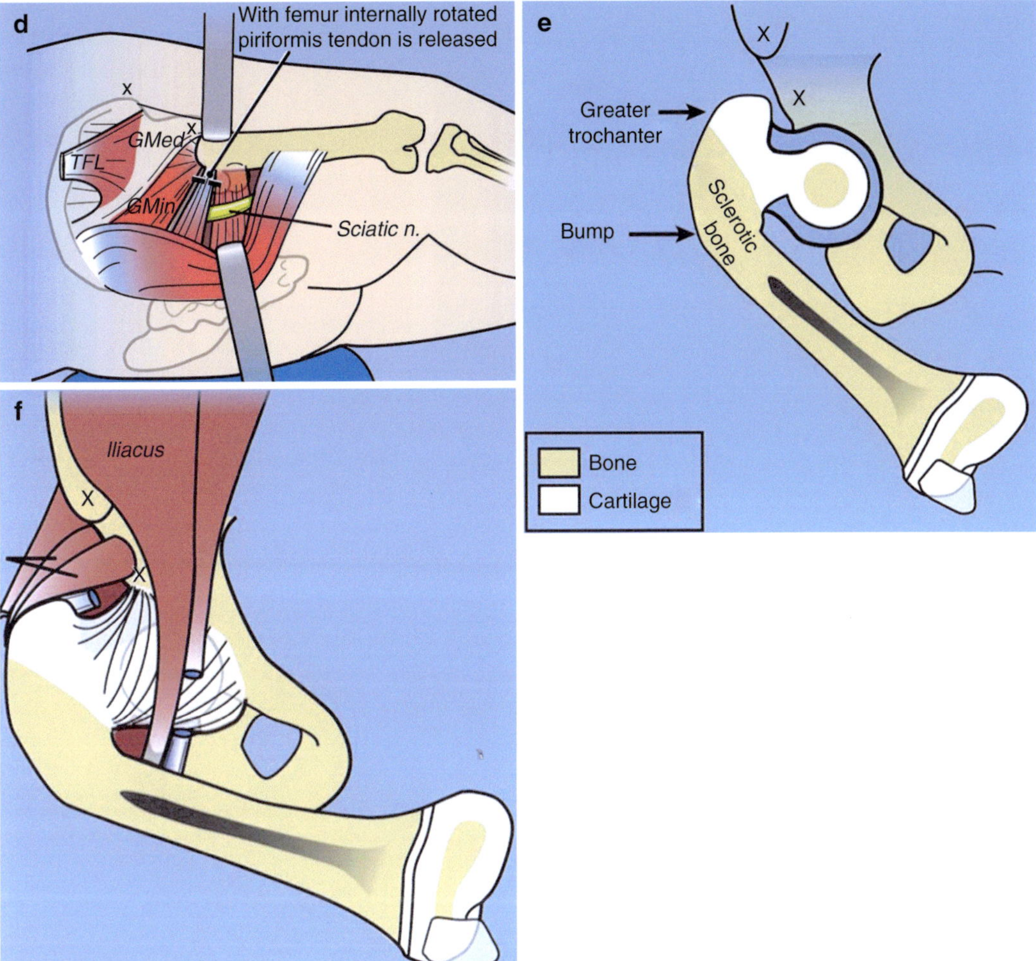

Fig. 13.3 (continued)

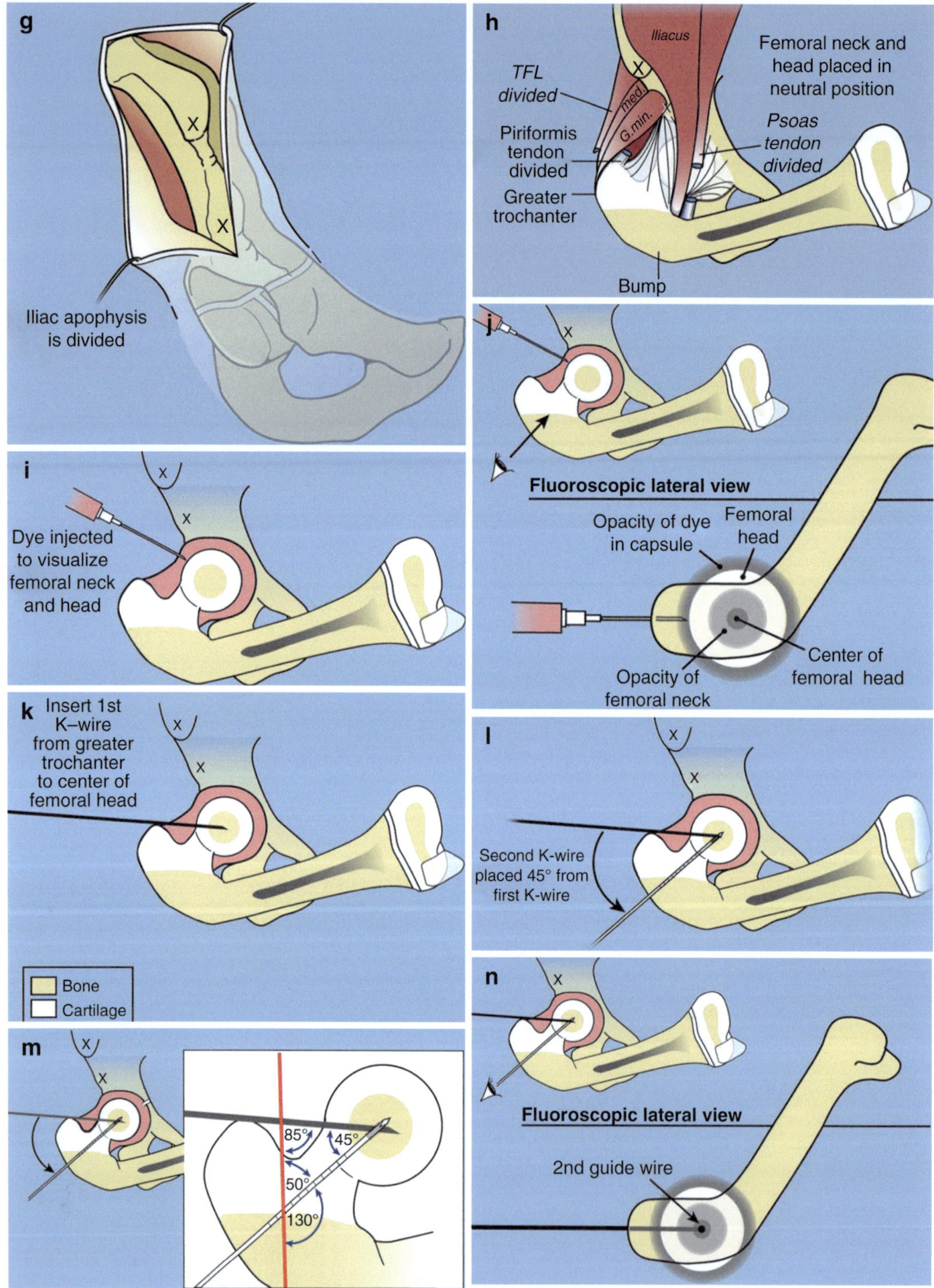

Fig. 13.3 (continued)

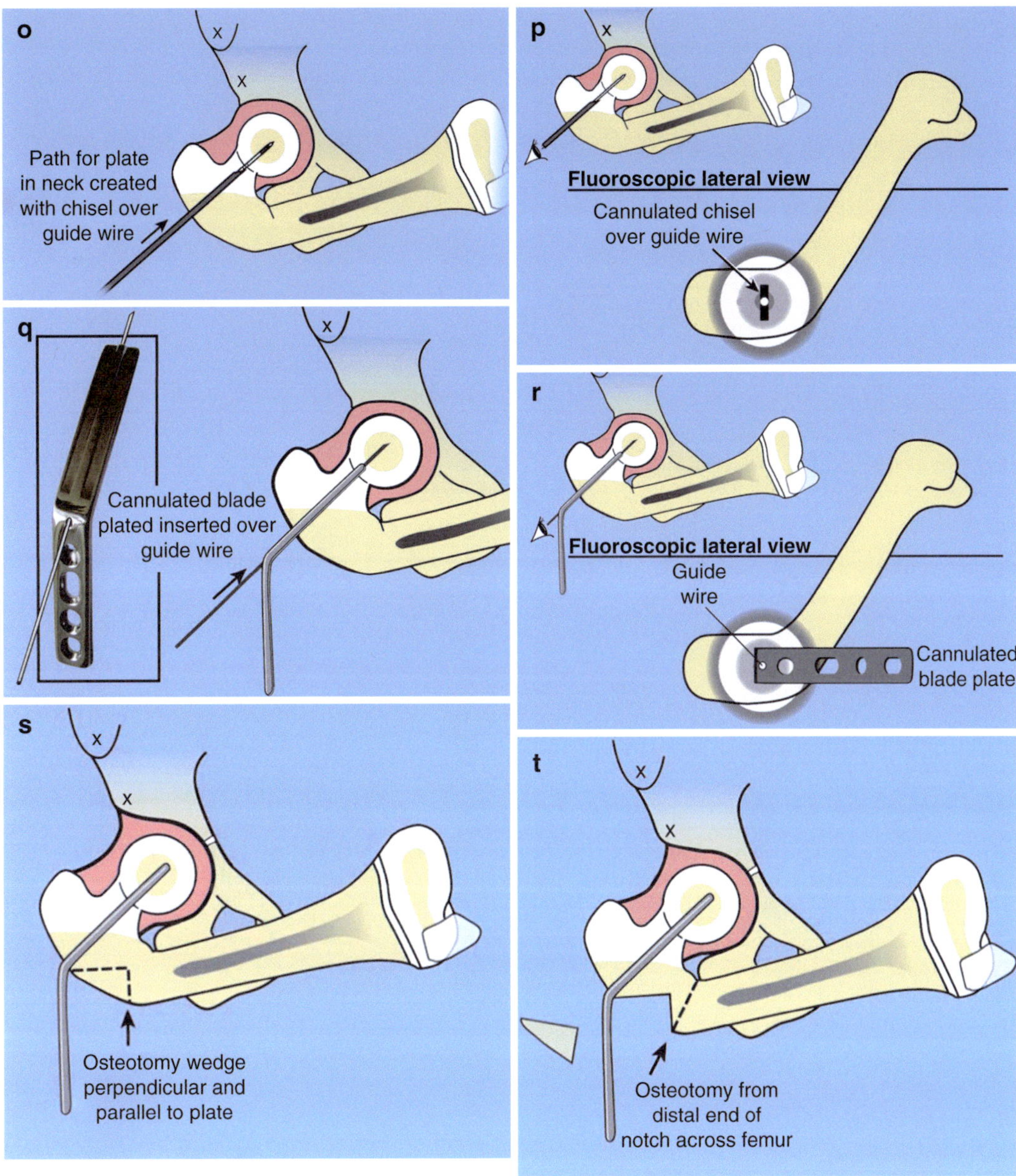

Fig. 13.3 (continued)

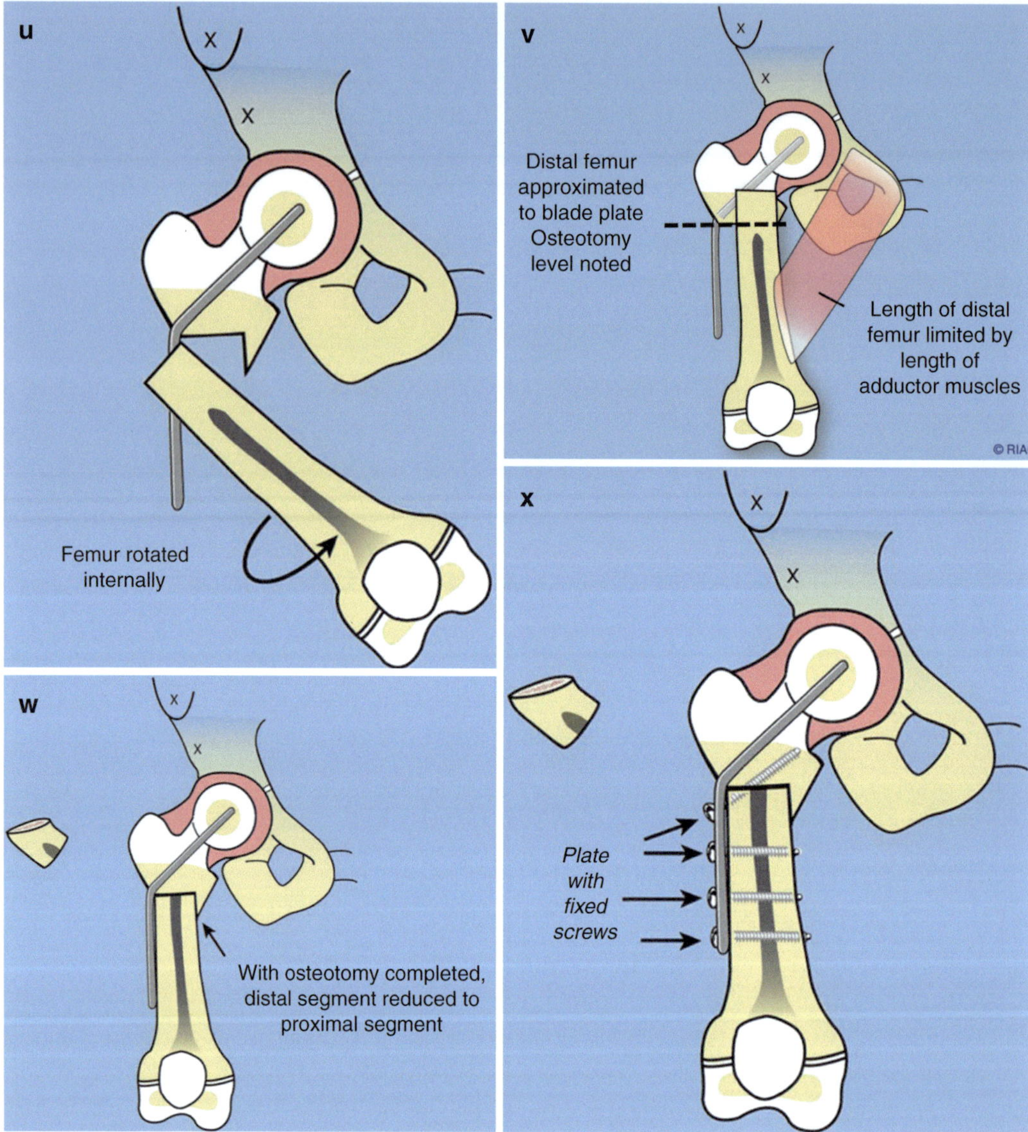

Fig. 13.3 (continued)

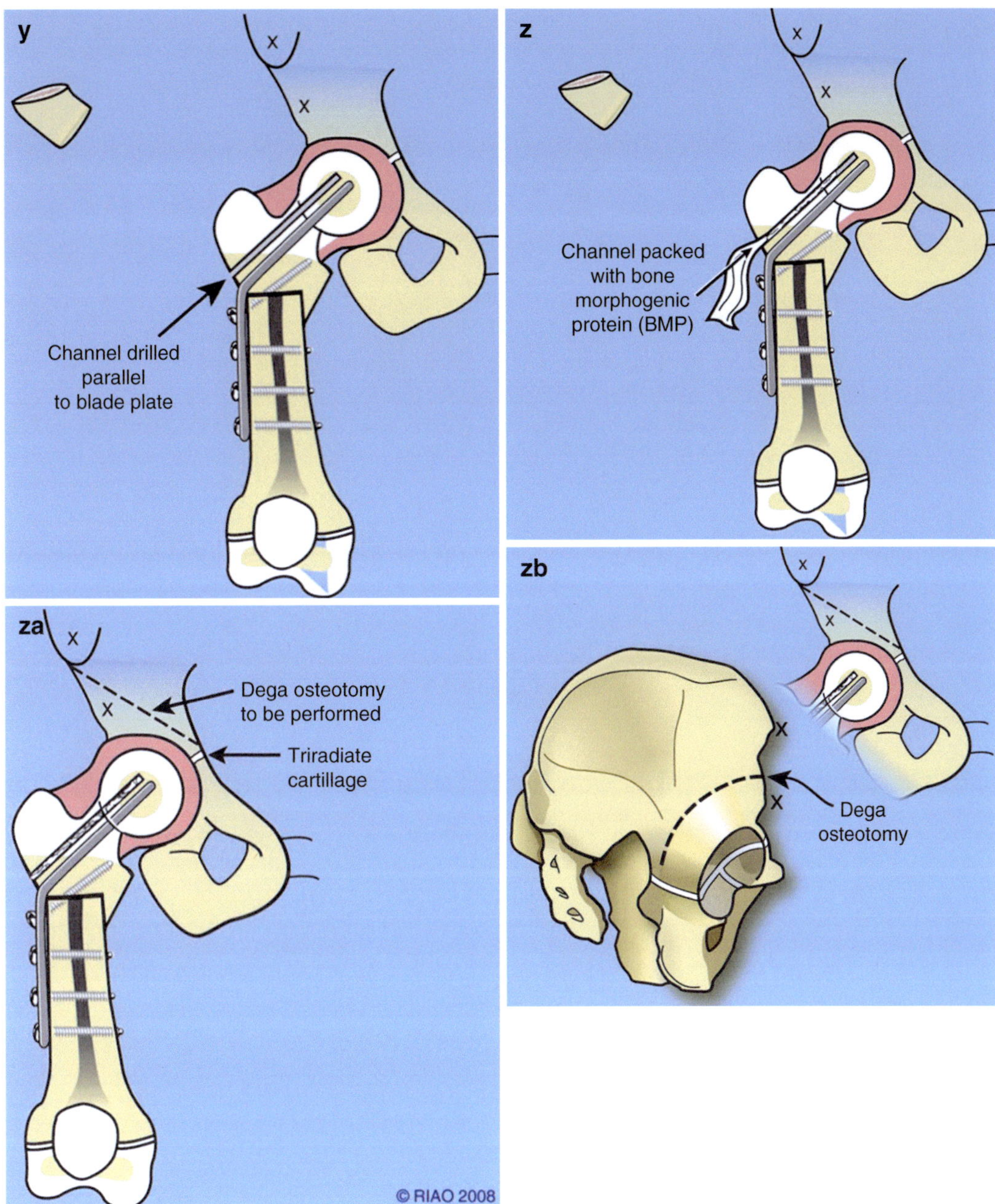

Fig. 13.3 (continued)

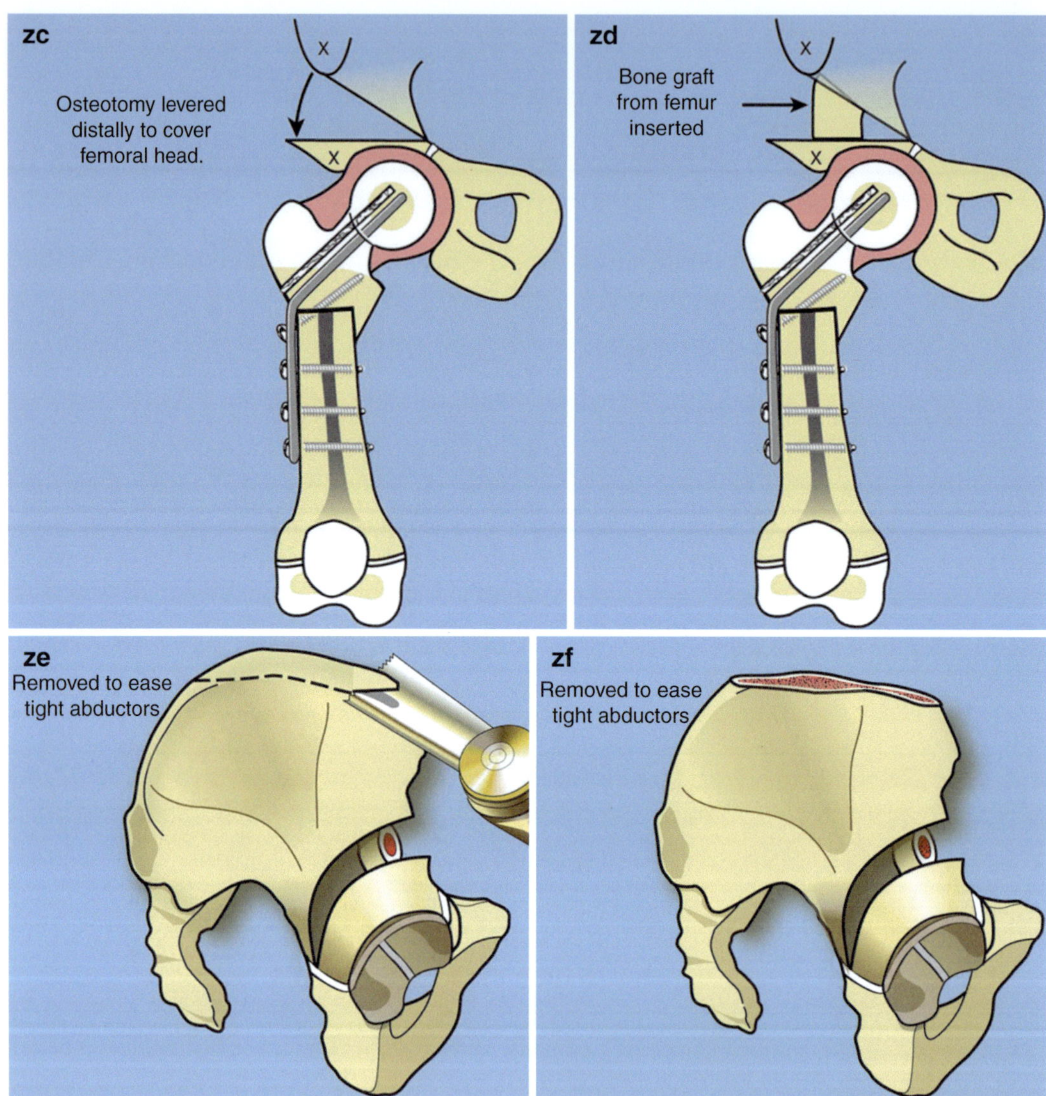

Fig. 13.3 (continued)

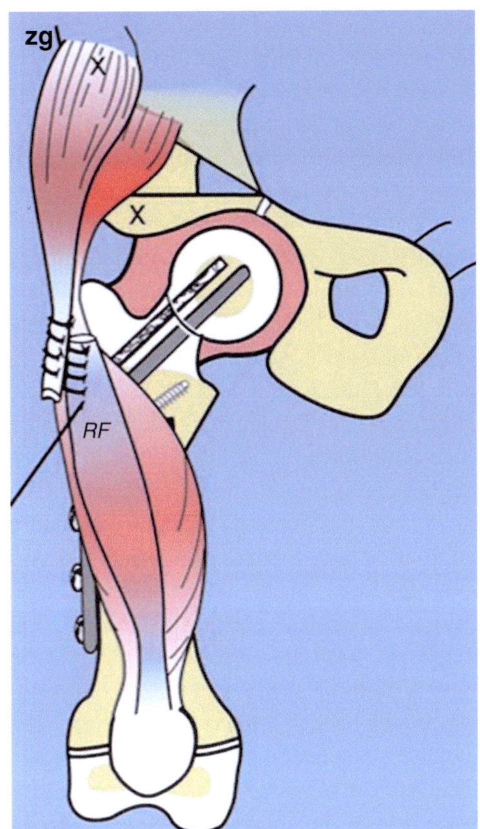

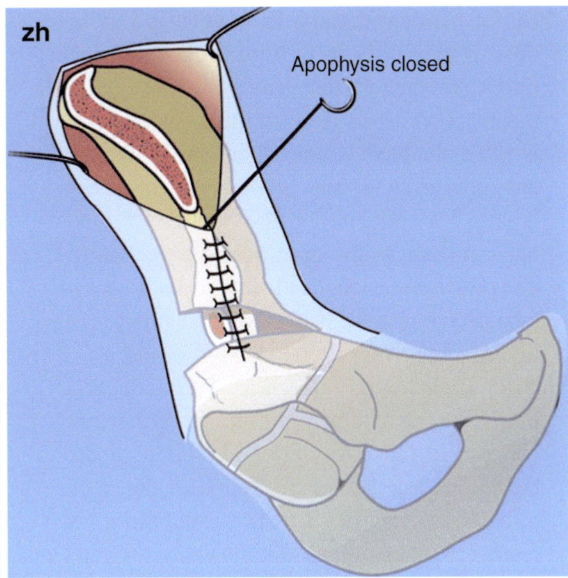

Fig. 13.3 (continued)

to the rectus is the iliopsoas muscle. The iliocapsularis muscle (capsular origin head of iliopsoas muscles) can also be seen here. The femoral nerve lies on the anteromedial surface of the iliopsoas muscle. Before looking for the psoas tendon, the femoral nerve should be identified and decompressed below the inguinal ligament. The posterior aspect of the iliopsoas muscle belly is now elevated from lateral to medial. The psoas tendon is located on the posteromedial surface in the substance of the muscle. The tendon is exposed and cut. Any remaining flexion contracture of the hip is due to the sartorius, gluteus medius and minimus (the part of these muscles originating anterior to the center of rotation of the femoral head in the sagittal plane), and the anterior fascia of thigh. If the anterior thigh fascia is tight, it can be released, taking care not to injure the neurovascular structures. Before releasing the anterior fascia, the lateral femoral cutaneous nerve should be identified and decompressed. It runs inside the fascia covering the sartorius muscle just medial to the anterior superior iliac spine. The next flexors to release are the gluteus medius and minimus muscles. This is accomplished by the abductor muscle slide technique (see step 6).

Step 5: *External rotation contracture release* (Fig. 13.3d). The piriformis tendon is contracted and prevents internal rotation of the hip. It should be released off of the greater trochanter. The greater trochanter should be identified by palpation. The gluteus medius muscle posterior border is very distinct and proceeds down to the greater trochanter where it inserts. Deep to the medius is the gluteus minimus and just distal to the minimus is the piriformis muscle. Its tendon can be palpated through its muscle. It may be difficult to identify the piriformis from the minimus. Care should be taken to avoid dissection at the distal border of the piriformis tendon. This is where the medial femoral circumflex branch anastomoses with the inferior gluteal artery branch. The entire piriformis is transected about one cm from its insertion onto the trochanter. The sciatic nerve can be identified and if necessary decompressed. It is more posterior to the trochanter and runs deep to the piriformis.

Step 6: *Abductor muscle slide*. The abductors may not appear to be tight on first inspection because of the coxa vara. Adduction of the hip into a true AP of the hip with the neck oriented normally in the acetabulum is restricted by the gluteus medius and minimus since the fascia lata has already been cut. Furthermore, the Dega osteotomy which lengthens the height of the ilium makes the abductors even tighter. There are two options to lengthen the abductor mechanism: lengthen it at the tendon end or slide its origin distally. At the tendon end, the conjoint tendon of the glutei and quadriceps can be released and then later reattached to the greater trochanter. I did this for 10 years and found that it lead to permanent weakness due to the change in muscle tendon length ratio. The second option is to detach the abductors from their origin and let them slide distally. This avoids changing the muscle tendon length ratio and avoids weakening the hip abductors. Since switching to the abductor slide, it has eliminated the problem of weakness, lurch, or Trendelenburg gait. To do this in the growing child, we split the iliac apophysis from the anterior inferior iliac spine to the anterior superior iliac spine and then posteriorly along the rest of the iliac crest. It is important to expose the apophysis along the entire length of the desired split. There is a tendency not to elevate the apophysis posteriorly enough. This starts with the reflection of the subcutaneous tissues in step 2 when the anterior and posterior flaps are elevated. The proximal and posterior extent of the dissection should be just beyond the highest point of the apophysis

laterally. The anterior extent is just distal to the anterior inferior iliac spine which is exposed for the release of the rectus femoris tendon. The abdominal external oblique muscle is peeled off of the apophysis to expose it along its entire length. The external oblique muscle insertion overlaps the apophysis more laterally and posteriorly than anteriorly. Once the apophysis is bare, it can be split from anterior to posterior. This should be done with a number 15 blade. To know where to split, pinch the apophysis between thumb and index finger of the hand not holding the knife. Then push down on the knife blade until you feel bone. It is important to try and stay in the middle of the apophysis along its entire length. It is also important to push down hard with the knife blade until one feels bone. Using a periosteal elevator, "pop off" the apophysis from the ilium. This should be done at multiple sites to get the entire apophysis to peel back as a unit from the ilium. The apophysis and lateral periosteum are reflected distally, thus relaxing the abductor muscles. Since part of the abductors acts as flexors of the hip, the abductor slide helps eliminate any remaining flexion deformity of the hip. The medial half of the apophysis is reflected medially with the iliacus muscle. This effectively produces a flexor slide effect for additional treatment of flexion contracture of the hip.

Step 7: *Elevation of quadriceps*. The quadriceps are now elevated off of the femur in a subperiosteal fashion. Since the femur is so short, the exposure may extend as far as the distal femoral physis. Proximally, the vastus lateralis should be elevated off of part of the cartilage of the greater trochanteric apophysis by sharp dissection.

Step 8: *Arthrogram*. A hip arthrogram is now performed using a 20 gauge spinal needle. This will outline the femoral head, acetabulum, and femoral neck.

Step 9: *Guidewire insertion*. Since the abduction, flexion, and rotation contractures have all been released, the femoral head and neck can now be placed in a neutral orientation to the pelvis by extending and maximally adducting the lower limb over top the other side. A guidewire should now be drilled up the center of the femoral neck to guide the insertion of a fixed angle fixation device. Since the femoral neck is unossified and short, it is very difficult to drill a guidewire at the correct angle up the femoral neck. The goal is to create a 130° neck shaft angle and a medial proximal femoral angle (MPFA) of 85°. In the normal femur, the angle between the neck shaft line and the tip of the greater trochanter to center of femoral head line is 45°. The first guidewire is inserted from the tip of the greater trochanter to the center of femoral head. Since the tip of the trochanter cannot be seen radiographically in young children because it is cartilaginous, the tip of the trochanter is located by palpation using the wire tip. From this point the wire is then drilled towards the center of the femoral head as shown in the arthrogram. The image intensifier is placed into the lateral view and the leg rotated until a "bull's eye" is seen. This "bull's eye" is formed by the overlapping shadows of three circles. The outermost circle is the dye surrounding the femoral head. The middle circle is the dye surrounding the femoral neck. The innermost circle is the ossific nucleus of the femoral head. All three circles should be seen concentrically. A second wire should be drilled into the center of this "bull's eye" at a 45° angle to the first wire. Using another wire of the same length as the second wire, measure the amount of wire inside the femoral neck by placing it alongside the second wire and measuring the difference in length between the two wires. This will be the length of the blade of the blade plate to be used.

Step 10: *Insert cannulated chisel.* The cannulated chisel for the blade plate should now be hammered up the femoral neck guided by the second guidewire. The chisel should be rotated until it is perpendicular to the back of the edge of the posterior aspect of the greater trochanter. This will guide it to the correct angle in the sagittal plane.

Step 11: *Plate insertion.* Bang the chisel out of the femur and reinsert the guidewire. Insert the appropriate length 130° blade plate along this wire to the depth of the bend of the plate. Make sure on the image intensifier that the tip of the blade is not too deep into the femoral head. Check its position on AP and lateral as well as

using the approach withdrawal technique with live fluoroscopy. If the plate is suspected of being too long, then replace it with one with a shorter blade. If the cannulation of the plate is off center, there is greater risk of protrusion into the joint.

Step 12: *First osteotomy.* The femur should be osteotomized with a saw perpendicular to the plate starting at the bend in the plate. The depth of this cut is incomplete and when the deformity angle is very large may be parallel to the lateral cortex. To guide this cut drill a wire perpendicular to the plate. Keep the plane of the saw blade perpendicular to the plate. The width of the perpendicular cut surface is as wide as the width of the femur diaphysis.

Step 13: *Second osteotomy.* A subtrochanteric osteotomy should be made oriented less than 90° to the first osteotomy to minimize the bone protruding medially.

Step 14: *Peel the femur off of the periosteum medially and cut the periosteum.* After the second osteotomy the distal femur can be peeled off of the surrounding periosteum. The periosteum medially is very thick and restricts correction of the varus and rotation deformity. Cut the periosteum by carefully separating it from the surrounding muscle. The profunda femoris and its perforators pass immediately under this periosteum and care should be taken to avoid injury to these vessels. Cutting the periosteum allows the thigh to stretch longitudinally reducing the amount of shortening required of the femur.

Step 15: *Shortening of the femur.* The distal femur is now mobile and can be valgusized and rotated internally. The distal femur is too long to fit end to end with the proximal femoral cut. The two ends should be overlapped. A mark should be made at the point of overlap. The distal femur should be osteotomized at this level. A wire is drilled perpendicular to the femur at the level of the osteotomy. A saw is used to cut the femur at this site. The segment of bone that is removed is stored on the back table in saline. It will be used as a bone graft for the Dega osteotomy.

Step 16: *Fixation of the distal femur.* The femur is now brought to the plate. The bone ends should oppose without tension. The femur is rotated internally to correct the external torsion deformity. To adjust the femur to the correct anteversion, the guidewire should be reinserted into the cannulation of the plate. This wire shows the orientation of the femoral neck. The knee should be flexed to 90° and the angle between the wire and the frontal plane of the femur as judged by the perpendicular plane to knee flexion is observed. This wire should appear at least 10° anteverted relative to the knee. The most distal hole in the plate can now be drilled with the femur held in this rotation. The drill hole should be made at the distal edge of the hole to compress the osteotomy. A depth gauge is used to measure the hole and a screw is inserted. Two more screw holes are drilled and screws inserted into the plate. The most proximal hole in the plate is designed to drill parallel to the blade of the plate. The wire in the plate cannulation is used to guide the drill bit. This screw helps secure the plate to the proximal femur. The other three screws secure the plate to the distal femur. In type 1b cases the blade of the plate goes across the proximal physis into the femoral head as does this oblique screw. In type 1a cases with a horizontally oriented growth plate, neither the blade nor the screw should cross the growth plate of the upper femur. In type 1a cases with a vertically oriented growth plate, the blade but not the screw should cross the physis.

Step 17: *Insertion of bone morphogenetic protein (BMP)*. In type 1b neck cases, BMP should be inserted into the upper femur to stimulate ossification of the cartilaginous neck of the femur. A wire is drilled proximal and parallel to the guidewire in the cannulation of the plate. A 3.8 mm hole is then drilled overtop this guidewire. The drill hole should extend all the way into the ossific nucleus. BMP-2 (Infuse-Wright Medical) is then inserted in this hole. The BMP-2 is on collagen sponges, which can be pushed into the hole using the tip of a 3.2 mm drill bit in one hand and a forceps in the other hand.

Step 18: *Pelvic osteotomy*. The type of pelvic osteotomy depends on the age of the patient and the degree of dysplasia. In the majority of patients under age 6, I prefer to use the Dega osteotomy to treat the dysplastic acetabulum. In older patients and especially if there is a high grade of dysplasia, I use a periacetabular triple osteotomy (PATO) in children and the Ganz periacetabular osteotomy (PAO) when the triradiate cartilage is closed or nearing closure.

Step 19: *Iliac wing osteotomy and repair of the iliac apophysis*. After the pelvic osteotomy, the apophysis can be sutured back together. Due to the abductor muscle slide, the lateral apophysis cannot reach the top of the iliac crest. Part of the crest has to be resected to allow repair of the apophysis. The bone removed can be inserted into the Dega osteotomy or used to bone graft a PATO or PAO as well as the subtrochanteric femoral osteotomy.

Step 20: *Muscle repairs and transfers*. The TFL muscle should be sutured down to the greater trochanter to act as a hip abductor. The rectus femoris tendon should be sutured to the side of the TFL. The quadriceps should be sutured to the region of the linea aspera. The gluteus maximus should be advanced back to the posterior border of the TFL.

Step 21: *Closure*. If no knee releases or reconstruction are required, the wound can now be closed. The interval between the TFL and the sartorius should be sutured closed with care not to suture the lateral femoral cutaneous nerve. Since there is no fascia lata, the deepest layer is the fat layer. This layer is called the underlayer. It should be sutured with a number one Vicryl. A Hemovac drain should be inserted before closing this layer. If a super-knee procedure is performed, a second more medial drain is also used. I prefer to bring the drains out proximally and anteriorly. The drains are usually secured with a clear adhesive sterile dressing (e.g., Tegaderm, 3M, Minnesota). It is important to close the wound in a fashion that the opposite layers get sutured at the same level. The next layer is Scarpa's fascia. It is closed with a 2-0 Vicryl running stitch. The deep dermal layer (subcutaneous layer) is closed with a 3-0 Vicryl and the skin is closed using a subcuticular stitch with 4-0 Monocryl. Sterile dressings are now applied.

Step 22: *Final radiographs*. After the drapes are removed, an AP pelvis to include the femur is obtained. A lateral of the femur relative to the knee joint is also obtained. These X-rays are reviewed before proceeding to the spica cast.

Step 23: *Spica cast.* All infants are placed in a spica cast. The position of the limbs in the cast is important. The operated upon limb should be placed in full hip and knee extension. The opposite limb can be in a flexed, abducted, and externally rotated position. The cast should include the entire affected side but with the foot left free. The opposite side should stop short of the knee joint. The cast should be bivalved before leaving the operating room. In most cases the cast can be converted to a removable spica cast after 5 days.

13.5 Knee Considerations

The knee in CFD may range from a normal stable undeformed knee to an unstable, contracted, deformed joint. The most common deformity of the knee is valgus. The valgus deformity of the knee is usually nonprogressive. The distal femoral physis is usually closer to the knee joint on the lateral side. This is often attributed to hypoplasia of the lateral femoral condyle. CFD cases often have a variable degree of anteroposterior and rotatory instability of the knee related to absent or hypoplastic cruciate ligaments. In some cases, the tibia dislocates anterior or posterior on the femur during extension or flexion, respectively. Furthermore, there may be rotatory instability present. One study has related the radiographic appearance of the tibial spines to the degree of hypoplasia of the anterior cruciate ligament (Manner et al. 2006). The patella is usually hypoplastic and may be maltracking laterally. In some cases it dislocates with flexion. Finally, many cases of CFD have a fixed flexion deformity of the knee.

13.5.1 Indications for Preparatory Surgery of the Knee Prior to Lengthening

Isolated anteroposterior instability is not necessarily an indication for surgery. Grade 3 instability (no endpoint on anterior and posterior drawer tests) will usually become symptomatic as the child gets older. If the child is going to undergo a superhip procedure or Dega osteotomy prior to lengthening, and since the fascia lata is going to be excised, it makes sense to rebuild the knee ligaments and not "waste" the fascia lata. In some children there is a "catch" or "locking" sensation in the knee when going from extension to flexion. This is due to contracture of the iliotibial band. This catching feeling may even be painful and may require a trick motion to release it. In more severe cases, the tibia actually subluxes or dislocates anteriorly on the femur and reduces at about 30° of flexion. Once again the culprit is the iliotibial band combined with an aplasia of the anterior cruciate ligament (ACL). In older patients, the posterior aspect of the tibia may be rounded contributing to anterior dislocation of the tibia on the femur. Whether this is a secondary change due to chronic dislocation or a primary deformity is not clear since the tibia is not ossified posteriorly in infancy.

Patellar hypoplasia and instability is very common. The patella frequently maltracks laterally with flexion. In some cases it even dislocates with flexion. This is due to a combination of factors: valgus distal femur, hypoplastic or absent patellar groove, contracture of the lateral retinaculum with the tight iliotibial band, and external rotatory instability of the tibia on the femur due to cruciate deficiency which lateralizes the patellar tendon insertion. Patellar maltracking or subluxation should be corrected prior to lengthening.

Flexion contracture of the knee is another congenital deformity that may be present and which should be corrected before proceeding with lengthening. When the femur is very short, the acute angle created by the posterior thigh muscles gives the appearance of a flexion contracture. The definition of a flexion contracture however is a flexed angle between the anterior cortical line of the femur and tibia in maximum extension. When the contracture is more than 15°, it should be corrected surgically. Knee flexion contracture can be due to bony or soft tissue causes. In CFD the most common is intra-articular capsular contracture. There may be some extra-articular contribution due to contracture of the hamstring muscles and gastrocnemius muscles. Release of these muscles alone rarely corrects the contracture, while capsular release without complete hamstring release corrects the contracture. In some cases, there is a true bony flexion of the distal femur that may need to be corrected by osteotomy.

The knee reconstruction I developed in 1994 (Paley 1998) is called the superknee procedure. The superknee is a conglomerate procedure combining two or more of the following five procedures, three of which were previously described by other authors and two of which was developed by me: (1) Langenskiöld procedure (Langenskiöld and Ritsila 1992) for congenital dislocation of the patella, (2) MacIntosh procedure (Amirault et al. 1988) for ACL deficiency including extra- and intra-articular anterior cruciate ligament reconstruction using the fascia lata, (3) Grammont procedure (Grammont et al. 1985) for recurrent dislocation of the patella, (4) Paley procedure also referred to as the reverse MacIntosh (Amirault et al. 1988) to prevent external rotatory instability and to act as an extra-articular posterior cruciate ligament, and (5) Paley anterior approach to posterior capsulotomy of the knee. The combinations of these five procedures may be performed at the same time as a pelvic osteotomy or superhip procedure.

The superknee procedure is a combination of some or all of these components including extra- and intra-articular knee ligament reconstruction, patellar realignment, posterior capsulotomy, and knee flexor tendon releases. Typically, the superknee consists of the MacIntosh extra- and intra-articular ACL reconstruction, the reverse MacIntosh (Paley) PCL extra-articular reconstruction, the Grammont patellar tendon realignment, lateral release of the patella, and in some cases the modified Langenskiöld (Paley) procedure for patellar reduction. If performed with a superhip procedure, the incision is a distal extension of the superhip incision. If performed as an isolated procedure, a small second incision can be made to cut the fascia lata at its origin, thus reducing the length of the proximal extent of the midlateral thigh incision. If the superknee is performed without the superhip procedure, the entire surgery can be performed under tourniquet control. The release of the posterior capsule is performed only when there is a significant knee flexion contracture ($\geq 15°$).

13.5.2 Superknee Procedure (Ligamentous Reconstruction Only) (Fig. 13.4)

Step 1: *Fascia lata harvest*. The knee is exposed through a long S-shaped incision ending just distal to the tibial tuberosity distally and midlateral proximally. The anterior margin of the fascia lata (iliotibial band) and the posterior margin where it blends with the intermuscular septum are incised longitudinally. The fascia lata is transected at its musculotendinous junction with the tensor fascia lata and reflected distally until its insertion onto the tibia (Gerdy tubercle).

Step 2: *Ligamentization of fascia lata*. The fascia lata should be split into two longitudinal strips to make two ligaments. The posterior half is tubularized using nonabsorbable suture and the Krackow whipstitch (Krackow et al. 1988)

Fig. 13.4 Superknee surgical technique including MacIntosh and Paley reverse MacIntosh illustrations. Superknee procedure (Paley Knee Reconstruction 1). (**a**) Through a midline lateral incision ending at the tibial tuberosity, reflext the entire width of the fascia lata (iliotibial band) distally. Leave it attached distally to Gerdie's tubercle. (**b**) Divide the harvested fascia into an anterior (FL1) and posterior (FL2) half. (**c**) Pass FL1 under the lateral collateral ligament. (**d**) Make a rent in the lateral intermuscular septum and pass FL1 through this. (MacIntosh Procedure; extra-articular ACL). Make a drill hole into the epiphysis of the proximal tibia from medial to the patellar tendon to the center of the knee joint. (**e**) Pass FL1 through the hole in the epiphysis. (**f**) Secure FL1 with an ACL type ligament screw. (Intra-articular ACL). (**g**) Pass FL2 under the patellar tendon. (**h**) Pass FL2 under the medial retinaculum and loop it around the adductor magnus tendon. (**i**) Suture it back to itself (Reverse MacIntosh; extra-articular PCL). (**j**) Suture FL1 to FL2 to further secure fixation of these ligaments and to allow immediate early motion

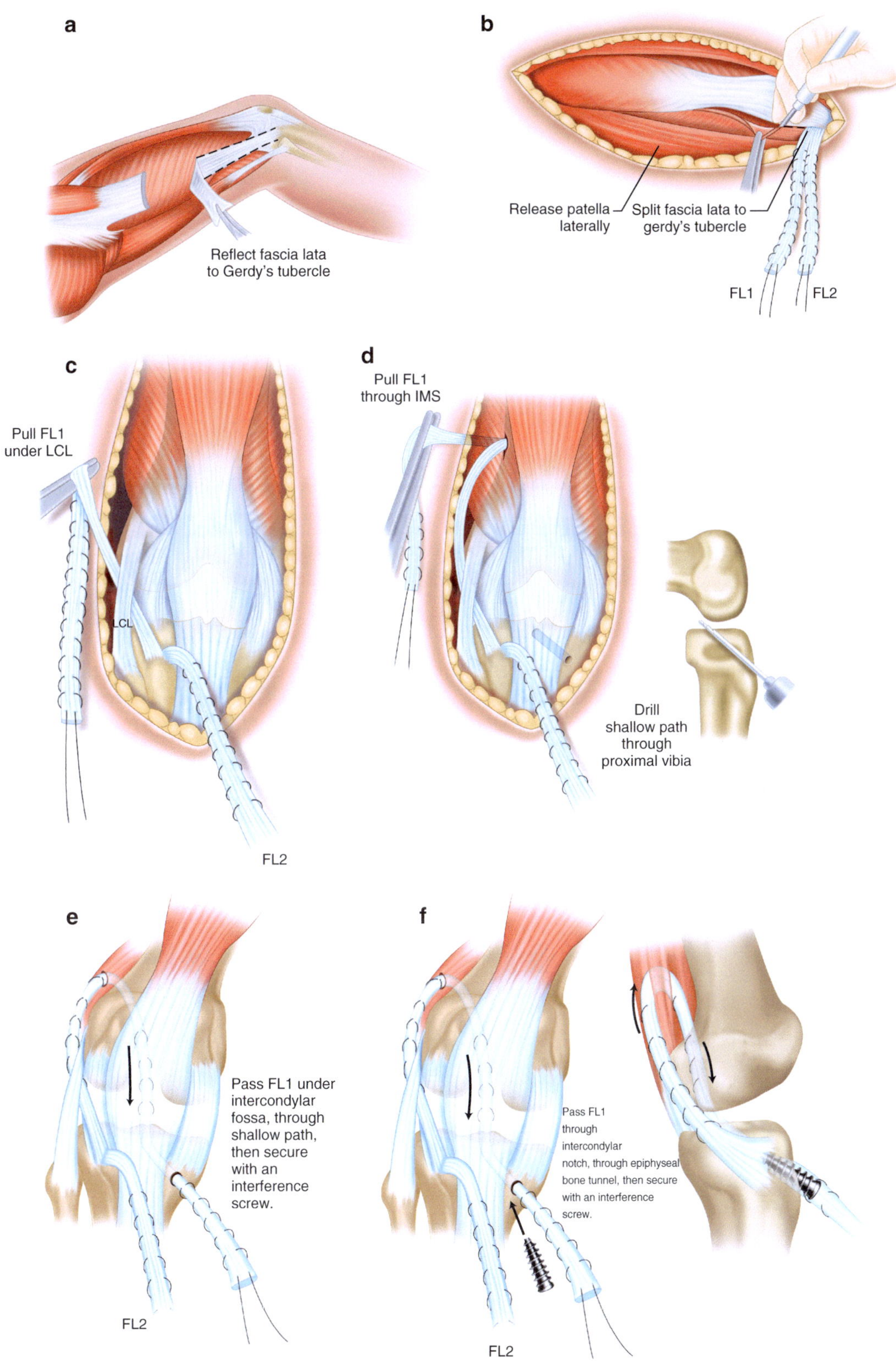
a
Reflect fascia lata
to Gerdy's tubercle
b
Release patella
laterally
Split fascia lata to
gerdy's tubercle
FL1
FL2
c
Pull FL1
under LCL
LCL
FL2
d
Pull FL1
through IMS
Drill
shallow path
through
proximal vibia
e
Pass FL1 under
intercondylar
fossa, through
shallow path,
then secure
with an
interference
screw.
FL2
f
Pass FL1
through
intercondylar
notch, through epiphyseal
bone tunnel, then secure
with an interference
screw.
FL2

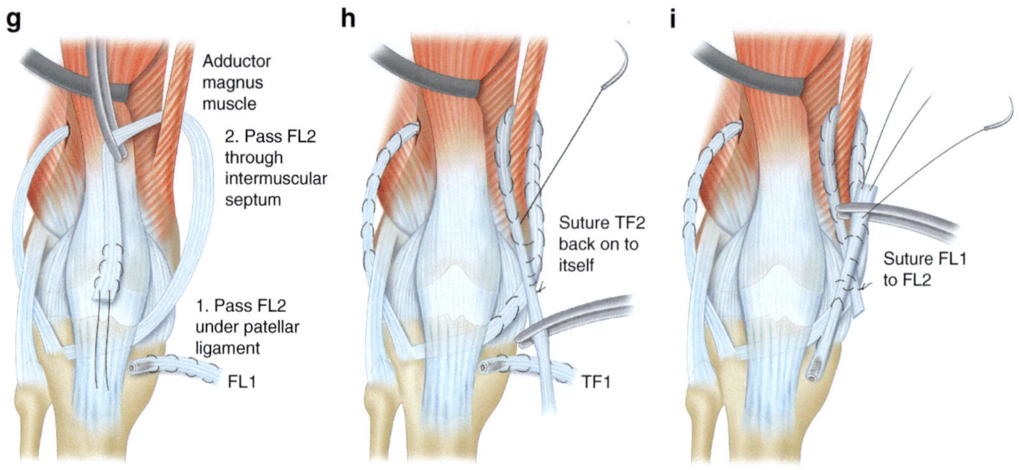

Fig. 13.4 (continued)

from distal to proximal. The medial half is left flat.

Step 3: *Lateral release and Grammont patellar tendon realignment*: If the patella tracks laterally but is not dislocated or dislocating, a lateral release and patellar tendon transfer should be performed to move the tendon medially. The lateral capsule and edge of the vastus lateralis should be cut to, but not through the synovium. The vastus lateralis is elevated from the lateral intermuscular septum and distal femur. If it is still acting as a major lateral tether of the patella, its tendon should be detached from the patella and then transferred medially at minimal tension. The lateral release is extended distally to the lateral aspect of the patellar tendon. This longitudinal deep incision should be extended past the tibial tuberosity along the crest of the tibia incising the proximal tibial periosteum. A parallel periosteal, para tendonous deep incision is made medial to the patellar tendon. Using sharp dissection with a knife blade, the patellar tendon is elevated off the tuberosity trying not to remove any cartilage if possible. Once the tendon is detached, the periosteal extension of the tendon is elevated with the tendon so that the detached tendon remains tethered distally. This procedure (described by Grammont in German) is the pediatric equivalent of the Elmslie-Trillat (Grammont et al. 1985) procedure in adults. The patellar tendon can now be displaced medially and sutured medial to the tuberosity with an absorbable suture.

Step 4: *Extra-articular PCL reconstruction (reverse MacIntosh)*. To prevent the tibia from rotating externally, which leads to subluxation of the patella and of the tibia on the femur posteriorly, a medial extra-articular ligament can be created using the medial half of the fascia lata. This creates a strap going around the medial tibia tethering it to the medial distal femur. This is the opposite direction of the extra-articular ligament created with the posterior half of the fascia lata (described in the next step). The lateral extra-articular ligament was described by David MacIntosh (one of my former professors from Toronto) for ACL reconstruction. In his honor and memory and in recognition of his idea of a lateral extra-articular ligament, I refer to the medial extra-articular ligament procedure that I innovated as the reverse MacInstosh or extra-articular PCL procedure. To anchor this ligament to the medial femur, it is necessary to elevate the skin flap in a medial direction. The anterior skin flap is kept as thick as possible and is reflected medially until the posterior border of the vastus medialis can be visualized. The medial intermusclar septum (very rudimentary) and the adductor magnus tendon are located posterior to the vastus medialis muscle. Care should be taken dissecting in this area to isolate and not damage the saphenous nerve as it exits from the quadriceps as the terminal branch of the femoral nerve. A subperiosteal tunnel is created around the adductor magnus tendon. The anterior limb of the fascia lata is now passed under the patella tendon, through a tunnel of superficial medial retinaculum and looped around the adductor magnus insertion (from posterior to anterior) and then sutured to itself with nonabsorbable suture. To ensure that this new ligament is isometric, a suture anchor can be inserted into the distal femoral epiphysis, just distal to the physis at the posterior junction of the physis with the posterior cortex (this point corresponds to the center of rotation of the knee). I like to use an absorbable anchor for this. The suture from this anchor is then tied around the fascia lata in 90° of knee flexion while the ligament is under tension. After that the part that is looped around the adductor magnus can be sutured to itself using this suture again. This extra-articular ligament should always be tensioned with the knee in 90° of flexion. If it is tensioned in extension, it may restrict flexion. The excess ligament is saved and sutured to the remaining end of the new ACL as it exits the tibia in the next step.

Step 5: *MacIntosh extra- + intra-articular ACL reconstruction*. David MacIntosh described first an extra-articular ligament reconstruction for the ACL-deficient knee and later a combined extra- and intra-articular reconstruction with the "over-the-top" technique. This method although no longer used in sports medicine is a very useful technique for congenitally deficient knees. In CFD the instability pattern is different than in an isolated tear of the ACL. There is more rotary instability in CFD. Therefore, a purely intra-articular ligament reconstruction is insufficient. In my early experience, we made this mistake and had a lot of recurrent instability. The combination of extra- and intra-articular ACL ligament reconstruction is ideal for CFD. Having stud-

ied under MacIntosh and having learned this procedure directly from him, it was natural for me to think about its application in the CFD cruciate-deficient knee. I have modified this procedure slightly to adapt it to the skeletally immature knee. It can now be safely done as young as 2 years of age.

The lateral collateral ligament (LCL) is identified using Grant's test. The leg is put in a figure four position, which allows the tensioned LCL to be easily palpated. I dissect the LCL while it is under tension and identify its anterior and posterior borders. An extra-articular tunnel is created under the LCL. The posterior limb of the fascia lata is passed through the LCL tunnel from anterior to posterior. A subperiosteal dissection is done in the over-the-top region preserving the intermuscular septum attachment. A curved tonsil clamp introduced through the "over-the-top" tunnel is used to perforate the posterior knee capsule centrally. Next, a drill hole needs to be made in the anterior tibial epiphysis to anchor the ligament to bone. Drill a guidewire through the anterior tibial epiphysis using image intensifier guidance. The wire should start proximal to the proximal tibial physeal line, lateral to the patellar tendon. The wire should be directed proximal and posterior to exit into the center of the knee about half way back on the tibia. As these patients don't have a true notch and a notchplasty is not an option in children, it is better that the ligament insert more posterior on the tibia than in the normal knee. This avoids damage to the ligament with knee extension. Once the wire is confirmed to be in the correct position in both the AP and lateral views, a hole is drilled with a cannulated ACL reamer. The diameter of the reamer chosen is matched to the diameter of the tubularized fascia lata ligament being passed (use the ligament sizers to determine this). A suture passer is then passed through the tibial epiphyseal tunnel and out the capsular perforation through the "over-the-top" tunnel laterally. The suture connected to the fascia lata is looped through the suture passer and pulled through the knee to exit anteriorly through the epiphyseal tunnel. The tubularized fascia lata is now pulled through the knee capsule and out the epiphyseal tunnel. As was done on the medial side, a suture anchor is placed into the supracondylar region to help anchor the extra-articular ligament and to support the over-the-top point. The extra-articular ligament should be tensioned in full knee extension. Once it is secured, the rest of the graft is anchored to the bony tibial epiphyseal tunnel using an absorbable headless interference screw. It too should be tensioned in full knee extension to prevent a flexion contracture of the knee. As the patient's epiphysis grows, the ligament becomes more taut. Therefore, one does not need to worry that it is not tight enough. I like to secure the ligament by suturing the posterior fascia lata graft to the anterior graft.

13.5.3 Superknee Procedure with Patellar Realignment for Dislocated/Dislocating Patella (Fig. 13.5)

13.5.3.1 Langenskiöld Patellar Realignment

If the patella is dislocated or dislocating, a modified version of the Langenskiöld (Langenskiöld and Ritsila 1992) procedure is performed before the ligament reconstruction. First the capsule is incised and separated from the patella and synovium medially and laterally. On the medial side the two layers are separated all the way to the medial gutter. The medial capsule is cut transversely at its distal end. The patellar tendon and the quadriceps are also separated from the synovium distally and proximally, respectively. The synovium is now incised circumferentially around the patella, separating the patella from

the synovium completely. The quadriceps tendon is left attached to the patella proximally, and the patellar tendon remains attached to the patella distally. The synovium is separated from these structures. The synovium now has a patella-sized hole in it. The synovium is sutured closed in a longitudinal direction. This leaves the patella temporarily as an extra-articular bone. The patellar tendon is elevated from the apophysis by sharp dissection after circumscribing a medial and lateral incision extending distally into the periosteum (Grammont procedure). After the tendon is elevated, it is shifted medially at least a centimeter (in the original Langenskiöld, it is detached from the tuberosity). A longitudinal incision is made in the synovium centered over the knee and the patella is sutured to the edges of this new hole in the synovium, and the synovium is sutured to the patella circumferentially. The medial capsule with the vastus medialis is now advanced over the top of the patella and stitched to its lateral border. The lateral capsule is left open. If the Paley reverse MacIntosh procedure is used, the fascia lata should not be fixed in place until after the Langenskiöld repair is completed.

13.5.4 Superknee Procedure with Knee Flexion Deformity (Fig. 13.6)

Knee flexion contracture release: If there is a knee flexion deformity >15°, it can be treated by posterior capsular release. This is often done in combination with a superhip procedure or one of the

Fig. 13.5 Superknee surgical technique including Grammont, modified Langenskiöld, and Paley reverse MacIntosh procedure illustrations. Modified Langenskiold and Grammont Procedures (one variant of the superknee or Paley Knee Reconstruction). (**a** and **b**) Through a midlateral incision, lengthen the biceps tendon and reflect distally the fascia lata to Gerdie's tubercle. The patella is laterally dislocated. Cut through its capsule medially and laterally. Do not cut through the synovium. (**c**) Separate the capsule from the synovium circumferentially around the patella. (**d**) Cut the synovium at its attachment to the patella, separating the patella, quadriceps muscle and patellar tendon from synovium. (**e**) Suture closed the hole in the synovium. (**f**) Release the patellar tendon from the apophysis by sharp dissection. Strip the tendon off distally with a sleeve of periosteum (Grammont procedure). (**g**) Centralize the patella on the synovium in knee extension and mark out its borders. (**h**) Incise the synovium to make a new hole for the patellar articular surface to re-enter the knee joint. (**i** and **j**) Suture the edge of the patella to the synovium. (**k**) Advance the medial capsule with the vastus medialis overtop the patella and suture to the lateral edge. Suture the medial edge of the patellar tendon to the tibia after displacing it medially. (**l** and **m**) Pass fascia lata under patellar tendon and retinaculum and around the adductor magnus tendon and suture back to itself (extra-articular ligament: Reverse MacIntosh)

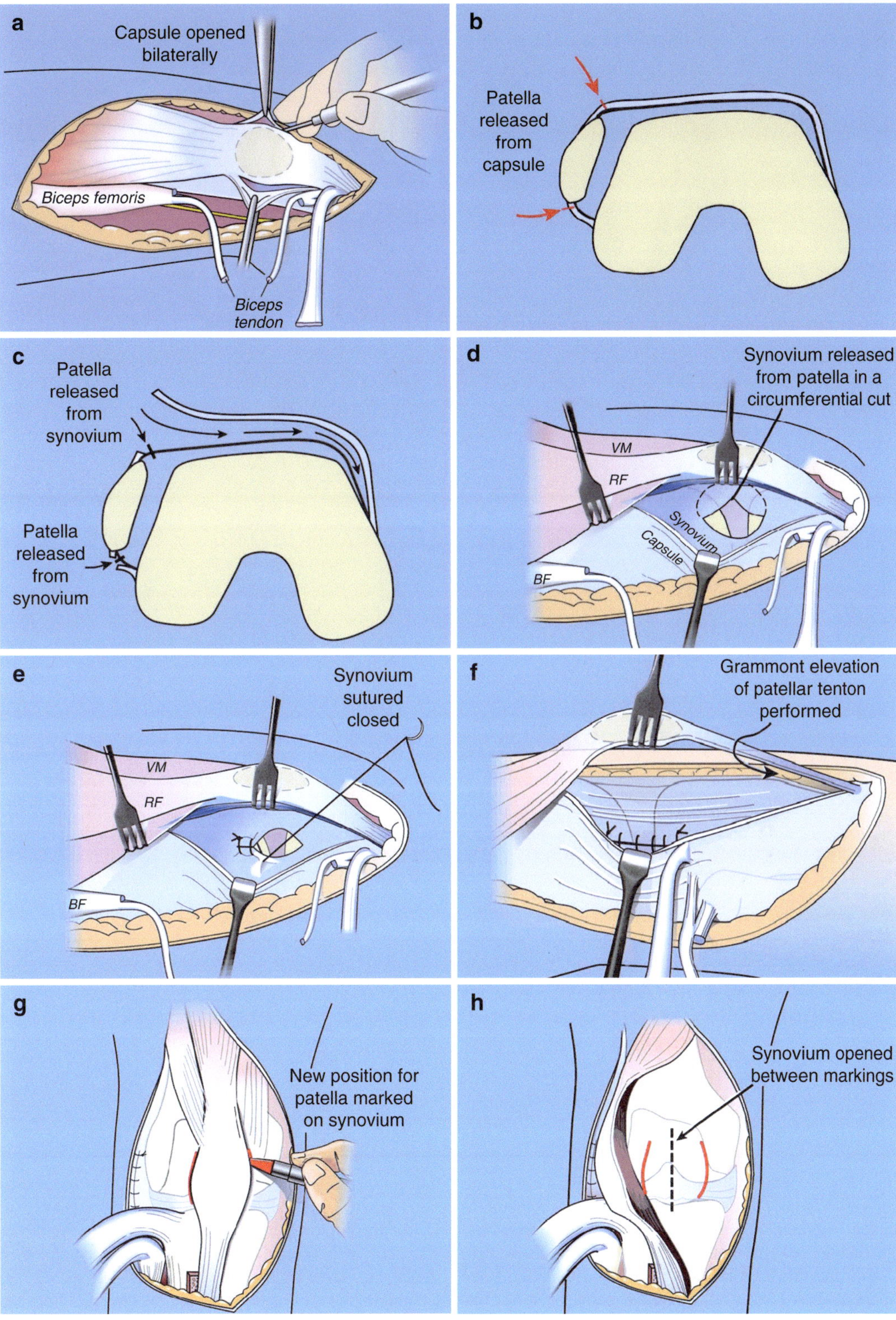
a
Capsule opened bilaterally
Biceps femoris
Biceps tendon
b
Patella released from capsule
c
Patella released from synovium
Patella released from synovium
d
Synovium released from patella in a circumferential cut
VM
RF
Synovium
Capsule
BF
e
Synovium sutured closed
VM
RF
BF
f
Grammont elevation of patellar tenton performed
g
New position for patella marked on synovium
h
Synovium opened between markings

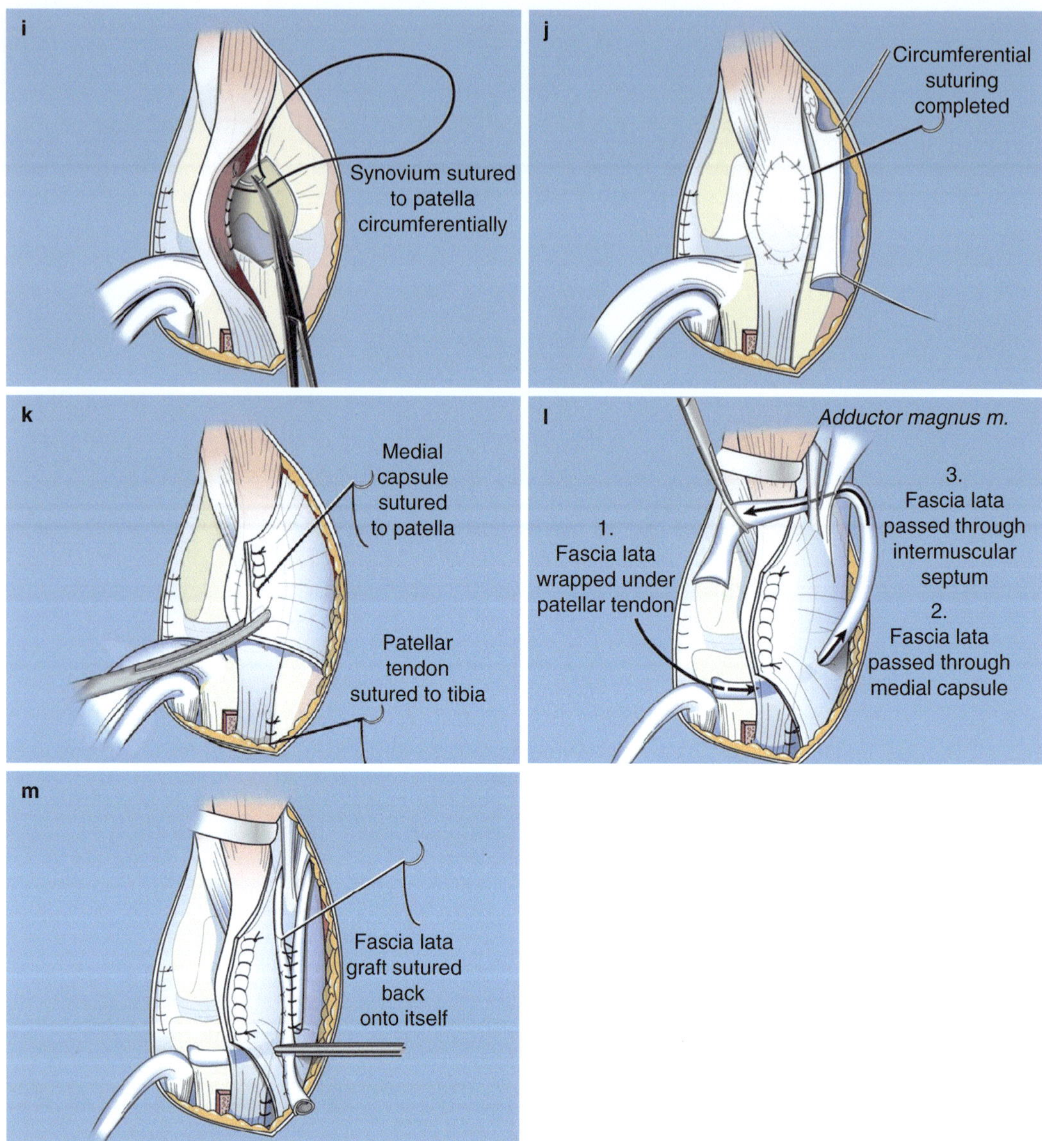

Fig. 13.5 (continued)

Fig. 13.6 Superknee surgical procedure including posterior capsulotomy, fascia lata, biceps and gastrocnemius tendon lengthening, and peroneal nerve decompression illustrations. (**a**) Through a lateral incision expose the fascia lata and release it distally. Do a z-lengthening of the biceps tendon. Identify the common peroneal nerve. (**b**) Decompress the peroneal nerve and its branches. Expose and release the lateral head of gastrocnemius tendon from the femur. Incise the lateral capsule. (**c**) Through a medial incision expose and divide the medial head of gastrocnemius tendon. (**d**) Incise the posteromedial capsule. (**e**) Dissect the popliteal fossa contents away from the posterior capsule on both lateral and medial sides and then divide the posterior capsule from lateral to medial. (**f**) Complete the posterior capsulotomy by dividing the medial capsule. (**g**) The posterior capsule is now fully divided. (**h**) The knee can now be extended fully and the biceps tendon repaired

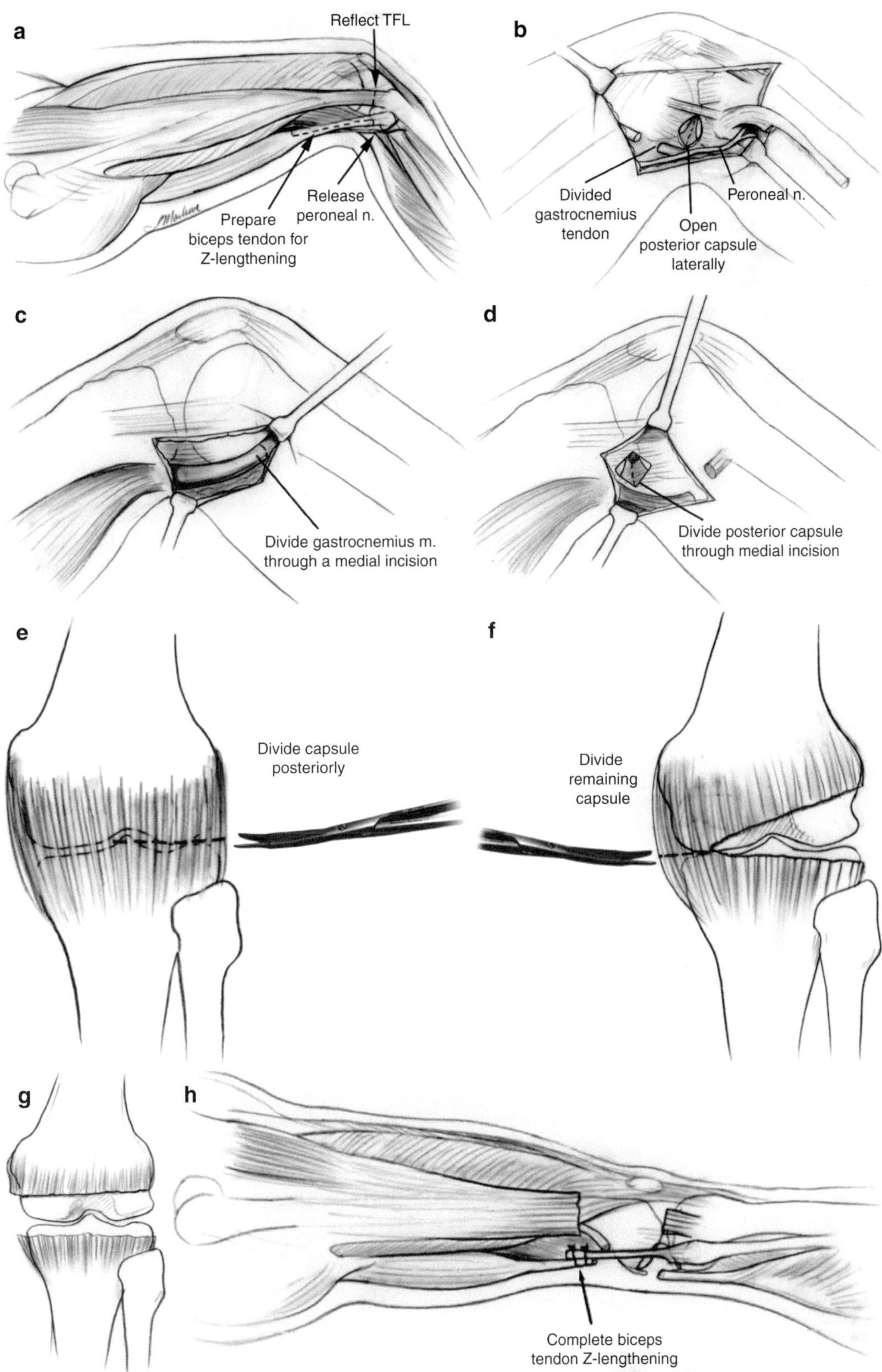

a
Reflect TFL
Prepare biceps tendon for Z-lengthening
Release peroneal n.

b
Divided gastrocnemius tendon
Open posterior capsule laterally
Peroneal n.

c
Divide gastrocnemius m. through a medial incision

d
Divide posterior capsule through medial incision

e
Divide capsule posteriorly

f
Divide remaining capsule

g

h
Complete biceps tendon Z-lengthening

knee reconstruction procedures described above. To avoid direct surgical and indirect stretch injury to the peroneal nerve, this nerve should be identified and decompressed at the neck of the fibula. Next, the biceps tendon should be Z-lengthened.

The common peroneal nerve can be palpated in most people over the neck of the fibula. A fascial incision is made through the superficial fascia that covers the nerve. Define the proximal and distal borders of the nerve. It is not necessary to remove the fat over the nerve. Follow the common peroneal nerve until it disappears into the lateral compartment. Make a transverse incision over the lateral compartment fascia and expose the muscle of the lateral compartment. Retract the muscle of the lateral compartment medially to expose the underlying arcade of fascia covering the common peroneal nerve. This is the decompression of the first tunnel. The common peroneal nerve can be seen dividing into deep and superficial branches, the superficial running down in the lateral compartment, and the deep branch going in the direction of the anterior compartment of the leg.

Extend the transverse compartment fasciotomy across to the anterior compartment. Notice the intermuscular septum separating the two compartments and confluent with the fascia overlying both compartments. Dissect the muscle of both sides of the septum. Be careful not to cut any superficial sensory branches of the nerve that may ascend the septum and innervate the skin overlying the compartments. With the septum exposed on its medial and lateral aspects, cut it from anterior to posterior. Be careful to stop as soon as the septum ends. Immediately below the septum a band of fat can often be seen. This fat band contains the deep peroneal nerve. This completes the decompression of the deep peroneal nerve (second tunnel). Extend the decompression of the common peroneal nerve under the biceps muscle. With the nerve protected and visualized, Z-lengthen the biceps muscle and tendon. In congenital cases, there is little tendon and mostly muscle. The biceps muscle consists of two parts: the short and long heads. To avoid damage to this muscle, the short head should be dissected off of the periosteum of the femur. Try and keep as much of the muscle together for the Z-lengthening and reflect this part proximally and isolate as much of the tendon by sharp dissection off of the muscle and reflect this part distally.

The lateral head of the gastrocnemius should be released from the femur. It has a very broad insertion of muscle and tendon. The lateral capsule can now be identified. Dissect the contents of the popliteal fossa away from the posterior capsule. To confirm that it is the posterior capsule, incise it posterolaterally and enter the knee joint. With the knee flexed the only vascular structure that one should see at the level of the knee joint is the central geniculate artery. This can be dissected free and cauterized. Care should be taken to make sure that the dissection does not inadvertently go distal to the level of the knee joint. If the dissection is behind the tibia instead of the knee joint line, the anterior tibial vessels may be encountered or injured. The rest of the popliteal soft tissues can be carefully dissected off of the capsule all the way to the medial side. The capsule can be cut under direct vision. A head lamp may be useful for this part. Once the capsule is open, try and extend the knee joint. If there is still too much resistance, then the medial side should be exposed. When performing a superknee with ligament repair, a medial skin flap needs to be elevated. If the posterior capsulotomy is being performed without the rest of the superknee, then the dissecting scissors can be inserted from lateral to medial until they can be seen under the medial skin. A separate small skin incision can be made medially to visualize the medial capsule. The medial head of the gastrocnemius is identified as the only structure with a muscle inserting proximally. The medial head should be cut from the femur, being careful not to injure the femoral vessels that lie just lateral to the medial head of gastrocnemius. The capsule is dissected free of the medial popliteal fossa to communicate with the lateral dissection. The capsule can then be cut under direct vision from both sides. The knee FFD can be corrected by extending the knee. The collateral ligaments are left intact. If after the capsulotomy the medial hamstrings are felt to be tight, they can be lengthened through the medial part of the dissection. I prefer to recess the aponeurosis of the semitendinosus and semimembranosus tendons rather than do a Z-lengthening.

After doing the knee capsular release, the knee is examined for instability. If it is unstable, then the ligamentous reconstruction of the super-knee procedure is carried out as in Fig. 13.4.

The above hip and knee problems must all be addressed before beginning femoral lengthening procedures. These are called preparatory surgery for lengthening. By performing preparatory surgery, we prevent complications that occur during lengthening: Pelvic osteotomy prevents hip subluxation/dislocation; proximal femur reconstruction (superhip) prevents worsening of coxa vara, proximal migration of femur, and dislocation of hip; patellar realignment prevents patellar dislocation and extension contracture of knee; ACL-PCL reconstruction prevents knee subluxation/dislocation and late problems of knee instability in adolescence; and fascia lata excision prevents knee stiffness and contracture, pressure on joint and physis, valgus deformity, and patellar subluxation.

13.6 Rehabilitation After Superhip and Superknee Surgery

13.6.1 Preoperative

An evaluation can be performed preoperatively when warranted to establish a relationship and determine any special concerns that the patient may have while in the hospital. Evaluation should include past medical and surgical history, pain level, preoperative range of motion (ROM), strength, sensation, limb length discrepancy and/or deformity, posture, coordination, and mobility including transitions and gait. Initiation of an exercise program may be needed prior to surgery to address deficits identified. The preoperative visit is also useful to educate the family and patient on what to expect after surgery and establish realistic postoperative goals.

13.6.2 Acute

The goal of inpatient PT after a superhip/knee surgery is to teach the parents how to manage with a child in a spica cast. Necessary skills include bed mobility, carrying and holding their child, transfers to wheel chair and car seat, equipment procurement (wheel chair, safety belt for car seat, sliding board if needed), and perineal hygiene (diaper vs. toilet) including how to keep the spica cast clean.

13.6.3 First 6 Weeks After Surgery

After the patient is discharged, they return to the hospital to have the spica cast made into a removable cast. The spica can be removed for gentle passive range of motion (PROM) of flexion and extension and abduction of the involved hip and flexion and extension of the knee not to exceed 0–90°. Therapist should be very gentle and not push the extremes of motion. It is important to support the limb both proximally and distally at all times when performing PROM. Parents will also be instructed in PROM techniques with hand-over-hand training and video recordings for reinforcement of proper technique at home.

13.6.4 After 6 Weeks

The spica cast is discontinued after 6 weeks. If the 6-week radiographs show adequate bony healing, then the patient can progress to weight bearing and active range of motion as well as gait training. A PT evaluation is performed after the SPICA cast is removed and includes assessment of strength, range of motion (ROM), proprioception, motor planning, mobility, transitions, gait, and developmental milestones. Treatment will aim to gently restore passive and active (P/A) ROM in order to regain independent mobility including rolling, transitions, standing, and walking with assistive device as needed. A gradual return to independent walking with a shoe lift will occur.

The goal at this stage is to regain mobility, strength, and gait training and restore range of motion. The end goal is to restore the child to normal function before they proceed with limb lengthening.

13.7 Femoral Lengthening of Type 1 CFD

13.7.1 Choice of Osteotomy Level for Lengthening of the Congenital Short Femur

Distal osteotomy for lengthening has the advantage of a broader cross-sectional diameter for better bone formation and less deforming forces from the adductors and hamstrings. If distal femoral valgus is present, it can be corrected using a distal lengthening osteotomy. Distal osteotomy lengthening is closer to the knee joint and therefore applies greater forces to the knee joint. This increases the risk of knee stiffness and subluxation. These risks can be reduced by articulating across the knee joint with extension of the fixator to the tibia. Proximal osteotomies have less effect on the knee, but are more prone to poor bone formation and consolidation in patients with CFD. There is also a higher rate of fracture after removal of external fixation in the proximal than in the distal lengthening groups. Proximal osteotomies have a greater effect on the hip joint and produce a much higher risk of adduction contracture, hip subluxation, and dislocation. Extension of the external fixator across the hip is more complex and less desirable than articulated distraction of the knee. For all of these reasons, I prefer to lengthen at the distal femur in patients with CFD.

The external rotation deformity of the femur with CFD should be corrected only by using a proximal osteotomy. The quadriceps muscle is in a normal relationship to the knee joint and because most of the quadriceps muscle originates distal to the level of a proximal femoral osteotomy, a proximal femoral internal rotation osteotomy does not change the orientation of the quadriceps relative to the knee joint. A distal osteotomy leaves the bulk of the quadriceps muscle attached proximally in a lateral position and rotates the knee medially, thus increasing the effective Q angle and increasing the tendency to lateral subluxation/dislocation of the patella. Varus deformity of the hip or proximal femoral diaphysis is corrected using a proximal valgus osteotomy, whereas valgus deformity of the knee is corrected using a distal varus osteotomy.

If the femur has undergone previous hip preparatory surgery such as superhip reconstruction or combination of Dega and proximal femoral osteotomy for milder cases, the proximal femoral deformities will already have been corrected and no proximal osteotomy is required at the time of lengthening. If hip preparatory surgery was not required, but there is external femoral torsion and perhaps mild proximal varus, then a proximal internal rotation-valgus osteotomy of the femur is carried out together with a distal lengthening osteotomy.

The distal femoral lengthening osteotomy should also acutely correct the valgus and any mild flexion deformity of the knee. For valgus correction alone no peroneal nerve decompression is required. However, if a flexion deformity is to be corrected acutely, the peroneal nerve should be decompressed just prior to the correction at the same surgery. As noted above, this distal region of the femur has a wider cross-sectional area than the proximal femur and is not in the zone of sclerotic poorly healing bone. Therefore, the regenerate bone in the distal femur is wider and stronger and subjected to axial deviation muscular forces than the proximal femur.

In older children with a wider medullary canal, implantable limb lengthening or lengthening over nail can be performed. A proximal osteotomy can be used for lengthening with nails because there is little risk of refracture and bone does not extend external fixation treatment time since the internal rod supports the bone until bone consolidation is complete. Intramedullary nailing in children adds the risk of disturbance of growth of the apophysis and avascular necrosis of the femoral head. To avoid the latter, we use a greater trochanteric starting point and a nail with a proximal bend (e.g., trochanteric entry femoral, or humeral or tibial). To avoid a coxa valga deformity, we prefer to use this technique in patients with some coxa vara. A theoretical apophysiodesis created by the nail can lead to gradual correction of residual coxa vara. I state theoretical because I have not observed this complication yet. Fixator only lengthening is the method we usually use for the first lengthening. LON or implantable lengthening is used for the second or third lengthening if the anatomic dimensions of the femur permit.

13.7.2 Soft Tissue Releases for Lengthening in Cases of CFD

Soft tissue releases are essential in conjunction with lengthening to prevent subluxation and stiffness of knee and hip. If a preparatory hip-knee surgery has already been performed, then the fascia lata and rectus femoris and in some cases biceps have already been lengthened. There is no need to repeat soft tissue releases that were already performed.

If soft tissue releases have not been performed, they should be carried out at the time of the lengthening surgery. If there is no contracture or tightness at the time of the index procedure, the soft tissue releases can either be performed at the index procedure or delayed until these soft tissues become contracted (6 weeks later). I usually prefer to do the soft tissue releases at the time of the index surgery to avoid an additional anesthetic.

Before surgery, the range of motion of the hip and knee should be evaluated using muscle lengthening tests and the presence of contractures or limitation identified. The muscle lengthening tests are the straight leg raising test (popliteal angle) for the hamstrings, the prone knee flexion test (Ely test) for the rectus femoris, hip abduction range for the adductors, and hip adduction range with knee and hip in extension for the fascia lata. One can also do an Ober test for the fascia lata. If a patient is able to straight leg raise so that the hip is at $90°$ of flexion and the knee is in full extension (popliteal angle $=0°$), the hamstring muscles are not tight and require no treatment before lengthening. If there is a popliteal angle $>0°$, the hamstrings are already tight and will lead to contractures during lengthening. The medial and lateral hamstrings should be fractionally lengthened through a single midline posterior incision proximal to the knee, to reduce the popliteal angle to $0°$.

If the patient is able to fully flex the knee while prone without the pelvis flexing at the hip, the rectus femoris is not tight (negative Ely test). I still prefer to release the rectus femoris (RF) from the anterior inferior spine since it will still become tight during lengthening. Obviously, if the Ely test is positive before surgery (pelvic flexion with prone knee bend), the RF should be released through a small anterior inguinal incision.

If hip abduction is limited, especially with proximal lengthening, percutaneous adductor tenotomies should be performed of the adductor longus and gracilis tendons. During lengthening, if more severed adduction contracture or hip subluxation develops, an open more extensive adductor release (including adductor brevis). Distal adductor magnus release has been described for congenital femoral lengthening (ref Richard Gross). I have not found this to be useful or necessary. For distal femoral lengthening, it is not necessary to release the hip adductors in most cases. For proximal lengthening, adductor release is very important.

In every case of CFD lengthening, the FL should be lengthened if it has not already been excised previously. The entire fascia lata is transected at the level of the proximal pole of the patella. I prefer to make a 3 cm longitudinal incision at the posterior edge of the FL where it connects with the intermuscular septum. The FL is transected by dissecting anterior to the incision. By making the incision more posterior, the biceps muscle can be easily exposed by retracting the incision posteriorly. The lateral biceps can be safely recessed.

Proximal release of the FL is almost never done at the index procedure. If however hyperlordosis develops, the fascia lata is released as it passes over the greater trochanter through a small lateral incision. This is almost never done at the index procedure but is performed during the lengthening or in conjunction with frame removal, to treat the hyperlordosis, abduction contracture, and hip flexion contracture secondary to the lengthening. We have noticed that patients who have undergone the superhip never develop this complication, while those who have just had distal incision of the fascia lata may develop this complication. They also have less difficulty maintaining knee range of motion during lengthening. We assume this is due to the fascia lata resection. We are therefore opting for limited incision complete FL resection in nonsuperhip patients. This can be achieved through two or three small incisions with tunneling between them.

13.7.2.1 Botulinum Toxin Injection

Botulinum toxin should be injected into the quadriceps to a limit of ten units of Botox per kg body weight. I prefer to limit the volume of the saline into which we mix the Botox to avoid systemic toxicity. I therefore usually inject with a total of 3–5 cc. The effect of Botox has been shown to be helpful in prevention of muscle contracture in an animal model of lengthening (Sam Rosenfeld). In humans I have observed that the role of Botox is to decrease muscle stretch pain especially due to muscle spasm and during physical therapy. The Botox should be injected only to the quadriceps muscles both because the amount allowable during one injection is only sufficient for the quadriceps and also because the quads are the primary muscle to have spasm during therapy.

13.7.3 Knee Instability Consideration

Almost all cases of CFD can be assumed to have hypoplastic or absent cruciate ligaments, with mild to moderate anteroposterior instability. Some also have medial-lateral and torsional instability. Despite this, the knee tracks normally preoperatively, and there is no indication to perform ligamentous reconstruction in most cases. The significance of the knee instability to lengthening is the tendency of the knee to subluxate with lengthening. Knee subluxation with lengthening is usually posterior or posterolateral (posterior plus external rotation of the tibia on the femur), but can also be anterior. Knee extension usually reduces posterior subluxation before lengthening. Therefore, to prevent posterior subluxation, some surgeons recommend splinting the knee in extension throughout the distraction phase (1). This promotes knees stiffness while protecting the knee from subluxation. I prefer to protect the knee by extending the external fixation to the tibia with hinges. The hinges permit knee motion while preventing posterior as well as anterior subluxation. They also prevent pressure being transmitted to the knee joint cartilage. Hinges are an integral part of circular external fixators such as the Ilizarov device. They are now also integral parts of some monolateral external fixators (e.g., Orthofix LRS, Smith and Nephew Modular Rail System).

A less common knee instability is anterior subluxation/dislocation of the tibia on the femur. This type of dislocation occurs as the knee goes into extension. It is important to document at which angle of flexion the knee relocates (conversely at which angle short of full extension the knee dislocates). These dislocations can be due to anterior deficiency of the distal femur (the lateral radiograph of the knee shows a lack of the anterior protuberance of the femoral condyles) or posterior deficiency or rounding of the posterior tibial plateaus. The posterior rounding of the tibial plateau is the more common bony deficiency. The treatment of such instability is by the superknee procedure combined with a posterior elevation osteotomy of the tibial plateau. In growing children, the osteotomy is epiphyseal, while in skeletally mature patients, it starts in the metaphysis.

13.7.4 Distal Femoral Lengthening-Ilizarov Fixator Technique

All the acute soft tissue releases are performed first. If soft tissue releases are to be performed on a delayed basis, proceed directly with the frame application. If a proximal femoral derotation, valgus, and/or extension osteotomy is needed, the proximal pin is inserted into the proximal femur with the hip in the position in which it will lie after the correction. For example, for an internal rotation osteotomy, the proximal pin should be inserted with the knee in external rotation. For a valgus osteotomy, the proximal pin should be inserted with the hip adducted. For an extension osteotomy, the proximal pins should be inserted with the hip flexed. For correction of varus, flexion, and external rotation, the femur should be externally rotated and crossed over the other thigh to adduct and flex the hip. This places the hip in the true neutral position. The first half-pin is from lateral to medial in the frontal plane, parallel to the line from the tip of the greater trochanter to the center of the femoral head. The plan is to attach the proximal arch parallel to the line from the tip of the trochanter to the center of the femoral head, the middle ring perpendicular to the mechanical axis of the shaft of the femur (7° to the shaft), and the distal ring parallel to the knee joint line. After the osteotomies, when all the rings and arch are parallel, the mechanical axis of each segment will be aligned and the joint orientation of the hip and knee will be parallel.

A second proximal half-pin is inserted on the proximal arch from 30° anterolateral to the first pin. The proximal arch is perpendicular to the floor with the leg crossed over and rotated as described above for correction of deformity. Two Ilizarov rings properly sized for the distal femur are applied to a distal femoral reference wire, which is parallel to the knee joint. For young children, we obtain arthrograms to better outline the cartilaginous femoral condylar line. The arthrogram is also useful to visualize the posterior femoral condyles for hinge placement. Conical washers or hinges are used between the two distal rings because of the valgus of the distal femur. The rings are at the valgus deformity angle to each other. A lateral half-pin is inserted into the mid-segment of the femur. This pin is at 7° to the shaft of the bone. At that point, the proximal subtrochanteric osteotomy can be performed. This is done percutaneously by making multiple drill holes and then using an osteotome. The osteotomy is internally rotated, laterally translated, and then angulated into valgus and extension to correct all components of the deformity. The order of correction is important to achieve the necessary displacement without loss of bone-to-bone contact and stability. Two additional half-pins are inserted and fixed onto the distal ring, one from posteromedial and one from posterolateral between the quadriceps and the hamstring muscles. One more middle pin is inserted. In small children, all half-pins are inserted by using the cannulated drill technique. This involves insertion of a wire first, then a cannulated drill, and then a half-pin. This technique permits very accurate placement of large diameter pins in narrow bones to avoid eccentric placement. Eccentric placement of drill holes and half-pins in the femoral diaphysis can lead to fracture. The distal femoral osteotomy is performed percutaneously, with multiple drill holes and an osteotome. The only wire used is removed to avoid tethering of the quadriceps and fascia lata.

13.7.4.1 Knee Hinges

The last step is to extend the fixation to the tibia using hinges. The center of rotation of the knee is located at the intersection of the posterior femoral cortical line and the distal femoral phy-seal line (1) in the plane where the two posterior femoral condyles are seen to overlap on the lateral view. For younger children, it is helpful to inject arthrographic dye into the knee to visualize the posterior femoral condyles. It is important that the distal femoral ring, which is parallel to the knee, appears to be perpendicular to the X-ray beam. The medial and lateral skin is marked at the location of the planned hinge placement. A single half-ring is attached to two threaded rods from the hinges. This half-ring is oriented perpendicular to the tibia with the knee in full extension. The first half-pin is inserted from anterior to posterior into the tibia. After fixing this pin to the proximal tibial half-ring, the knee is flexed and extended through a range of motion. If this range feels frictionless (perform a drop test: drop the tibia and see if it flexes without any catch), a second and third tibial half-pin are added. Finally, a removable knee extension bar is inserted between the distal femoral and the tibial half-ring.

13.7.5 Distal Femoral Lengthening-Orthofix Fixator Technique

One needs to start by identifying the center of rotation axis of the knee joint (see description of this above). A 1.8 mm wire is drilled into the lateral edge of the physis at the intersection of the posterior cortex of the femur with the physis in line with the plane of overlap of the posterior femoral condyles. The Orthofix LRS (pediatric or adult depending on the size of the child) is lined up with the hinge axis through its most distal hole. A commercially available sandwich clamp is used or if one is not available an extra lid is used in the pin clamp to create a second layer of pin holes more anteriorly. The fixator bar is lined up with the shaft of the femur and the most proximal-most half-pin inserted. The distal-most pin is then drilled one hole proximal to the center of rotation pin. The LRS without sandwich clamps is then used to place the rest of the pins (three proximal and three distal). If there is a distal femoral valgus that is to be corrected, an acutely swivel clamp is used for distal pin placement. When using a pediatric LRS, the three-hole pin clamp contains two half-pins only, since one hole is used up for the knee center of rotation. A third pin is added using Ilizarov cubes connected via these two pins. Before reapplying the sandwich clamps, the osteotomy is performed and the distal valgus corrected acutely. After the correction the fixator can be exchanged for one with straight clamps and with the sandwich attachments. All the pins should be in the upper deck of the double-decker sandwich clamps. The only pin in the lower deck is the knee axis pin. This pin does not enter the patient's leg. It is a 6 mm segment of pin which protrudes laterally. A Sheffield clamp from Orthofix is applied to this pin to act as a hinge. It is locked in place by putting a cube lateral to it with a set screw to prevent it moving outward. Conical washers are used between the Sheffield clamp and the LRS to prevent stiction friction. The Sheffield clamp is left partially loose to permit motion. A 1/3 Sheffield arch is attached to the clamp arching towards the tibia. An antero-posterior pin is inserted and the drop test (see above) is performed. If there is friction, the Sheffield clamp should be loosened. If friction persists adjust the connection of the pin to the Sheffield arch. If friction persists the axis pin may need to be bent slightly to alter the axis of rotation. Once the drop test is negative, two more oblique pins are inserted into the tibia and connected to the Sheffield arch using cubes. A removable knee extension bar is fashioned from Ilizarov parts to be used especially at night time. If there is an unstable hip, an axis pin for the hip can also be fashioned and attached from the proximal clamp. The same Sheffield clamp and arch arrangement are used. Two pins are placed in the pelvis from the anterior inferior and superior spines extending posteriorly. These are fixed to the Sheffield clamp to prevent proximal subluxation of the hip during lengthening. As one can see, the same principles are applied when using monolateral as with circular fixation, i.e., hinge fixation across joints when there is a joint at risk.

13.7.6 Distal Femoral Lengthening-Modular Rail System (Smith and Nephew, Memphis) (Figs. 13.7 and 13.8) **Technique**

This external fixator was designed by me specifically for the CFD patient. It is able to articulate

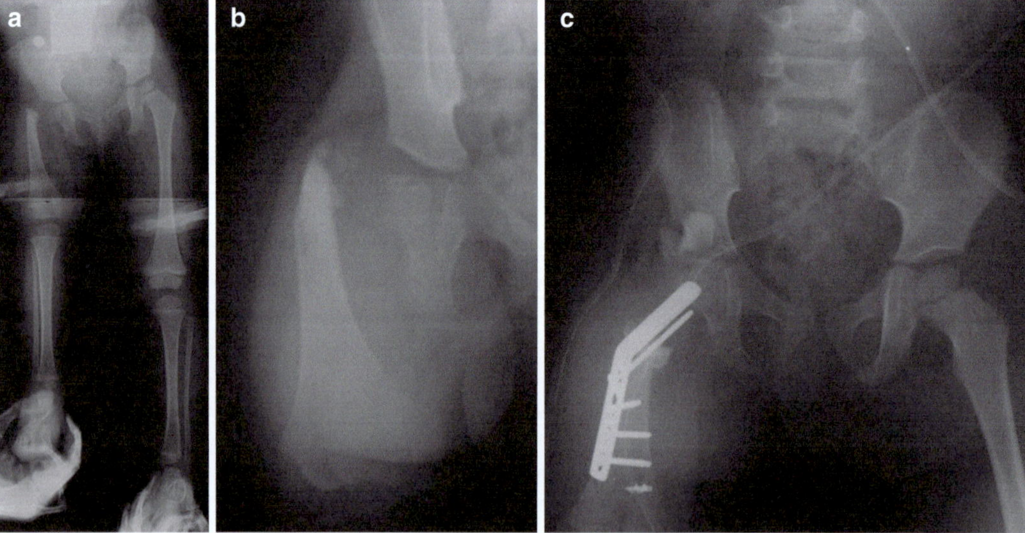

Fig. 13.7 CFD Paley type 1b with delayed ossification of femoral neck (**a, b**). Superhip procedure at age 2 including insertion of BMP in femoral neck (**c**). The neck is fully ossified by age 3 (**d**). First lengthening performed at age 4 with Smith and Nephew Modular Rail System external fixator with articulation across the knee joint (**e, f**). Eight centimeters of lengthening achieved (**g**). Removal of external fixator with Rush rodding of bone to prevent fracture (**h**)

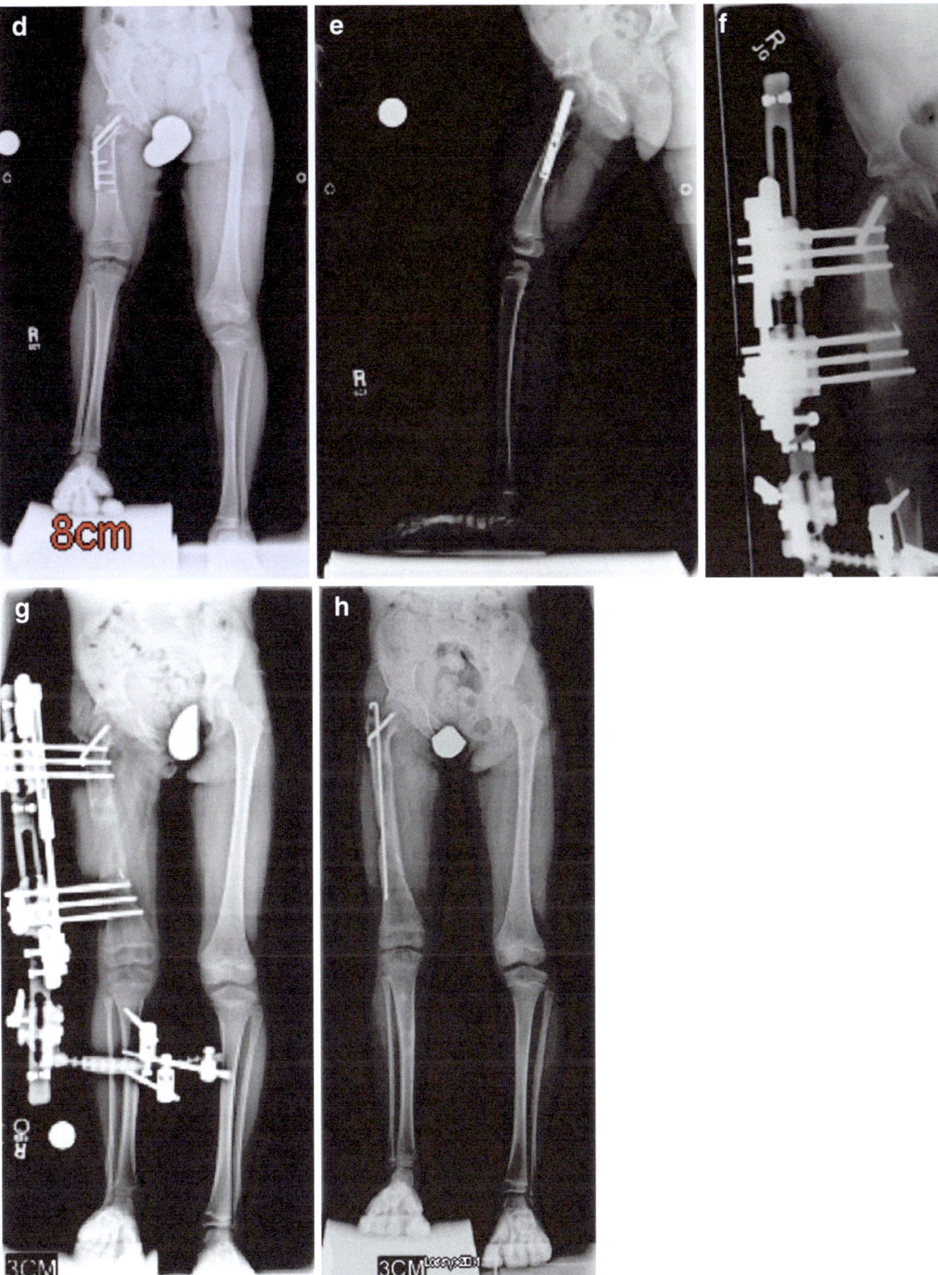

Fig. 13.7 (continued)

and span across the hip and knee joint either separately or at the same time. It also has clamps that allow fixation in the oblique plane in addition to the frontal plane producing delta fixation.

Step 1: Preconstruct the external fixator using pediatric or adult rail segments, two pin clamps, knee hinge, and tibial rail segment.

Step 2: Inject radiocontrast solution into the knee joint.

Step 3: Bring the image intensifier to the lateral projection and rotate the femur until the posterior aspect of the medial and lateral femoral condyles overlap.

Step 4: Insert a 2 mm Steinmann pin into the center of rotation (COR) of the knee joint. The

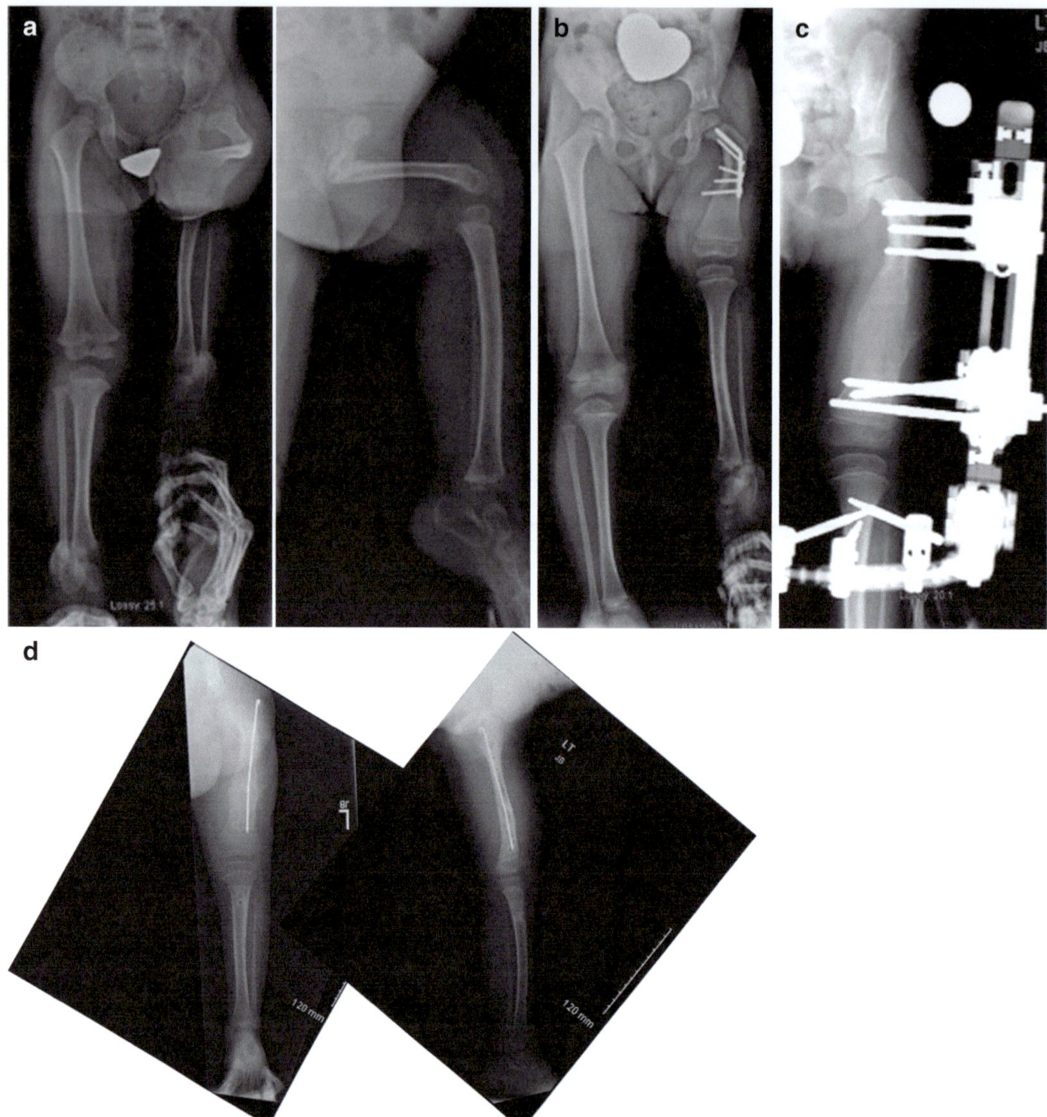

Fig. 13.8 A two-year-old girl with CFD Paley type 1b with delayed ossification and severe angulation of the subtrochanteric level of the femur (**a**). The deformity is fully corrected and the femur is healed after the superhip sur-gery (**b**). Lengthening of the femur was performed at age 4 years (**c**). X-rays after lengthening of the femur 7 cm and insertion of Rush rod (**d**)

COR is defined as the point of intersection of the posterior femoral cortex with the distal femoral physis. In adults it is the intersection of Blumensaat's line with the posterior cortex of the femur. Confirm on the AP view that the pin is parallel to the joint line.

Step 5: If there is no valgus or flexion deformity, proceed to drilling a 1.8 mm wire into the proximal femur parallel to the Steinmann pin. This wire should be as proximal as possible in the femur but distal to the trochanteric apophysis. Confirm the location of this wire making sure that it is located in the mid-diaphysis or slightly posterior to the midline. Drill a hole using a cannulated drill appropriate to the pin size preferred (e.g., 4.8 mm for a 6 mm pin, 3.8 mm for a 4.5 mm pin, 3.2 mm for a 3.5–4.5 mm pin).

Step 6: Insert a pin of the appropriate thread length corresponding to the diameter of the bone at that level. It is better not to leave threads outside of the near cortex to obtain the maximum bending strength out of each pin. The bending strength of the pin is related to the smallest diameter protruding from the near cortex.

Step 7: Mount the preconstructed MRS onto the Steinmann pin and the proximal half-pin. The Steinmann pin goes through the cannulation in the hinge of the fixator.

Step 8: Drill a 1.8 wire through the distal-most pin hole of the clamp. I prefer to use an overhang clamp to minimize the distance from the most distal pin to the hinge. This pin should be just proximal to the physis. Overdrill the wire with a cannulated drill and insert the pin.

Step 8: As long as the other pin clamp holes line up with the bone, use all three to fix the bone. All the pins should be parallel to each other.

Step 9: Make sure that the distal pin clamp is locked down to the fixator with red bolts (7 mm). Slide off the fixator from the pins.

Step 10: Make a 7 mm incision just proximal to the most proximal-distal pin. Drill the femur at this level with multiple drill holes. Complete the osteotomy using a sharp osteotome.

Step 11: Reapply the fixator to the pins. Make sure the osteotomy did not displace. If it did, adjust it in the frontal plane. If AP clamps are being used, drill at least one hole for posterolateral oblique pin proximally and distally. The total number of pins per segment should be 3 or 4 depending on the size of the femur and the thigh being lengthened.

Step 12: Drill a hole in the upper tibia from anterior to posterior using a 3.2 mm drill bit. Insert a pin into this hold. Make sure that the drill hole is distal to the tip of the proximal tibial apophysis.

Step 13: Connect the tibial pin to an arch mounted off of the tibial rail extension using a cube. Test the motion of the knee to confirm that the knee moves freely. By placing the first tibial pin in the sagittal plane, anteroposterior adjustment of the tibia in case of subluxation can be done. Apply a set screw to the pin once the knee motion is free. To confirm it is free, do the "drop test." If the leg drops with no friction from 0 to 90°, then the hinge is perfect.

Step 14: Apply two more pins in different orientation in the proximal tibia.

Step 15: Inject Botox to the quadriceps muscles.

Step 16: Apply a knee extension bar constructed from Ilizarov parts. This includes a post proximally and a twisted hinge distally. Off of each of these, insert a post and fixate it with a 20 or 30 mm socket. Connect a threaded rod between the two posts. The knee extension bar should be placed in maximum extension of the knee and locked down so that the rod length cannot be changed. The patient uses the bar all night long and half the time during the day. It is easily removable for exercise.

Step 17: Apply a distractor.

Step 18: Apply sterile dressings.

Step 19: Obtain final radiographs before leaving the operating room.

Modification for valgus ± flexion deformity of the distal femur

Step 5a: Insert a wire into the distal femur using the MRS as a guide. This wire should be parallel to the Steinmann pin. Use a cannulated drill and then insert a half-pin.

Step 6a: Drill a wire into the proximal femur at about 7° to the shaft. This proximal wire should subtend a valgus angulation with the distal pin. It should be in the same rotational orientation as the distal pin.

Step 7a: Perform an osteotomy of the distal femur at the planned level leaving enough room to add two more pins distal to the osteotomy.

Step 8a: Correct the valgus deformity by making the pins parallel to each other in the frontal plane. Reapply the external fixator to the pins.

Step 9a: If there is also a flexion deformity of the knee, extend the knee using the tibia to lever the osteotomy into extension.

Step 10a: Add the remaining frontal plane pins.

Step 11a: Add the remaining AP clamp pins.

Step 12–19: same as before.

13.7.7 Rehabilitation and Follow-Up During Lengthening

Femoral lengthening requires close follow-up and intensive rehabilitation to identify problems and maintain a functional extremity. Clinically, the patient is assessed for hip and knee range of motion, nerve function, and pin site problems.

Radiographically, the distraction gap length, regenerate bone quality, limb alignment, and joint location are assessed.

Knee flexion should be maintained as close to 90° as possible. The minimum goal is >45°. If knee flexion is ≤45°, the lengthening should be stopped or at least slowed and the knee rehabilitated more. If after a few days the knee flexion improves, lengthening may resume. It is critical to never sacrifice function for length. More length can be obtained with subsequent lengthenings, but we cannot recreate a new knee joint. Therefore, everything should be done to preserve the knee joint and its motion. A flexion contracture may develop during lengthening. To prevent this, a knee extension bar may be used at night and part time during the day. A fixed flexion deformity (FFD) of the knee places it at risk of posterior subluxation. Subluxation of the knee can be suspected clinically based on a change in shape of the front of the tibia relative to the kneecap. Posterior subluxation of the tibia presents with a very prominent kneecap and a depression of the tibia relative to the kneecap (ski hill sign). Extension of the external fixation across the knee with hinges prevents posterior subluxation (1).

Hip motion may become more limited with lengthening. Adduction and flexion contractures are the most significant because they can lead to hip subluxation and dislocation. Release of the adductors and the rectus and the tensor fascia lata during lengthening may need to be considered to allow further lengthening and to prevent hip subluxation.

Weight bearing (WB) is permitted all throughout the lengthening. In younger lighter children walking without support can be achieved immediately because the fixator is so stiff relative to the patient's weight. When the child is older and heavier, they prefer to walk with crutches or a walker until there is sufficient consolidation. We therefore permit WB as tolerated (WBAT) as long as they have normal proprioception.

13.7.8 Fixator Removal and Rodding of Femur (Figs. 13.7 and 13.8)

The fixator can be removed once the regenerate bone is fully healed radiographically. The regen-erate bone should show no gaps (interzone closed) and evidence of corticalization on three or four cortices of the AP and lateral views.

The external fixator should be removed under anesthesia as an outpatient procedure. Remove all the middle pins and leave only the most distal and proximal pin in place. Using image intensifier radiography, first drill or ream a hole for a Rush rod and then insert a Rush rod into the femur from the greater trochanter to the distal femoral physis. The hooked tip of the rod should embed into the tip of the greater trochanter for ease of later removal.

13.8 Specific Complications and Their Treatment for Congenital Femoral Deficiency Lengthening (Paley 1990)

13.8.1 Nerve Injury

Nerve injury from surgery or distraction is unusual with femoral lengthening. To avoid peroneal nerve injury from the pins, the posterolateral pin should not enter posterior to the biceps tendon. During distraction, if the patient complains of pain in the dorsum of the foot or asks for frequent massage of the foot, this is most likely referred pain from stretch entrapment of the peroneal nerve. More advanced symptoms include hyper- or hypoesthesia in the distribution of the peroneal nerve or weakness of the extensor hallucis longus muscle. A nerve conduction study may show evidence of nerve injury but, in most cases since too many fibers are conducting normally, will likely be negative. Quantitative sensory testing using the Pressure Sensitive Sensory Device (PSSD), if available, is the most sensitive test to assess for nerve involvement (Nogueira et al. 2003). Near nerve conduction using very fine electrodes is also very accurate. If the nerve problem is identified early, it can be treated by slowing the rate of distraction. If despite slowing the distraction, symptoms continue or motor signs develop, the peroneal nerve should be decompressed at the neck of the fibula, including transverse fasciotomy of the lateral and anterior compartment and release of the intermuscular septum between these compartments. Paley (2005b); Nogueira and Paley (2011) found that peroneal nerve decompression is efficacious for the treatment of peroneal nerve injury secondary to lengthening.

13.8.2 Poor or Failure of Bone Formation

Hypotrophic regenerate formation requires slowing of the distraction rate. The rate can be slowed to ¾, ½, or ¼ mm per day. If the regenerate bone does not improve, a decision needs to be made as to whether lengthening may be continued knowing that the bone defect being created may need to be bone grafted. Biphosphonate infusion (e.g., zoledronic acid) can be used to prevent bone resorption while permitting bone formation. At the end of lengthening if the distraction gap does not fill, it can be bone grafted.

13.8.3 Incomplete Osteotomy and Premature Consolidation

Lack of separation of the osteotomy site after a week of distraction may be due to an incomplete osteotomy or at least a periosteal hinge that will not separate. Continued distraction can lead to an acute separation of the bone ends. There may be an audible pop associated with this. Such an acute separation is usually very painful. This pain continues unabated until the bone is acutely shortened by a few millimeters. It is important to advise the patient of this. If the bone does not separate or if the patient or parents wish to avoid a painful separation, a reosteotomy should be performed.

13.8.4 Hip Subluxation/Dislocation

Hip instability is judged radiographically. A break in Shenton's line or increased medial-lateral, head-teardrop distance indicates subluxation of the hip. Although the diagnosis is radiographic, the hip usually has an adduction and flexion contracture and may also exhibit stiffness to flexion-extension. Hip subluxation does not usually occur if there is adequate coverage of the femoral head. However, adduction and flexion contracture predisposes the hip to subluxation even in the presence of adequate coverage.

If hip subluxation occurs during lengthening or consolidation phases, the patient should urgently be taken to the operating room for soft tissue releases of the adductor longus and gracilis and in some cases the tensor fascia lata (assuming the rectus femoris has already been lengthened). A closed reduction of the hip should be performed by abducting the hip. If the hip will not reduce, the distraction gap should be shortened to loosen the hip joint. The external fixator should be extended to the pelvis with or without a flexion-extension hinge. With a hinge a hip extension bar should be added to prevent flexion contracture. The pelvic fixation consists of at least two anterolateral pins between the two tables and between the anterior inferior and superior spines and two pins more lateral. The femur should be in 15–20° of abduction to the pelvis to maintain the reduction.

13.8.5 Knee Subluxation/Dislocation

CFD knees usually have hypoplastic or absent cruciate ligaments. In the knee, posterior or anterior subluxation can be monitored on the lateral view full knee extension radiograph (Paley 2005c). Posterior subluxation is the most common, although in most cases, this is combined with an external rotation subluxation (posterolateral rotatory subluxation). If the fascia lata and biceps are intact, tension in these structures is the culprit.

Limb length equalization should be based on full length standing radiographs. Limb alignment is assessed for the femur and tibia separately and in combination. Separately, the joint orientation of the knee should be measured using the malalignment test (Paley 2005c, d). Axial deviation from lengthening (procurvatum and valgus for distal femoral lengthening and procurvatum and varus for proximal lengthening) is identified and corrected at the end of the distraction phase, when the regenerate bone is still malleable. When there is malalignment of the femur and tibia, the femoral malalignment is corrected to a normal distal femoral joint orientation. The femur is not over- or under-corrected to compensate for the tibial deformity. The tibia should be corrected separately, either during the same treatment or at a later treatment. Complete failure of bone formation is very unusual. Partial defects are not uncommon. The most common location is lateral. Dynamization of the fixator should be carried out and bone growth stimulators (our preference is the Exogen) can be used. Resection of the fibrous tissue in these defects and cancellous bone grafting may become necessary to reduce the external fixation time and prevent fracture after frame removal.

13.8.6 Fracture

Fractures associated with limb lengthening can be divided into those that occur while the external fixator is still on, those that occur at the time of removal, and those that occur after removal. Fractures can also be classified as to their location: regenerate or remote. The incidence of all these types of fractures associated with CFD lengthening was 34 % compared to 9 % for noncongenital femoral lengthening. In many cases this was despite the use of a spica cast after removal.

Since this rate was unacceptably high, we started prophylactically Rush rodding the femur at the time of removal. This new protocol virtually eliminated the complication of refracture after lengthening.

13.8.7 Hip and Knee Joint Luxation

Hip joint subluxation or dislocation is a dreaded complication associated specifically with congenital femoral lengthenings. The hip joint is often mildly or moderately dysplastic in patients with CFD. The acetabular dysplasia has a different pattern than that of DDH. The femoral head is usually uncovered laterally rather than anterolaterally. If the CE angle is less than 20°, the hip joint is considered at risk for dislocation

(Suzuki et al. 1994). The other parameter to look at is the orientation of the sourcil (dome). The sourcil should be horizontal. If it is inclined laterally, then the hip joint is potentially unstable even if the CE angle is greater than 20. It is always safer to err on the side of performing a pelvic osteotomy than to end up with a hip luxation.

During lengthening the hip abduction and flexion range of motion should be checked. Hip luxation always occurs together with adduction or flexion contractures of the hip. Hip luxation is diagnosed radiographically. The earliest signs are widening of the medial head teardrop distance and a break in Shenton's line.

Once luxation is diagnosed, distraction must stop. If it is early in the lengthening process, the patient can be taken to the OR, the hip reduced acutely, and the external fixator extended to the pelvis to stabilize the hip. Lengthening can proceed under such protection. If this occurs after at least 5 cm of lengthening, it is wiser to stop the lengthening completely and reduce the luxation by means of an abduction cast or fixator. Adductor, flexor release may be required including the proximal tensor fascia lata.

13.8.7.1 Knee Luxation

As previously noted, most cases of CFD have hypoplastic or absent cruciate ligaments. Most patients have a more dominant instability pattern (e.g., posterior vs. anterior vs. posterolateral). The tendency towards flexion contracture during lengthening predisposes the tibia to posterior subluxation. If the fascia lata remains intact the knee will sublux posterolaterally. Extension contracture leads to patella alta and anterior or anteromedial subluxation. Knee subluxation depends on the level of the lengthening. Proximal femoral lengthening is less likely to sublux the knee while distal femoral lengthening is more likely to sublux the knee. Proximal femoral lengthening has a narrower and often less well-formed regenerate bone with a much higher risk of fracture than distal femoral lengthening. Prevention of knee subluxation involves a combination of soft tissue release of the distal fascia lata together with extension of the external fixator to the tibia. The latter is best done with hinges to permit and maintain knee motion. One of the problems is that if the tibia is left unfixed with distal femoral lengthening without release of the fascia lata, the knee will begin to sublux after only 2–3 cm. If fascia lata release is performed without fixation to the tibia, the knee will start to sublux after about 4 cm. To permit greater lengthening and to protect the knee from pressure and subluxation, it is best to articulate across the knee. This protects the cartilage of the knee and physis from undue forces. In the past extending the frame across the knee with hinges was considered something that could only be done with circular external fixation. With the modularity of monolateral external fixators, the same can be achieved with monolateral external fixators. It is important to preserve the principal of articulated fixation to the tibia with all lengthenings of congenitally short femurs of 5 cm or more whether one prefers a monolateral or circular fixator. The biggest mistake is to become a slave to the fixator rather than the fixator becoming a slave to the surgeon. I have seen so many knee subluxations and dislocations secondary to lengthening without soft tissue releases and without protection of the knee by means of articulated distraction. One approach that has been used to protect the knee is to keep the knee in full extension without bending throughout the lengthening. While this may avoid subluxation in most cases, it may also result in a stiff knee.

13.8.8 Joint Stiffness and Contracture

The tendency is for the knee to lose flexion during lengthening. This is combined with the tendency for a flexion contracture. These problems can occur together or separately. Although the transfixing pins or wires may contribute to difficulty in flexion, lengthening with internal distractors (e.g., ISKD) still leads to loss of knee flexion with increased length. Stiffness of the knee is preventable. Surgical release/lengthening of specific soft tissues (fascia lata, rectus femoris) reduces the joint reactive forces on the knee due to lengthening. Physical therapy is essential to successful CFD lengthening. This is especially true for the

knee. I am not prepared to lengthen most CFD cases if they cannot organize outpatient PT.

If the knee gets stiff to flexion despite adequate rehab, then a quadricepsplasty should be performed. When there is a concomitant flexion contracture, I will choose either open or closed treatment: Closed requires an external fixator and gradual distraction. Open means posterior capsule release. Physical therapy including dynamic splinting can be used first to obtain extension of the knee before considering any type of quadricepsplasty.

Joint stiffness due to damage to the articular surface occurs due to unprotected compressive forces across the knee joint combined with immobility and subluxation. This irreversible complication can be prevented by means of distraction across the knee joint combined with protection against subluxation and maintenance of knee joint range of motion.

13.9 Treatment CFD Types 2 and 3

13.9.1 Treatment CFD Type 2a

Type 2a differs from type 2b by the presence of a mobile femoral head. If there is a mobile femoral head, an attempt should be made to obtain union between the femoral head and upper femur. Attempts at connecting these together are often met with failure or stiffness of the hip. I have developed a new way of reliably achieving union between the upper femur and the femoral head with the creation of a new femoral neck.

13.9.1.1 Superhip 2 Procedure for Treatment of a Mobile Proximal Femoral Pseudarthrosis (Figs. 13.9 and 13.10)

The same approach as the superhip is used. The operation remains the same until the subtrochanteric osteotomy. Before performing the osteotomy, the region of the femoral neck is dissected. The level of the acetabulum is identified with the image intensifier and the femoral head and acetabulum are identified. The capsule of the femoral head is opened. The femoral head is moved in the acetabulum using a needle as a joystick through its cartilage. If there is a cartilaginous femoral neck, it is excised down to the ossific nucleus of the femoral head. If there is no neck, the cartilage of the head is cut back to the ossific nucleus to expose the bone. The femoral neck is made from the proximal femur and greater

trochanter segment. This segment is rotated 135° on a soft tissue pedicle so that the greater trochanter goes distal and lateral and the distal cut end of the subtrochanteric osteotomy is fixed to the ossific nucleus of the femoral head. The subtrochanteric osteotomy is made by taking a trapezoidal segment of femur out. The distal cut is at

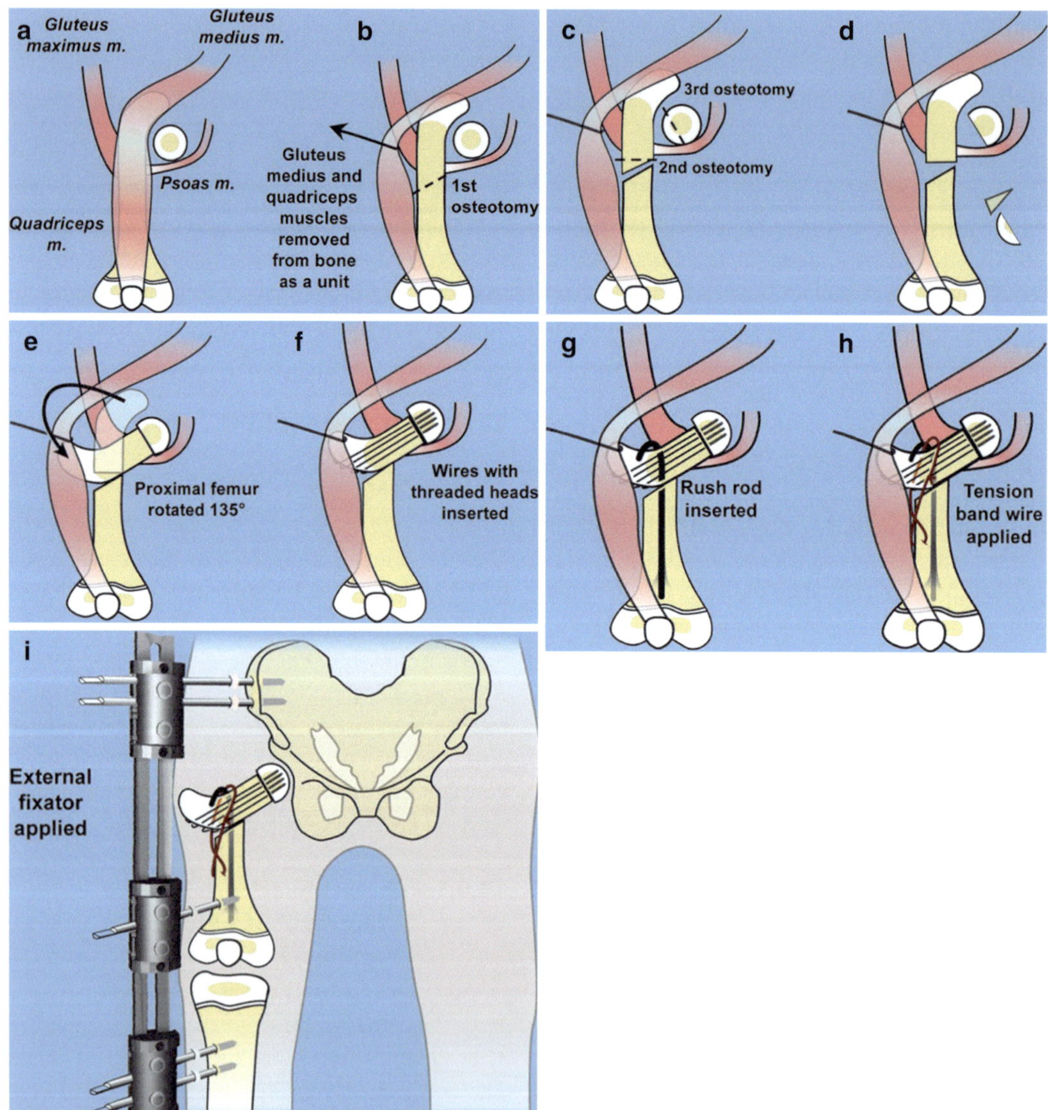

Fig. 13.9 Superhip 2 surgical technique illustrations. (**a**) Paley type 2 CFD. (**b**) The vascular pedicle of the proximal femur is the psoas and gluteus maximus. The hip abductors and quadriceps are removed. Alternatively in the newer method we now use, the quadriceps is left as the pedicle and all the rest of the muscles are removed and later reattached. (**c**) The proximal femur is osteotomized and the femoral head is exposed. (**d**) The femoral head and proximal femur are prepared to be connected together. (**e**) Rotate the proximal femur 135°. (**f**) Fixate the new neck to the head using threaded Steinman pins. (**g**) Use a Rush rod to fix the shaft to the new neck. (**h**) Compress using a tension band wire. (**i**) Neutralize the limited fixation of the femoral head to neck by an external fixator from the pelvis to the femur to the tibia

45° to the shaft of the femur, while the proximal cut is perpendicular. All of the soft tissue is dissected off the trochanteric segment except the gluteus maximus and the psoas tendon. Care should be taken next to the psoas tendon not to injure the profunda artery and other perforators at its inferior edge. The trochanteric segment is pre-drilled with a 1.8 mm wire in four places around its periphery. This bone is also drilled at 45° to its long axis for insertion of a Rush rod. This is drilled in a way to miss the four wire holes path. The distal femur diaphysis is also drilled with a 3.2 mm drill bit. The lateral cortical surface of the trochanteric segment which will be oriented inferiorly is slightly decorticated. The Rush rod is now fixed in place with the distal femur articu-

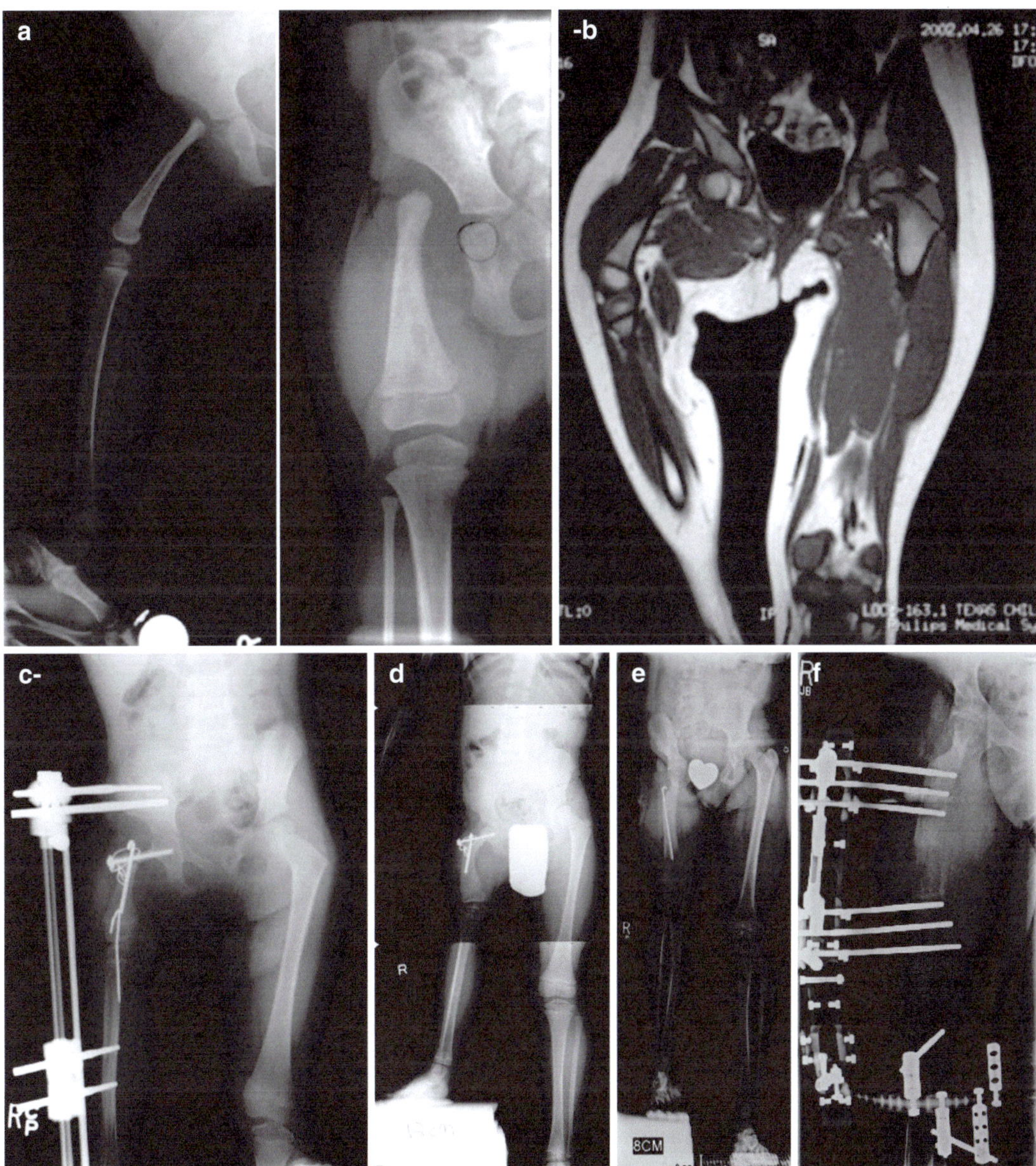

Fig. 13.10 X-ray (**a**) and MRI (**b**) of a girl with CFD Paley type 2a with a true pseudarthrosis of the femoral neck. X-ray after superhip 2 procedure with external fixator in place (**c**). The femoral neck is reconstructed and intact after removal of the external fixator (**d**). X-ray (**e**) after first lengthening surgery (6 cm). Second lengthening surgery (**f**). After (**g**) second lengthening surgery (8 cm). Two more lengthening surgeries are needed

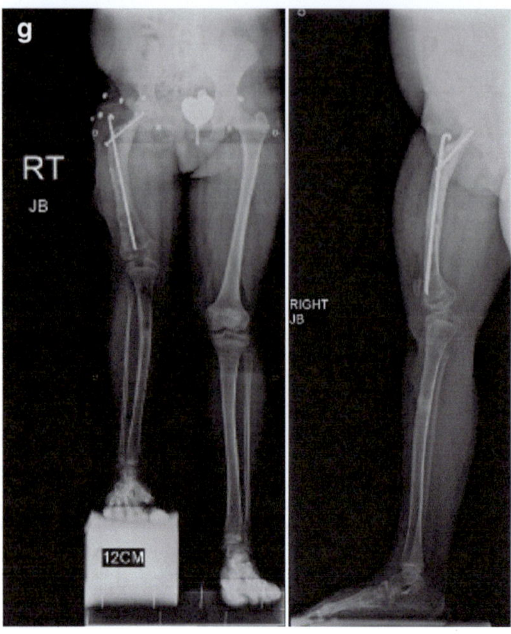

Fig. 13.10 (continued)

lating against the decorticated surface. A tension band wire is applied similar to the one described for the superhip. This new femoral neck which now subtends an angle of 135° to the femoral shaft is brought up in line with the femoral head. The cannulated wire is inserted into the femoral head and drilled with the 3.2 cannulated drill bit. An appropriately sized partially threaded 4.5 or 5.5 mm screw with washer is inserted to compress the femoral neck-head site. This osteosynthesis is stable for gentle abduction and adduction but cannot control flexion and extension since the single screw acts as a hinge for flexion and extension. An additional threaded k wire is inserted parallel to the screw into the femoral head. To neutralize the forces on the femoral neck-head junction, an external fixator is applied from the pelvis to the tibia. The external fixator is applied before closure to ensure that there is no loss of fixation. Two anterior external fixation pins are put into the pelvis between the anterior inferior and superior spines in an oblique anteroposterior direction following the orientation of the ilium. The tibial pins are also anteroposterior. A pediatric Orthofix LRS with cubes as needed to get fixation of the pelvic pins is applied for neutralization. Prior to closure any residual bone

graft can be morselized around the osteotomy site. The abductor-quadriceps muscle tendon unit followed by the tensor fascia lata is sutured to the greater trochanter. The rest of the closure is per routine. It is important to use suction drains to prevent a hematoma under the anterior flap. The fixator is removed after 3 months. Physical therapy for the hip joint can begin at that time.

13.9.2 Treatment CFD Type 2b

In this pathology, there is either a hypoplastic femoral head which is fused to the acetabulum (Fig. 13.11). If the fusion region is small (usually posteroinferior), it can be broken and converted and a superhip 2 performed. If the fusion area is large, the superhip 2 is not an option. What distinguishes this from the diaphyseal deficiency of type 3 is the cartilaginous cap of the greater trochanter which is present in type 2b. To reconstruct the hip without directly joining the proximal femur to the femoral head requires a pelvic support osteotomy. The treatment of type 2b cases is accomplished by combining a pelvic support osteotomy proximally with a distal femoral lengthening and realignment osteotomy (Fig. 13.8). This combination is called the *Ilizarov hip reconstruction*. Pelvic support osteotomy is usually enough to prevent proximal migration of the femur during lengthening for noncongenital pathologies (Rozbruch et al. 2005). For congenital pathologies, the fixation should be extended to the pelvis to prevent proximal migration of the femur.

In young children with very short femora, the femur may be too small to perform both the pelvic support and the distal lengthening osteotomies. Furthermore, the valgus component of the pelvic support osteotomy will remodel straight within a year in most cases. In such cases, pins are extended to the pelvis to prevent proximal migration during lengthening. Lengthening is then performed through a distal femoral osteotomy, much in the way described previously. In older children, the pelvic support osteotomy is performed at the level at which the proximal femur crosses the ischial tuberosity in the maximum cross-legged X-ray. The amount of valgus

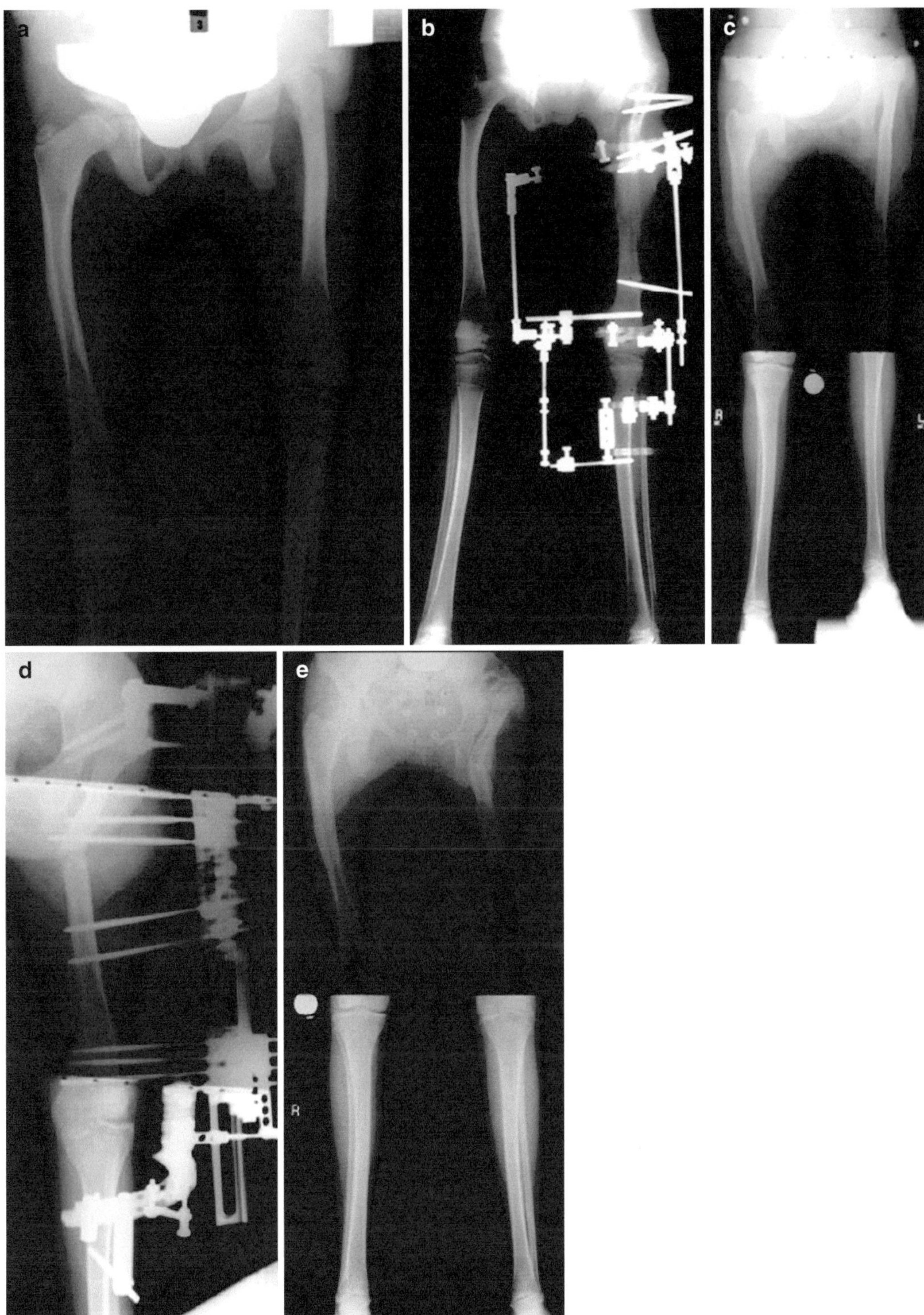

Fig. 13.11 X-ray (**a**) of 10-year-old girl with Paley type 2c CFD (absent femoral head). She was treated by pelvic support osteotomy (**b**) and distal femoral lengthening (13 cm). The pelvic support angulation remodeled and the leg length difference was 10 cm at skeletal maturity (**c**). At age 16 she underwent a second pelvic support osteotomy with 10 cm lengthening (**d**). Final radiographic result showing limb length equalization. She has excellent function (**e**)

is equal to the total amount of adduction of the hip plus 15° overcorrection. The proximal osteotomy should also be internally rotated and extended. The amount of rotation is judged by the position of the knee relative to the hip in maximum adduction. The amount of extension depends on the amount of hip FFD. The level of the distal osteotomy is planned by extending the line of the tibia proximally and seeing where it intersects a line perpendicular to the pelvis passing through the mid-proximal segment of femur. The distal osteotomy is usually mid-diaphyseal. The external fixator must still be extended to the tibia with hinges, as previously discussed.

13.9.3 Treatment Type 3a: Diaphyseal Deficiency, Knee ROM >45°

Deficiency of the proximal femur with absent femoral head, greater trochanter, and proximal femoral metaphysis results in a mobile pseudarthrosis and a very short femoral remnant. Some cases have a mobile knee with ≥45° of motion (type 3a), usually with a 45° knee flexion deformity, whereas others have a stiff knee with <45° range of motion (type 3b) and usually a greater flexion deformity. The most predictable and reliable treatment option in these cases remains prosthetic reconstruction surgery (PRS) (e.g., rotationplasty or Syme's amputation). LRS has a role in these cases and can equalize LLD. Because the numbers of these patients treated by LRS is small, the ultimate functional result for these cases is still not predictable or reliable.

13.9.3.1 LRS Approach for Diaphyseal Deficiency Cases: Type 3a

LRS is most applicable to type 3a cases in which there is a functional range of knee motion present (Fig. 13.12). In type 3 cases, a knee flexion deformity is usually present. In addition, a hip flexion contracture is present. Both of these are treated by soft tissue release using the same approach as that described above for type 1 cases. The fascia lata is reflected proximally, and the quadriceps and abductors are elevated off the proximal femur. The psoas tendon is absent, but the rectus and sar-

torius are present. Any fibrous femoral anlage is resected, and frequently, some of the cartilaginous femoral anlage may need to be trimmed. The proximal femur is freed from these attachments, including the hip capsular remnants, permitting it to move proximally without a soft tissue tether. This is important, especially for the acute correction of the knee contracture. The long lateral incision is extended distally and the peroneal nerve decompressed and protected. Because the femur is so short, it is advisable to explore the peroneal nerve before the proximal release and then follow it proximally to the hip joint region. This will prevent injury to the sciatic nerve as it passes very near the dissection around the hip capsular remnant. The medial and lateral approach knee flexion contracture release of the posterior capsule is performed, and the knee joint is fully extended. A 2 mm Steinmann pin is drilled across the knee joint from the femur into the tibia to maintain full knee extension. During the same operation, a monolateral fixator is placed from the pelvis to the femur and tibia. The most important and strongest pelvic pin is one from the anterior inferior iliac spine oriented towards the greater sciatic notch (using the cannulated drill technique). Another pin from the lateral side in the supra-acetabular region is attached to the fixator. One pin is used in the distal femur and two in the tibia. The fixation is kept in place for 6 weeks to maintain knee and hip extension. Range of motion exercises are then begun to regain the knee motion in its new more functional arc (arc extending to full knee extension).

After the preparatory work described above, the femur is lengthened. The external fixator is placed from the pelvis to the femur to the tibia. The femur is lengthened up to 8 cm. The knee joint is distracted, but since no knee or hip hinges are used when the femur is so short, there is little need for physical therapy during this first lengthening. The goal of this first lengthening is to convert a type 3a femur to a type 2b femur. The rest of the treatment is for type 2b, with serial lengthenings and finally a pelvic support osteotomy combined with the final lengthening. Since the predicted discrepancy ranges between 30 and 40 cm, at least four lengthenings and an epiphysiodesis are required to equalize limb lengths.

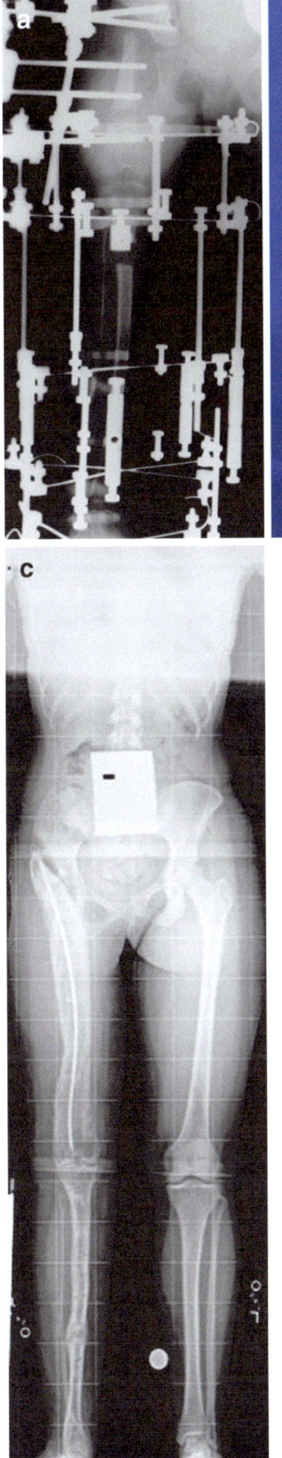

Fig. 13.12 CFD Paley type 3A in a patient whose parents refused a rotationplasty. She was treated at age 7 with a lengthening of the femur and tibia for a total of 12.5 cm (**a**). At age 10 she underwent the same treatment again and achieved another 12.5 cm of lengthening. At age 14 when she was skeletally mature, she underwent a pelvic support osteotomy together with a 10 cm femur lengthening (**b**). At age 18 she underwent her fourth femoral plus lengthening of 12.5 cm. She had a final tibial lengthening of 2.5 cm to correct the deformity and equalize her lengths (**c**). She has excellent clinical function

13.9.3.2 Prosthetic Reconstructive Surgery Approach to CFD with Diaphyseal Deficiency: Type 3

Prosthetic fitting is possible without any surgery. The difficulties with this approach are the FFD of the hip and knee and the need to put the foot in equinus. For better prosthetic fitting, a Syme's or Boyd amputation of the foot can be performed to create a residual limb that can more easily be fitted. Furthermore, surgical correction of the hip and knee flexion contractures, as described above, can also help with prosthetic fitting. In some cases, even a pelvic support osteotomy may be considered to decrease limp and stabilize the hip joint.

The other approach to PRS is with rotationplasty (Alman et al. 1995). Torode and Gillespie (1983) popularized the Van Nes rotationplasty for patients with CFD. They used a long oblique incision. The goal was to fuse the residual knee and rotate the limb 180° so that the foot is pointed backward and the ankle could function as a knee joint. This was most applicable to cases in which the ankle was already at the level of the opposite knee joint. Brown (2001) modified the rotationplasty approach using a racquet-like incision, performing the rotation between the femoral remnant and the pelvis. He then fused the femur to the lateral aspect of the ilium, thus converting the knee into a hip joint and the ankle into a knee joint. This provided improved hip stability over that provided by the Van Nes rotationplasty. One problem with the Brown method is excessive shortening of the hip muscles and lateralization of the hip and lower limb.

I modified the Brown technique by combining it with a Chiari osteotomy of the pelvis and fusing the femoral remnant to the cancellous roof of ilium (Figs. 13.13 and 13.14). I also don't remove any of the detached muscles and I take care to transfer all of them as distal as possible. I refer to this procedure as the Paley-Brown rotationplasty to distinguish it from the original published version. Furthermore, great care is taken to appropriately shorten the knee muscles so that they can function adequately as hip flexors and extensors. Finally, reattach the tensor fascia lata to the tibia to serve as a hip abductor. Because the knee in these patients is often contracted (as much as 90°), release the posterior. Decompress the peroneal nerve to prevent injury and allow greater rotation. Because the tibia in these patients typically has an internal rotation deformity, a supramalleolar osteotomy should also be performed to derotate the tibia and fibula. Although epiphysiodesis can be done at a second surgery, I prefer to achieve this with the same screws used for fixation of the femur to the pelvis (fig). The modified Brown rotationplasty provides very functional results with better hip function and stability than does the Van Nes rotationplasty.

13.10 Age Strategies

The majority of type 1 CFD cases require at least two lengthenings. As the expected discrepancy at skeletal maturity increases, the number of lengthenings required to equalize LLD increases. Generally, we prefer to perform the first lengthening when the patient is between the ages of 2 and 4 years. We have found that children between the ages of 4.5 and 6 or 7 years often are not at the optimal age psychologically to deal with limb lengthening. Their cognitive level is insufficient to understand why their parents allowed someone to do this to them, despite that they are beginning to be more independent and may appear to be mature enough to handle the process. The younger children do much better because their cognitive level accepts everything their parents decide without questioning it. Children at this age group seem to understand too little and too much at the same time. They don't connect their recognition that they have a short leg with the solution of limb lengthening. Beyond the age of 6 or 7 years, the child enters the age of reason and begins to understand that he or she is different from other children and that he or she has a problem for which there is a solution. They learn to accept the solution by reason rather than by faith. Their cooperation is voluntary rather than coerced. The amount of lengthening that can be performed in the femur at any one stage is usually between 5 and 8 cm. This lengthening amount seems to be independent on the initial length of the femur and age of the child. Generally, 5–8 cm can be performed safely in toddler (age 2–4 years), as well as in older chil-

Fig. 13.13 Paley modified Brown rotationplasty surgical technique. (**a**) Paley type 3 CFD with external rotation of the lower limb. Further rotation to achieve a rotationplasty requires about 135°. (**b**) The femoral artery and vein are preserved. The femoral, sciatic, peroneal and posterior tibial nerves are all decompressed. All of the muscles are disconnected distally. (**c**) The proximal femur is cut. A Chiari osteotomy is performed. (**d**) The Chiari is displaced medially. (**e**) Screws are used to fuse the femur to the pelvis and to epiphysiodesis the distal femoral physis. (**f**) After fixation the muscles are all reattached distally

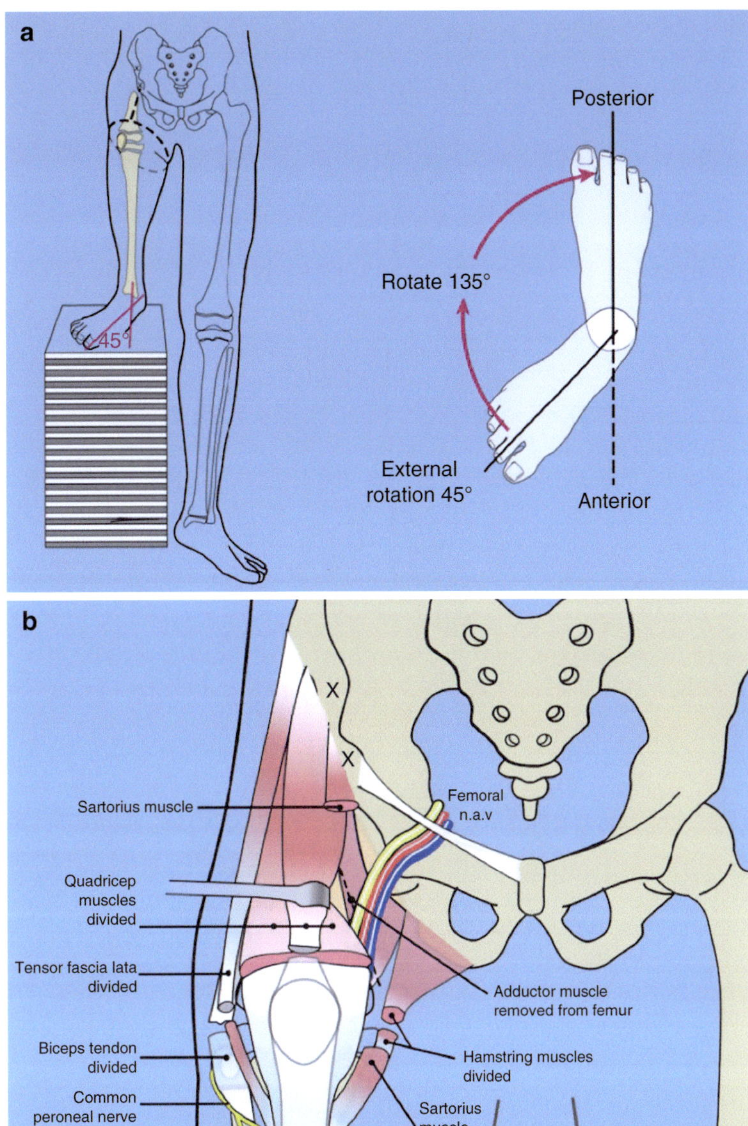

Fig. 13.13 (continued)

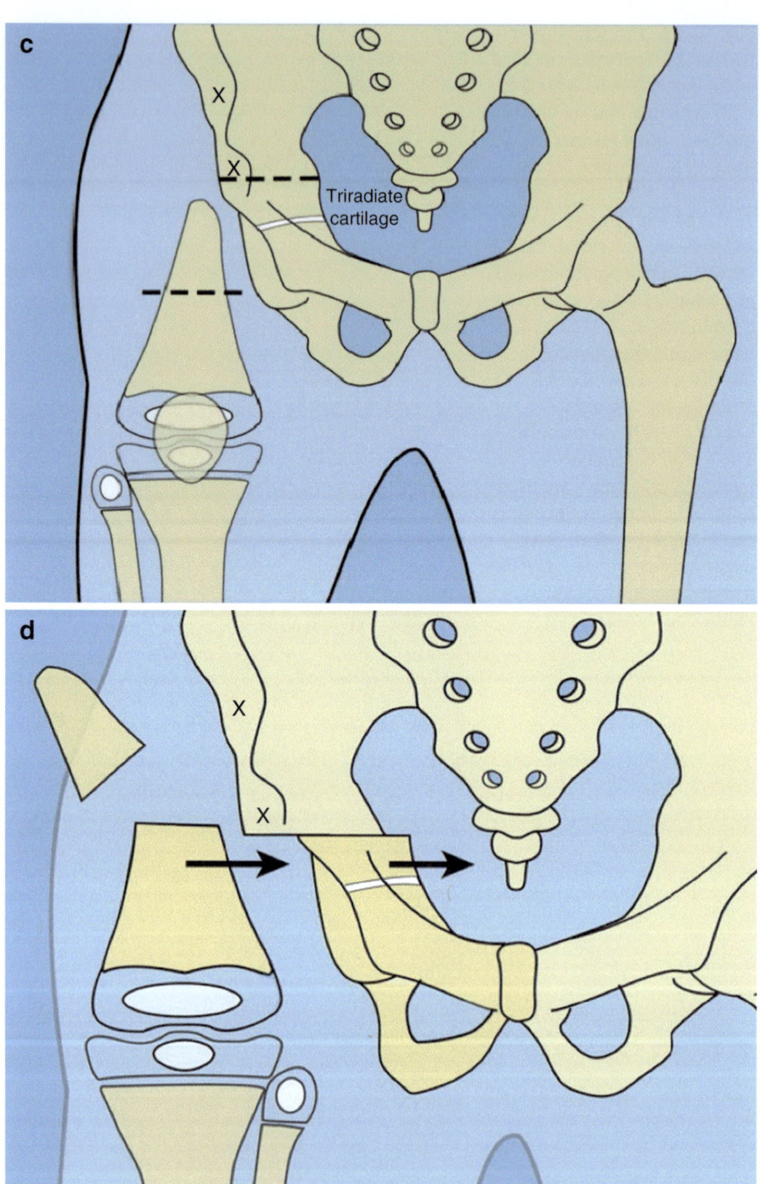

Fig. 13.13 (continued)

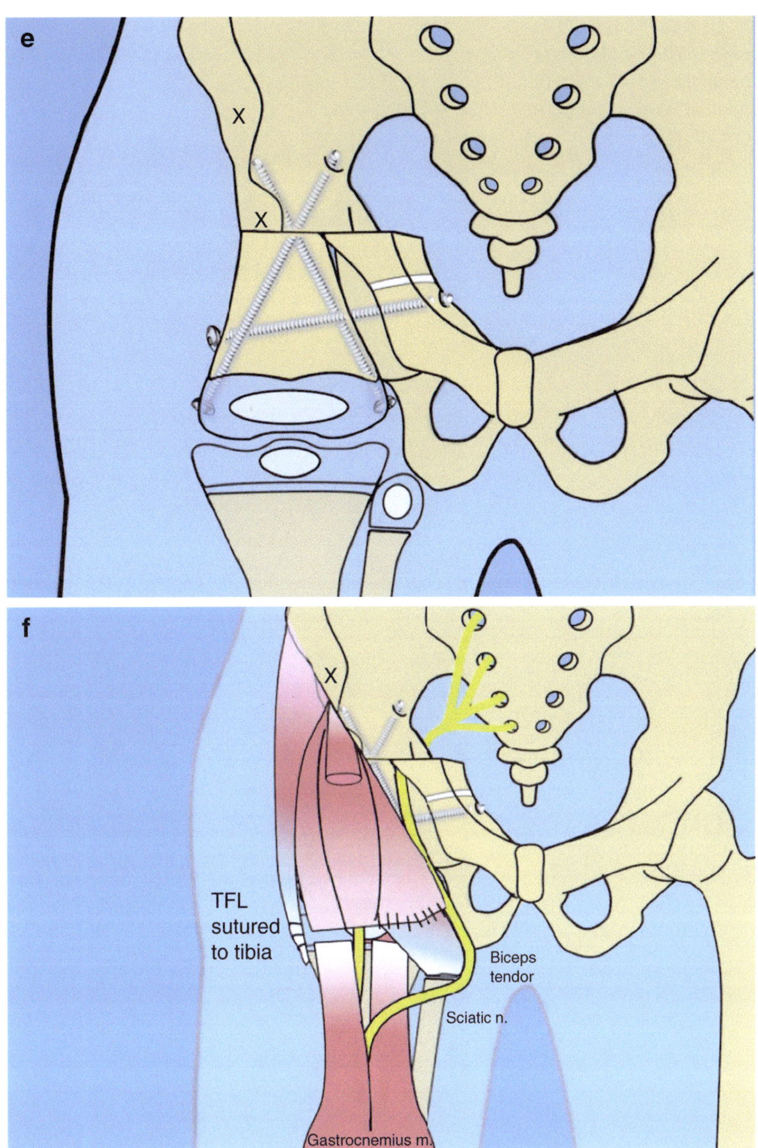

dren and adults. Combined femoral and tibial lengthenings allow greater total lengthening amounts. Tibial lengthening ≤5 cm can be combined with a 5 cm femoral lengthening. Lengthening of the femur in children younger than 6 years may be associated with sustained growth stimulation. By beginning lengthening at a young age, we are able to reduce one or more levels of prosthetic/orthotic need. This means going from a hip-knee-ankle-foot orthosis to an ankle-foot orthosis and shoe lift or from an ankle foot orthosis and shoe lift to a shoe lift only or from a shoe lift to no lift. The complication rate in this young age group is no higher than in older children, in our experience.

We have also lengthened adults (age 15–60 years) with CFD whose parents refused PRS for them when they were children. We were able to successfully equalize their leg lengths with one or two lengthenings, depending on the discrepancy (the most severe case underwent 25 cm of equalization with two LON treatments) (Fig. 13.11).

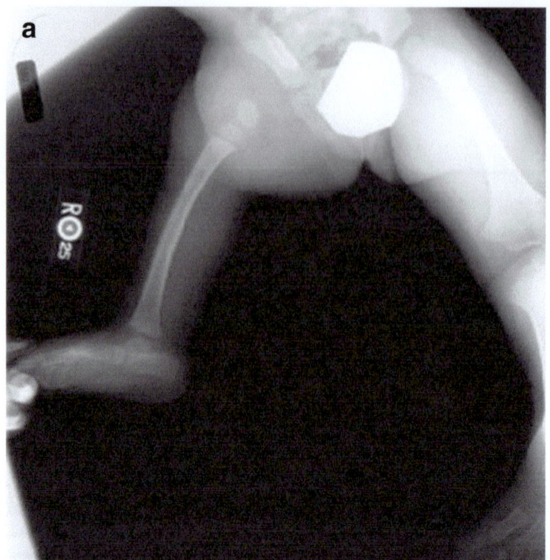

Fig. 13.14 X-ray of Paley type 3b CFD with fibular hemimelia (**a**). X-ray after rotationplasty age 4 (**b**) and age 10 (**c**)

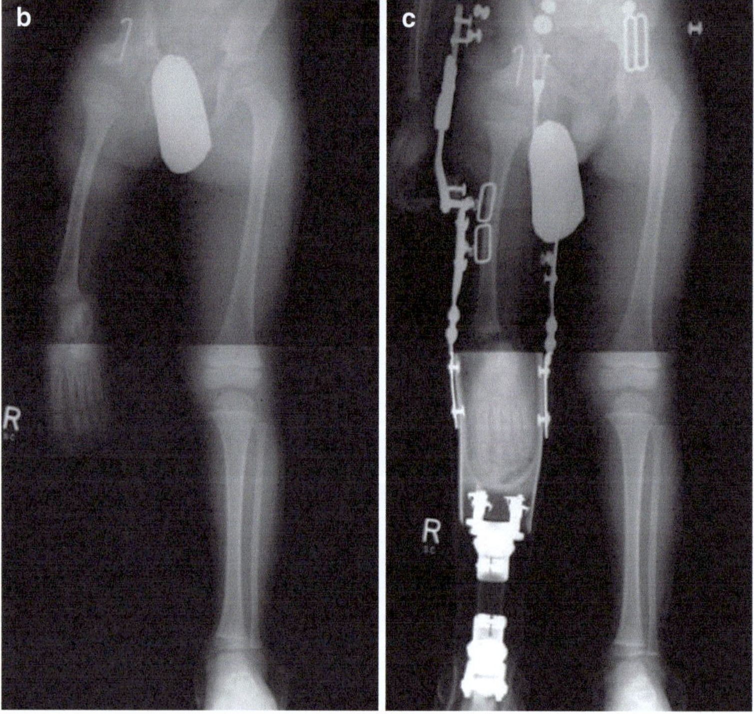

Therefore, adult CFD residua are not contraindications to treatment.

The frequency of lengthening should be spread out to no less than every 3 years and preferably every 4 years. The strategy of rule of 4 is a good guiding strategy. Assuming that a preparatory surgery is done between ages 2 and 3 years, the first lengthening can be done between ages 3 and 4 years. The second lengthening would occur around age 8 years and the final third lengthening around age 12 years. For psychosocial reasons it is preferable to complete all the lengthenings by age 14 when the child starts high school education. If a forth lengthening is required, it is done around age 16 years.

13.10.1 Role of Epiphysiodesis and Hemiepiphysiodesis

Epiphysiodesis is used as an adjuvant method to equalize limb length discrepancy. It should be calculated into the total strategy of equalization surgeries. Epiphysiodesis should be used for up to 5 cm of LLD equalization. Judicious use in some cases may avoid the need for one lengthening (e.g., predicted LLD = 12 cm; plan 7 cm lengthening before age 4 and 5 cm epiphysiodesis around puberty). Calculation of the timing of epiphysiodesis can be achieved quickly and accurately using the multiplier method (Paley et al. 2000).

Hemiepiphysiodesis is very useful to correct the valgus deformity of the knee from distal femoral or proximal tibial origins. I prefer to use the epiphysiodesis plate devices the concept of which was developed by Peter Stevens (Burghardt et al. 2008). Correction of the valgus deformity of the femur permits implantable lengthening of the femur since there is no angular deformity.

References

Alman BA, Krajbich JI, Hubbard S (1995) Proximal femoral focal deficiency: results of rotationplasty and Syme amputation. J Bone Joint Surg Am 77:1876–1882

Amirault JD, Cameron JC, MacIntosh DL, Marks P (1988) Chronic anterior cruciate ligament deficiency: long-term results of MacIntosh's lateral substitution reconstruction. J Bone Joint Surg Br 70:622–624

Brown KL (2001) Resection, rotationplasty, and femoro-pelvic arthrodesis in severe congenital femoral deficiency: a report of the surgical technique and three cases. J Bone Joint Surg Am 83:78–85

Burghardt RD, Herzenberg JE, Standard SC, Paley D (2008) Temporary hemiepiphyseal arrest using a screw and plate device to treat knee and ankle deformities in children: a preliminary report. J Child Orthop 2(3):187–197

Grammont PM, Latune D, Lammaire IP (1985) Treatment of subluxation and dislocation of the patella in the child: Elmslie technic with movable soft tissue pedicle (8 year review) [in German]. Orthopade 14:229–238

Grudziak JS, Ward WT (2001) Dega osteotomy for the treatment of congenital dysplasia of the hip. J Bone Joint Surg Am 83-A(6):845–854

Krackow KA, Thomas SC, Jones LC (1988) Ligament-tendon fixation: analysis of a new stitch and comparison with standard techniques. Orthopedics 11(6):909–917

Langenskiöld A, Ritsila V (1992) Congenital dislocation of the patella and its operative treatment. J Pediatr Orthop 12:315–323

Manner HM, Radler C, Ganger R, Grill F (2006) Dysplasia of the cruciate ligaments: radiographic assessment and classification. J Bone Joint Surg Am 88(1):130–137

Millis MB, Hall JE (1979) Transiliac lengthening of the lower extremity. A modified innominate osteotomy for the treatment of postural imbalance. J Bone Joint Surg 61A:1182

Nogueira MP, Paley D (2011) Prophylactic and therapeutic peroneal nerve decompression for deformity correction and lengthening. Oper Tech Orthop 21:180–183

Nogueira MP, Paley D, Bhave A, Herbert A, Nocente C, Herzenberg JE (2003) Nerve lesions associated with limb-lengthening. J Bone Joint Surg Am 85-A(8): 1502–1510

Paley D (1990) Problems, obstacles, and complications of limb lengthening by the Ilizarov technique. Clin Orthop Relat Res (250):81–104. Review

Paley D (1998) Lengthening reconstruction surgery for congenital femoral deficiency. In: Herring JA, Birch JG (eds) The child with a limb deficiency. AAOS, Rosemont, pp 113–132

Paley D (2005a) Chapter 12. Six -axis deformity analysis and correction. In: Principles of deformity correction, 1st edn. 2002. Corr. 3rd printing 2005. Springer, Heidelberg, Germany, pp 411–436

Paley D (2005b) Chapter 10. Lengthen consideration: gradual versus acute correction of deformities. In: Principles of deformity correction, 1st ed. 2002. Corr. 3rd printing 2005. Springer, Heidelberg, Germany, pp 269–289

Paley D (2005c) Chapter 3. Radiographic assessment of lower limb deformities. In: Principles of deformity correction, 1st edn. 2002. Corr. 3rd printing 2005. Springer, Heidelberg, Germany, pp 31–60

Paley D (2005d) Chapter 2. Malalignment and malorientation in the frontal plane. In: Principles of deformity correction, 1st edn. 2002. Corr. 3rd printing 2005. Springer, Heidelberg, Germany, pp 19–30

Paley D, Bhave A, Herzenberg JE, Bowen JR (2000) Multiplier method for predicting limb-length discrepancy. J Bone Joint Surg Am 82-A(10):1432–1446

Pappas AM (1983) Congenital abnormalities of the femur and related lower extremity malformations: classification and treatment. J Pediatr Orthop 3(1):45–60

Rozbruch SR, Paley D, Bhave A, Herzenberg JE (2005) Ilizarov hip reconstruction for the late sequelae of infantile hip infection. J Bone Joint Surg Am 87(5): 1007–1018

Salter RB (1978) The classic. Innominate osteotomy in the treatment of congenital dislocation and subluxation of the hip by Robert B. Salter, J. Bone Joint Surg. (Brit) 43B:3:518, 1961. Clin Orthop Relat Res (137):2–14

Sanpera I Jr, Sparks LT (1994) Proximal femoral focal deficiency: does a radiologic classification exist? J Pediatr Orthop 14:34–38

Suzuki S, Kasahara Y, Seto Y, Futami T, Furukawa K, Nishino Y (1994) Dislocation and subluxation during femoral lengthening. J Pediatr Orthop 14: 343–346

Torode IP, Gillespie R (1983) Rotationplasty of the lower limb for congenital defects of the femur. J Bone Joint Surg Br 65:569–573

Congenital Pseudarthrosis of the Tibia: Redefined (Congenital Crural Segmental Dysplasia)

14

Michael Weber

Contents

M. Weber, MD, PhD
Professor Weber's German Institute
of Orthopaedic Excellence, NMC- Healthcare-
International, Abu Dhabi, UAE

Faculty Member of RWTH-University, RWTH-
University-Aachen, Aachen, Germany
e-mail: weber.bone.lengthening@gmail.com

14.1   Introduction

Congenital pseudarthrosis of the tibia is a rare disorder with an incidence of 1 in 140,000 live births and associated with neurofibromatosis type 1 (NF-1) in 50 % of the cases (Andersen 1972; Baker et al. 1992; Camurati 1930; Hefti et al. 2000; Hendersen and Clegg 1941; Keret et al. 2000; Marie et al. 1997; Murray and Lovell 1982; Paget 1891; Peltier 1982; Pho et al. 1985).

14.2   Pathology

Our morphological investigations (light microscopy, transmission electron microscopy and immunohistochemistry) of the area of tibial pseudarthrosis revealed cells of neurogenic origin surrounding the vessels in the thickened periosteum comparable to those cells forming the neural myelin sheath (Fig. 14.1).

This phenomenon leads to a constriction of the vessels and reduction of the perfusion in periosteum and bone (Fig. 14.1). It results in a degenerative fibrosis of the periosteum giving rise to a vicious cycle and decreases the vascular perfusion of the bone. The consequence is fracture of the weakened bone and a subsequent nonunion (Boyd 1982; Camurati 1930; Hermanns et al. 1999; Hermanns-Sachweh et al. 2005; Morrissy 1982; Weber 2006). My theory is supported by a remarkable animal experiment of Wright and co-authors (Wright et al. 1991).

M. Kocaoğlu et al. (eds.), *Advanced Techniques in Limb Reconstruction Surgery*,
DOI 10.1007/978-3-642-55026-3_14, © Springer Berlin Heidelberg 2015

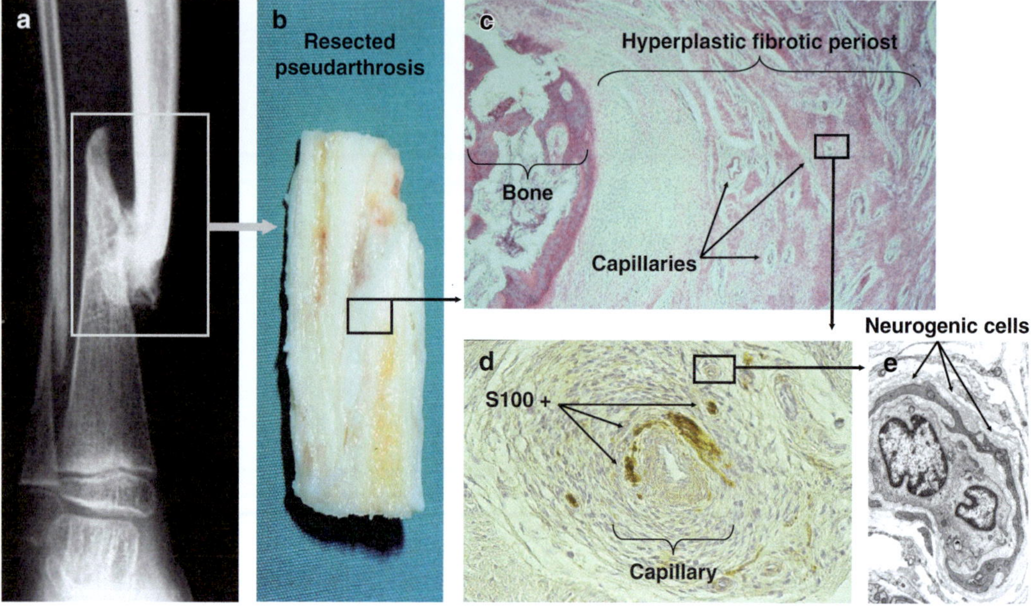

Fig. 14.1 Illustration of the pathological anatomy demonstrated for CCSD type Vb. (**a**) X-ray of tibial and fibular pseudarthrosis with sclerosis of more than 30 %. (**b**) Resected tibial pseudarthrosis. The rectangular field shows the area were specimen was taken out for histological examination. (**c**) Light microscopically hyperplastic fibrotic periosteum is evident. (**d**) Immunohistochemical staining (S-100) shows neurogenic cells surrounding the capillaries in the periosteum. (**e**) Electron microscopically the capillaries are obliterated by surrounding neurogenic cells (Hermanns et al. 1999 and 2005)

14.3 New Definition: Congenital Crural Segmental Dysplasia (CCSD)

The old term congenital pseudarthrosis of the tibia is wrong because:

- The pseudarthrosis of the tibia occurs in 90 % of all cases not until the first years of life (Andersen 1973; Hefti et al. 2000; Murray and Lovell 1982).
- The pseudarthrosis is not restricted to the tibia but affects in 60 % of all cases also the fibula.
- The fibula is affected alone with a pseudarthrosis in 19 % without affection of the tibia (Keret et al. 2000).
- Own researches on aetiology and pathogenesis provide an entirely new image view of this disease based on results of light microscopy, immunohistology and electron microscopy (Fig. 14.1) (Hermanns et al. 1999; Hermanns-Sachweh et al. 2005).

14.4 Clinical Evaluation

1. Postpartum without pseudarthrosis (90 %).
2. Postpartum with pseudarthrosis (10 %).
3. Forms 1 and 2 which have had unsuccessful prior surgery.
4. The diagnosis of CCSD should be considered in children who in the absence of trauma present with a fracture or nonunion or procurvatum and varus deformity of the lower leg, especially if the deformity is increasing.
5. The diagnosis is also supported by the presence of neurofibromatosis (incidence of 50 %).

14.4.1 Diagnostic Tools

The new own technique of radiological measurement of the extent of sclerosis, independent of different tibial lengths and magnification factor, and a method to determine the extent of resection ensures a successful healing process. Furthermore,

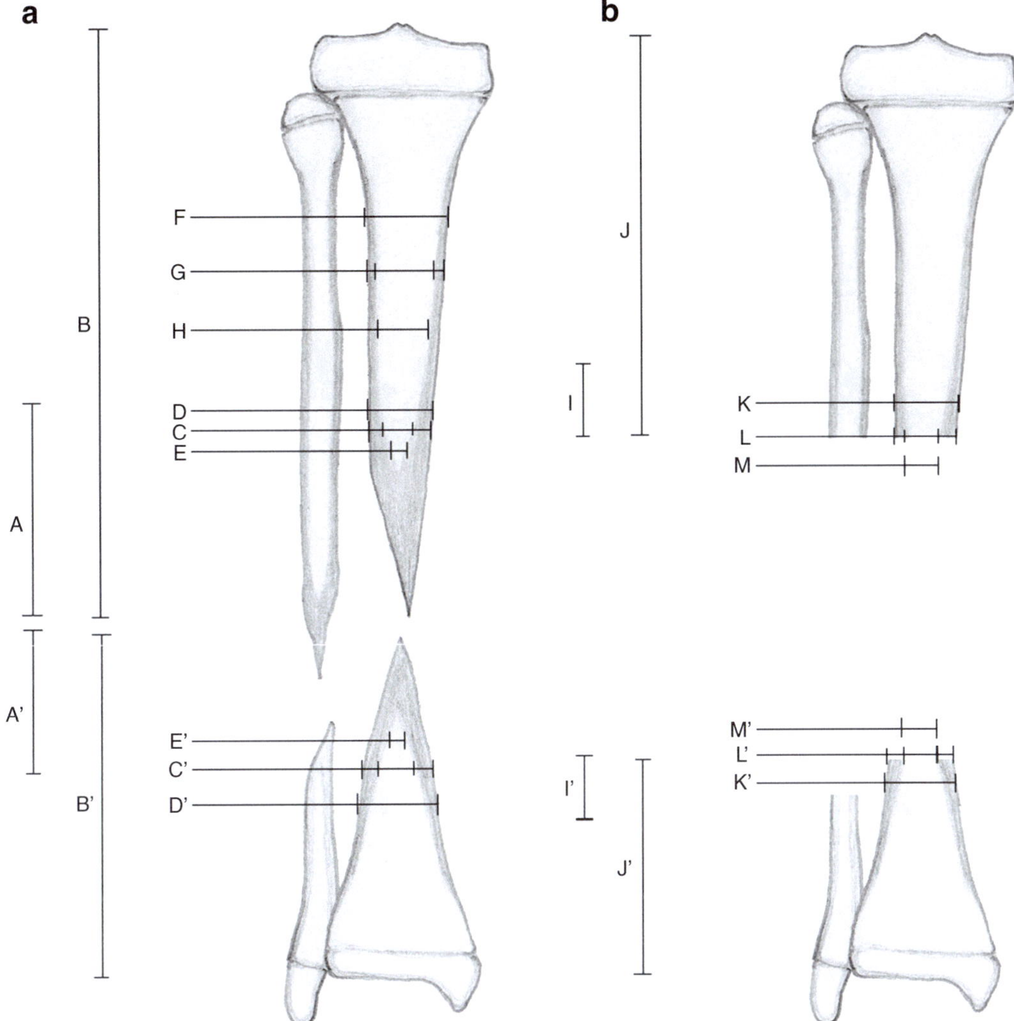

Fig. 14.2 (**a**) Illustration to the method for evaluation of the preoperative/postoperative extension of sclerosis. (*A*) Length of the diaphyseal sclerosis proximal of the pseudarthrosis. (*A'*) Length of the diaphyseal sclerosis distal from the pseudarthrosis. (*B*) Length of the tibia proximal of the pseudarthrosis. (*B'*) Length of the tibia distal of the pseudarthrosis. (*C*) Width of the cortical sclerosis at the level of the pseudarthrosis, proximal. (*C'*) Width of the cortical sclerosis at the level of the pseudarthrosis, distal. (*D*) Width of the tibial diaphysis at the level of the pseudarthrosis, proximal. (*D'*) Width of the tibial diaphysis at the level of the pseudarthrosis, distal. (*E*) Width of the medullary canal at the level of the pseudarthrosis, proximal. (*E'*) Width of the medullary canal at the level of the pseudarthrosis, distal. (*F*) Width of the diaphysis near the metaphysis, proximal. (*G*) Width of the cortical sclerosis near the metaphysis, proximal*. (*H*) Width of the medullary canal near the metaphysis, proximal. * The width of the cortex was measured when at this level sclerosis was no longer present. (**b**) Illustration to the method for evaluation of the postoperative extension of the sclerosis. (*I*) Length of the diaphyseal sclerosis proximal of the resection. (*I'*) Length of the diaphyseal sclerosis distal of the resection. (*J*) Length of the tibia proximal to the resection. (*J'*) Length of the tibia distal to the resection. (*K*) Width of the diaphysis at the level of resection, proximal. (*K'*) Width of the diaphysis at the level of resection, distal. (*L*) Width of the cortical sclerosis at the level of resection, proximal. (*L'*) Width of the cortical sclerosis at the level of the resection, distal. (*M*) Width of the medullary canal at the level of resection, proximal. (*M'*) Width of the medullary canal at the level of resection, distal

it allows to collect data pre- and postoperatively for comparison with own results and the results of other authors (Fig. 14.2) (Andersen 1972; Boyd 1982; Edvardsen 1973; Mahnken et al. 2001). Length extent of sclerosis (%)=length of sclerosis: length of bone × 100. Width extent of sclerosis

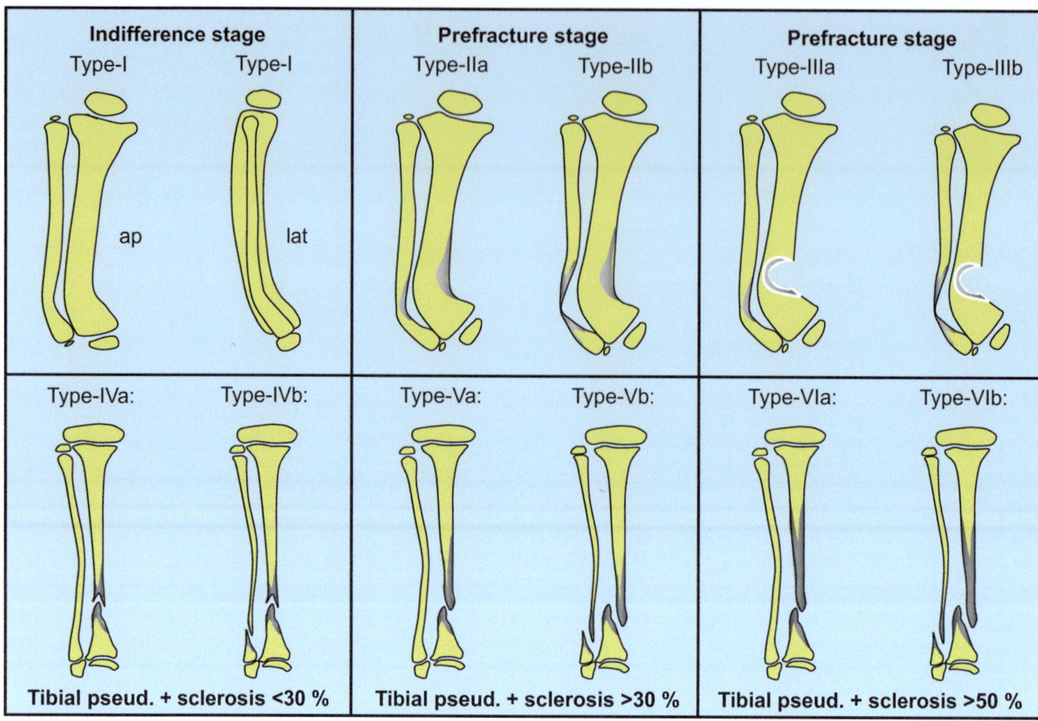

Fig. 14.3 Diagram of the different CCSD types according to Weber Classification (Weber 2006)

(%) = width of sclerosis: width of diaphysis × 100. In our clientele the resection of >90 % of the sclerotic bone ensures a healing rate of 93 %.

MRI: to detect the thickened periosteum and confirm the diagnosis. It is also useful in planning the extent of surgical resection of the lower leg segment (Mahnken et al. 2001).

14.4.2 Classification According to Weber (2006)

This new classification (Fig. 14.3) (Weber 2006) shows several advantages in comparison to older classifications (Andersen 1972, 1973; Boyd 1982; Boyd and Sage 1958; Crawford and Bagamery 1986):

- Severity of disease increases with the types.
- Relation to treatment and prognosis is given.
- Independence from time of diagnosis (any stage).
- Only X-rays are needed for classification.
- The important role of fibula is respected.

Type I is a stage of *indifference*.
It is characterised by the typical procurvatum-varus deformity of the lower leg without fracture or pseudarthrosis and without progression of the deformity.

Types II and III are the stages of *prefracture*.
It is characterised by impending fracture of increasing deformity in type II and cystic lesion in type III.

Types IV to VI describe the stages of *pseudoarthrosis* of the tibia.
The differences between types IV, V and VI are in the extent of the longitudinal sclerosis.

Subtypes of types II–VI
(a) Fibula without fracture.
(b) Fibula with fracture (different stages: persisting fibular fracture/pseudarthrosis with hypoplasia/dislocation of the lateral malleolus including a subluxation of the distal talofibular joint/increasing valgus deformity of the ankle).

14.4.3 Scoring

The score system (Weber 2006) (Tables 14.1 and 14.2) which leads to six different classes gives the advantage to compare different cases of different

Table 14.1 Classification and score system of CCSD

CCSD type			Score
I	Indifference stage, procurvatum-varus deformity without progress, no fractures		32
IIa	Prefracture stage, progressive deformity, no fibular fracture		29
IIb	Prefracture stage, progressive deformity, + fibular fracture		26
IIIa	Prefracture stage, cystic lesion, no fibular fracture		23
IIIb	Prefracture stage, cystic lesion, + fibular fracture		20
IVa	Tibial pseudarthrosis, sclerosis <30 %, no fibular fracture		17
IVb	Tibial pseudarthrosis, sclerosis <30 %, + fibular fracture		14
Va	Tibial pseudarthrosis, sclerosis between 30–50 %, no fibular fracture		11
Vb	Tibial pseudarthrosis, sclerosis between 30–50 %, + fibular fracture		8
VIa	Tibial pseudarthrosis, sclerosis >50 %, no fibular fracture		5
VIb	Tibial pseudarthrosis, sclerosis >50 %, + fibular fracture		2
Leg length discrepancy	0–20 %	In comparison to the healthy leg	2
	21–40 %		1
	>41 %		0
Contracture of the upper ankle joint	No		2
	Mild		1
	Severe		0
Contracture of the knee joint	No		2
	Mild		1
	Severe		0
Localisation of pseudarthrosis	Middle	Third of lower leg	4
	Middle-distal		2
	Distal		0
Deformity of the upper ankle joint	0–5°	In comparison to standard	2
	6–10°		1
	>11°		0
Osteoporosis	No		2
	Mild		1
	Severe		0
Number of preoperations	0		2
	1–4		1
	>4		0
Compliance of the child	Good		2
	Moderate		1
	Bad		0
Compliance of parents	Good		2
	Moderate		1
	Bad		0
Muscle function	Good		2
	Moderate		1
	Bad		0

authors according to their results of treatment due to evaluation of the main problems of the disease:

1. Different types of the Weber Classification (types I to VI = high to less points)
2. Extent of length deficiency
3. Amount of contractures at knee and ankle
4. Location of pseudarthrosis
5. Deformity of ankle joint
6. Extent of osteoporosis
7. Number of previous operations
8. Compliance of patient and parents
9. Muscle function

Table 14.2 Six different classes of CCSD according to the scores

Class	Score
6	0–9
5	10–18
4	19–27
3	28–36
2	37–45
1	46–54

Class 1 to 6 = good case to worst case

14.5 Treatment Options

14.5.1 Conservative Treatment

Conservative treatment is indicated only when there is no fracture and no progression of the deformity (**Type I**):

1. **Ankle-Foot Orthesis** = lower leg/foot orthotic device with isometrical hinges at upper ankle joint (indications: if the apex of the deformity is typically located in the middle to the distal third of the lower leg and no increase of deformity can be detected or fracture risk is low).
2. **Knee-Ankle-Foot Orthesis** = a knee-ankle-foot orthotic device with isometrical hinges at the knee and upper ankle joint (indications: if the deformity is located more proximally, if increasing deformity of lower leg can be detected and if increasing fracture risk is given).
3. Alternative therapeutic modalities such as pulsating electromagnetic fields (Basset et al. 1977; Basset and Schink-Ascani 1991; Crossett et al. 1989) have been used; however, their therapeutic success is not proven yet (Fern et al. 1990, Gordon et al. 1986).

14.5.2 Time of the Surgical Treatment

I disagree with a frequently expressed opinion that a surgery should not be performed before the end of puberty. The delay of surgical treatment until puberty leads to the development of significant problems as follows:

- Hypoplasia (foot, entire leg)
- Muscle atrophy
- Increasing leg length discrepancy
- Osteoporosis
- Contractures
- Dislocation of the lateral malleolus including
- Subluxation of the distal talofibular joint
- Increasing valgus deformity of the ankle

14.5.3 Surgical Techniques

Instruments
1. Image intensifier
2. Ring fixators
3. Weber-Cable Device
4. Intramedullary rods

In concordance with the results of the EPOS multicenter study, I prefer the use of ring fixators due to the best stability and variability (Grill et al. 2000).

According to our pathological-anatomical studies and my clinical experience, I recommend following principles of surgical treatment:

- Complete resection of pseudarthrosis.
- Complete resection of the affected periosteum.
- Complete resection of the sclerotic bone.
- Internal bone transport (cable technique) if resected bone is (approximately) > 3 cm in children and > 5 cm in adults.
- Acute docking and external callus distraction at metaphysis if resected bone is (approximately) < 3 cm in children and < 5 cm in adults.
- Correct the axis (after resection of sclerotic bone + pseudarthrosis).
- Do not use circulatory disturbing techniques.
- Autologous bone graft is useful (docking area).
- Callus distraction has additional favourite effects (correction of axis, lengthening, angio-neogenesis, osteoneogenesis).
- Intramedullary roding especially of the docking area reduces the risk of refracture after removal of fixator.

1. **CCSD Type IIa** (progressive deformity of the lower leg without fibular fracture despite conservative orthotic treatment. The principle of treatment is prevention of a fracture) (Figs. 14.4, 14.5 and 14.6)

    (a) Complete resection of the affected periosteum and transplantation of non-affected autologous periosteum with or without autologous and/or homologous bone graft of the tibia and fibula is performed (during

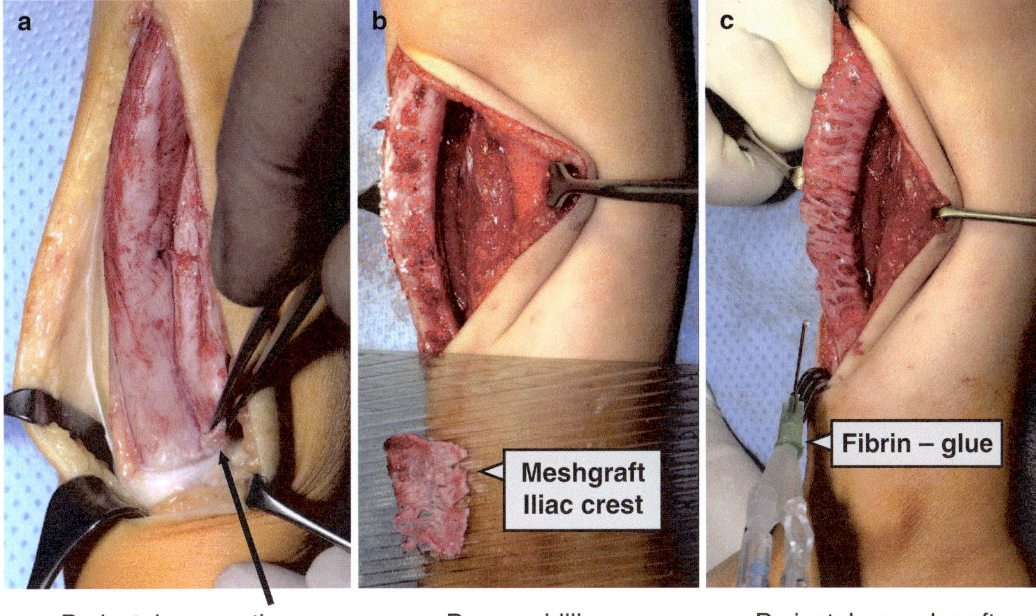

Fig. 14.4 One-year-old boy, score: 49, class: I, type IIa in Weber-classification. Resection of the pathological periosteum and substitution with autogenous meshed healthy periosteum. (**a**) Removal of hyperplastic perios-teum. (**b**) Drilling of bowed tibia. (**c**) Surrounding the bowed tibia with the mesh-grafted healthy periosteum and fixation with fibrin glue

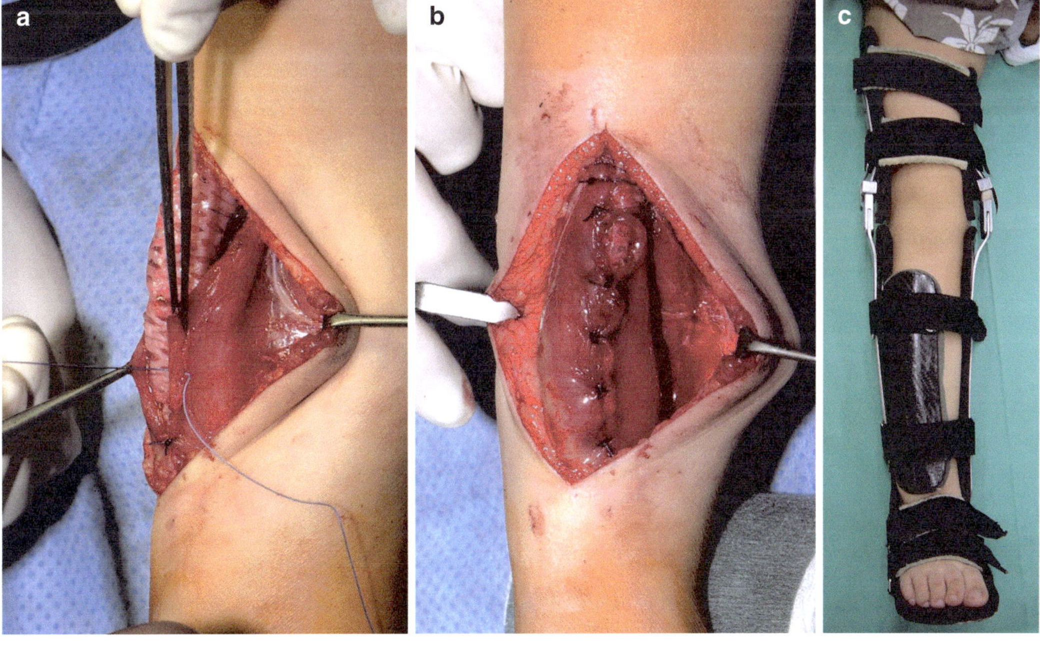

Fig. 14.5 (**a**, **b**) Covering of the periosteal graft with local muscle tissue. (**c**) Orthoprosthetic care; important is the support of the bowed area with counter-pressure by memory foam-covered shell

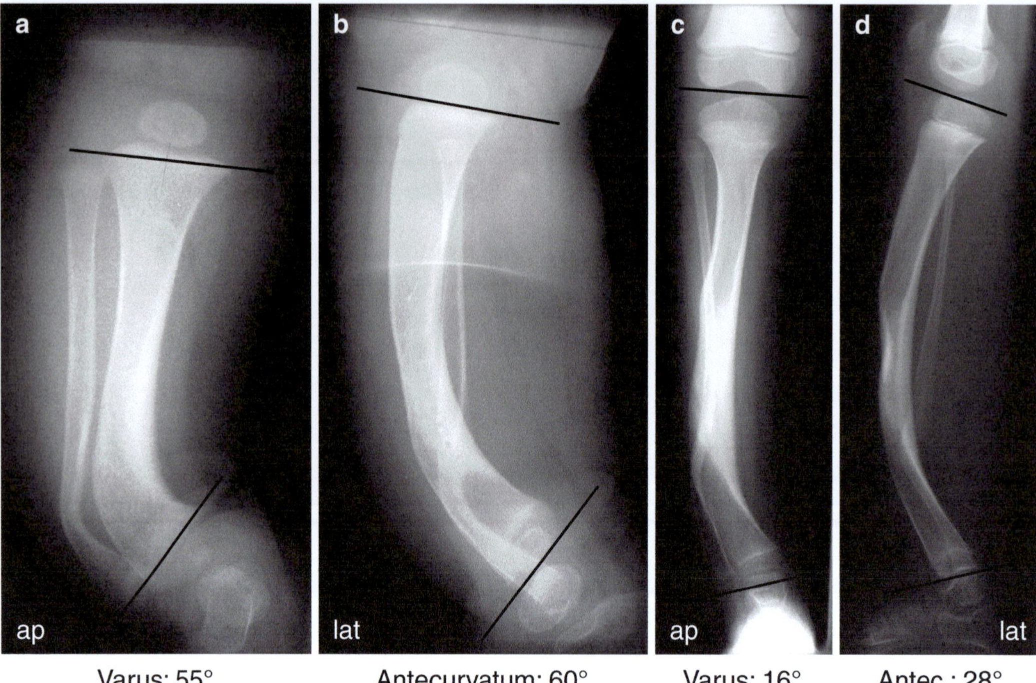

Fig. 14.6 (**a–d**) Radiologic course up to 4 years after the periosteal transplantation with enormous improvement of the deformity

this procedure the affected periosteum is resected in its entire circumference and longitudinal extension).

(b) The sclerotic bone is drilled with a diameter of 2 mm in multiple locations; the drilled bone is left in situ and if required additionally augmented with autologous and/or homologous bone graft (especially at concave part of bony deformity).

(c) The affected area will be enveloped with healthy meshed periosteum (from the contralateral iliac crest) and fixed with fibrin glue.

(d) If no sufficient size of periosteum is available to cover the bone completely, the concave side only of the procurvatum and varus deformity should be covered with the healthy periosteum (the best source of periosteal tissue is a contralateral iliac crest where simultaneously autologous bone graft is harvested).

(e) The periosteum is then covered with muscle and the skin is closed in layers.

(f) The child should avoid weight bearing without a brace at all times (during growth).

2. **CCSD Type IIb** (progressive deformity of the lower leg with fibular fracture despite a conservative orthotic treatment)

(a) The principle of the treatment is nearly identical with type IIa.

(b) The only difference is that the fibular fracture must be fixed to avoid a hypoplasia and dislocation of the lateral malleolus.

(c) Initially, the pathological (sclerotic) part of both fibular ends should be amply resected including the affected periosteum. If the fibula is very small, the sclerotic bone end can be left in situ but has to be treated with own special autologous bone graft wrapping technique (see below). Afterwards, two operative techniques can be applied:

I. The autograft or allograft bone is inserted for the augmentation of the fracture/pseudarthrosis. After

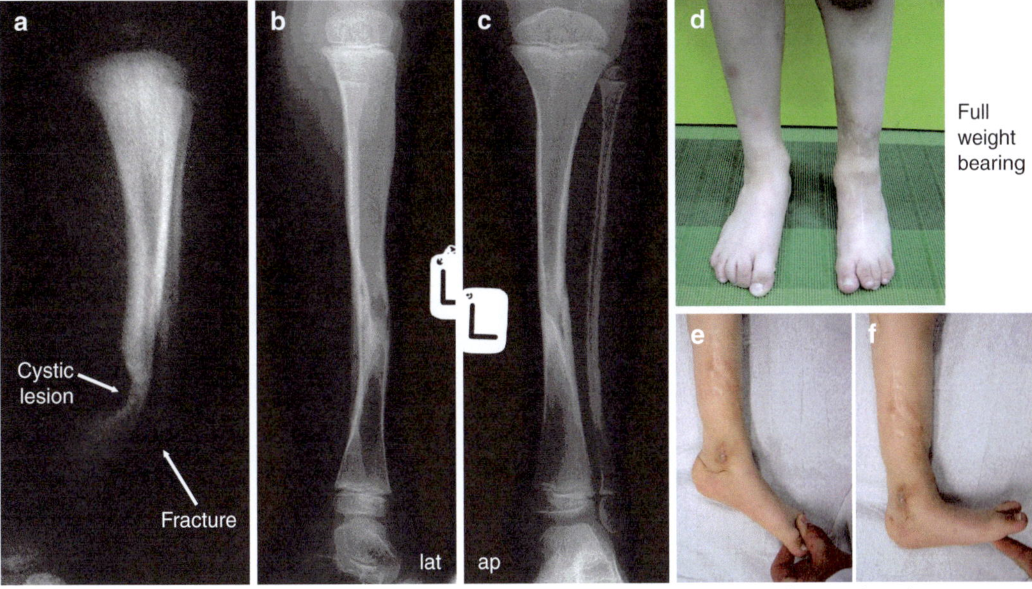

Fig. 14.7 Six-month-old boy; score: 30, class: III, type IIIb in Weber-classification. Clinical course of the type IIIb treatment with resection-osteosynthesis and proximal lengthening is shown. Primary operation of a 6-month-old boy. Operation technique (see Fig. 14.9). (**a**) X-ray, ap, showing the cystic lesion of tibia and the fractured fibula. (**b**, **c**) X-ray postoperatively with complete healing of docking area and remodelling of medullary canal. (**d**, **e**, **f**) Postoperative clinical pictures

that, bone graft and fibular ends are wrapped with a healthy periosteum. If the fibula is of sufficient size, a central intramedullary wire should be inserted through the fibular fragments. The author recommends using a unicortical graft with cancellous bone from the iliac crest (in this case the healthy periosteum is left in place attached to the bone originally).

II. Own wrapping technique: unicortical bone grafting (iliac crest) with multiple non-complete incisions at the cortical side with a saw enables the transplant to bend like a roll. The fibular fragments are wrapped by the bone transplant with the spongious part externally (Fig. 14.8). Fibular atrophy complicates the preparation of a conforming cylinder of a corresponding small radius. In this situation, several cortical-cancellous streaks are placed like planks of a barrel surrounding the position of augmentation. In this case, the periosteum can be left attached to the bone and the spongious part of the transplant should be attached to the fibula.

3. **CCSD Type IIIa** (prefracture stage with distinct cystic lesion without fibular fracture)
   (a) Resection of the cystic and entire sclerotic tibial segment.
   (b) Resection of the entire hyperplastic and fibrotic periosteum.
   (c) Internal bone transport using Weber-Cable Technique (see CCSD Type IVa) (Weber 1998, Weber et al. 1999) (Fig. 14.10).
   (d) DO NOT cut the intact fibula (increasing risk for nonunion).

4. **CCSD Type IIIb** (prefracture stage with distinct cystic lesion with fibular fracture) (Fig. 14.7)
   (a) Resection of the cystic and entire sclerotic segment.

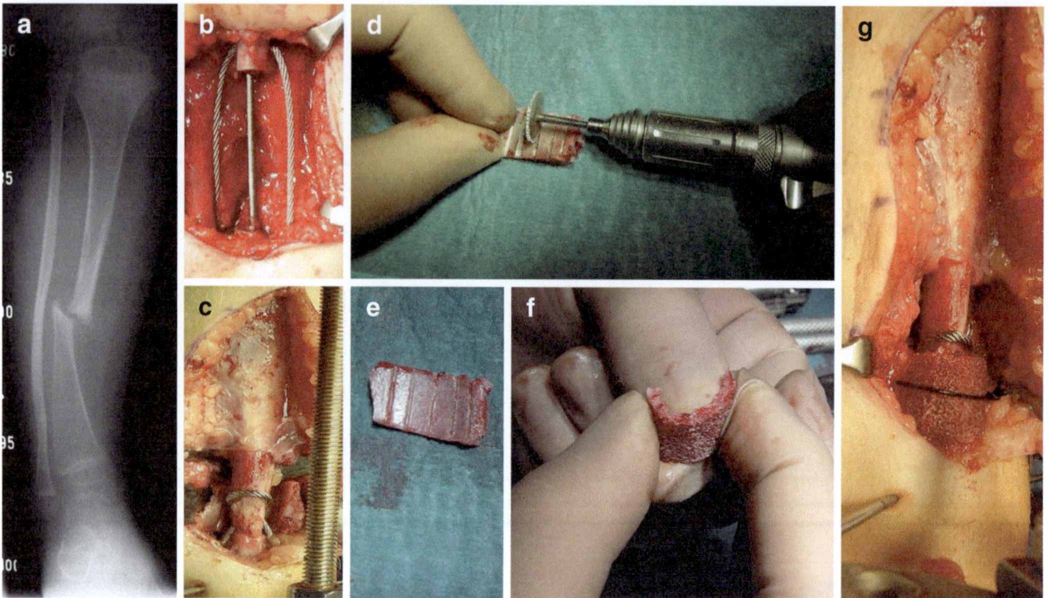

Fig. 14.8 Three-year-old boy; score: 35, class: III, type IVa in Weber-classification. Wrapping technique for the augmentation of the docking site following internal bone transport using the cable technique demonstrated at type IVa. (**a**) X-ray, ap: pseudarthrosis at mid to distal third of tibia. (**b**) Operative situs after resection of tibial pseudarthrosis, application of cable and insertion of intramedul- lary rod as preparation for internal bone transport. (**c**) Preparation of docking area for bone grafting. (**d**) Sawing of unicortical bone transplant from the iliac crest. (**e**, **f**) Prepared bone transplant can be bent around the finger. (**g**) The cortical part of bone graft is wrapped around the tibial docking area with the spongious part outside for better organisation

(b) Resection of the entire hyperplastic and fibrotic periosteum.

(c) Performing acute compression of the bone ends with autologous and/or homologous bone grafting (see wrapping technique) and a simultaneous proximal lengthening of the lower leg if the resected pseudarthrosis or bone segment is less than 30 % in children (about 5 cm) or less then 20 % in adults (about 3 cm).

Two Options

1. End-to-end osteosynthesis of refreshed bone ends with additionally fixation with Ilizarov wires intramedullary (Fig. 14.13).

2. Dowel technique with insertion of the sharpened proximal bone ends into the drilled medullary canal of distal bone ends (Fig. 14.9).

(d) Performing segmental bone transport using the Weber-Cable Technique (Fig. 14.10) (if more than 30 % of the length of the lower leg if the resected pseudarthrosis or bone segment is more than 30 % in children (about 5 cm) or more than 20 % in adults (about 3 cm).

(e) Fibular fracture has been treated as CCSD type IIb.

5. **CCSD Type IVa** (tibial pseudarthrosis and sclerosis with less than 30 % of tibial length without fibular pseudarthrosis) (Figs. 14.8 and 14.10)

(a) Resection of nonunion and entire sclerotic segment of both ends.

(b) Resection of the entire hyperplastic and fibrotic periosteum.

(c) Internal bone transport using Weber-Cable Technique (Weber 1998; Weber 2006; Weber et al. 1999).

(d) Fixation of the transport segment with the cable in a Bunnell-like technique inserted via two crossed but not reconvening drill holes with a loop over the bone to prevent a cut through. Leading

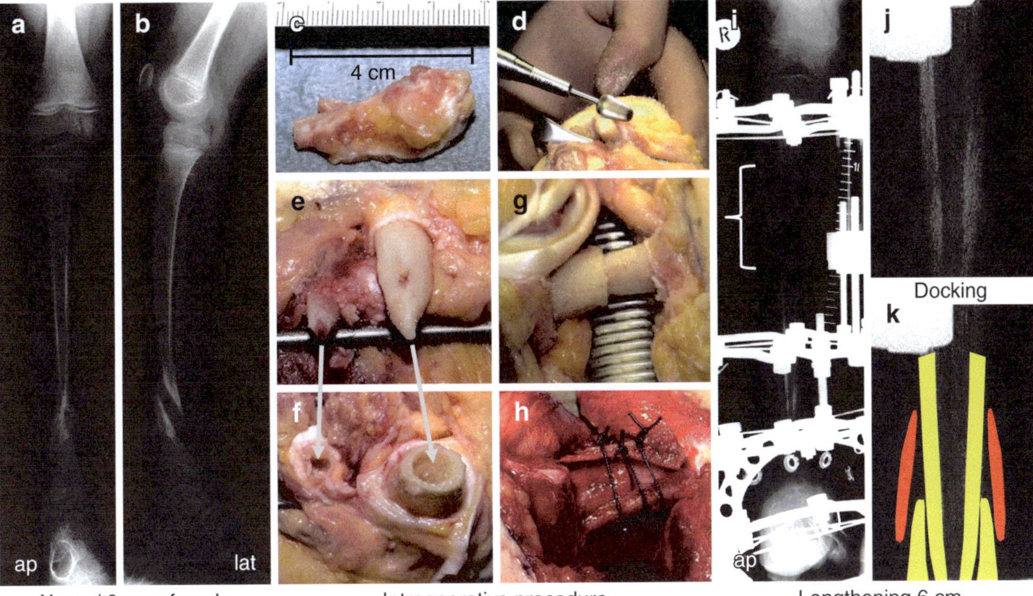

Fig. 14.9 Six-year-old girl; score: 25, class: IV, type IVb in Weber-classification. Technique of the performed resection-osteosynthesis with proximal lengthening, shown at type IVb. (**a**, **b**) X-ray of pseudarthrosis at tibia and fibula in the distal third of lower leg. (**c**–**h**) The dowel technique is demonstrated in its sequence: (**c**) resected pseudarthrosis, (**d**) piercing of the proximal ends of the resection with the air drill, (**e**–**g**) insertion of the pierced bone ends into the corresponding distal ends of the resection with the dowel technique and (**h**) wrapping technique of the docking site with cancellous bone facing the resected pseudarthrosis and spongious bone outside for better organisation. (**i**) X-ray after 6 cm lengthening. (**j**) Docking area postoperatively. (**k**) Schematic drawing of docking area with invaginated tibial bone ends (*yellow*) and bone transplant wrapped docking area (*red*)

out of the cables medially and laterally distally to the docking area through the soft tissue in alignment with the mid of the bone. Two intramedullary Ilizarov wires ensure a precise docking and can be left in place after removal of the fixator as internal splinting. The cables are routed over pulleys and attached to the distractors. Distraction frequency, distraction rate and distraction speed are applied as usual.

6. **CCSD Type IVb** (tibial pseudarthrosis and sclerosis with less than 30 % of tibial length with fibular pseudarthrosis) (Fig. 14.9).
   (a) Resection of sclerotic bone ends of both tibial and fibular nonunion.
   (b) Resection of the entire hyperplastic and fibrotic periosteum.
   (c) Osteosynthesis of both refreshed bone ends (acute docking).

   I. End-to-end technique: compression osteosynthesis combined with intramedullary stabilisation by two Ilizarov wires or rods (Baker et al. 1992).
   II. Dowel technique: inserting one fragment into the medullary cavity of the other fragment like solid internal splinting (Fig. 14.9). This can be combined with intramedullary roding also, if there is enough space (Fig. 14.13).
   (d) Simultaneous proximal lengthening of both tibia and fibula.

7. **CCSD Type Va** (tibial pseudarthrosis and sclerosis between 30–50 % of tibial length without fibular pseudarthrosis).
   The principle and procedure of the treatment are the same as described for CCSD type IVa (Figs. 14.8 and 14.10).

8. **CCSD Type Vb** (tibial pseudarthrosis and sclerosis between 30–50% of tibial length

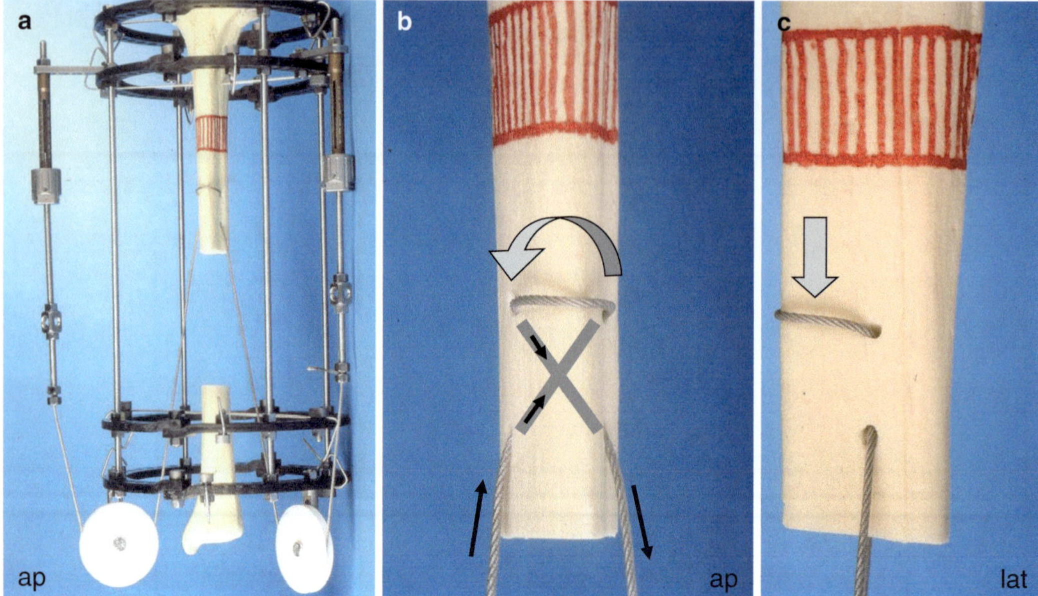

Fig. 14.10 Weber-Cable Technique applied at Ilizarov ring fixator demonstrated with a saw bone. (**a**) The cable is fixed at the distal bone end of the transport segment and led out in the median level of the distal tibial fragment distally of the docking area. The cable is guided to the pulleys and from the pulleys to the distractors. (**b**) The cable is inserted from one side of the crossed drill holes with a loop over the ventral half of the bone and led out to the other drill hole. Both drill holes should not meet inside the crossing. This can be prevented by leaving the first drill bit in the bone while drilling the second drill hole. (**c**) The lateral view of the Bunnell-like fixation of the transport segment shows the loop over the bone which prevents the cut through of the cable. For fixations like this only 2 cm of the bone is needed to be exposed

with fibular pseudarthrosis) (Figs. 14.11, 14.12 and 14.13).

(a) Resection of sclerotic bone ends of both tibial and fibular nonunion.

(b) Internal bone transport using Weber-Cable Technique (as in type IVa).

(c) Splinting the medullary canal with a K-wire (if possible).

(d) Bone grafting (wrapping technique) after docking of bone transport.

9. **CCSD Type VIa** (tibial pseudarthrosis and sclerosis with more than 50 % of tibial length without fibular pseudarthrosis).

Treatment procedure as described in CCSD type IVa.

10. **CCSD Type VIb** (tibial pseudarthrosis and sclerosis with more than 50 % of tibial length with fibular pseudarthrosis).

Treatment procedure as described in CCSD type IVb.

Technical Note

If pseudarthrosis of the distal tibia is very close to the ankle joint, the external fixator has to be extended to the foot for better stabilisation. A transfixation of the ankle joint by wires or rods is not necessary. This assembly can also been used to treat ankle joint contractures after consolidation of the docking area.

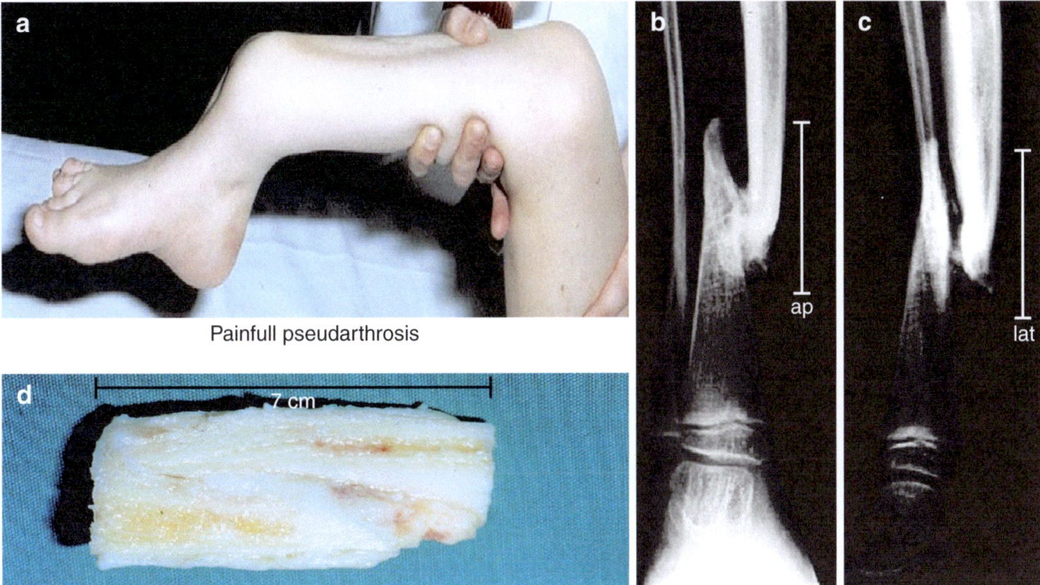

Fig. 14.11 Five-year-old boy; score: 20, class: IV, type Vb in Weber-classification. The resection distance of 7 cm requires a bone transport (see Fig. 14.10). (**a**) Painful pseudarthrosis. (**b, c**) X-rays of lower leg pseudarthrosis at distal third. Line: see amount of resection to remove all sclerotic bone. (**d**) See amount of resected tibial pseudarthrosis and sclerosis

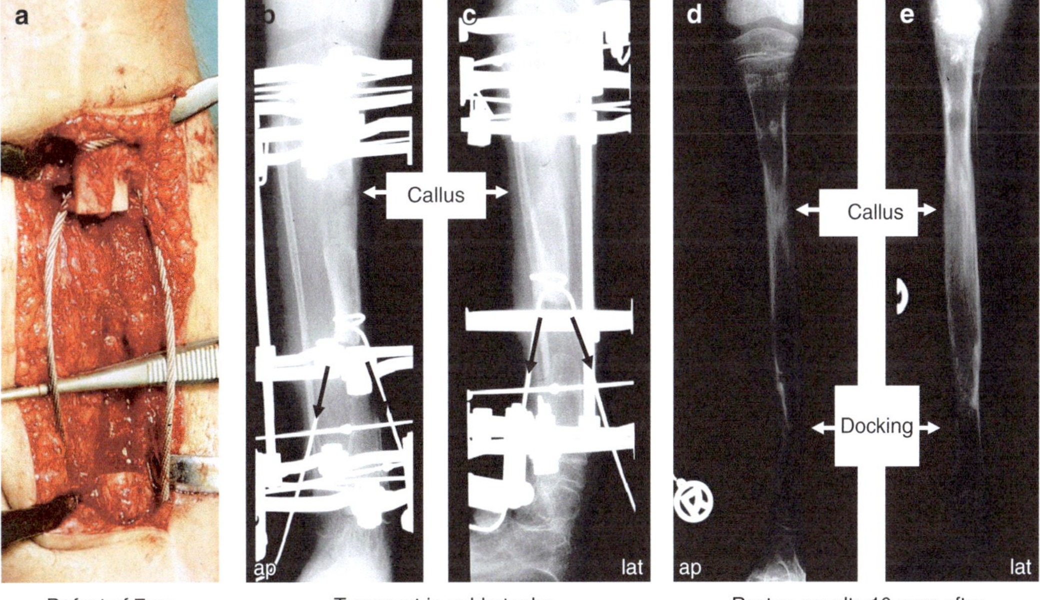

Fig. 14.12 Same patient as in Fig. 14.11. Intraoperative and postoperative photographs of the cable technique are demonstrated. (**a**) Operative situs after resection of the pseudarthrosis and sclerotic tibial bone and application of cable. Note only 2 cm of the bone end is needed for appli- cation of cable. (**b, c**) X-rays showing ongoing internal bone transport with Weber-Cable Technique. (**d, e**) X-rays 10 years after surgery. Note the recanalisation of the med- ullary canal as clear sign of healing of pseudarthrosis

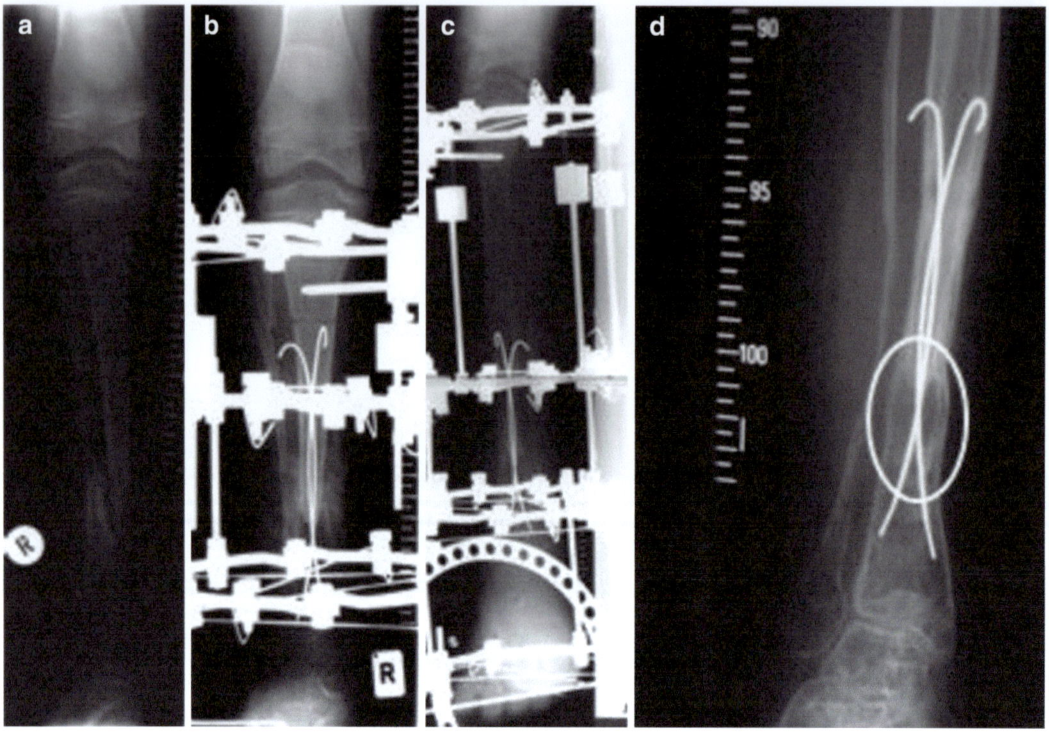

Preoperative | Before and after lengthening | Ilizarov wires in place after removal of fixator, circle = docking area

Fig. 14.13 Weber type IVb CCSD after resection-osteosynthesis in dowel technique and proximal lengthening. The intramedullary Ilizarov wire guidance of the docking site stabilises the tibia even after the removal of the fixator. The circle marks the docking site (dowel technique) with bone grafting. (**a**) X-ray preoperatively with sclerosis less than 30 % of tibial length in distal third. (**b**) Intraoperative X-ray showing acute docking after pseudarthrosis resection in dowel technique, intramedullary roding and corticotomy at proximal tibia and fibula. (**c**) X-ray after lengthening. (**d**) The intramedullary Ilizarov wires stays in place for protection of docking area after removal of fixator. Note recanalisation of docking area (*circle*) as clear sign of healing of pseudarthrosis

14.6 Treatment of Other Problems Seen with CCSD

A. **Valgus deformity of ankle joint** (Fig. 14.14a).
   (a) Growth disturbance of the lateral tibial epiphysis.
   (b) Fibular pseudarthrosis (shortening and atrophy of lateral malleolus).

   Treatment Options

   1. Temporary epiphysiodesis of the medial distal growth plate of the tibia until the normalisation of the wedge-shaped distal tibia epiphysis occurs.
   2. Dome osteotomy for acute correction of the joint line valgus deformity after completion of the growth (Fig. 14.14).
   3. Tibiofibular synostosis proximally to the growth plate for the stabilisation of the ankle joint if the fibular pseudarthrosis cannot be healed (Fig. 14.15).

B. **Contractures** originate due to immobilisation, bracing of the adjacent joint of the lower leg or usage of orthoprosthetics without hinges at the joints.

   Treatment Options

   Extension of the external fixator to the adjacent joint to treat a contracture.

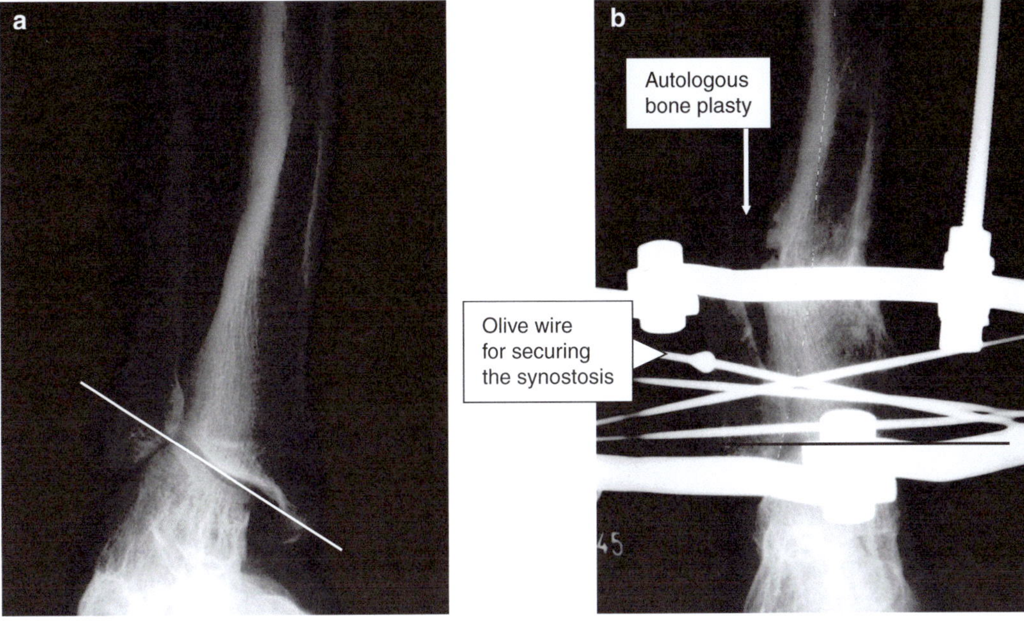

Fig. 14.14 Former CCSD type Vb after healing of pseudarthrosis: correction of typical valgus deformity at ankle joint by dome osteotomy. Stabilisation with ring fixator for simultaneous lengthening. (**a**) Ankle deformity with remaining fibular fracture. (**b**) Acute correction of deformity by dome osteotomy and performing tibiofibular synostosis

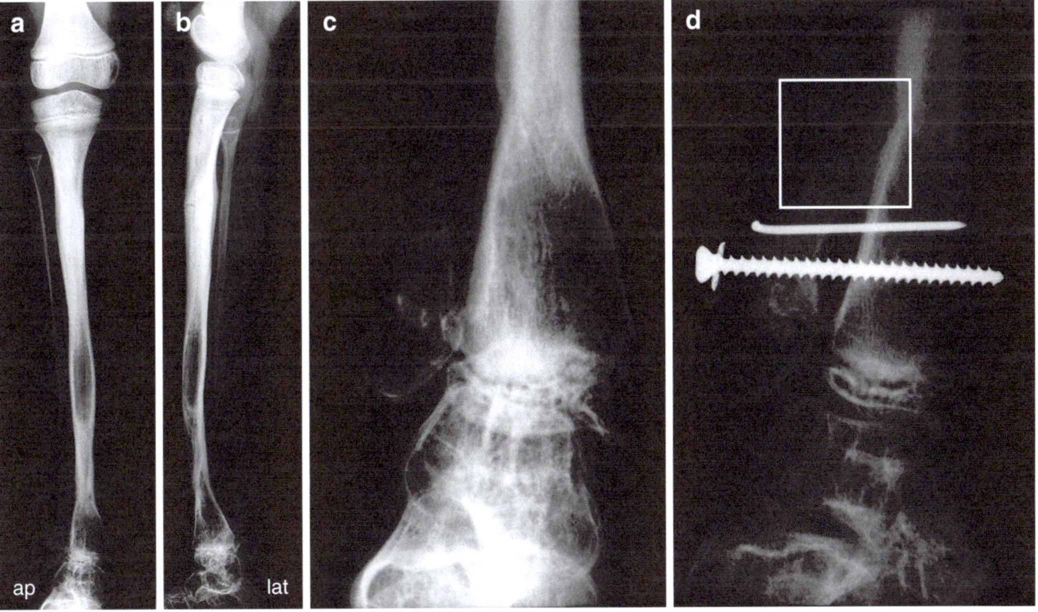

Fig. 14.15 Stabilisation of the ankle joint by tibiofibular synostosis demonstrated in former CCSD type IVb. (**a, b**) Successfully treated tibial pseudarthrosis. Note the recanalisation of medullary canal. Severe atrophy of the fibula is seen due to long-term fibular pseudarthrosis. (**c**) X-ray of the ankle joint shows the remnant of malleolus externus. (**d**) X-ray of tibiofibular synostosis. The frame shows the area of the bone grafting

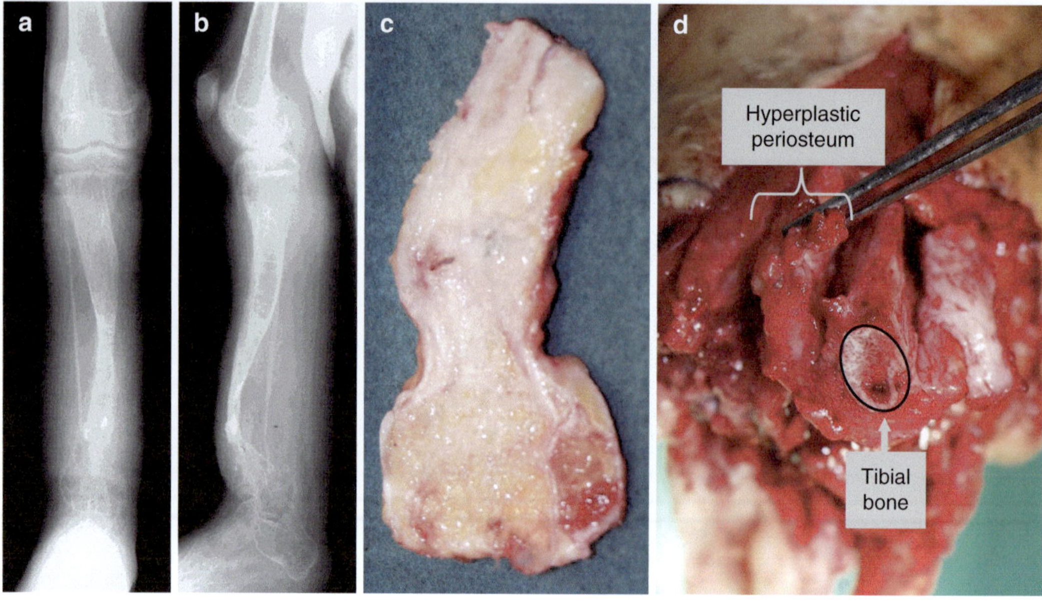

Fig. 14.16 CCSD type VIb, score: 5, class:VI in a 14-year-old, mentally retarded boy unsuccessfully treated 12 times alio loco. He spent 2 years in hospitals. Amputation was inevitable due to poor bone stock with severe osteoporosis, fusion of ankle joints, LLD of > 10cm and refusal of parents for further limb reconstruc-tion. (**a, b**) X-rays show the severe sclerosis (>50 %) and atrophy of tibia and fibula. (**c**) Resected distal lower leg with ankylosed ankle joint and severe osteomalacia. (**d**) The proximal tibial stump end shows the small calibre of bone in comparison to hyperplastic periosteum

C. **Reconstruction of lower leg is impossible due to poor bone stock**.

Treatment Options

The fibular transfer from the contralateral healthy leg should be preserved for those cases only where the internal bone transport is not possible due to lack of anatomical substance.

In cases of multiple unsuccessful surgeries, an amputation can be inevitable (Aitken and Frantz 1953; Andersen 1976a, b; Edvardsen 1973; McCarthy 1982; Tudisco et al. 2000; van Nes 1966). In such circumstances we prefer an amputation of lower leg with Weber Stump Plasty using neurovascular pedicled heel (Weber 2001, 2002) (Figs. 14.16, 14.17, 14.18 and 14.19). The advantages of this technique in comparison to conventional amputation are:

- No stump problems (no stump piercing)
- Axial lengthening of the stump by heel docking and further growth of the calcaneal apophysis
- Uneventful wound healing by vascular pedicled autologous transplant
- Full end bearing of the stump with physiological sensitivity and blood flow
- Uneventful prosthetic fitting
- Stump lengthening possible

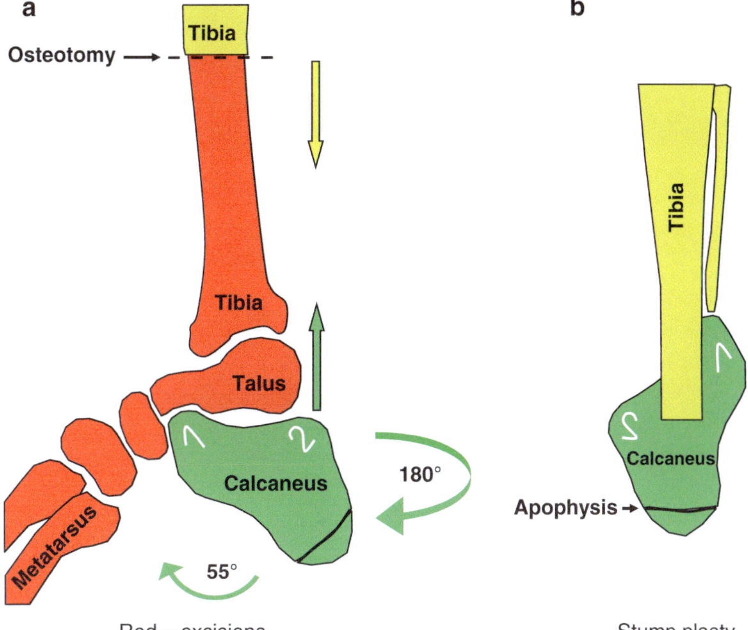

Fig. 14.17 Schematic drawing of Weber Stump Plasty (Weber 2001, 2002). (**a**) Red colour indicates the resected areas. The calcaneal bone (*green*) is turned 55° posteriorly, 180° of its longitudinal axis, and inserted with its Chopart joint area into the tibial bone end. (**b**) Result is a heel stump plasty with longitudinal alignment of apophyseal growth plate

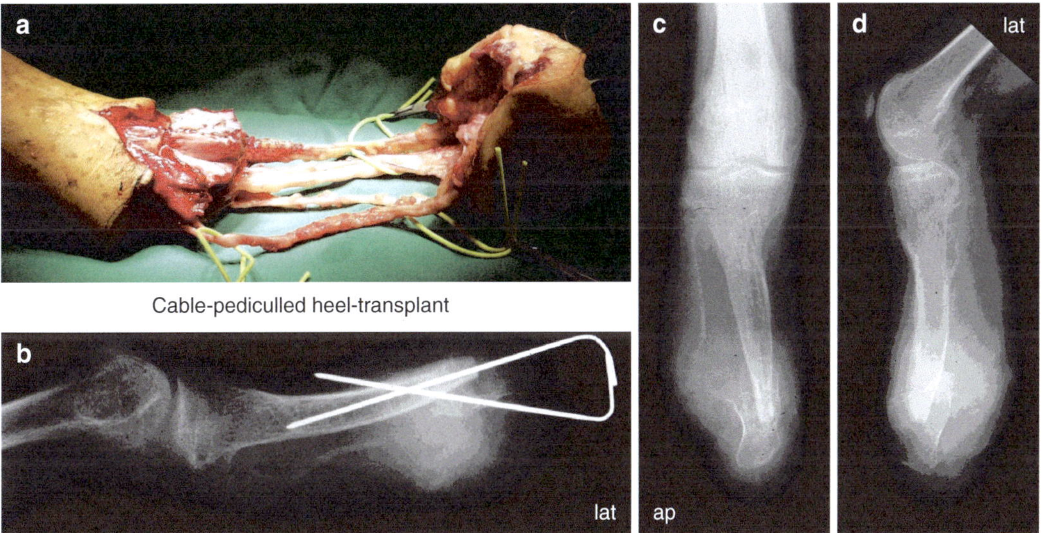

Fig. 14.18 CCSD type VIb same patient as Fig. 14.16. (**a**) Preparation of heel with the three neurovascular bundles. (**b**) X-ray shows the osteosynthesis of the heel to the tibia by two K-wires. (**c**, **d**) X-rays after consolidation of osteosynthesis and removal of K-wires

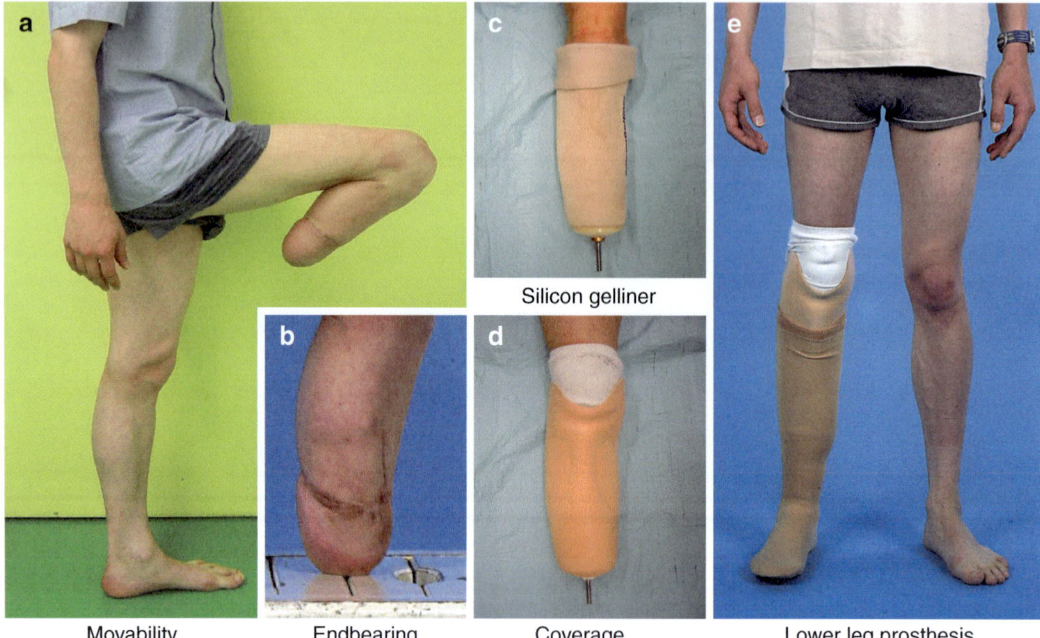

Fig. 14.19 Clinical outcome of other case. (**a**) Full ROM of knee joint. (**b**) Unproblematic full end bearing of stump plasty without protection. (**c, d**) Prosthetic fitting in Botta techniques with silicon inliner. (**e**) With the applied prosthesis the patient is able to play soccer as a goal keeper in the league

14.7 Complications

1. Lymphedema and disturbance of blood supply, persistent soft tissue bulging due to too much acute compression (not respecting the recommendation of performing an internal bone transport if more than 30 % in children and 20 % in adults are resected of the lower leg) or the consistence of the soft tissue envelope (scars) is not put into consideration.
2. Refracture (resection of pseudarthrosis and/or sclerotic bone has to complete like a tumour resection. Insufficient resections are related with healing disturbance and refracturing).
3. In fibular transfer a high rate of embolisation of micro anastomoses, fibular fracture as well as valgus deformity of ankle joint and lateral instability of knee joint at the Donor site has to be expected. It has to be considered also that the transplanted fibula has to be lengthened (multiple times) for achieving leg length equality. In case of no fully transformation of fibula to the size of a tibia a live long bracing of the leg is needed.

References

Aitken GT, Frantz CH (1953) The juvenile amputee. J Bone Joint Surg Am 35-A:659–664

Andersen KS (1972) Congenital angulation of the lower leg and congenital pseudarthrosis of the tibia in Denmark. Acta Orthop Scand 43:539–549

Andersen KS (1973) Radiological classification of congenital pseudarthrosis of the tibia. Acta Orthop Scand 44:719–727

Andersen KS (1976a) Congenital pseudarthrosis of the leg. Late results. J Bone Joint Surg Am 58:657–662

Andersen KS (1976b) Congenital pseudarthrosis of the tibia and neurofibromatosis. Acta Orthop Scand 47:108–111

Baker JK, Cain TE, Tullos HS (1992) Intramedullary fixation for congenital pseudarthrosis of the tibia. J Bone Joint Surg Am 74:169–178

Bassett CAL, Pilla AA, Pawluk RJ (1977) A non-operative salvage of surgically-resistant pseudarthroses and non-unions by pulsing electromagnetic fields - A preliminary report. Clin Orthop 124:128–142

Bassett CAL, Schink-Ascani M (1991) Long-term pulsed electromagnetic field (PEMF) results in congenital pseudarthrosis. Calcif Tissue Int 49:216–220

Boyd HB (1982) Pathology and natural history of congenital pseudarthrosis of the tibia. Clin Orthop Relat Res 166:5–13

Boyd HB, Sage FP (1958) Congenital pseudarthrosis of the tibia. J Bone Joint Surg Am 40-A:1245–1270

Camurati M (1930) Les pseudartrosi congenite della Tibia. Chir Organi Mov 15:1–162

Crawford AH Jr, Bagamery N (1986) Osseous manifestations of neurofibromatosis in childhood. J Pediatr Orthop 6:72–88

Crossett LS, Beaty JH, Betz RA, Warner W, Clancy M, Steel HH (1989) Congenital pseudarthrosis of the tibia-Long-term follow-up study. Clin Orthop 245: 16–18

Edvardsen P (1973) Resection osteosynthesis and Boyd amputation for congenital pseudarthrosis of the tibia. J Bone Joint Surg Br 55:179–182

Fern ED, Stockley L, Bell MJ (1990) Extending intramedullary rods in congenital pseudarthrosis of the tibia. J Bone Joint Surg (Br) 72-B:1073–1075

Gordon L, Weulker N, Jergesen H (1986) Vascularized fibular grafting for the treatment of congenital pseudarthrosis of the tibia. Orthopedics 9:825–830

Grill F, Bollini G, Dungl P, Fixsen J, Hefti F, Ippolito E, Romanus B, Tudisco C, Wientroub S (2000) Treatment approaches for congenital pseudarthrosis of tibia: results of the EPOS multicenter study. European Paediatric Orthopaedic Society (EPOS). J Pediatr Orthop B 9:75–89

Hefti F, Bollini G, Dungl P, Fixsen J, Grill F, Ippolito E, Romanus B, Tudisco C, Wientroub S (2000) Congenital pseudarthrosis of the tibia: history, etiology, classification, and epidemiologic data. J Pediatr Orthop B 9:11–15

Hendersen M, Clegg R (1941) Pseudarthrosis of the tibia: report of a case. Proc Staff Meetings Mayo Clin 16: 769–774

Hermanns B, Senderek J, Wilke M, Weber M (1999) Periostal proliferations in bone lesions of congenital pseudarthrosis of the tibia have morphological features of Neurofibromatosis type-I. Pathol Res Pract 195:266

Hermanns-Sachweh B, Senderek J, Alfer J, Klosterhalfen B, Buttner R, Fuzesi L, Weber M (2005) Vascular changes in the periosteum of congenital pseudarthrosis of the tibia. Pathol Res Pract 201:305–312. doi:10.1016/j.prp.2004.09.013

Keret D, Bollini G, Dungl P, Fixsen J, Grill F, Hefti F, Ippolito E, Romanus B, Tudisco C, Wientroub S (2000) The fibula in congenital pseudoarthrosis of the tibia: the EPOS multicenter study. European Paediatric Orthopaedic Society (EPOS). J Pediatr Orthop B 9:69–74

Mahnken AH, Staatz G, Hermanns B, Gunther RW, Weber M (2001) Congenital pseudarthrosis of the tibia in pediatric patients: MR imaging. Am J Roentgenol 177:1025–1029. doi:10.2214/ajr.177.5.1771025

Marie PJ, de Pollak C, Chanson P, Lomri A (1997) Increased proliferation of osteoblastic cells expressing the activating Gs alpha mutation in monostotic and polyostotic fibrous dysplasia. Am J Pathol 150: 1059–1069

McCarthy RE (1982) Amputation for congenital pseudarthrosis of the tibia. Indications and techniques. Clin Orthop Relat Res 166:58–61

Morrissy RT (1982) Congenital pseudarthrosis of the tibia. Factors that affect results. Clin Orthop Relat Res 166:21–27

Murray HH, Lovell WW (1982) Congenital pseudarthrosis of the tibia. A long-term follow-up study. Clin Orthop Relat Res 166:14–20

Paget J (1891) Studies of old case books. Longman's Green and Company, London

Peltier L (1982) Vorwort zu Paget (1891) s. dort. Clin Orthop Relat Res 166:2

Pho RW, Levack B, Satku K, Patradul A (1985) Free vascularised fibular graft in the treatment of congenital pseudarthrosis of the tibia. J Bone Joint Surg Br 67: 64–70

Tudisco C, Bollini G, Dungl P, Fixen J, Grill F, Hefti F, Romanus B, Wientroub S (2000) Functional results at the end of skeletal growth in 30 patients affected by congenital pseudoarthrosis of the tibia. J Pediatr Orthop B 9:94–102

van Nes CP (1966) Congenital pseudarthrosis of the leg. J Bone Joint Surg Am 48:1467–1483

Weber M (1998) Segment transport des Knochens mittels Kabelrollen und flexiblem Draht - Eine neue Technik am Ringfixateur. Med Orth Tech 118:134–140

Weber M (2001) Eine neue Technik der Stumpfkappenplastik am Unterschenkel. Orthop Tech 4: 240–246

Weber M (2002) Neurovascular calcaneo-cutaneus pedicle graft for stump capping in congenital pseudarthrosis of the tibia: preliminary report of a new technique. J Pediatr Orthop B 11:47–52

Weber M (2006) Congenital leg deformities: congenital pseudarthrosis of tibia – congenital crural segmental dysplasia – redefined. In: Rozbruch SR, Ilizarov S, (eds) Limb lengthening and reconstruction surgery. Informa Healthcare, New York. pp 485–493

Wright J, Dormans J, Rang M (1991) Pseudarthrosis of the rabbit tibia: a model for congenital pseudarthrosis? J Pediatr Orthop 11:277–283

Weber M, Siebert CH, Heller KD, Birnbaum K, Kaufmann A (1999) Segmental transport utilizing cable wires and pulleys mounted on an Ilizarov frame –A new technique. J Bone Joint Surg (Suppl.) 81-B:148

Michael Weber

Contents

M. Weber, MD, PhD
Weber's German Institute of Orthopaedic Excellence,
NMC-Healthcare-International,
Electra Street, Abu Dhabi, UAE

RWTH-University, RWTH-University-Aachen,
Pauwelsstrasse, Aachen, Germany
e-mail: weber.bone.lengthening@gmail.com

15.1 Introduction

Tibial hemimelia is described as 'longitudinal reduction deficiency of tibia' with a variety of deformities at hip, femur, patella, tibia, fibula and foot. It has an incidence of 1/1,000,000 per live birth (Brown 1971; Weber et al. 2005). A wide range of treatment options is suggested, from conservative approach with orthotics to bone and soft tissue (re)constructive surgeries and amputation (Weber 2007). In this chapter, diagnostic approach, classification and (re)constructive surgery options are summarized. The main topic of this chapter focus on 'constructive surgical techniques' which includes motoric replacement techniques, callus distraction and my own new techniques of 'transformation surgery' and 'booster surgery'.

- Transformation surgery means the use of biological resources (anatomical structures) to create better functions. Once an anatomical structure has been transformed to a different function, automatically, this structure develops the form it needs accordingly (form follows function).

M. Kocaoğlu et al. (eds.), *Advanced Techniques in Limb Reconstruction Surgery*,
DOI 10.1007/978-3-642-55026-3_15, © Springer Berlin Heidelberg 2015

- The booster surgery means the enhancement of sleeping growth potentials of the cartilaginous anlage. In the literature, the cartilaginous anlage is not well recognized – it is a remnant of the tibial growth disturbance, which can be used to construct the missing tibial parts and the joints for five different types (IIIa, IVa, Va, VIa and VIIa).

15.2 Indications

Indications for conservative, surgical or amputating approaches are determined according mainly to the need of the patient and/or parents or guardians. The surgeon has to discuss all treatment options with the patient, parents or guardians, according to the following:

- Conservative treatment with orthesis and orthoprosthesis
- Surgical techniques that improve the use of orthesis and orthoprothesis
- Constructive surgery
- Amputation

The patients, parents and guardians should be informed of all steps, including possibilities of repetitive surgeries and possible complications in a neutral manner. If parents insist on a definitive solution with minimum surgery, amputations and prosthetic fitting are the preferred methods. Patients and parents have to be advised that amputation is not the conclusive solution and end of therapy, but, in contrast, the start of a lifelong deal of prosthetic fitting and adjustments which can require additional surgeries in case of stump complications. For bilateral cases, amputating approaches should be done cautiously as the energy consumption of the gait is much higher compared with unilateral amputation.

- The medical advice given to the patient/parents/guardians should start as early as possible to commence the best recommendable and suitable treatment option. Hence, the sooner the treatment starts, the better the functional outcome and clinical results can be expected. Especially in constructive surgery, the early treatment ensures a good biological response according to 'form follows function'.

Detailed indications will be discussed under surgical techniques of each type according to Weber classification (Fig. 15.1, Tables 15.1 and 15.2; Weber 2008).

15.3 Examination, Imaging and Classification

Tibial hemimelia was previously classified according to bony structure and X-rays (Jones et al. 1978; Kalamchi and Dawe 1985). However, tibial hemimelia is a combined malformation of soft tissue, cartilage, bone and joints with leg and foot deformities, leg shortening, joint contractures and muscle and joint dysfunction. For this reason, I suggested a more comprehensive classification and score, where the tibial defects are detected more precisely, the pathological anatomical terms are used correctly, the whole leg and its function is included, a scientific comparison of the treatment outcome of different types and results from different authors is possible and, consequently, a recommendation for therapeutic options is given (Fig. 15.1, Tables 15.1 and 15.2; Weber 2008).

Examination of the patient should include the complete leg (coxa-femur-patella-tibia-fibula-pes) obviously with specific importance of the tibia and the muscle function at the different leg levels. The condition is characterized mainly by knee and ankle deformities. Usually, a global instability of the knee and/or ankle with contracture is present, depending which joint is affected by tibial aplasia or agenesia. The fibula is usually nearly normal developed but can be hypoplastic, dysplastic or bowed. The fibular head is located proximally and dorsally to the femoral condyle in proximal tibial aplasia's (types I; IVa, b; Va, b; VIa, b and VIIa, b). The lateral malleolus is distally and dorsally positioned to the talus in distal tibial aplasias (types I; II; IIIa, b; Va, b; VIa, b; and VIIa, b). In biterminal tibial aplasias and tibial agenesis (types Va, b; VIa, b; and VIIa, b), the fibula shows an over length proximally and distally with dorsalization. In distal tibial aplasias the foot is positioned in varus (types: II; IIIa, b; Va, b; and VIIa, b), with or without equinus deformity. So more distinct the tibial aplasia, so more the deformity occurs. In tibial agenesia the deformities are the most. The foot can show adductus, supinatus and excavatus deformities as well as malformations in form of polydactyly, double foot, hypoplasia, aplasia, agenesis of

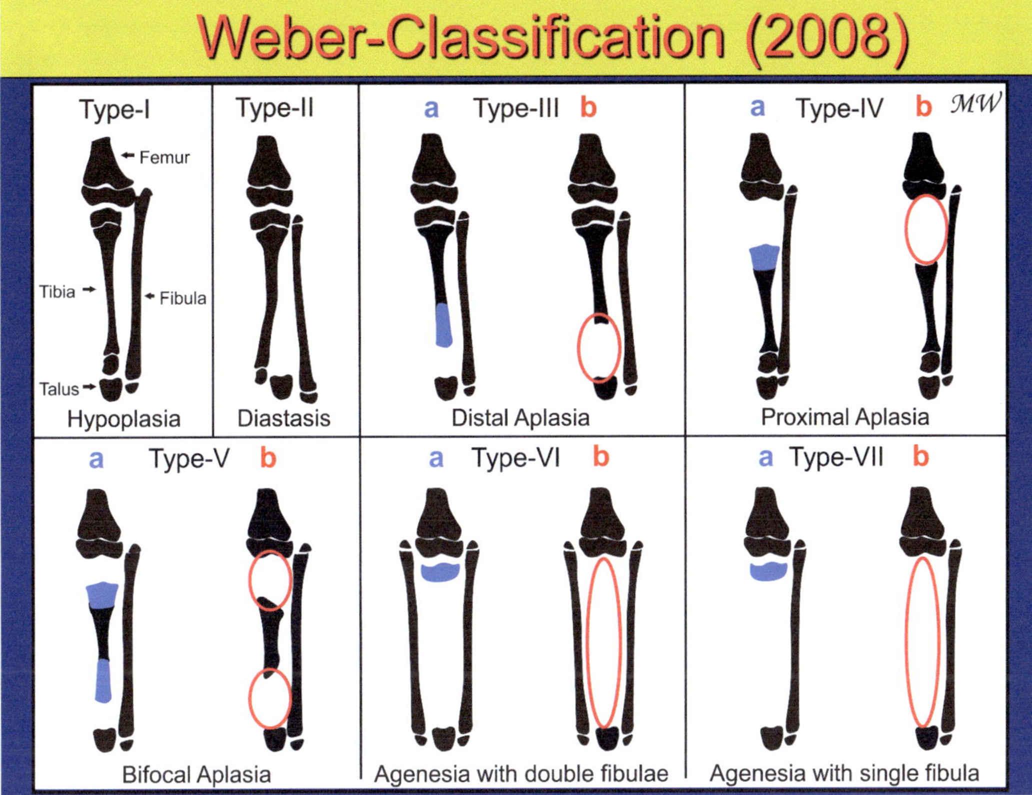

Fig. 15.1 Weber classification of tibial reduction defects in seven types and five subgroups (a=with cartilaginous anlage, b=without cartilaginous anlage) according to the severity of the malformation. *Black*=bone, *blue*=cartilaginous anlage and *red circle*=tibial defect without cartilaginous anlage. The figure represents a higher maturation level of the lower leg instead of the situation immediately after birth because of the possibility to give more detailed illustrations

digits and rays, synchondrosis and synostosis of the calcaneus and talus.

Precise diagnosis can be made using X-rays, CT scan, sonography and especially MRI. The intraoperative diagnostic of the anatomical structures, especially the course of tendons, is important for functional improvement. The patella (important for transformative knee arthroplasty) can be detected by ultrasound and MRI. The presence of a cartilaginous anlage, important for joint construction, can be detected by MRI; the use of gadolinium contrast in combination with MRI is useful. The muscle function and power as well as the amount of joint contractures should be detected at each joint level for planning of the surgical procedure (Tables 15.1 and 15.2).

- Custom-made analysis is important and means to use modern techniques (ultrasound, MRI, etc.), precise examinations and the intraopera-

tive view for analysing the biological resources, important for constructive surgery.

15.4 Procedures

This chapter is focused on constructive surgical techniques of the limb with motoric replacement, callus distraction, transformation and booster surgery rather than amputation and orthotic treatment methods. Each subgroup of the Weber classification (Weber 2008, Fig. 15.1) has its own treatment strategies which are explained below. The principle of the surgical procedure is to increase the function and the length of the affected leg and foot:

- Motoric replacement techniques are used to align tendon structures to their proper insertions.

Table 15.1 Score system with classification of tibial reduction defect of the leg

<table>
<tr><th colspan="9" align="center"><u>Score</u></th></tr>
<tr><td colspan="9">Name:</td></tr>
<tr><td>Anatomic region</td><td>Type</td><td>Sceletal defect</td><td>Score</td><td>X</td><td>Muscle-function</td><td>Type</td><td>Score</td><td>X</td></tr>
<tr><td>Coxa</td><td></td><td></td><td></td><td></td><td>(Hip)</td><td></td><td></td><td></td></tr>
<tr><td>co</td><td>I</td><td>Normal</td><td>2</td><td></td><td>Existent</td><td>+</td><td>2</td><td></td></tr>
<tr><td>co</td><td>II</td><td>Dysplasia</td><td>1</td><td></td><td>Partly absent</td><td>(+)</td><td>1</td><td></td></tr>
<tr><td>co</td><td>III</td><td>Subluxation</td><td>0</td><td></td><td>Absent</td><td>–</td><td>0</td><td></td></tr>
<tr><td>Femur</td><td></td><td></td><td></td><td></td><td>(Quadriceps/knee)</td><td></td><td></td><td></td></tr>
<tr><td>fe</td><td>I</td><td>Normal</td><td>2</td><td></td><td>Existent</td><td>+</td><td>2</td><td></td></tr>
<tr><td>fe</td><td>II</td><td>Distal hypoplasia</td><td>1</td><td></td><td>Partly absent</td><td>(+)</td><td>1</td><td></td></tr>
<tr><td>fe</td><td>III</td><td>Distal dysplasia</td><td>0</td><td></td><td>Absent</td><td>–</td><td>0</td><td></td></tr>
<tr><td>Patella</td><td></td><td></td><td></td><td></td><td></td><td></td><td></td><td></td></tr>
<tr><td>pa</td><td>I</td><td>Normal</td><td>3</td><td></td><td></td><td></td><td></td><td></td></tr>
<tr><td>pa</td><td>II</td><td>Dysplasia</td><td>1</td><td></td><td></td><td></td><td></td><td></td></tr>
<tr><td>pa</td><td>III</td><td>Agenesis</td><td>0</td><td></td><td></td><td></td><td></td><td></td></tr>
<tr><td>Tibia</td><td></td><td></td><td></td><td></td><td>(Foot/lower leg)</td><td></td><td></td><td></td></tr>
<tr><td>ti</td><td>**I**</td><td>**Hypoplasia**</td><td>22</td><td></td><td>Existent</td><td>+</td><td>2</td><td></td></tr>
<tr><td>ti</td><td>**II**</td><td>**Diastasis**</td><td>20</td><td></td><td>Partly absent</td><td>(+)</td><td>1</td><td></td></tr>
<tr><td>ti</td><td>**III**</td><td>**Distal aplasia**</td><td></td><td></td><td>Absent</td><td>–</td><td>0</td><td></td></tr>
<tr><td>ti</td><td>a</td><td><u>With</u> Cartilaginous anlage</td><td>18</td><td></td><td></td><td></td><td></td><td></td></tr>
<tr><td>ti</td><td>b</td><td><u>Without</u> Cartilaginous anlage</td><td>8</td><td></td><td></td><td></td><td></td><td></td></tr>
<tr><td>ti</td><td>**IV**</td><td>**Proximal aplasia**</td><td></td><td></td><td></td><td></td><td></td><td></td></tr>
<tr><td>ti</td><td>a</td><td><u>With</u> Cartilaginous anlage</td><td>16</td><td></td><td></td><td></td><td></td><td></td></tr>
<tr><td>ti</td><td>b</td><td><u>Without</u> Cartilaginous anlage</td><td>6</td><td></td><td></td><td></td><td></td><td></td></tr>
<tr><td>ti</td><td>**V**</td><td>**Biterminal aplasia**</td><td></td><td></td><td></td><td></td><td></td><td></td></tr>
<tr><td>ti</td><td>a</td><td><u>With</u> Cartilaginous anlage</td><td>14</td><td></td><td></td><td></td><td></td><td></td></tr>
<tr><td>ti</td><td>b</td><td><u>Without</u> Cartilaginous anlage</td><td>4</td><td></td><td></td><td></td><td></td><td></td></tr>
<tr><td>ti</td><td>**VI**</td><td>**Agenesis with double fibula**</td><td></td><td></td><td></td><td></td><td></td><td></td></tr>
<tr><td>ti</td><td>a</td><td><u>With</u> Cartilaginous anlage</td><td>12</td><td></td><td></td><td></td><td></td><td></td></tr>
<tr><td>ti</td><td>b</td><td><u>Without</u> Cartilaginous anlage</td><td>2</td><td></td><td></td><td></td><td></td><td></td></tr>
<tr><td>ti</td><td>**VII**</td><td>**Agenesis with single fibula**</td><td></td><td></td><td></td><td></td><td></td><td></td></tr>
<tr><td>ti</td><td>a</td><td><u>With</u> Cartilaginous anlage</td><td>10</td><td></td><td></td><td></td><td></td><td></td></tr>
<tr><td>ti</td><td>b</td><td><u>Without</u> Cartilaginous anlage</td><td>0</td><td></td><td></td><td></td><td></td><td></td></tr>
<tr><td>Fibula</td><td></td><td></td><td></td><td></td><td></td><td></td><td></td><td></td></tr>
<tr><td>fi</td><td>I</td><td>Normal</td><td>2</td><td></td><td></td><td></td><td></td><td></td></tr>
<tr><td>fi</td><td>II</td><td>Hypoplasia</td><td>1</td><td></td><td></td><td></td><td></td><td></td></tr>
<tr><td>fi</td><td>III</td><td>Dysplasia</td><td>0</td><td></td><td></td><td></td><td></td><td></td></tr>
<tr><td>Pes</td><td></td><td></td><td></td><td></td><td></td><td></td><td></td><td></td></tr>
<tr><td>pe</td><td>I</td><td>Normal</td><td>2</td><td></td><td></td><td></td><td></td><td></td></tr>
<tr><td>pe</td><td>II</td><td>3–4 rays</td><td>1</td><td></td><td></td><td></td><td></td><td></td></tr>
<tr><td>pe</td><td>III</td><td>1–2 rays</td><td>0</td><td></td><td></td><td></td><td></td><td></td></tr>
<tr><td colspan="2"></td><td align="right">Σ:</td><td>A</td><td></td><td></td><td></td><td align="right">Σ:</td><td>B</td></tr>
<tr><td colspan="4">**Score: A+B = + =**</td><td colspan="5"></td></tr>
</table>

Table 15.2 Five different classes of tibial reduction defects of the leg according to the scores

Class	Score
5	0–7
4	8–15
3	16–23
2	24–31
1	32–39

A plus sign (+) at the class number indicates the highest score number of the class; a minus sign (−) at the class number indicates the lowest score number of the class: e.g. score 7 = class 5+, score 8 = class 4−

- Soft tissue distraction as preparation of fibula pro tibia transformation and foot centralization.
- Callus distraction is performed to increase the length of the shortened bones and corrects deformities.
- Transformation surgery gives anatomical structures a new function.
- Booster surgery improves the growth of the cartilaginous anlage of the tibia and creates joints.

The use of ring fixators (Mini-Ilizarov, Maxi-Ilizarov and Taylor Spatial Frame) is preferred because they give the best stability and correction options. I use the different fixator types according to their advantages and combine them together to enhance their advantages.

- The postoperative functional results should be better than before surgery and better as a non-operated leg supported by an orthoprosthesis or prosthesis only.

The treatment can be divided generally into three stages: (1) a preoperative planning and preparation stage; (2) surgery and correction period; (3) removal of the fixator, preserving correction and restore function. All three stages are accompanied with intensive physiotherapy and ergotherapy to prevent or to treat contractures. A versatile and individual technical support by orthesis and orthoprosthesis is essentially at all stages of treatment especially at stage one and three. Especially after removal of the fixator, the callus should be protected from fracturing by a brace, by a cast or even better by an orthotic device. By wearing a custom-made brace, the risk of callus fracture during physiotherapy can be reduced.

- The type of treatment should not focus only on the operative possibilities and should

respect the wishes of the patients and/or parents/guardians.

15.4.1 Type I: Hypoplasia of the Tibia (Fig. 15.1)

This type is characterized by a complete osseous anlage of the tibia with distal and proximal joint. The tibia is shorter in contrast to the increased length of fibula. The treatment is focused on lengthening of tibia to its correct length in relation to fibula. It can be achieved with two ways: First, application of frame only to tibia and lengthening of tibia by callus distraction. This method applies great tension on soft tissues and can lead to joint subluxations, rarely at the ankle but mostly at the knee depending on the amount of lengthening. Therefore, lateral collateral ligament (ligamentum capitis fibulae) and other soft tissue releases (e.g. Achilles tendon) are necessary before lengthening. Second, this technique includes a montage of the frame over knee and ankle joint to preserve joint function whilst lengthening. Joint subluxation is avoided with this method, but joint stiffness becomes a problem after long-term immobilization. To prevent joint contracture, isometric mechanical hinges can be placed at the axes of the joints with slight acute distraction on the joint capsule of up to 5 mm and are used to mobilize the joints 6 weeks after the lengthening is stopped.

15.4.2 Type II: Distal Diastasis of the Tibia (Figs. 15.2, 15.3, 15.4, 15.5, and 15.6)

Insufficiency of the syndesmosis and transverse separation of tibia and fibula leads to subluxation/luxation of the ankle joint with proximalization of foot and talus between tibia and fibula (Figs. 15.2 and 15.6). For treatment, the foot is distracted with a foot integrating fixator to the level that the distal tibia can acutely be positioned over the talus without stress. Then, diastasis is corrected acutely with reconstruction of syndesmosis using anterior and posterior periosteal

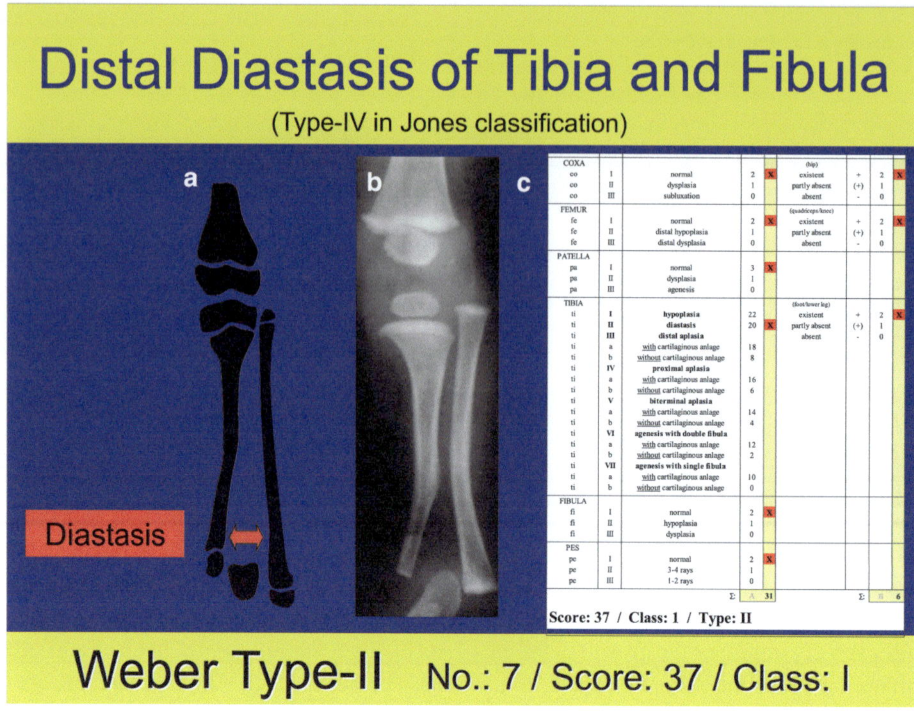

Region	Code	Grade	Description	Σ A	X	Function		Σ B	X
COXA						(hip)			
	co	I	normal	2	X	existent	+	2	X
	co	II	dysplasia	1		partly absent	(+)	1	
	co	III	subluxation	0		absent	-	0	
FEMUR						(quadriceps/knee)			
	fe	I	normal	2	X	existent	+	2	X
	fe	II	distal hypoplasia	1		partly absent	(+)	1	
	fe	III	distal dysplasia	0		absent	-	0	
PATELLA									
	pa	I	normal	3	X				
	pa	II	dysplasia	1					
	pa	III	agenesis	0					
TIBIA						(foot/lower leg)			
	ti	I	**hypoplasia**	22		existent	+	2	X
	ti	II	**diastasis**	20	X	partly absent	(+)	1	
	ti	III	**distal aplasia**			absent	-	0	
	ti	a	<u>with</u> cartilaginous anlage	18					
	ti	b	<u>without</u> cartilaginous anlage	8					
	ti	IV	**proximal aplasia**						
	ti	a	<u>with</u> cartilaginous anlage	16					
	ti	b	<u>without</u> cartilaginous anlage	6					
	ti	V	**biterminal aplasia**						
	ti	a	<u>with</u> cartilaginous anlage	14					
	ti	b	<u>without</u> cartilaginous anlage	4					
	ti	VI	**agenesis with double fibula**						
	ti	a	<u>with</u> cartilaginous anlage	12					
	ti	b	<u>without</u> cartilaginous anlage	2					
	ti	VII	**agenesis with single fibula**						
	ti	a	<u>with</u> cartilaginous anlage	10					
	ti	b	<u>without</u> cartilaginous anlage	0					
FIBULA									
	fi	I	normal	2	X				
	fi	II	hypoplasia	1					
	fi	III	dysplasia	0					
PES									
	pe	I	normal	2	X				
	pe	II	3-4 rays	1					
	pe	III	1-2 rays	0					
				Σ A 31				Σ B 6	

Score: 37 / Class: 1 / Type: II

Fig. 15.2 Leg no. 7. (**a**) Schematic drawing of tibial reduction defect Weber type II with tibiofibular diastasis and luxated foot. (**b**) Preoperative X-ray of treated leg with Weber type II. (**c**) Related score of leg (score: 37, class: I)

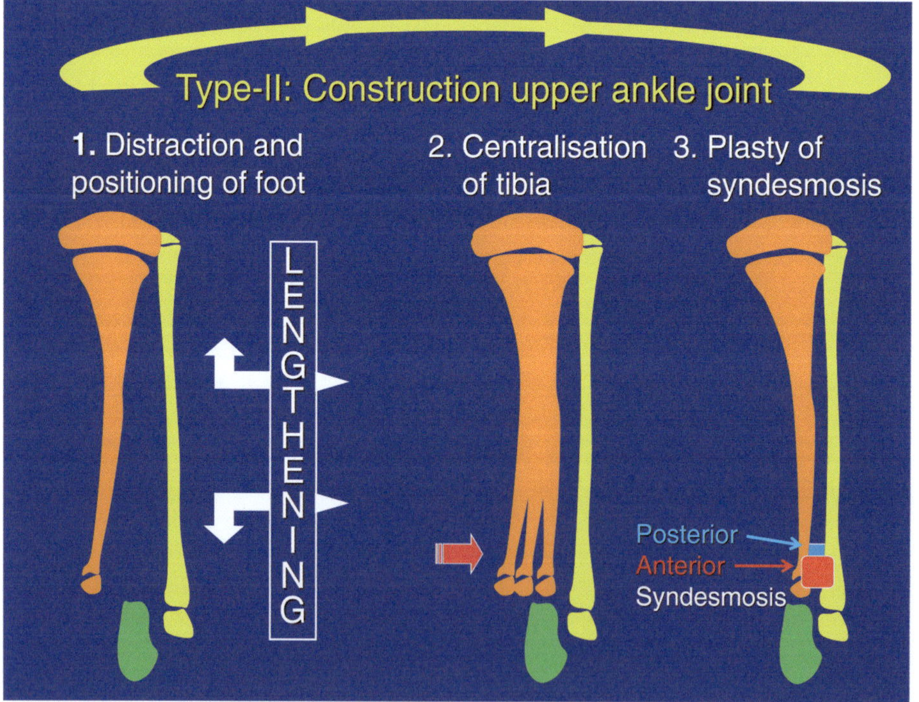

Fig. 15.3 Leg no. 7. Schematic drawing of surgical procedure for treatment of tibial reduction defect Weber type II of left leg. (*1*) Soft tissue distraction with correct positioning of the luxated foot. (*2*) Acute centralization of tibia to talus. (*3*) Protection of the centralized tibia from recurrence of diastasis by plasty of syndesmosis with perichondrial-periosteal flaps

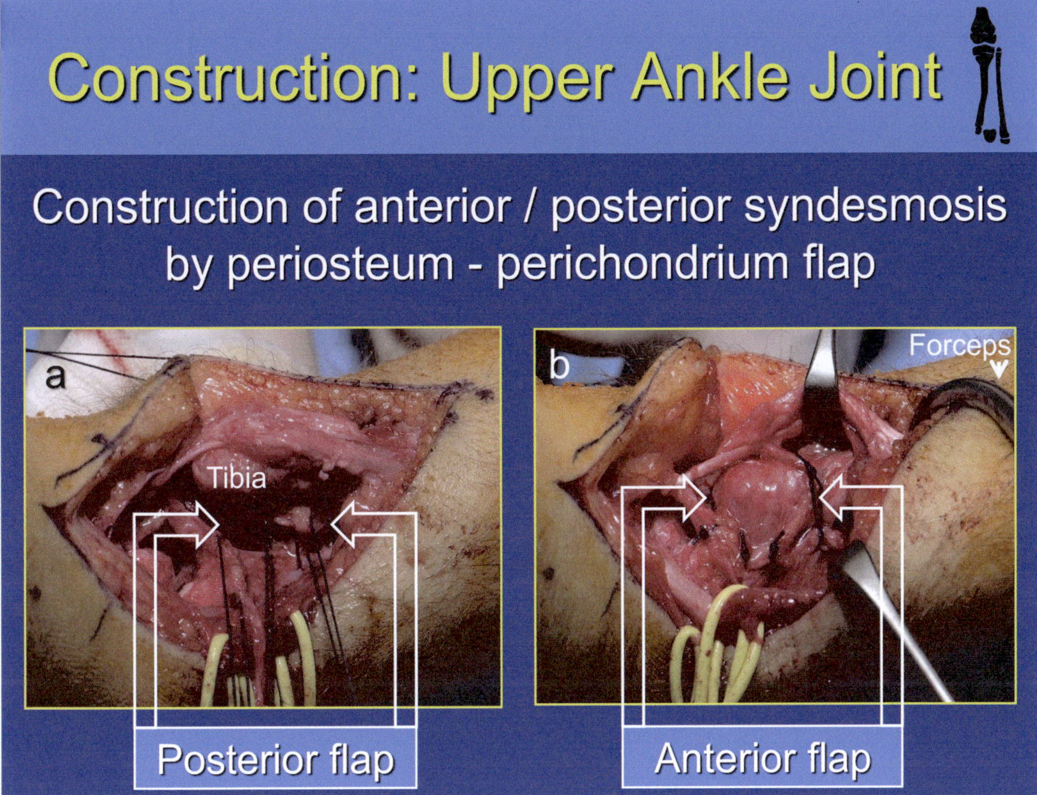

Fig. 15.4 Leg no. 7. Intraoperative pictures of ankle joint construction and procedure of syndesmosis plasty. (**a**) After preparation of joint capsule, construction of correct alignments of intra-articular tendons and holding them aside by vessel loops. The posterior perichondrial-periosteal flap is prepared from the dorsal part of the tibia and sutures inserted (*arrows*). (**b**) The tibia is positioned acutely with forceps and secured by an intramedullary K-wire through talus and tibia. The anterior perichondrial-periosteal flap is sutured to the anterior surface (*arrows*) of fibula after suturing of the posterior flap to the posterior surface of fibula

flaps, peroneal tendon plasty or allografts (Figs. 15.3 and 15.4). The tendons, which often are disoriented and can be aligned through the ankle joint, should be prepared and aligned properly. An axially placed wire secures ankle joint and tibia, whilst an olive wire preserves syndesmosis reconstruction during healing. After 6 weeks the wires can be removed and the upper ankle joint can be mobilized by the adjusted isometric mechanical hinges. Due to luxation of the foot with weight bearing of fibular tip and/or no weight load of the tibia, hyperplasia of distal fibular end and/or increase of hypoplasia of tibia occurs. So much the luxation of foot lasts, so more time it takes to recover proper structures after reposition of foot (Fig. 15.5).

15.4.3 Type IIIa: Distal Aplasia of the Tibia with Cartilaginous Anlage (Figs. 15.7, 15.8, and 15.9)

The proximal part of the tibia is ossified with normal knee joint, whilst the distal tibia is not ossified and a cartilaginous anlage is present without having contact with the talus (Figs. 15.7 and 15.9). The principle of the treatment is to bring the distal cartilaginous anlage in contact with the talus to form an ankle joint (Fig. 15.8). A proximal tibia osteotomy at the osseous part is performed and distracted until contact. Magnetic resonance imaging (MRI) can be used to measure required lengthening, and contact can be demonstrated with contrast

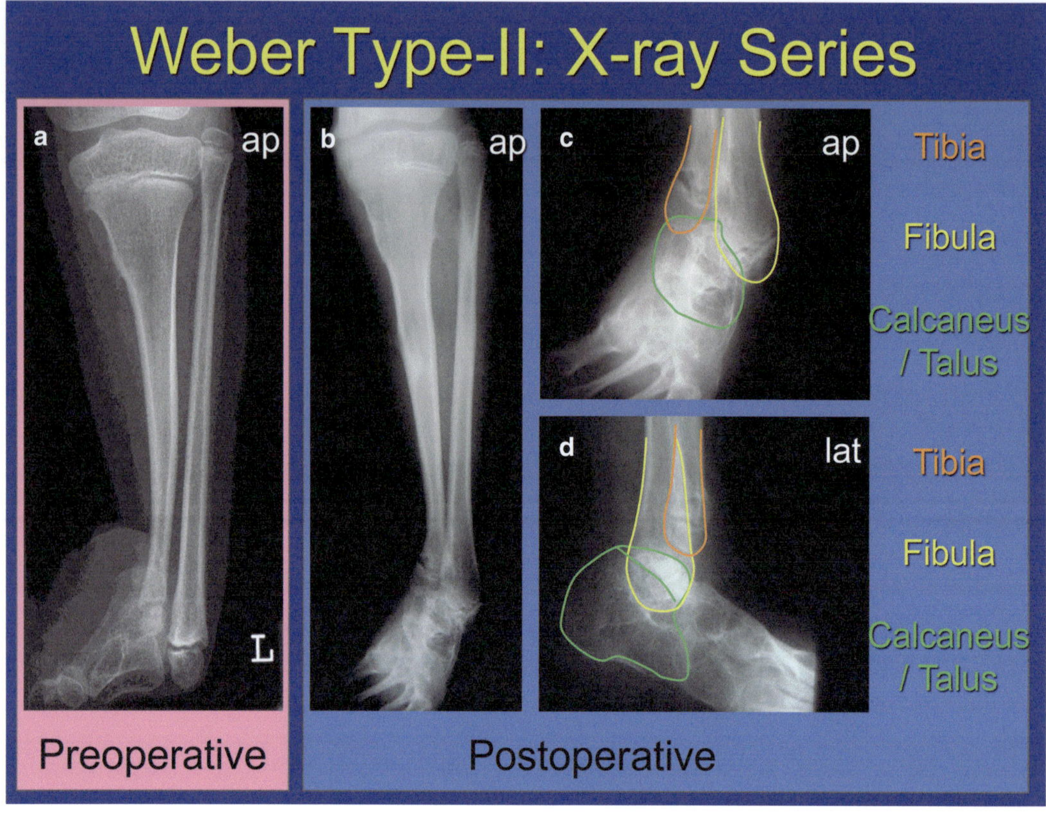

Fig. 15.5 Leg no. 7. X-ray series: (**a**) preoperative; (**b–d**) postoperative, after ankle construction with positioning of foot and distal tibia, alignment of extensor tendons and plasty of the syndesmosis ventrally and dorsally by perichondrial-periosteal flaps. (**a**) Diastasis of the left tibia and fibula distally with luxated foot according to Weber type II. Hyperplasia of distal fibula occurred due to the fact that the patient was walking on the tip of fibula. (**b**) Lower leg and foot ap. (**c**) Ankle ap. (**d**) Ankle lat: different coloured lines marking the contours of the corrected bones

arthrography. The new ankle joint is mobilized with isometric hinges mounted on the foot integrated fixator until callus maturation and removal of fixator (Fig. 15.9).

15.4.4 Type IIIb: Distal Aplasia of the Tibia without Cartilaginous Anlage (Figs. 15.10, 15.11, 15.12, 15.13, 15.14, 15.15, and 15.16)

The proximal tibia (which can occur in different lengths) is ossified and, distally, no cartilaginous anlage is attached. It is not possible to use distal tibia to form an ankle joint for this type (Figs. 15.10 and 15.13). The technique useful in this type is the transformation of the fibula to tibia. Distally, the fibula is used as an ankle joint by centralization to the foot at the talar neck. Proximally, the fibula is fused with tibial osseous anlage. Distraction is performed as the first step of the treatment. To avoid epiphyseolysis of the fibular head, lateral collateral ligament (LCL) has to be separated from the femur and the Achilles tendon has to be lengthened before distraction. After required distraction, fibular head is transposed acutely under tibial osseous anlage and foot underneath distal fibula. Proximally, the cartilaginous fibular head is cut at the surface to open the capillaries and connected to the tibia. The Ligamentum capitis fibulae (LCF) has to be divided and inserted medially and laterally onto the tibia, and perichondrial-periosteal flaps have to be prepared from the fibulae to ensure the osteochondrosynthesis (Fig. 15.11). Additionally,

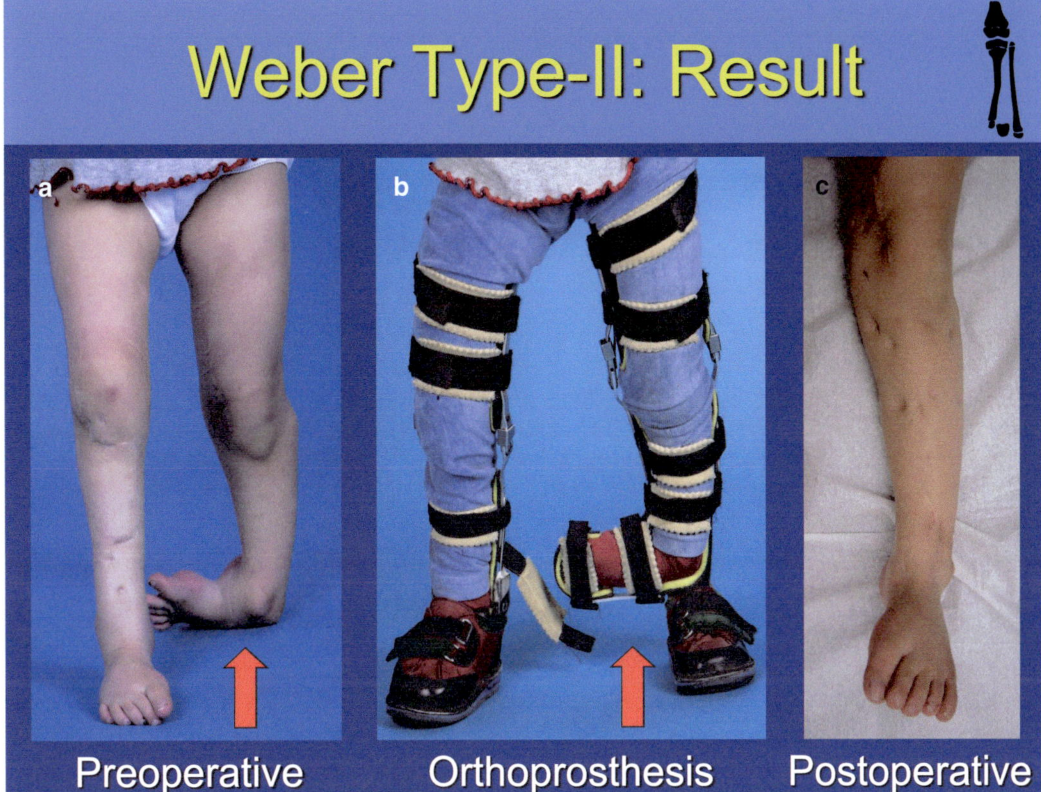

Fig. 15.6 Leg no. 7. Clinical pictures of the 6-year-old girl with diastasis of the left tibia and fibula distally with luxated foot according to Weber type II before (**a**, **b**) and after surgery (**c**). (**a**) The girl is walking with a luxated foot on the tip of the fibula. (**b**) The preoperative ortho-prosthesis could hardly enable the patient for walking. (**c**) After surgery the left leg was supported for further growth guidance by lower leg orthotics with Tamarack joints at ankle level. Later, the lower leg orthotics could be removed and normal shoes could be worn

an intramedullary wire is used to secure proximal fibular epiphysis and a transverse wire (anchor wire) to secure osteochondrosynthesis. The central fibular wire courses from proximal through the distal epiphysis into the foot and is connected outside at the fixator. Before the wire is attached to the fixator, it has to be pushed back into the proximal tibia to give additional stabilization for the osteochondrosynthesis (Fig. 15.12). The ankle joint can be stabilized in two ways. First option: bilaterally periosteal flaps from the fibula attached to the calcaneus (Figs. 15.14, 15.15, and 15.16). Second option: bilateral malleolus plasty (Weber et al. 2002). Before joint mobilization the central wire has to be removed. The knee and ankle joint are mobilized over isometrical hinges attached to the fixator (Fig. 15.13).

15.4.5 Type IVa: Proximal Aplasia of the Tibia with Cartilaginous Anlage (Fig. 15.1)

In this type, the distal tibia is ossified with a proximal connected cartilaginous anlage which has no contact to the femoral condyles. The treatment strategy is to bring the cartilaginous anlage into contact with the femoral condyles to form a knee joint. Therefore, an osteotomy is performed distally at the osseous part of tibia for callus distraction. The treatment procedure is the same as described for the proximal bone transport in type Va (Figs. 15.18, 15.19, 15.20, 15.21, and 15.22). For this purpose, a fixator is mounted at the lower limb integrating the upper limb. In case of a short distal tibial segment, an integration of the foot

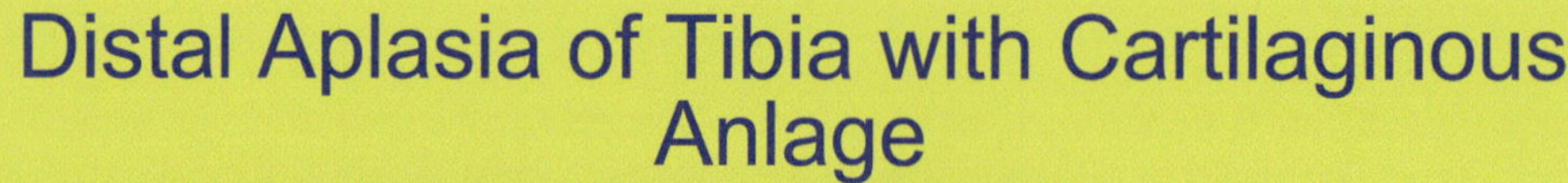

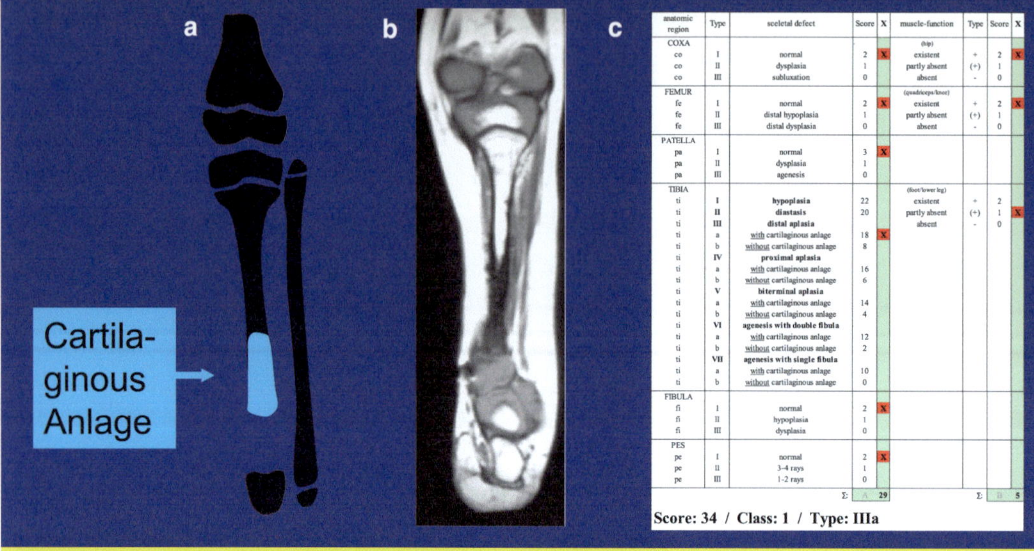

anatomic region	Type	sceletal defect	Score	X	muscle-function	Type	Score	X
COXA					(hip)			
co	I	normal	2	X	existent	+	2	X
co	II	dysplasia	1		partly absent	(+)	1	
co	III	subluxation	0		absent	-	0	
FEMUR					(quadriceps/knee)			
fe	I	normal	2	X	existent	+	2	X
fe	II	distal hypoplasia	1		partly absent	(+)	1	
fe	III	distal dysplasia	0		absent	-	0	
PATELLA								
pa	I	normal	3	X				
pa	II	dysplasia	1					
pa	III	agenesis	0					
TIBIA					(foot/lower leg)			
ti	**I**	**hypoplasia**	22		existent	+	2	
ti	**II**	**diastasis**	20		partly absent	(+)	1	X
ti	**III**	**distal aplasia**			absent	-	0	
ti	a	with cartilaginous anlage	18	X				
ti	b	without cartilaginous anlage	8					
ti	**IV**	**proximal aplasia**						
ti	a	with cartilaginous anlage	16					
ti	b	without cartilaginous anlage	6					
ti	**V**	**biterminal aplasia**						
ti	a	with cartilaginous anlage	14					
ti	b	without cartilaginous anlage	4					
ti	**VI**	**agenesis with double fibula**						
ti	a	with cartilaginous anlage	12					
ti	b	without cartilaginous anlage	2					
ti	**VII**	**agenesis with single fibula**						
ti	a	with cartilaginous anlage	10					
ti	b	without cartilaginous anlage	0					
FIBULA								
fi	I	normal	2	X				
fi	II	hypoplasia	1					
fi	III	dysplasia	0					
PES								
pe	I	normal	2	X				
pe	II	3-4 rays	1					
pe	III	1-2 rays	0					
			Σ: A	29			Σ: B	5

Score: 34 / Class: 1 / Type: IIIa

Fig. 15.7 Leg no. 50. (**a**) Schematic drawing of tibial reduction defect Weber type IIIa with tibial aplasia distally and with cartilaginous anlage of left leg. (**b**) Preoperative MRI of lower leg showing the cartilaginous anlage. (**c**) Related score of leg (score: 34, class: I). No type in the classifications of Jones et al. (1978), Henkel et al. (1978) and Kalamchi and Dawe (1985) available

into the fixator montage is recommended. Required distraction can be measured with MRI and demonstrated by contrast arthrography at knee joint. The knee joint is mobilized by isometrical mechanical hinges. Following callus maturation, fixator is removed and correction preserved with orthesis.

15.4.6 Type IVb: Proximal Aplasia of the Tibia without Cartilaginous Anlage (Fig. 15.1)

Distal tibia with ankle joint is formed, but proximal tibia is absent without cartilaginous anlage. Patella may be normally developed, underdeveloped or absent. In case no patella exists, the proximal fibular segment is transposed under femoral condyles and an osteosynthesis performed with the proximal tibial end. The fibular head should transform to a 'tibial plateau' during further growth under weight bearing (compare to type VIIb without patella). LCL is transformed as anterior cruciate ligament (ACL) to prevent fibular head dislocation. To achieve transposition, an initial distraction has to be performed and LCL has to be separated from femur to avoid epiphyseolysis of fibular head. The ring fixators have to be placed at thigh, fibula and foot. The soft tissue lengthening is finished until the fibular head can be transposed under the femoral condyles. Anterior S-shape approach to the knee with preservation of crural fascia is performed. The crural fascia can be transformed into collateral

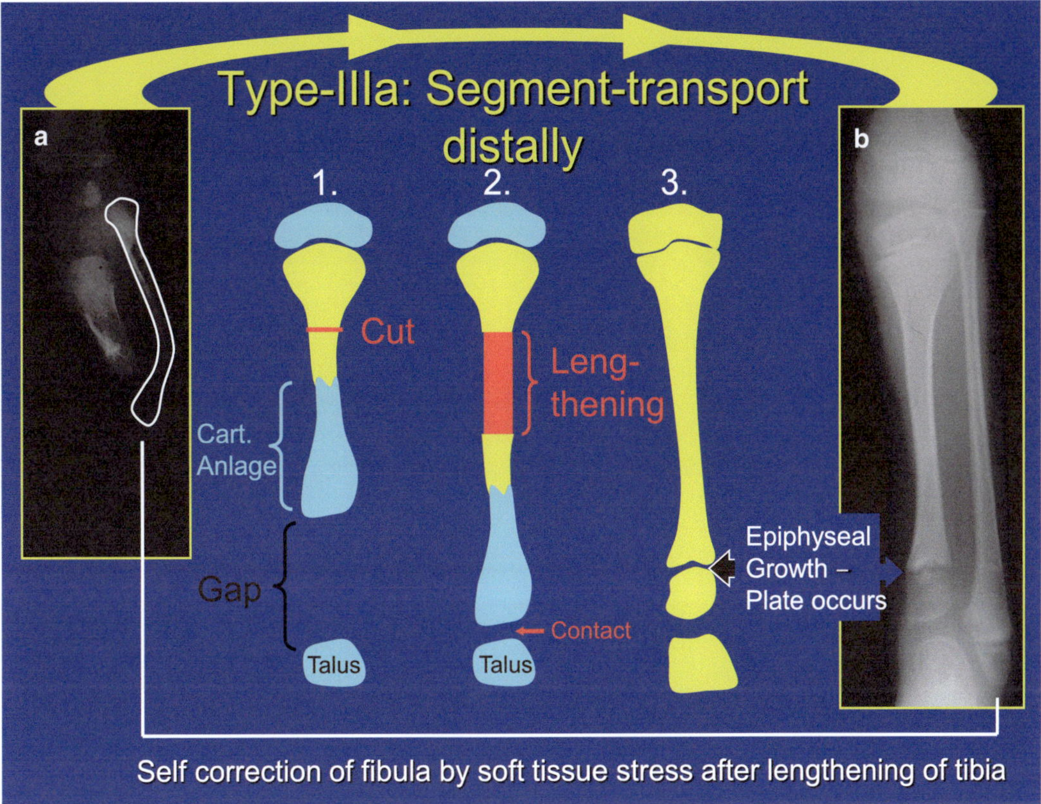

Fig. 15.8 Leg no. 50. Schematic drawing of operational procedure for treatment of tibial reduction defect Weber type IIIa. (*1*) Osteotomy at the bony part of the proximal tibia. (*2*) Callus distraction of the tibia to bring the cartilaginous anlage in contact with the talus. (*3*) Status after maturation of callus and development of tibial growth plate distally at area of former cartilaginous anlage. (**a**) Preoperative X-ray of left lower leg of a 3-year-old boy with severe bowing of fibula due to over length in relation to tibia. (**b**) X-ray of left lower leg with complete maturation of the cartilaginous anlage due to growth stimulating effect of callus distraction and weight bearing with epiphyseal growth plate of distal tibia and good ankle joint configuration 4 years after surgery

ligaments for stabilization of the knee joint. The LCF (or fascia lata, biceps tendon or capsule tissue) is passed through a drill hole from the central part of the femoral leading out to the lateral femoral condyle. The fibula has to be cut at the level of the proximal tibial end and an osteosynthesis of both bones will be performed. An axial intramedullary wire secures the proximal fibular epiphysis and, additionally, the osteosynthesis of fibula and tibia. Isometrical mechanical hinges allow early mobilization of the new knee joint.

In case a sufficient developed patella exists, it will be used as a 'substitution of the tibial plateau' (see type VIIb with patella). With this technique the patella is transformed into a tibial plateau which leads to much better function as the transformation of the fibular head (Weber 2002).

15.4.7 Type Va: Biterminal Aplasia of the Tibia with Cartilaginous Anlage (Figs. 15.17, 15.18, 15.19, 15.20, 15.21, and 15.22)

The central part of the tibia is ossified and even so the proximally and distally attached cartilaginous anlage without contact to femoral condyles and talus, respectively. In case of contact of the cartilaginous anlage to their joint partners, the fibula shows severe bowing (Fig. 15.17).

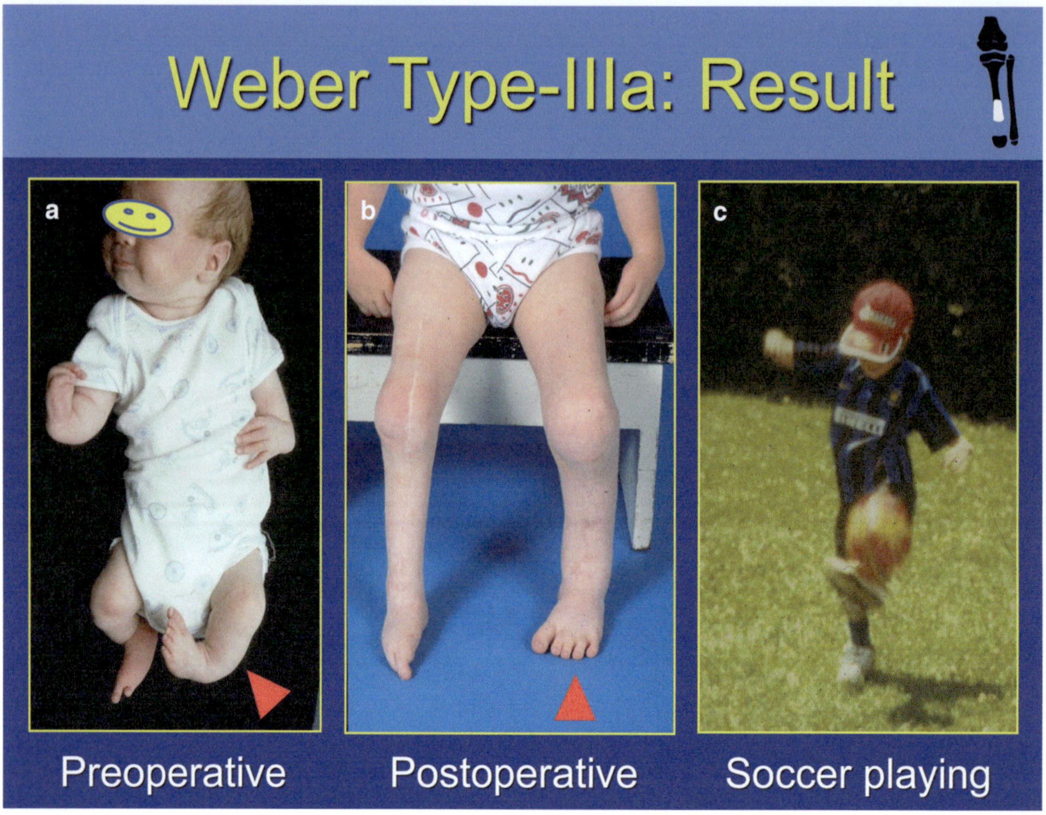

Fig. 15.9 Leg no. 50. Clinical results including orthoprosthesis care. (**a**) Preoperative, all four extremities show malformations: bilateral radial club hand and bilateral tibial reduction deficiency (see Spranger et al. 1996). (**b**) The left leg after surgery can take full weight load and shows nearly normal ROM of upper ankle joint. According to the procedure of the right leg see Figs. 15.29, 15.30, 15.31, 15.32, 15.33, and 15.34. (**c**) The boy is able to play soccer, skiing and skateboarding protected with orthotic devices

Both cartilaginous anlagen are used to create their adjacent joints by bringing them into contact with their joint partners via callus distraction of the central ossified tibia. This contact with the later weight load and the growth-enhancing effect of callus distraction leads to the booster effect of the created joints; these joints develop well (Figs. 15.18 and 15.22).

The first step is soft tissue distraction at knee and ankle level. The fixators are applied at thigh, lower leg and foot (Fig. 15.19). LCL and Achilles tendon (if shortened) is lengthened with Z-plasty. After required distraction is performed, the ossified anlage is osteotomized. The proximal tibial segment is transported towards femur to form a knee joint, and the distal tibial segment is transported towards the talus to form an ankle joint. Arthrography is used to evaluate successful docking (Fig. 15.20). Isometrical mechanical hinges are used to allow joint motion. The fixator is removed after consolidation of callus. The leg is fitted in a long leg orthotics with movable mechanical joints at knee and foot during growth of the child or a permanent stability of the joints is recognized. With the same technique a second (or more) lengthening can be performed (Figs. 15.21 and 15.22).

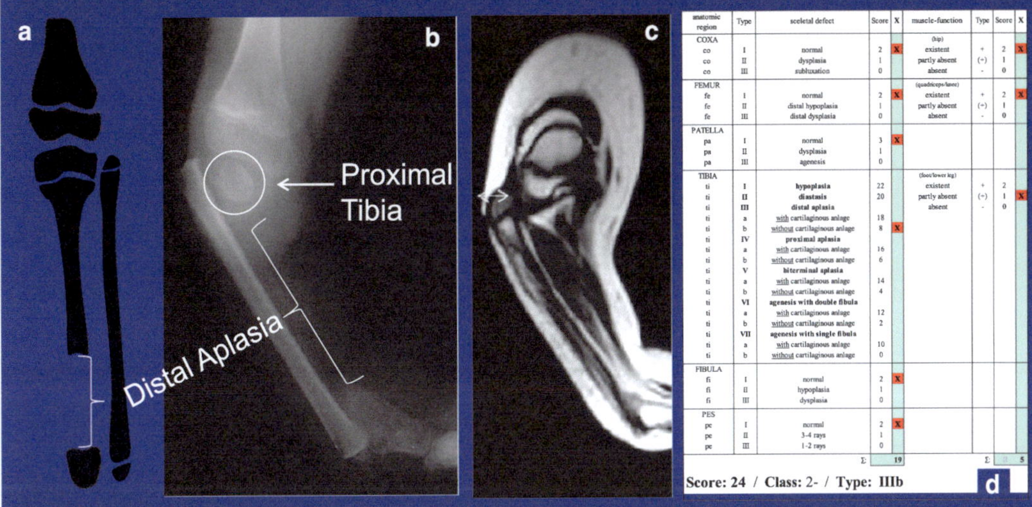

anatomic region	Type	sceletal defect	Score	X	muscle-function	Type	Score	X
COXA					(hip)			
co	I	normal	2	X	existent	+	2	X
co	II	dysplasia	1		partly absent	(+)	1	
co	III	subluxation	0		absent	-	0	
FEMUR					(quadriceps/knee)			
fe	I	normal	2	X	existent	+	2	X
fe	II	distal hypoplasia	1		partly absent	(+)	1	
fe	III	distal dysplasia	0		absent	-	0	
PATELLA								
pa	I	normal	3	X				
pa	II	dysplasia	1					
pa	III	agenesis	0					
TIBIA					(foot/lower leg)			
ti	I	**hypoplasia**	22		existent	+	2	
ti	II	**diastasis**	20		partly absent	(+)	1	X
ti	III	**distal aplasia**			absent	-	0	
ti	a	with cartilaginous anlage	18					
ti	b	without cartilaginous anlage	8	X				
ti	IV	**proximal aplasia**						
ti	a	with cartilaginous anlage	16					
ti	b	without cartilaginous anlage	6					
ti	V	**biterminal aplasia**						
ti	a	with cartilaginous anlage	14					
ti	b	without cartilaginous anlage	4					
ti	VI	**agenesis with double fibula**						
ti	a	with cartilaginous anlage	12					
ti	b	without cartilaginous anlage	2					
ti	VII	**agenesis with single fibula**						
ti	a	with cartilaginous anlage	10					
ti	b	without cartilaginous anlage	0					
FIBULA								
fi	I	normal	2	X				
fi	II	hypoplasia	1					
fi	III	dysplasia	0					
PES								
pe	I	normal	2	X				
pe	II	3-4 rays	1					
pe	III	1-2 rays	0					
			Σ	19			Σ	5

Fig. 15.10 Leg no. 59. (**a**) Schematic drawing of tibial reduction defect Weber type IIIb with tibial aplasia distally without cartilaginous anlage. (**b**) Preoperative X-ray of right lower leg showing the bony anlage of proximal tibia (*white circle*). (**c**) MRI of right leg demonstrates the aplasia of distal tibia without cartilaginous anlage. (**d**) Related score of leg (score: 24, class: 2−). Unclear which type it could be in the Jones classification (Jones et al. 1978)

15.4.8 Type Vb: Biterminal Aplasia of the Tibia without Cartilaginous Anlage (Figs. 15.14, 15.15, 15.16, 15.29, 15.30, 15.31, 15.32, 15.33, 15.34, 15.35, 15.36, 15.37, 15.38, 15.39, and 15.40)

This type is characterized by a centrally ossified tibia without a proximally or distally annexed cartilaginous anlage. This aplasia appears with or without patella.

This type can be approach in two ways: First, resection of the tibial anlage and continuing treatment as type VIIb. Second, biterminal segment transport as described in type Va. However, it should be put in consideration that in this situation no growth zones and no joint partners may be available. This would result in multiple lengthening procedures during the infantile growth and, additionally, in an unsafe situation in the region of the joints.

15.4.9 Type VIa: Agenesia of the Tibia with Cartilaginous Anlage and Double Fibula (Fig. 15.1)

This type is characterized by a completely absent tibia except a mostly proximally located cartilaginous anlage.

Fig. 15.11 Leg no. 59. Schematic drawing of operational procedure for treatment of tibial reduction defect Weber type IIIb. (*1*) Schematic situs. (*2*) Soft tissue lengthening after detachment of ligamentum capitis fibulae from femoral insertion and lengthening of Achilles tendon. (*3*) Centralization of fibular head and osteochondrosynthesis of fibular head into proximal tibia. The LCF is splitted longitudinally and attached medially and laterally to the tibia. Centralization of foot is performed (see Figs. 15.14, 15.15, and 15.16)

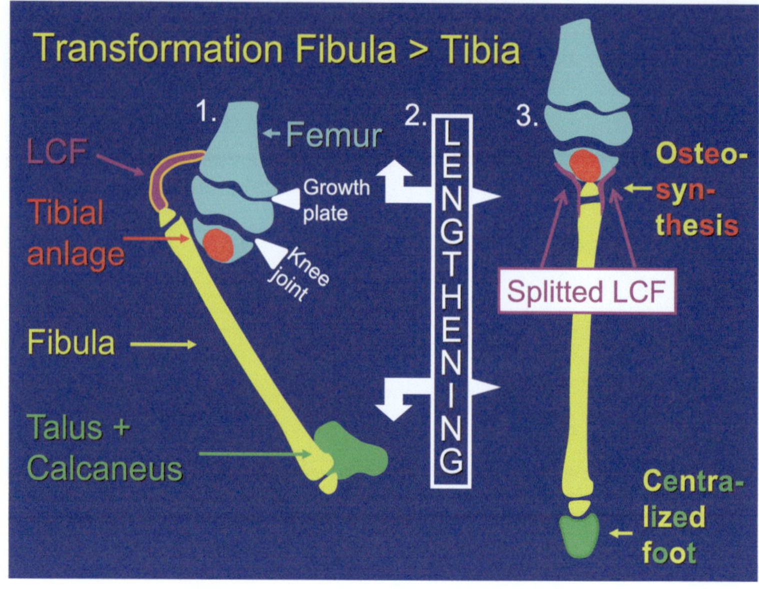

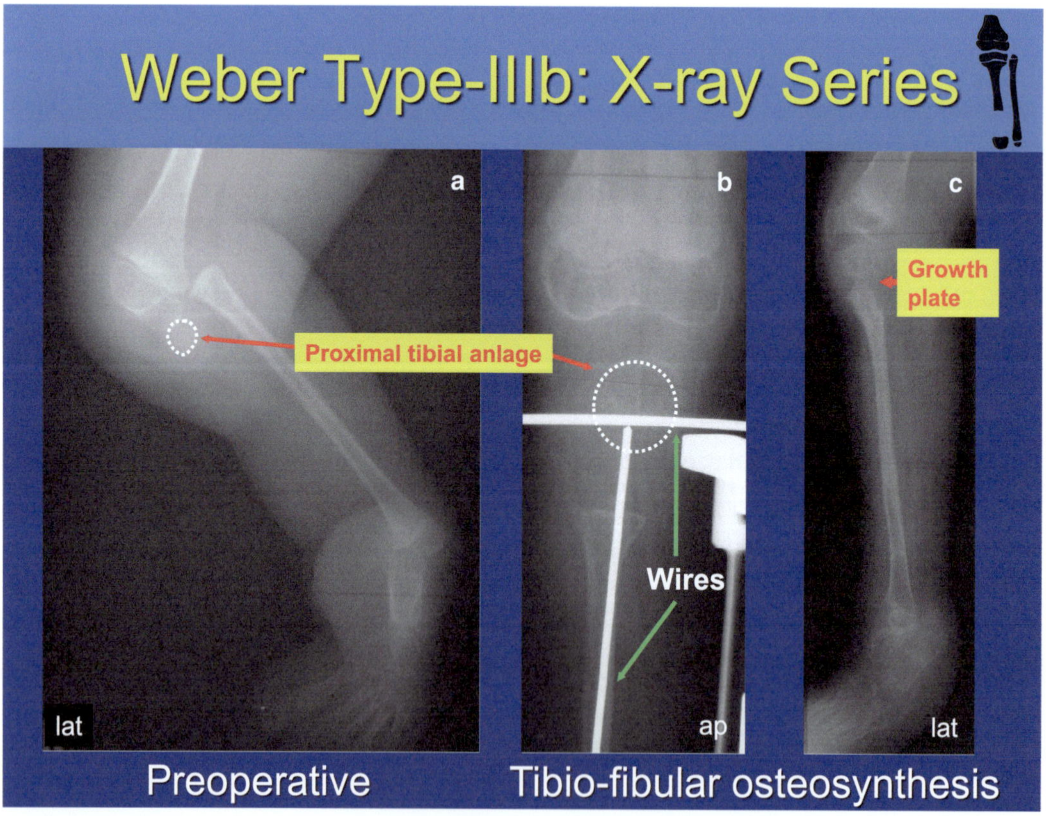

Fig. 15.12 Leg no. 59. X-ray series of a 6-year-old girl with tibial reduction deficiency Weber type IIIb. (**a**) Preoperative situation. (**b**) Transfixation of tibial anlage and fibular head by an axial fibular and a transverse wire through the bony proximal tibial anlage. (**c**) Result after surgery. Note the open growth plate of the former fibular head after the solid fusion between fibular head and proximal tibial anlage

Fig. 15.13 Leg no. 59. (**a**) The right leg before surgery showing the malformation of the lower leg with complete instability at knee level and luxated clubfoot. (**b**) The result after surgery shows correct axis of lower leg with slight reduction of knee flexion but full extension, normal ROM of upper ankle joint and corrected club foot

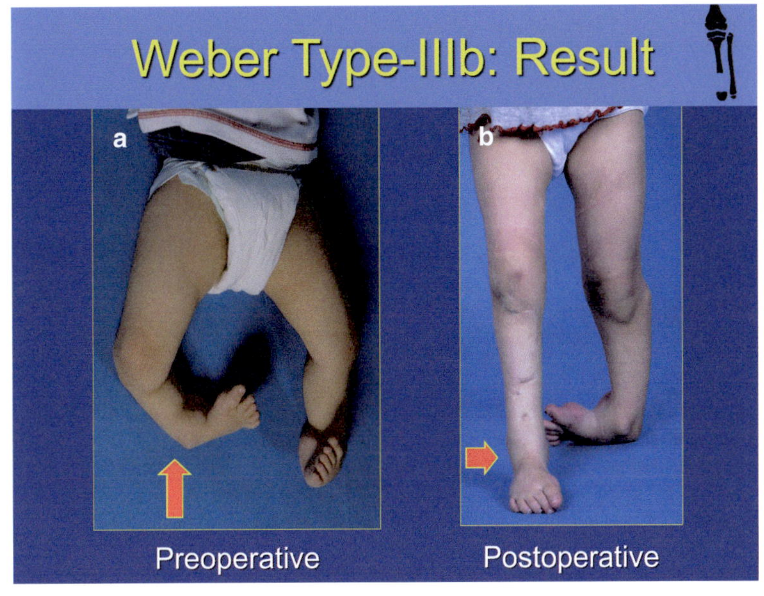

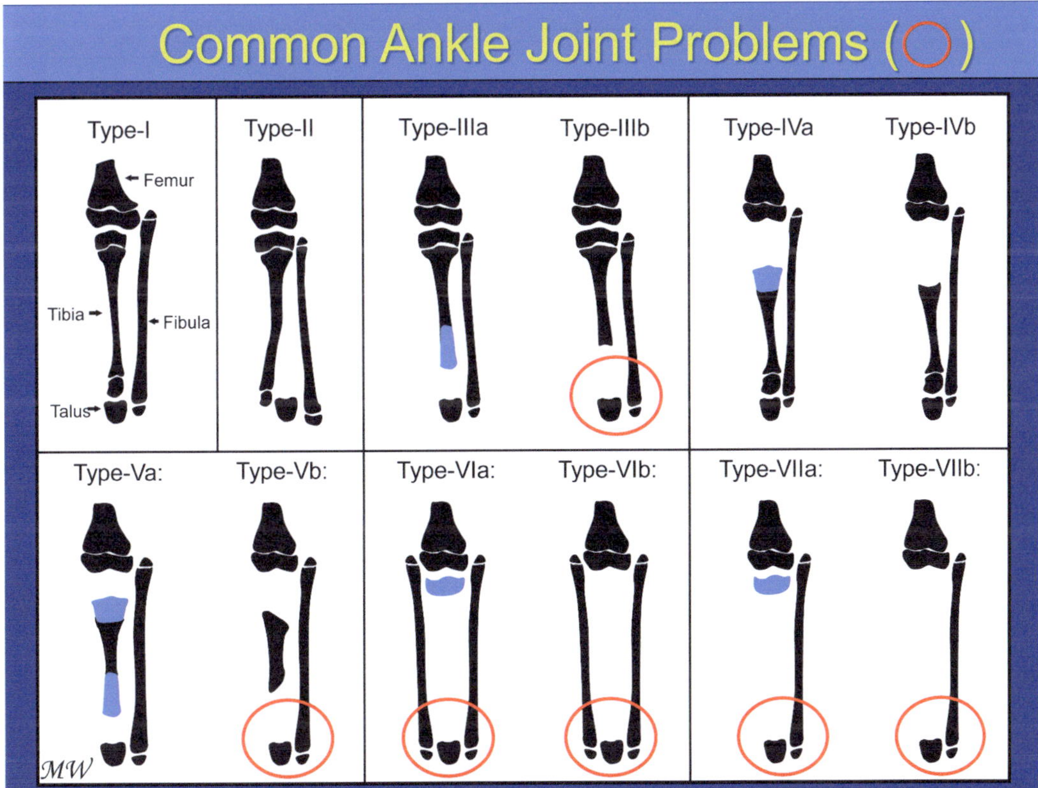

Fig. 15.14 Weber classification of tibial reduction deficiencies. The *red circles* are marking the common unstable ankle joint problems in different types (*IIIb*, *Vb* and *VI–VII*) which can be treated in two different ways (see Sect. 15.4.4): stabilization either by bilaterally malleolus plasty with transformation of iliac crest transplant into malleolus (Weber 2002) or bilaterally periosteal flaps transforming into collateral ligaments (see Figs. 15.16 and 15.17)

Fig. 15.15 Schematic drawing of ankle joint stabilization procedure for treatment of tibial reduction defects (Weber types IIIb, Vb and VI–VII) by transformation of bilaterally periosteal fibular flaps into collateral ligaments. (*1*) Schematic situs. (*2*) Soft tissue lengthening for centralization of foot. (*3*) Preparation of periosteal flaps from medially and laterally surface of distal fibula. The flaps are folded down and attached to calcaneus

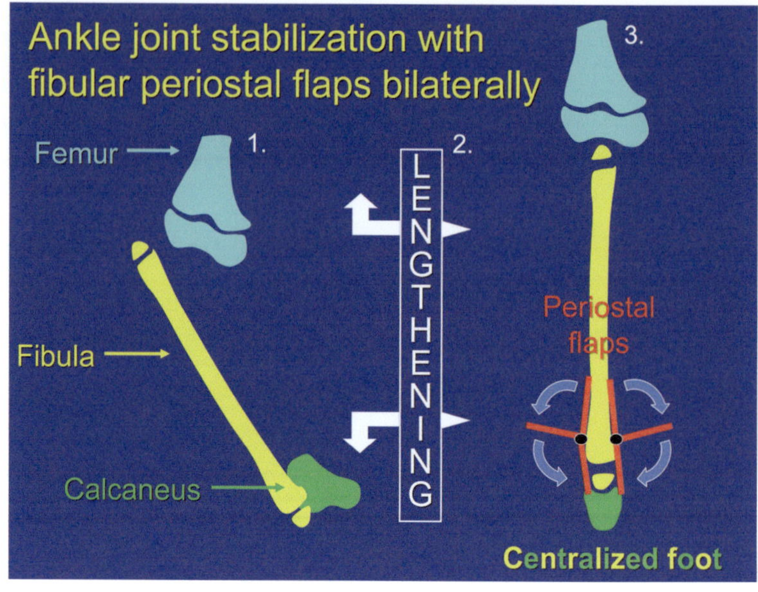

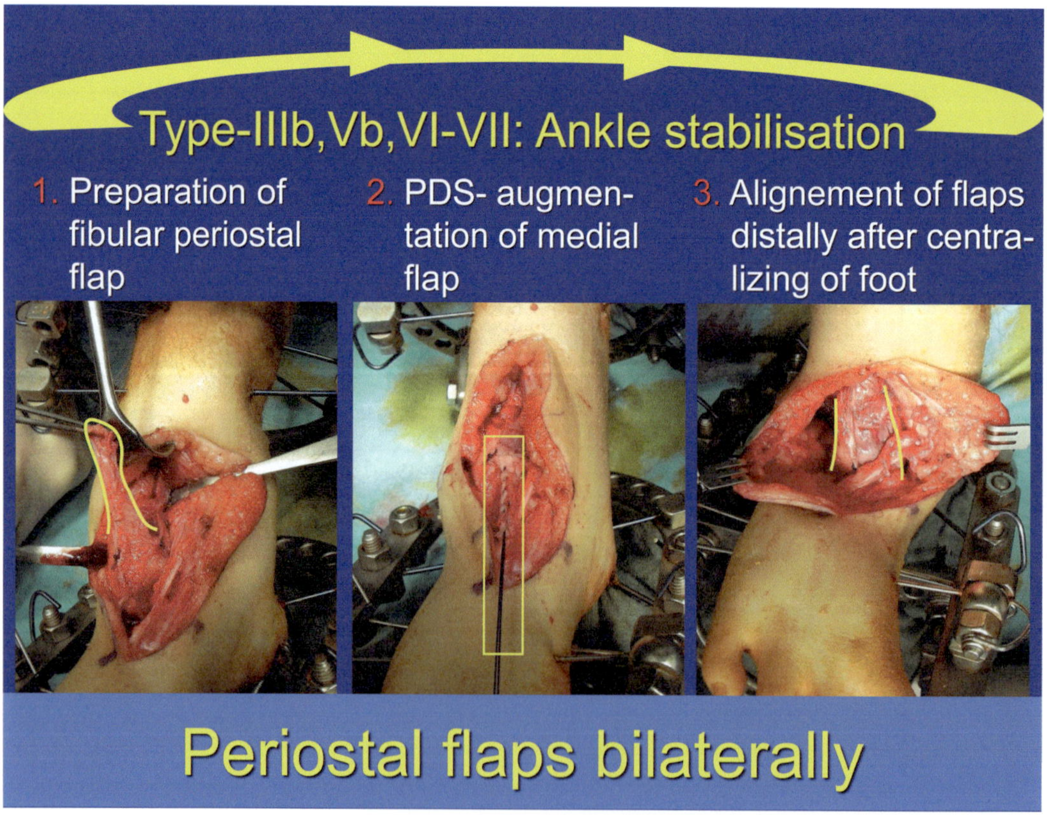

Fig. 15.16 Transformation of bilaterally fibular periosteal flaps into collateral ligaments at ankle joint. (*1*) Preparation of periosteal flap from distal fibula medially. (*2*) Augmentation of periosteal flap with PDS suture. (*3*) Situs after leading the bilaterally flaps down along the calcaneus subperiosteally. The PDS suture is leading through the skin of the foot and attached at the foot fixator with slight tension. After 6 weeks the PDS suture is cut off at the heel

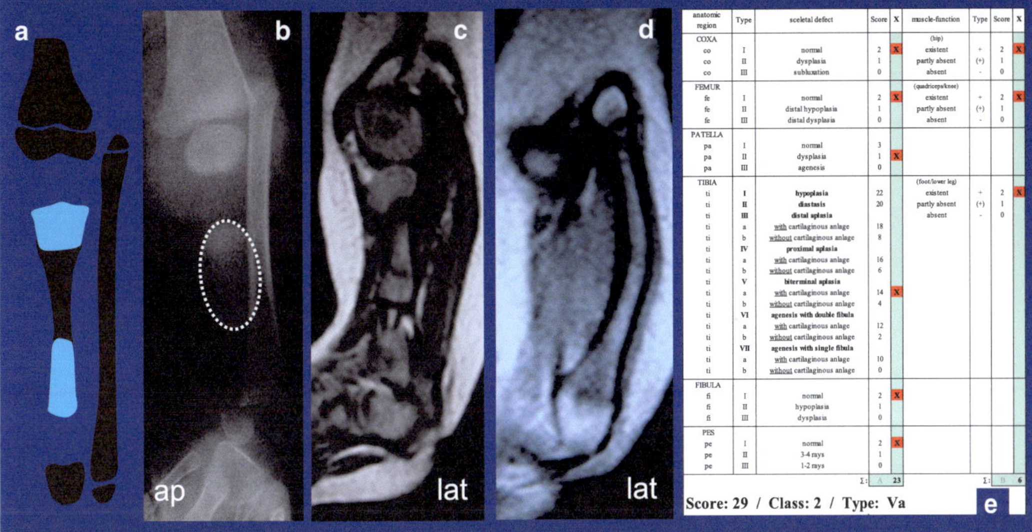

anatomic region	Type	sceletal defect	Score	X	muscle-function	Type	Score	X
COXA					(hip)			
co	I	normal	2	X	existent	+	2	X
co	II	dysplasia	1		partly absent	(+)	1	
co	III	subluxation	0		absent	-	0	
FEMUR					(quadriceps/knee)			
fe	I	normal	2	X	existent	+	2	X
fe	II	distal hypoplasia	1		partly absent	(+)	1	
fe	III	distal dysplasia	0		absent	-	0	
PATELLA								
pa	I	normal	3					
pa	II	dysplasia	1	X				
pa	III	agenesis	0					
TIBIA					(foot/lower leg)			
ti	**I**	**hypoplasia**	22		existent	+	2	X
ti	**II**	**diastasis**	20		partly absent	(+)	1	
ti	**III**	**distal aplasia**			absent	-	0	
ti	a	<u>with</u> cartilaginous anlage	18					
ti	b	<u>without</u> cartilaginous anlage	8					
ti	**IV**	**proximal aplasia**						
ti	a	<u>with</u> cartilaginous anlage	16					
ti	b	<u>without</u> cartilaginous anlage	6					
ti	**V**	**biterminal aplasia**						
ti	a	<u>with</u> cartilaginous anlage	14	X				
ti	b	<u>without</u> cartilaginous anlage	4					
ti	**VI**	**agenesis with double fibula**						
ti	a	<u>with</u> cartilaginous anlage	12					
ti	b	<u>without</u> cartilaginous anlage	2					
ti	**VII**	**agenesis with single fibula**						
ti	a	<u>with</u> cartilaginous anlage	10					
ti	b	<u>without</u> cartilaginous anlage	0					
FIBULA								
fi	I	normal	2	X				
fi	II	hypoplasia	1					
fi	III	dysplasia	0					
PES								
pe	I	normal	2	X				
pe	II	3-4 rays	1					
pe	III	1-2 rays	0					
			Σ:	A	23		Σ:	B	6

Score: 29 / Class: 2 / Type: Va

Fig. 15.17 Leg no. 49. (**a**) Schematic drawing of tibial reduction deficiency Weber type Va with bifocal tibial aplasia with cartilaginous anlage. (**b**) Preoperative X-ray of left lower leg showing the bony anlage of middle tibia (*white circle*). (**c**) MRI of left leg demonstrates the bifocal aplasia of tibia with cartilaginous anlage. (**d**) MRI of left leg showing complete and bended fibula. (**e**) Related score of leg (score: 29, class: 2). No type in the classifications of Jones et al. (1978), Henkel et al. (1978) and Kalamchi and Dawe (1985) available

The treatment of this type depends on the growth potential of the cartilaginous anlage. If the anlage is too rudimentary to function, it is resected and treatment continues as described for type VIb. If the cartilaginous anlage is substantial enough to form a knee joint, it should be preserved. Then, a maturation of the cartilaginous anlage can be expected following a transformation of fibula to tibia. Therefore, the fibula is transposed underneath the cartilaginous anlage with chondrodesis. The distal construction is planned according to the position of distal part of medial fibula. The medial fibula should articulate distally with the talus. If not, a technique appropriate for a diastasis should be chosen (see type II). If the level of the lateral fibula is correct and the lower limb not shortened, the transposition of the medial fibula underneath the cartilaginous anlage can be performed by a shortening osteotomy. In the case of shortening of the lower leg with over length of the fibulae, an equalization of length by a soft tissue distraction using a ring fixator should be performed. For this purpose, the same technique has to be used as applied for type VIIb.

15.4.10 Type VIb: Agenesia of the Tibia without Cartilaginous Anlage and Double Fibula
(Figs. 15.23, 15.24, 15.25, 15.26, 15.27, and 15.28)

This type is characterized by a totally lack of tibia, a double fibula and with or without patella.

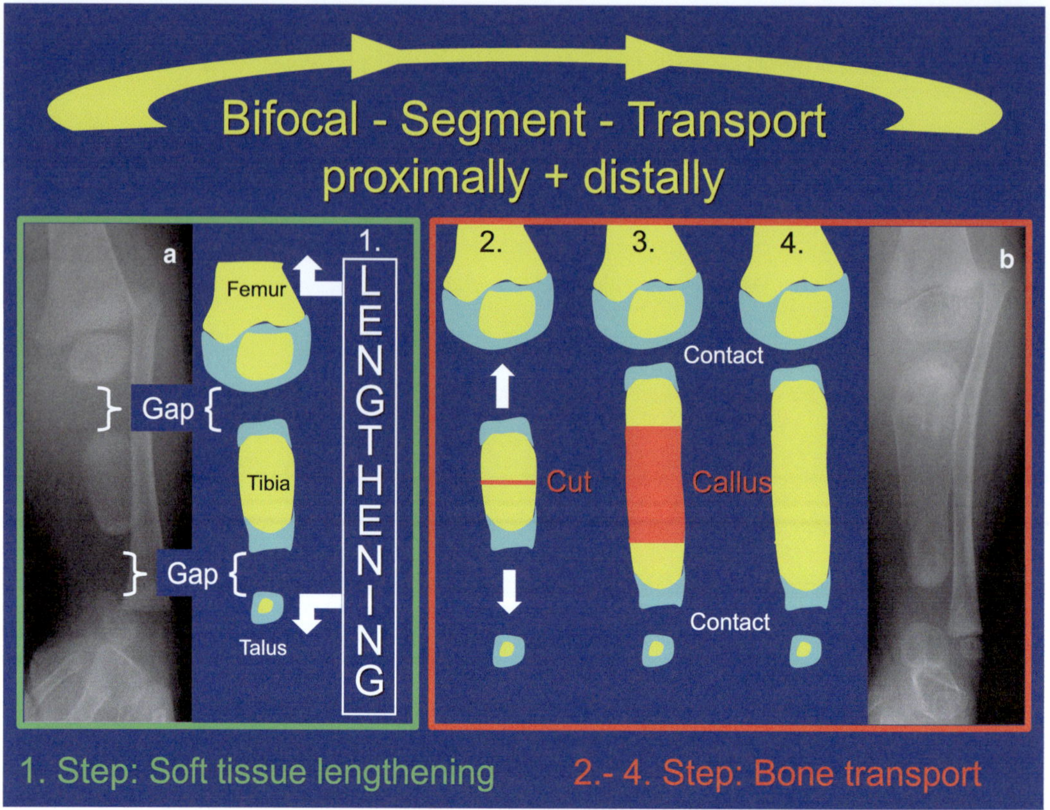

Fig. 15.18 Leg no. 49. Schematic drawing of operational procedure for treatment of tibial reduction defect Weber type Va. (*1*) Situation before procedure. (*2*) Osteotomy of tibial bone for callus distraction. (*3*) The gap between the cartilaginous anlage of the proximal tibia and the femoral condyles as well as distal tibia and the talus is closed by bidirectional bone transport to proximal and to distal. (*4*) Status after maturation of callus and contact of cartilaginous anlage. (**a**) X-ray shows the left lower leg before operation in a 10-month-old girl. (**b**) X-ray shows the same lower leg left 1 year after first lengthening

In case the patella is absent, both fibulae are used to form a tibial plateau. The LCF of the medial fibula is transformed as ACL and the LCF of the lateral fibula is transformed as posterior cruciate ligament (PCL). The talus is transposed under medial fibula. The lateral fibula distally functions as lateral malleolus. In case of a double foot with double talus, the medial talus has to be transposed under the medial fibula and the lateral talus has to be transposed under the lateral fibula after narrowing and fusion of the double foot. The stabilization of the ankle joint can be done with fibular periosteal flaps as substitute of collateral ligaments as described in type VIa (Figs. 15.14, 15.15, and 15.16). The difference to the procedure as described under type VIa is that the lateral collateral ligament will be constructed with the periosteal flap from the lateral surface of the distal lateral fibula and the medial collateral ligament will be constructed with the periosteal flap from the medial surface of the distal medial fibula. In case both fibulae are at risk of developing a diastasis, a syndesmosis plasty can be constructed by using periosteal flaps from the medial surface of the lateral fibula and from the lateral surface of the medial fibula (compare procedure of type II; Figs. 15.2, 15.3, 15.4, 15.5, and 15.6).

Initially, soft tissue distraction is performed with knee and ankle spanning ring fixator. Gradually, lateral and medial fibulae are pulled under the level of lateral and medial femoral condyles. During distraction, both LCF have to be

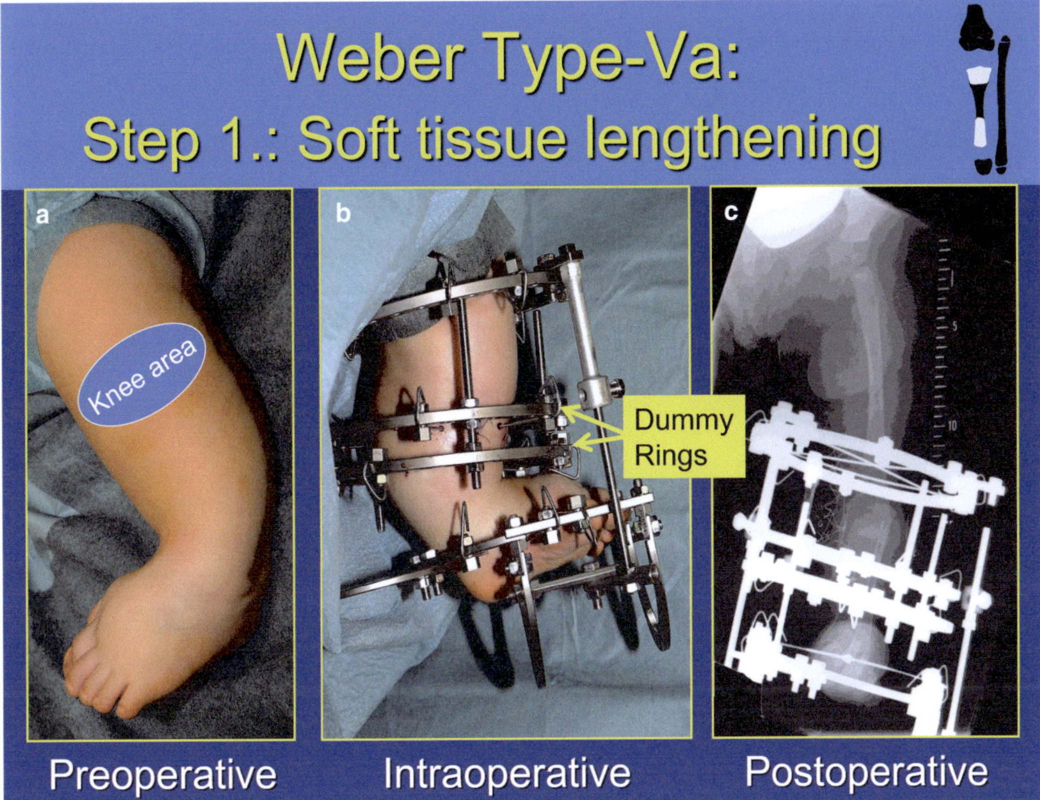

Fig. 15.19 Leg no. 49. First step of treatment of Weber type Va tibial defect with cartilaginous anlage is to lengthen the soft tissue at knee and ankle level. (**a**) Left leg before surgery with unstable knee and luxated six ray clubfoot. (**b**) Intraoperative situs after application of mini-ring fixator. Note the dummy ring between the proximal ring at femur and distal ring at foot. This ring will be used to perform the bifocal callus distraction. (**c**) X-ray after montage of fixator, the soft tissue lengthening takes place between femur and foot

released in a way that they can be used later as cruciate ligaments. After distraction is achieved, acute transposition of both fibular heads under the corresponding femoral condyles has to follow. In case the space below the femoral condyles is filled with soft tissue, it can be used to create menisci by cutting the soft tissue accordingly. Capsule and fascia remnants are used to construct LCL. LCF of the fibulae are used to construct cruciate ligaments. In case patella is present, it will be transformed to tibial plateau. The same technique should be used as described in type VIIb with patella. The only difference is that in this case both fibular heads have to be fusioned to the patella. The transformations of the ligaments are the same as described above.

15.4.11 Type VIIa: Agenesia of the Tibia with Cartilaginous Anlage and Single Fibula (Fig. 15.1)

This type is characterized by total absence of tibia except a mostly proximal cartilaginous anlage with single fibula. The treatment of this type depends on the growth potential of the cartilaginous anlage. If the anlage is too rudimentary to function, it is resected and treatment continues as described for type VIIb. If the cartilaginous anlage is substantial enough to form a knee joint, its maturation can be expected following fibular transformation to tibia as described in type VIa. The procedure for centralization of fibula to foot

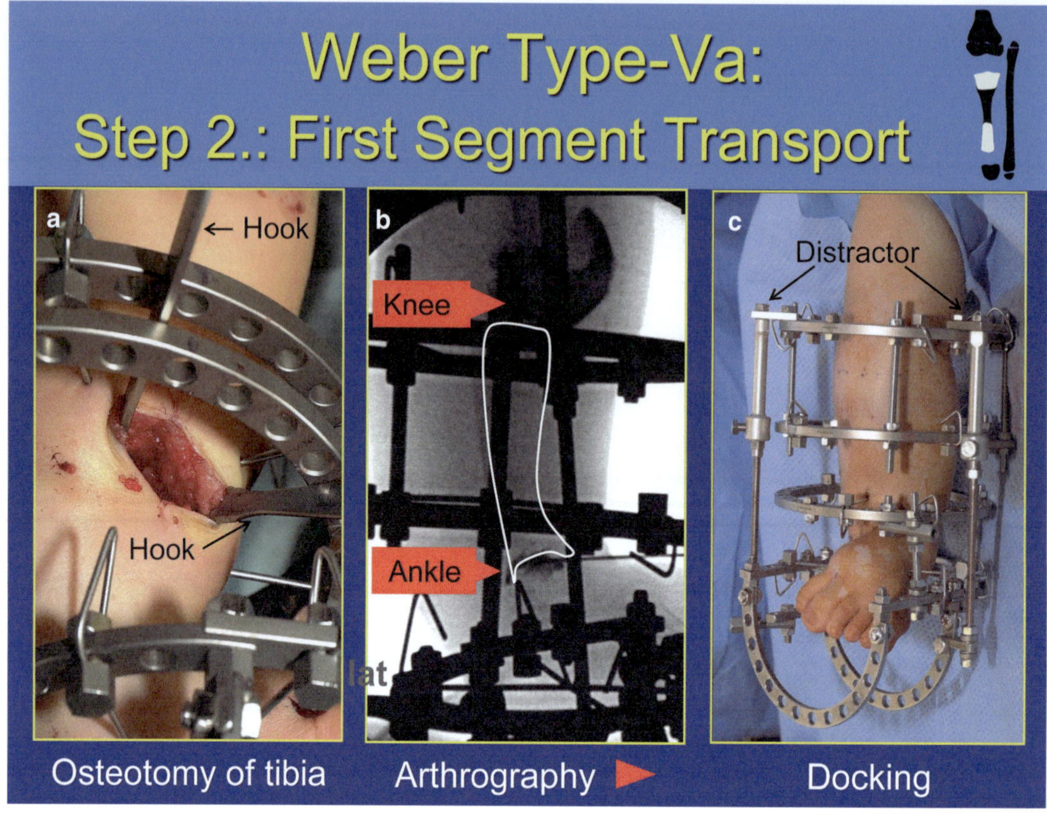

Fig. 15.20 Leg no. 49. Second step of treatment with bifocal bone transport by callus distraction of tibia is performed. (**a**) Osteotomy of tibial bone between the dummy rings. After osteotomy the bifocal bone transport is performed with the dummy rings. The dummy rings are working now as transport ring and are not connected to the rest of fixator. (**b**) Arthrography at knee and ankle shows docking of both segments. (**c**) After docking of tibial segments, the fixator is remounted for further lower leg lengthening. Note that the proximal transport ring is attached to the femoral ring and the distal transport ring is attached to the foot. With this montage luxation of constructed joints can be prevented

and creating ankle joint is the same as described in type IIIb (Figs. 15.14, 15.15, and 15.16).

15.4.12 Type VIIb: Agenesia of the Tibia without Cartilaginous Anlage and Single Fibula

(Figs. 15.29, 15.30, 15.31, 15.32, 15.33, 15.34, 15.35, 15.36, 15.37, 15.38, 15.39, and 15.40)

This type is characterized by a complete absent tibia with or without patella.

The first step is to distract lower leg for transposition of fibula into tibia and centralization of distal fibula to foot. For creating an ankle joint, the same procedure is used as in type IIIb (Figs. 15.14, 15.15, and 15.16).

If a sufficient patella is present, it has to be transformed into a tibial plateau and inserted into the centralized fibular head. The caudally transposition of the patella is performed by transverse double visor flaps of the knee capsule shifted towards each other. Thus, the patella is transformed into a 'tibial plateau' and the fibula into a 'tibia' (Figs. 15.29, 15.30, 15.31, 15.32, 15.33, and 15.34; Weber 2002)

The approach is performed by an S-like skin section beginning proximo-laterally, integrating the scar of the former incision for the preparation of the LCF, crossing the region genu horizontally to the medial side and from this point

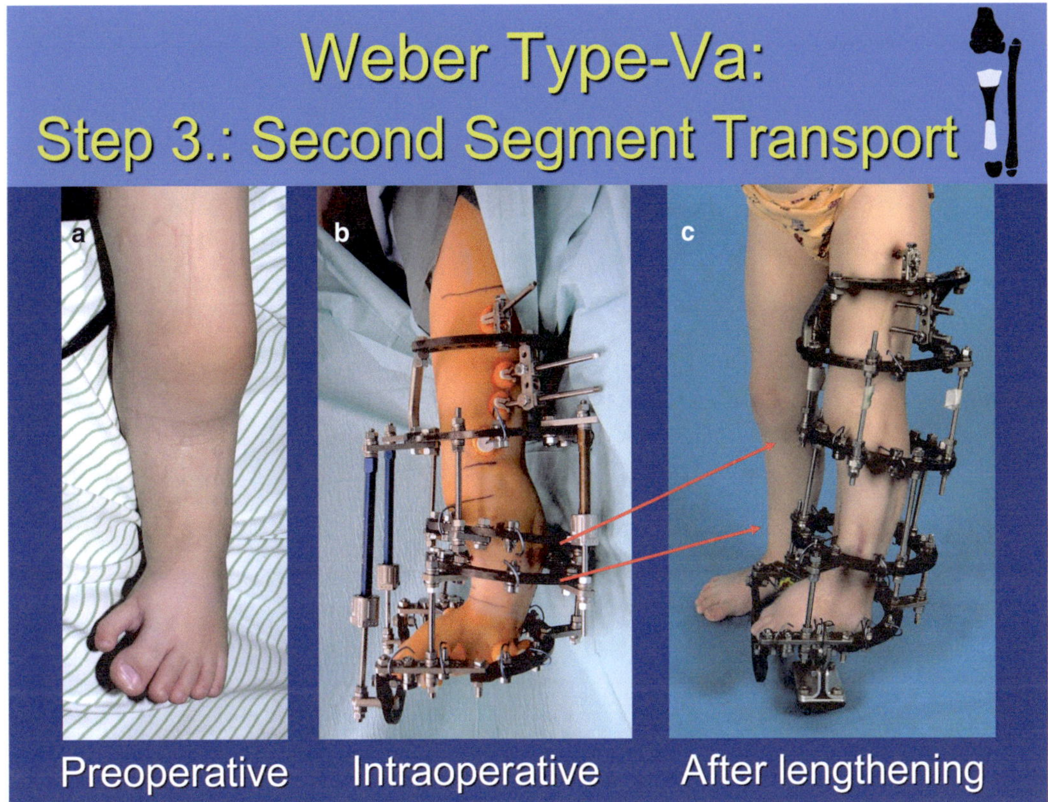

Fig. 15.21 Leg no. 49. Third step of treatment with second bifocal bone transport by callus distraction of tibia is performed, same procedure as first bone transport see Fig. 15.20. (**a**) Leg after first lengthening, the additional sixth ray was amputated later. After the first lengthening, the knee instability, ankle instability and club foot deformity could be solved. (**b**) Montage of maxi-ring fixator for second segment transport of tibia in the same way as in the first transport. (**c**) Leg after stop of lengthening. Note the achieved length between the dummy rings before (in **b**) and after lengthening indicated by *arrows*

disto-medially with a subfascial preparation of the skin. Following this step, the suture augmented LCF is prepared and disconnected from its insertion to the femur. Afterwards, the quadriceps tendon is cut and lengthened in Z-plastic manner. Following this step, the knee joint capsule is incised three times in a horizontal way. The first incision is carried out at the proximal fold of the knee capsule, the second one is made directly at the distal patellar pole and the third incision follows the distal fold of the knee capsule. Thus, two visor flaps are created which are laterally and medially pedicled. The proximal visor flap which includes the patella is shifted distally and the distal visor flap is transposed proximally. The capsule flaps are sutured with one another at the contact points.

As a result of this reversal shifting of the visor flaps, the patella is adjusted under the femoral condyles. When a cruciate ligament plasty should not be performed, the head of the fibula is prepared and rabbet into the centre of the patella at their ventral surface. During this process the perichondrium of the head of the fibula is incised in an H-manner resulting in two door-like perichondrial flaps. In the same way – but rotated 90° – the perichondrium of the patella is centrally incised. The perichondrium and the capsule tissue of fibula and patella, respectively, are sutured together after the cartilage surface of patella and fibula facing each other is cut. Thus, the patella is converted into a 'tibial plateau' and the fibula into a 'tibia' (form follows function).

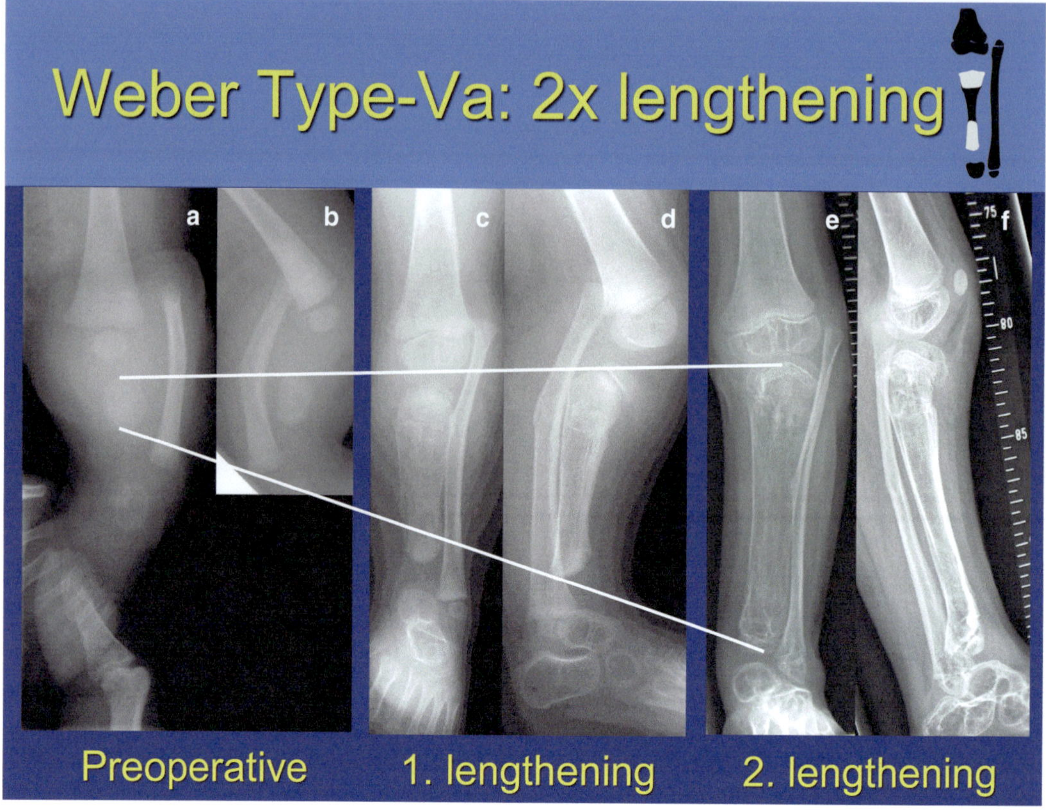

Fig. 15.22 Leg no. 49. X-ray series before lengthening (**a**, **b**), after first lengthening (**c**, **d**) and after second lengthening (**e**, **f**) showing a total lengthening of tibial bone of 400 % (see *white lines*). **a**, **c** and **e** = ap views; **b**, **d** and **f** = lateral views

The fibular epiphysis is secured with a central Ilizarov wire up to the patella to prevent epiphyseolysis. The patella is anchored with a horizontal tangentially oriented Ilizarov wire and integrated into the montage of the lower limb.

By this procedure a chondrodesis is secured. If simultaneously a cruciate ligament plastic using the LCF (or soft tissue structures attached to the head of the fibula, e.g. fascia lata, capsule etc.) is intended, a tunnel is drilled through the centre of the patella and the ligament is leading through the tunnel. At the favoured point of insertion (centrally located between both femoral condyles or in the case of a femoral dysplasia in the centre of the femoral joint surface), a drill hole transepiphyseal through the medial femoral condyle is performed and the LCF (ACL) trans osseous laterally sutured with sufficient tension. The remaining procedure is obtained like the technique without substitution of the cruciate ligament. The tendon of the quadriceps muscle is sutured in Z-plastic manner before closure of arthrotomy and skin. Two hinges are positioned on the ring fixator at the isometric axis of the constructed knee joint. Thus, a mechanical stress of the chondrodesis between fibula and patella is prevented and the newly constructed knee joint is guided.

The LCF can be used as additional anchor for the chondrodesis between the fibula head and patella or as substitution of the cruciate ligament leading out through the patella and transepiphyseal through the femoral condyle.

If a patella is absent (Figs. 15.35, 15.36, 15.37, 15.38, 15.39, and 15.40), the principle of the operation is a transposition of the fibular head to the femoral condyle to induce a hypoplasia of the head of the fibula and to shape a

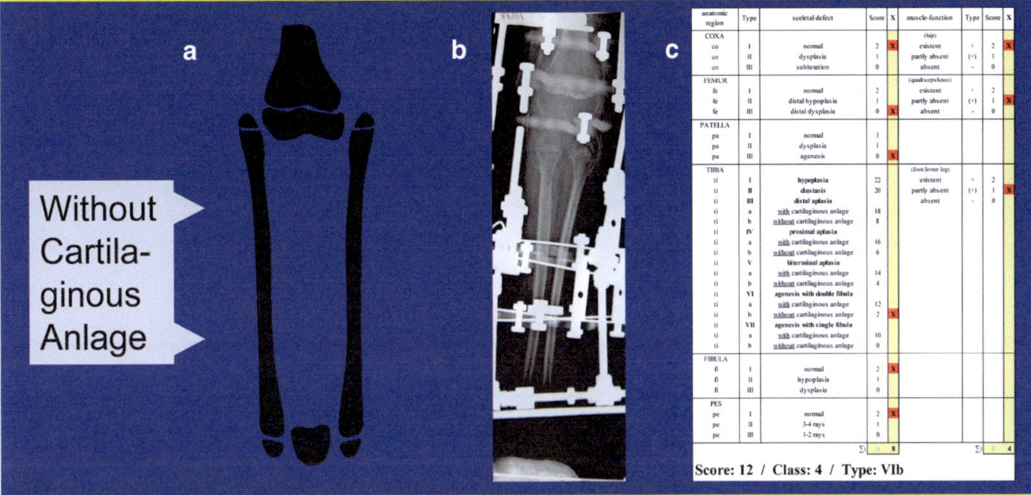

anatomic region	Type	sceletal defect	Score	X	muscle-function	Type	Score	X
COXA					(hip)			
co	I	normal	2	X	existent	+	2	X
co	II	dysplasia	1		partly absent	(+)	1	
co	III	subluxation	0		absent	-	0	
FEMUR					(quadriceps/knee)			
fe	I	normal	2		existent	+	2	
fe	II	distal hypoplasia	1		partly absent	(+)	1	X
fe	III	distal dysplasia	0	X	absent	-	0	
PATELLA								
pa	I	normal	3					
pa	II	dysplasia	1					
pa	III	agenesis	0	X				
TIBIA					(foot/lower leg)			
ti	I	hypoplasia	22		existent	+	2	
ti	II	diastasis	20		partly absent	(+)	1	X
ti	III	distal aplasia			absent	-	0	
ti	a	with cartilaginous anlage	18					
ti	b	without cartilaginous anlage	8					
ti	IV	proximal aplasia						
ti	a	with cartilaginous anlage	16					
ti	b	without cartilaginous anlage	6					
ti	V	biterminal aplasia						
ti	a	with cartilaginous anlage	14					
ti	b	without cartilaginous anlage	4					
ti	VI	agenesis with double fibula						
ti	a	with cartilaginous anlage	12					
ti	b	without cartilaginous anlage	2	X				
ti	VII	agenesis with single fibula						
ti	a	with cartilaginous anlage	10					
ti	b	without cartilaginous anlage	0					
FIBULA								
fi	I	normal	2	X				
fi	II	hypoplasia	1					
fi	III	dysplasia	0					
PES								
pe	I	normal	2	X				
pe	II	3-4 rays	1					
pe	III	1-2 rays	0					
			Σ:	A 8			Σ:	B 4

Fig. 15.23 Leg no. 54. (**a**) Schematic drawing of tibial reduction deficiency Weber type VIb with tibial agenesis and double fibula and without cartilaginous anlage. (**b**) Intraoperative X-ray of right lower leg after centralization of both fibulae and feet. (**c**) Related score of leg (score 12, class 4). No type in the classifications of Jones et al. (1978), Henkel et al. (1978) and Kalamchi and Dawe (1985) available

form of substitution of the tibia plateau (form follows function). A cruciate plasty prevents a dislocation of the fibular head using the LCF or soft tissue structures attached to the fibular head. The foot is transposed to the distal end of the fibula.

If no sufficient patella is present, the principle of the treatment is the same as described for tibia type IVb. The remaining therapy of the ankle joint is the same as described above (Figs. 15.14, 15.15, 15.16, and 15.17).

15.5 Complications

There are many complications reported in the literature, depending on the type and preferred treatment technique. Soft tissue distraction creates great tension on the LCL, which may lead to epiphyseolysis of fibular head. For prevention of epiphyseolysis, LCL has to be detached from femoral insertion and prepared until fibular head insertion before distraction. The LCL can be augmented with suture along the pedicles to avoid unwanted soft tissue fusion and to relieve re-preparation. It is not possible to recognize growth plate orientation before maturation of the growth plates. Secondary deformities may develop, requiring corrective osteotomies. Failed centralization of the foot or improperly used orthesis may lead to luxation. Then, re-centralization and malleolus plasty have to be performed. Intensive physiotherapy is essential. Noncompliance may require reapplication of the frame for joint contractures. Growth plate arrest is a known complication of joint spanning frames.

To avoid it, frame has to be loosened every 6 weeks to relieve the resulting growth tension. Anatomical peculiarities like atypical alignment of both the soft tissues and tendons and fusions of the knee capsule with adjacent cartilaginous tissues are the additional factors complicating surgery.

The many complications arising in conservative treatments (orthoprosthesis care) as there are inappropriate application and indication with loss of precious time for constructive operative techniques as well as the presentation of complications following amputations will not be discussed in this overview.

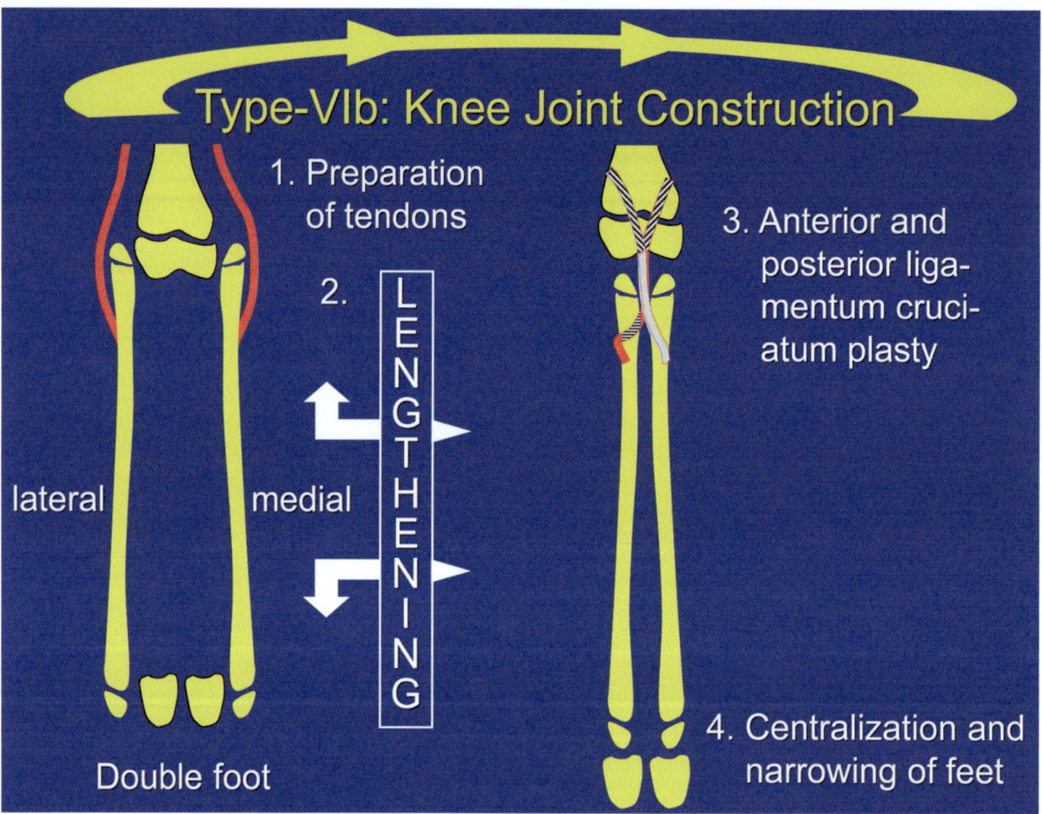

Fig. 15.24 Leg no. 54. Schematic drawing shows operational procedure for treatment of tibial reduction deficiency Weber type VIb. (*1*) Preparation of LCF with detachment of the femoral insertion. (*2*) Soft tissue lengthening at knee and foot level as preparation for centralization. (*3*) Transformation of LCFs into anterior and posterior cruciatum ligaments after transforming fibulae into tibia. (*4*) Centralization and narrowing of foot. Due to the complexity of narrowing and fusion of a double foot, it can be recommended to do this surgery as the first step

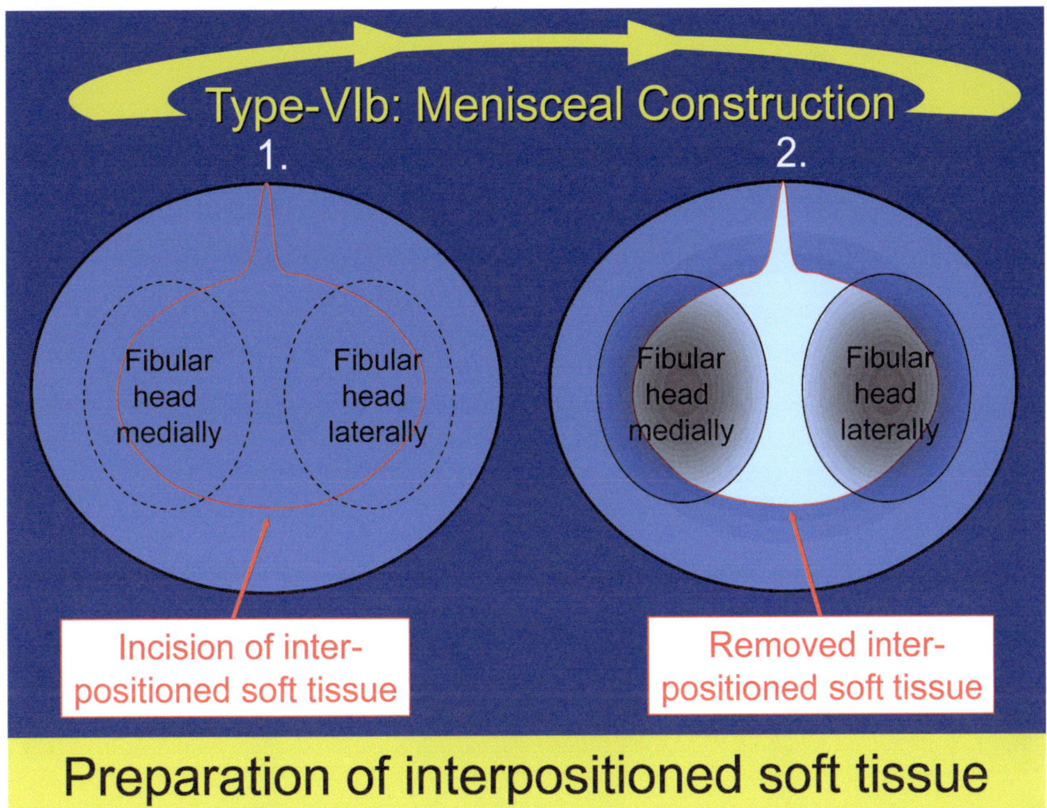

Fig. 15.25 Leg no. 54. Schematic drawing shows meniscal construction by shaping of the intracapsular soft tissue of knee. (*1*) Circular incision of the interpositioned tissue (*light blue*) between fibular heads and femoral condyles (*red circle*). (*2*) Constructed medial and lateral meniscus, which are connected posteriorly

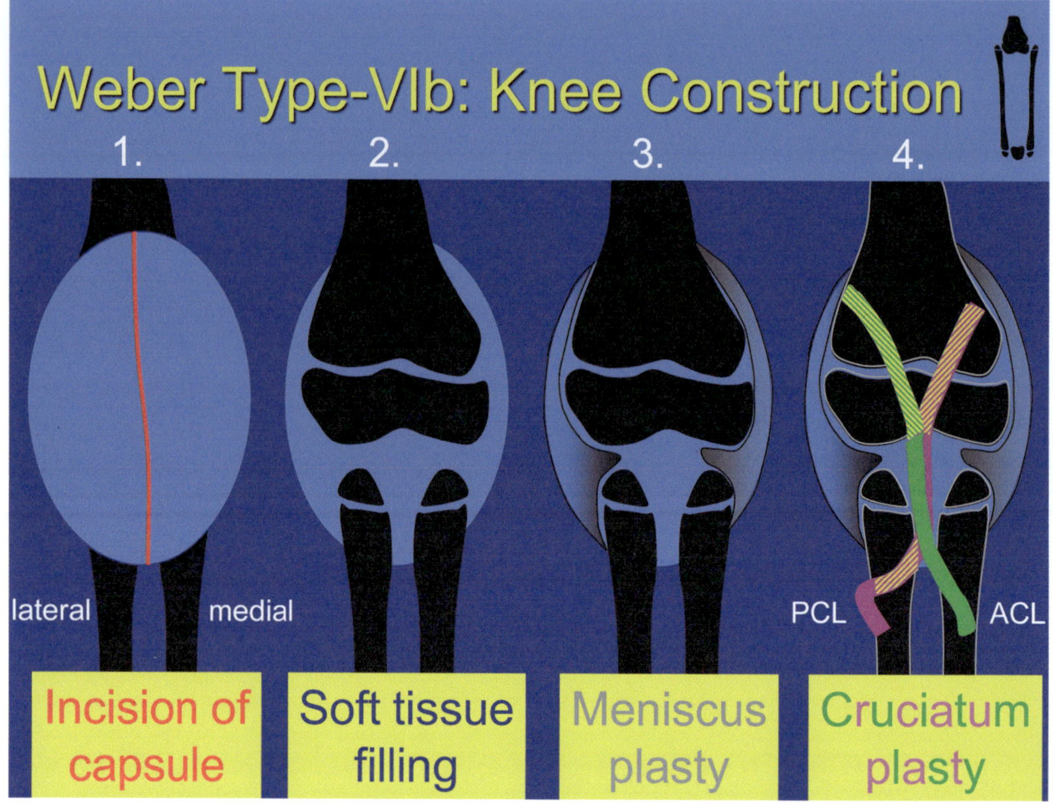

Fig. 15.26 Leg no. 54. The schematic drawing shows the different steps of knee joint construction. (*1*) Incision of knee capsule. (*2*) Identification of intracapsular soft tissue filling. (*3*) Construction of medial and lateral meniscus by shaping of the intracapsular soft tissue. (*4*) Construction of ACL (*green*) and PCL (*pink*) by using the LCF of each fibula (*hatched lines* = intraosseus course of ligaments). The PCL is leaded posterior of the lateral fibula through the knee joint into the medial femoral drill hole. The ACL is leaded anterior of the medial fibula through the knee joint into the lateral femoral drill hole

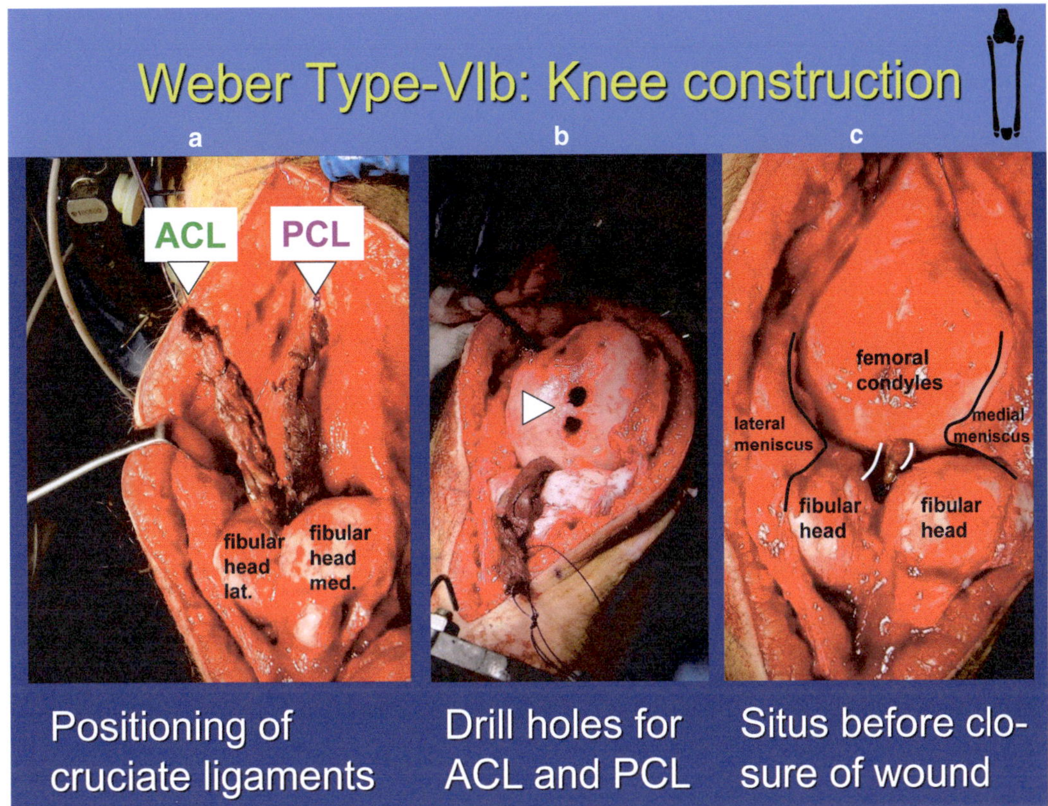

Fig. 15.27 Leg no. 54. Intraoperative pictures of knee construction. (**a**) Positioning of ACL and PCL between both fibular heads. (**b**) Drill holes (*arrow*) for the ACL and PCL at femoral condyles. (**c**) Operative situs after knee joint construction before closure of wound

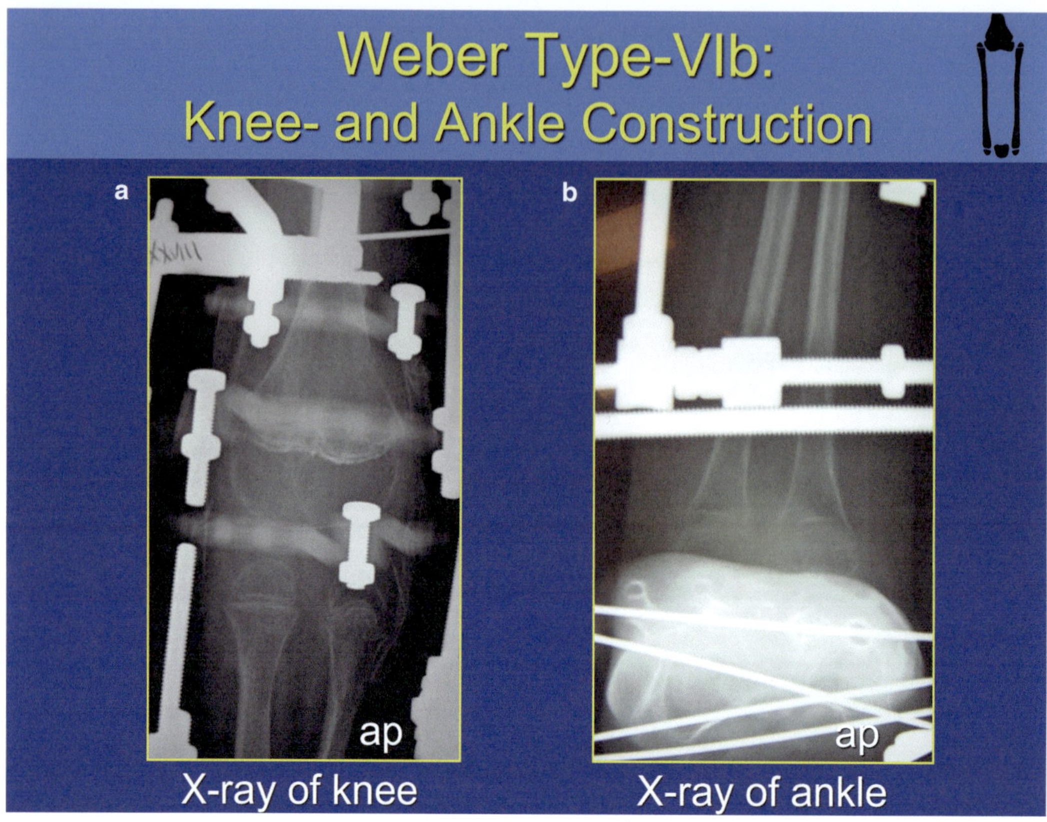

Fig. 15.28 Leg no. 54. Postoperative X-rays of constructed knee joint (**a**) and ankle (**b**)

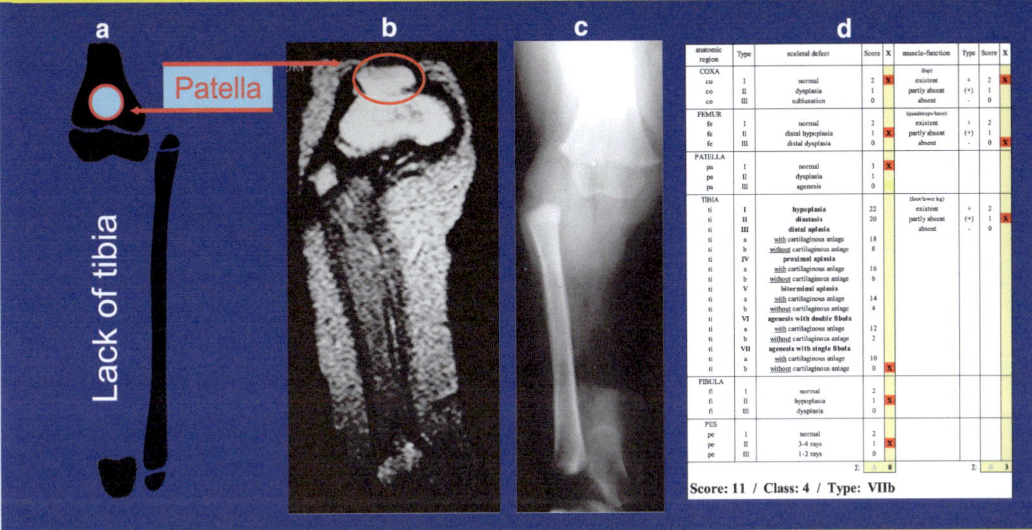

anatomic region	Type	sceletal defect	Score	X	muscle-function	Type	Score	X
COXA					(hip)			
co	I	normal	2	X	existent	+	2	X
co	II	dysplasia	1		partly absent	(+)	1	
co	III	subluxation	0		absent	-	0	
FEMUR					(quadriceps/knee)			
fe	I	normal	2		existent	+	2	
fe	II	distal hypoplasia	1	X	partly absent	(+)	1	
fe	III	distal dysplasia	0		absent	-	0	X
PATELLA								
pa	I	normal	3	X				
pa	II	dysplasia	1					
pa	III	agenesis	0					
TIBIA					(foot/lower leg)			
ti	I	hypoplasia	22		existent	+	2	
ti	II	diastasis	20		partly absent	(+)	1	X
ti	III	distal aplasia			absent	-	0	
ti	a	with cartilaginous anlage	18					
ti	b	without cartilaginous anlage	8					
ti	IV	proximal aplasia						
ti	a	with cartilaginous anlage	16					
ti	b	without cartilaginous anlage	6					
ti	V	biterminal aplasia						
ti	a	with cartilaginous anlage	14					
ti	b	without cartilaginous anlage	4					
ti	VI	agenesis with double fibula						
ti	a	with cartilaginous anlage	12					
ti	b	without cartilaginous anlage	2					
ti	VII	agenesis with single fibula						
ti	a	with cartilaginous anlage	10					
ti	b	without cartilaginous anlage	0	X				
FIBULA								
fi	I	normal	2					
fi	II	hypoplasia	1	X				
fi	III	dysplasia	0					
PES								
pe	I	normal	2					
pe	II	3-4 rays	1	X				
pe	III	1-2 rays	0					
			Σ	A 8			Σ	B 3

Score: 11 / Class: 4 / Type: VIIb

Fig. 15.29 Leg no. 57. (**a**) Schematic drawing of tibial reduction deficiency Weber type VIIb with patella. (**b**) MRI of right lower leg shows fibula and the patella (*red circle*) which has the important role in knee construction. (**c**) X-ray of lower leg with luxated foot and over length of fibula due to impaction into thigh soft tissue. (**d**) Related score of leg (score: 11, class: 4). Due to the existing patella and the utmost benefit for knee construction belongs this type still to class 4 and not to class 5

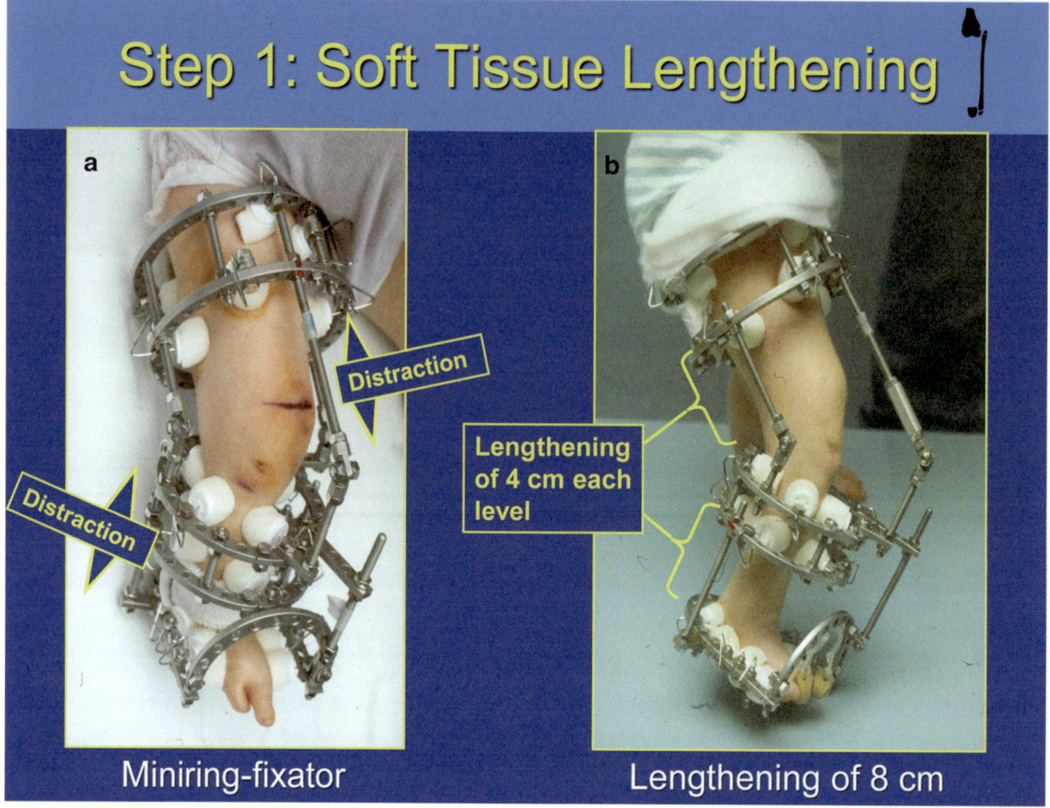

Fig. 15.30 Leg no. 57. First step of treatment is a soft tissue lengthening after Achilles tendon lengthening and detachment of LCF at its femoral insertion, as precondition for centralization of fibula under femoral condyles and foot under fibular end distally. See schematic drawing in Fig. 15.37. (**a**, **b**) The mini-ring fixator should be applied in a way that the knee and ankle region is free for further surgical approaches according knee and ankle construction

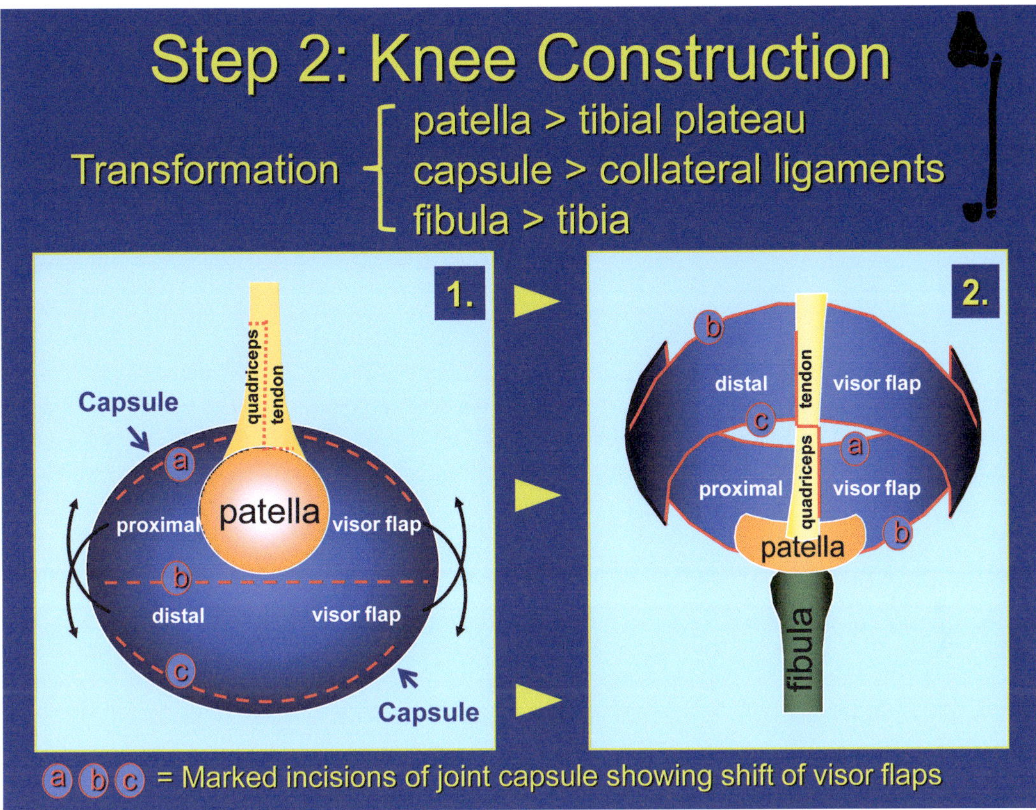

Fig. 15.31 Leg no. 57. In the second step, the knee arthroplasty is performed (Weber 2002). Schematic drawing of knee construction transforming patella into tibial plateau, the knee capsule – beside its original function – into collateral ligaments and the fibula into tibia. (*1*) Drawing of the incisions (*red dotted lines a, b, c*) into capsule (*blue circle*) required for creation of two visor flaps based medially and laterally. The quadriceps tendon is lengthened in Z-plastic manner and sutured end to end after visor flaps shift. (*2*) In order to bring the patella into the position of a tibial plateau, the visor flaps has to be crossed contra rotating and sutured. The patella is fusioned to the fibular head by chondrodesis (see Fig. 15.33)

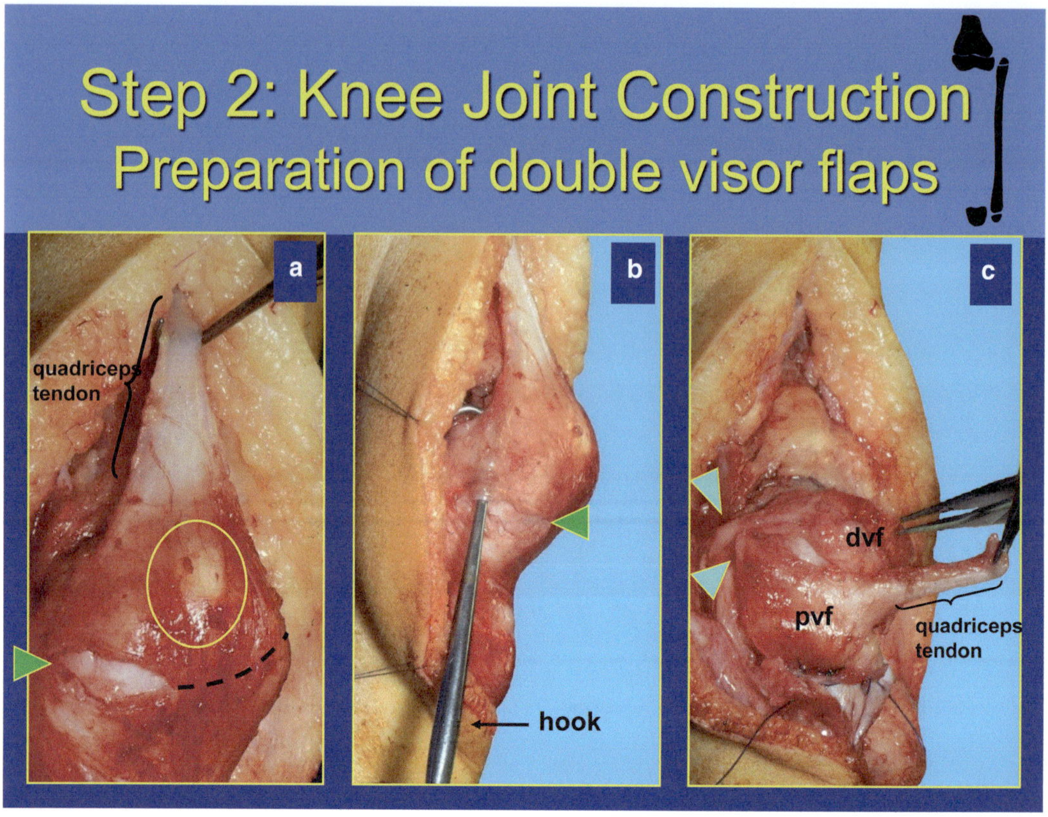

Fig. 15.32 Leg no. 57. Step 2: Intraoperative pictures of performing the knee construction. (**a**) Preparation of quadriceps tendon for Z-plastic. Start of intermediate incision (*green arrow*) under the patella which has to be continued (*dotted line*). The *yellow circle* marks the patella. (**b**) The hook is inserted under the pedicle of the proximal visor flap laterally. The pedicles of the visor flaps guarantee the blood supply and the collateral stability of the transformed patella into tibial plateau. The *green arrow* marks the middle incision. (**c**) Situs after completed visor flap shifts. The distal visor flap (*dvf*) is shifted proximally and the proximal visor flap (*pvf*) with the patella included distally. The *arrows* indicate the crossing over of the flap pedicles

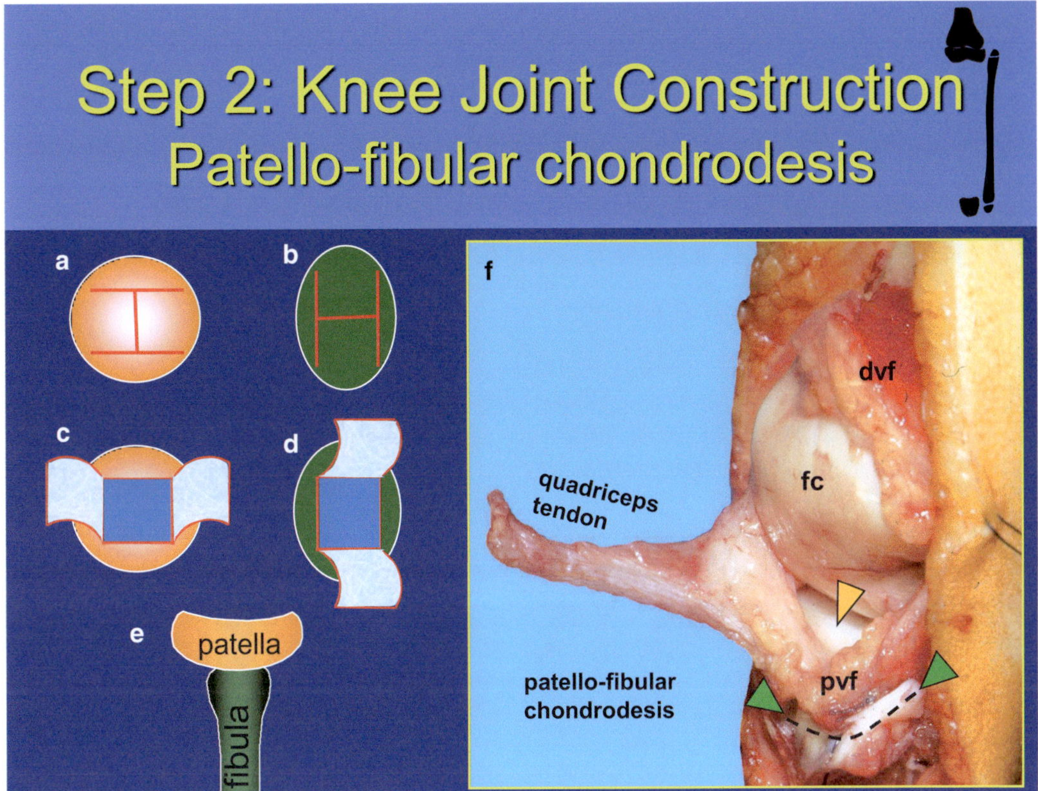

Fig. 15.33 Leg no. 57. Step 2: (**a–e**) Schematic drawing of chondrodesis between fibular head and patellar surface, *orange* = patella, *green* = fibula. (**a**, **b**) Contra rotating (90°) H-like incision of perichondrium of patella and fibula. (**c**, **d**) Double door-like preparation of perichondrial flaps. *Light blue fields* are representing the opened cartilage tissue. (**e**) Chondrodesis between fibular head and centre of patella after suturing of the perichondrial flaps of patella to the fibula and the perichondrial flaps of the fibula to the patella. (**f**) Situs after visor flap shifts with patella-fibular chondrodesis (*green arrows* and *dotted line*). The *yellow arrow* indicates the patellar joint surface working now as tibial plateau. *dvf* distal visor flap, *pvf* proximal visor flap and *fc* femoral condyles

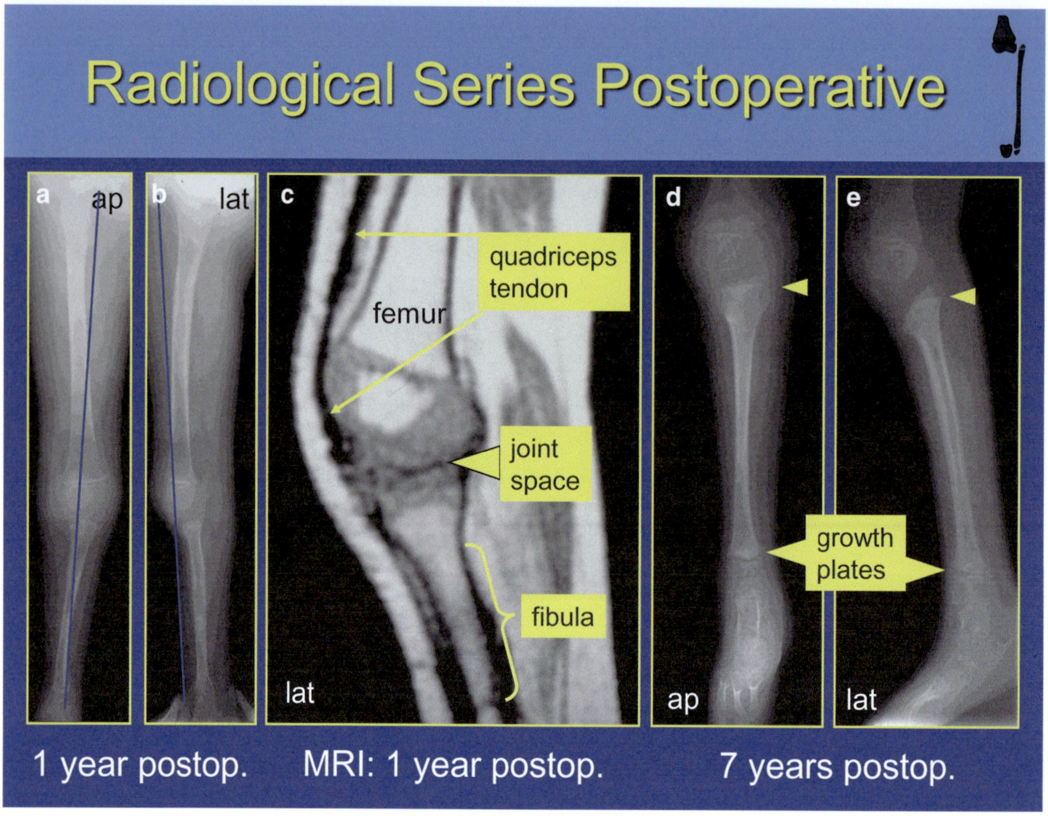

Fig. 15.34 Leg no. 57. Postoperative radiological series shows the results after performing the knee and ankle construction and after transformation of fibula into tibia. (**a, b**) X-rays, 1 year postoperative, demonstrating correct axis in both views and a severe hyperplasia of transformed fibula (form follows function). (**c**) MRI, 1 year after surgical procedure, demonstrating successful knee joint construction with complete fusion between fibular head and patella, clear joint space and insertion of quadriceps tendon into tibial plateau (former patella). (**d, e**) X-rays, 7 years after surgical procedure, demonstrating massive hyperplasia of former fibula, open epiphyseal growth plates (*arrows*) and building of metaphysis proximally and distally

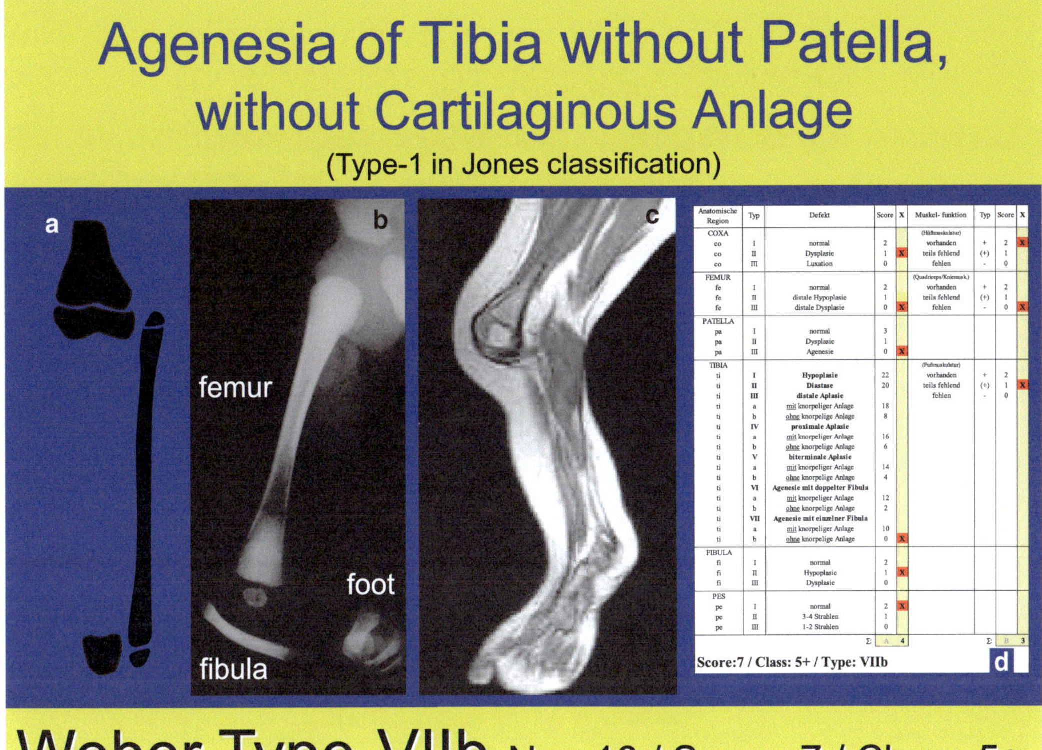

Anatomische Region	Typ	Defekt	Score	X	Muskel- funktion	Typ	Score	X
COXA					(Hüftmuskulatur)			
co	I	normal	2		vorhanden	+	2	X
co	II	Dysplasie	1	X	teils fehlend	(+)	1	
co	III	Luxation	0		fehlen	-	0	
FEMUR					(Quadriceps/Kniemusk.)			
fe	I	normal	2		vorhanden	+	2	
fe	II	distale Hypoplasie	1		teils fehlend	(+)	1	
fe	III	distale Dysplasie	0	X	fehlen	-	0	X
PATELLA								
pa	I	normal	3					
pa	II	Dysplasie	1					
pa	III	Agenesie	0	X				
TIBIA					(Fußmuskulatur)			
ti	I	Hypoplasie	22		vorhanden	+	2	
ti	II	Diastase	20		teils fehlend	(+)	1	X
ti	III	distale Aplasie			fehlen	-	0	
ti	a	mit knorpeliger Anlage	18					
ti	b	ohne knorpelige Anlage	8					
ti	IV	proximale Aplasie						
ti	a	mit knorpeliger Anlage	16					
ti	b	ohne knorpelige Anlage	6					
ti	V	biterminale Aplasie						
ti	a	mit knorpeliger Anlage	14					
ti	b	ohne knorpelige Anlage	4					
ti	VI	Agenesie mit doppelter Fibula						
ti	a	mit knorpeliger Anlage	12					
ti	b	ohne knorpelige Anlage	2					
ti	VII	Agenesie mit einzelner Fibula						
ti	a	mit knorpeliger Anlage	10					
ti	b	ohne knorpelige Anlage	0	X				
FIBULA								
fi	I	normal	2					
fi	II	Hypoplasie	1	X				
fi	III	Dysplasie	0					
PES								
pe	I	normal	2	X				
pe	II	3-4 Strahlen	1					
pe	III	1-2 Strahlen	0					
			Σ A	4			Σ B	3

Score:7 / Class: 5+ / Type: VIIb   **d**

Fig. 15.35 Leg no. 16. (**a**) Schematic drawing of tibial reduction deficiency Weber type VIIb without patella. (**b**) X-ray of right lower leg with transverse fibula and luxated foot. (**c**) MRI of right lower leg shows fibula and no patella. (**d**) Related score of leg (score: 7, class: 5+)

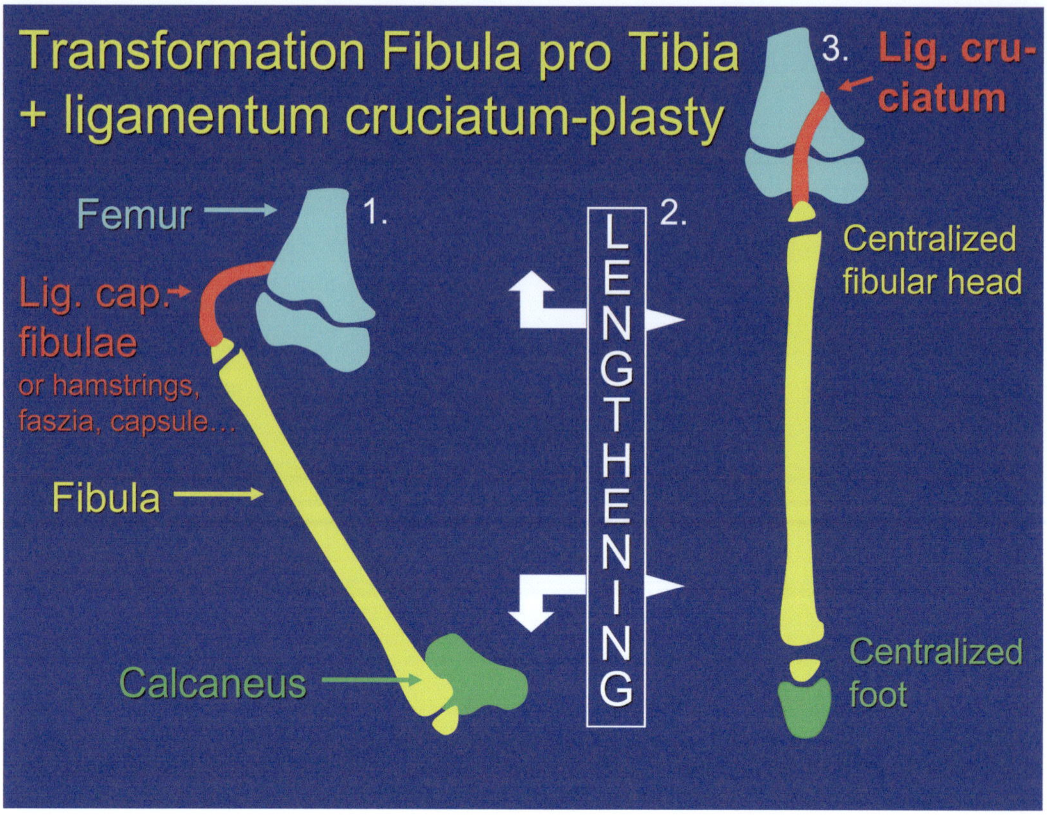

Fig. 15.36 Leg no. 16. Schematic drawing of operational procedure for treatment of tibial reduction defect Weber type VIIb without patella. (*1*) Situation before operation with luxation of fibula and foot and preparation of the ligamentum capitis fibulae (LCF) for use as ligamentum cruciatum. (*2*) Soft tissue lengthening at knee and ankle level for preparation of fibular centralization under femoral condyles and foot under distal fibula. (*3*) Situation after transformation of fibula into tibia, LCF into ACL and centralization of foot with bilaterally fibular periosteal flaps for stabilization (see Figs. 15.14, 15.15, and 15.16)

Fig. 15.37 Leg no. 16. X-rays before surgery. (**a**) Total lack of tibia without patella bilaterally and luxated club feet. (**b**) Lateral view of right lower leg

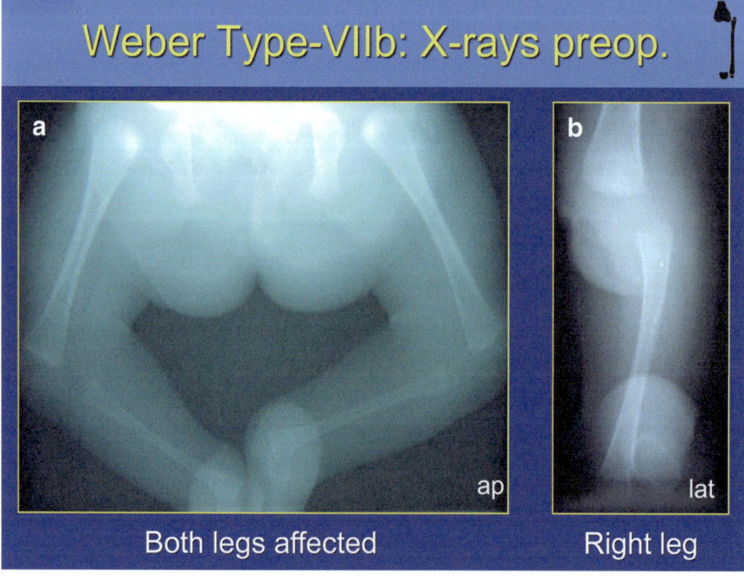

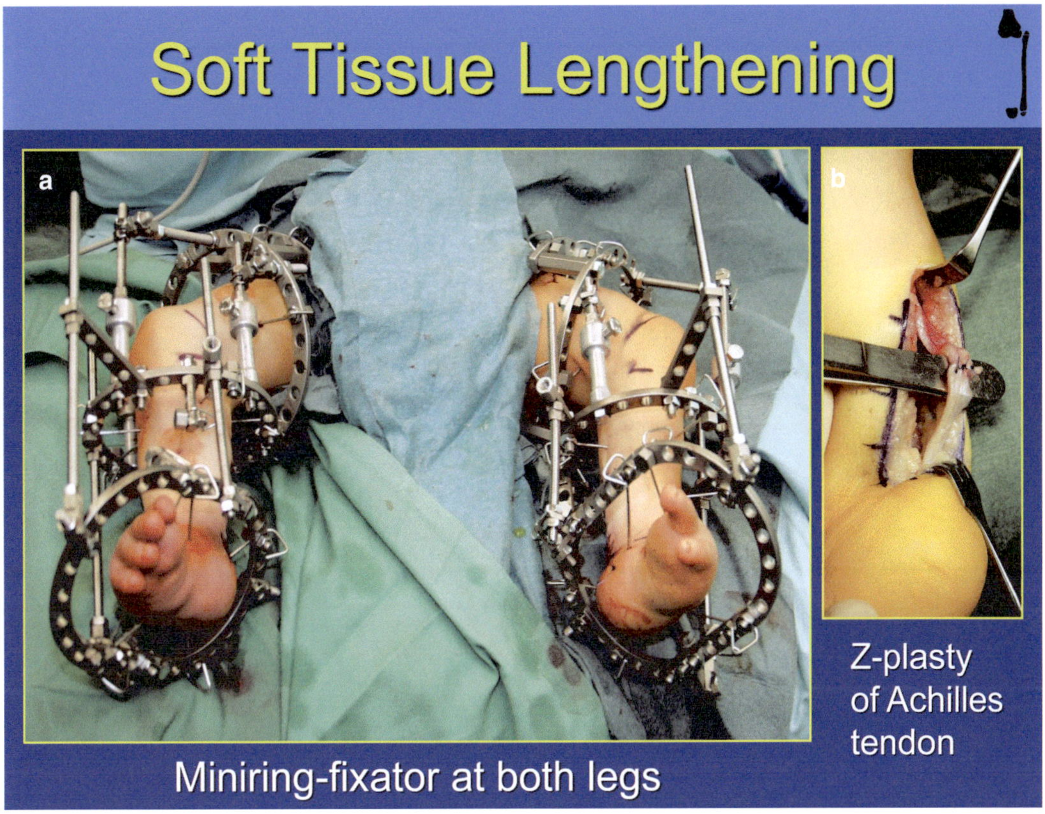

Fig. 15.38 Leg no. 16. (**a**) Intraoperative picture after application of mini-ring fixators bilaterally for soft tissue lengthening as preparation of fibular transformation into tibia and correction of club feet. (**b**) Z-plasty of Achilles tendon

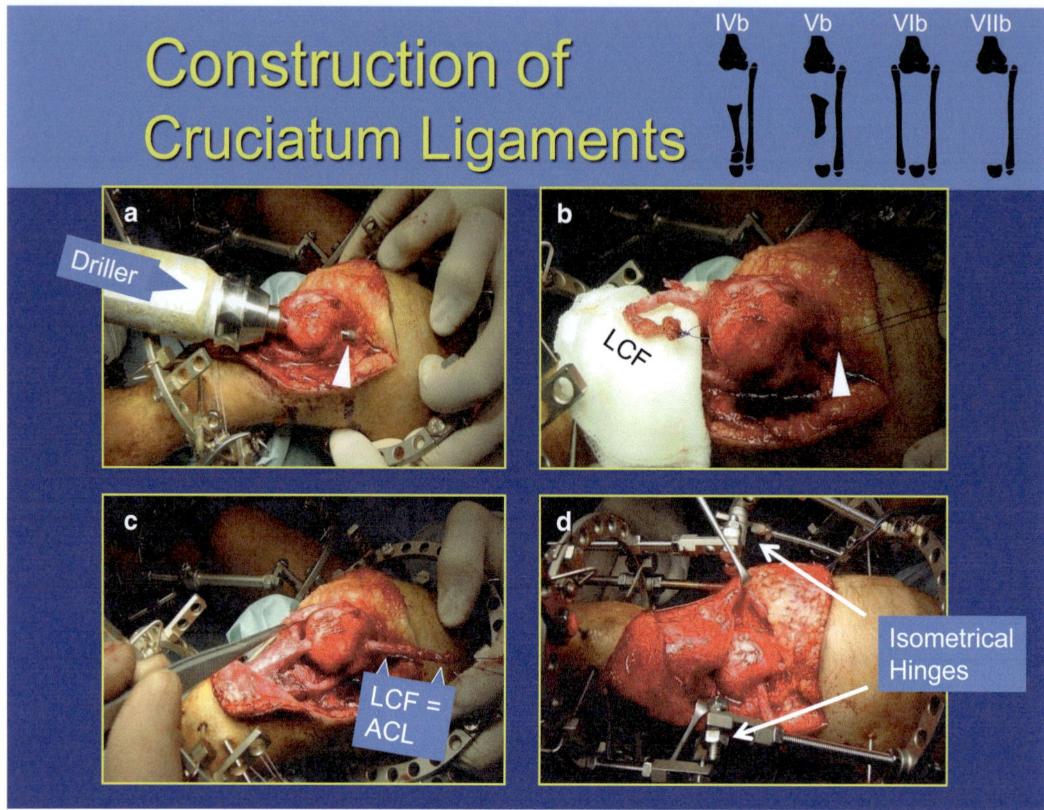

Fig. 15.39 Leg no. 16. Technique of cruciatum plasty in four steps (**a–d**). (**a**) Drilling of a transepiphyseal tunnel from the apex of the dysplastic distal femoral epiphysis to the lateral aspect of the femur is performed (the *arrow* indicates the apex of the diamond hollow driller). (**b**) The LCF is prepared for pulling through the tunnel by attached suture (*arrows*). (**c**) The LCF is pulled through the drill hole. Isometrical mechanical hinges (see **d**) are mounted to keep the position in place. For detection of isometrical position, the LCF can be used. If no movement of the LCF can be detected after extension and flexion of knee joint, the hinges are correctly positioned. (**d**) After correct application of the hinges, the LCF is fixed at the femur and working now as ACL

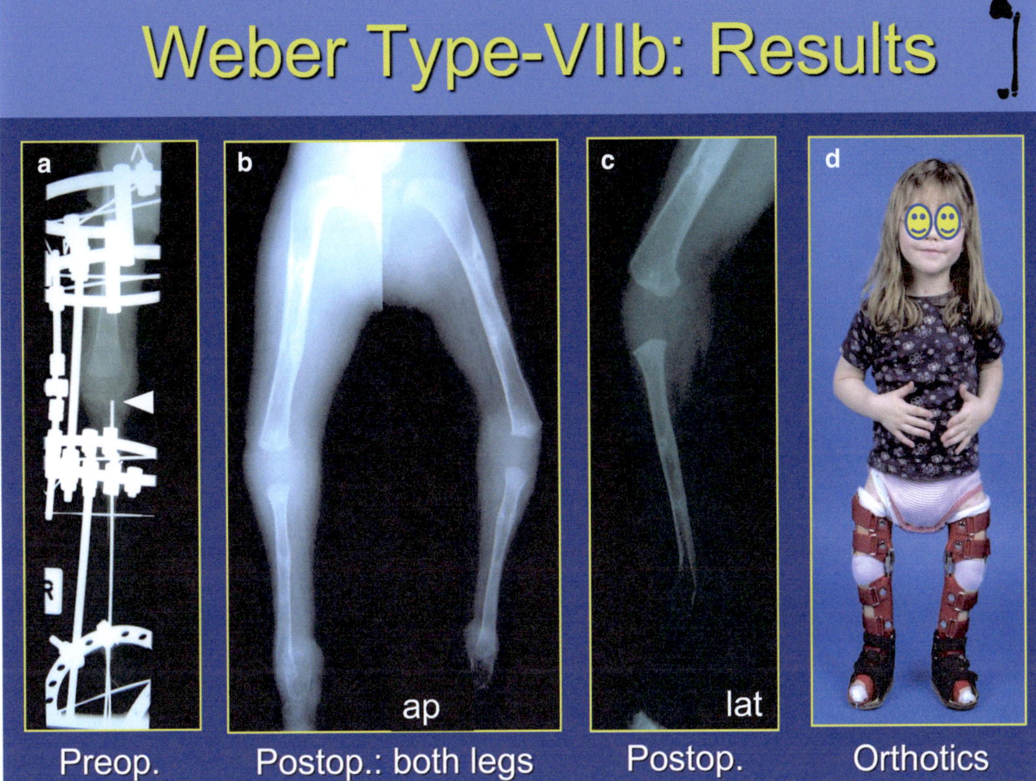

Fig. 15.40 Leg no. 16. (**a**) Postoperative X-ray. Note the axial wire of the fibula protecting against epiphyseal dislocation. (**b**, **c**) X-rays show hyperplasia of fibula and developing of metaphysis at fibular ends. (**d**) The 6-year-old girl is able to walk with orthotics bilaterally without use of crutches. The ROM of knee joints is limited especially in comparison to cases where the patella can be transformed into tibial plateau

References

Brown FW (1971) The Brown operation for total hemimelia tibia. In: Aitken GT (ed) Selected lower-limb anomalies. National Academy of Sciences, Washington, pp 20–28

Henkel HL, Willert HG, Gressmann C (1978) Eine internationale Terminologie zur Klassifikation angeborener Gliedmassenfehlbildungen. Arch Orthop Trauma Surg 93:1–19

Jones D, Barnes J, Lloyd-Roberts G (1978) Congenital aplasia and dysplasia of the tibia with intact fibula. Classification and management. J Bone Joint Surg Br 60:31–39

Kalamchi A, Dawe R (1985) Congenital deficiency of the tibia. J Bone Joint Surg Br Vol 67:581–584

Spranger S, Weber M, Tröger J, Tariverdian G, Opitz JM (1996) Bilateral radial deficiency with lower limb involvement. Am J Med Genet 63:193–197

Weber M (2002) A new knee arthroplasty versus Brown's procedure in congenital total absence of the tibia: a preliminary report. J Pediatr Orthop B 11: 53–59

Weber M (2007) Congenital leg deformities: tibial hemimelia. In: Rozbruch SR, Ilizarov S (eds) Limb lengthening and reconstructive surgery. Informa Healthcare, New York, pp 429–447

Weber M (2008) New classification and score for tibial hemimelia. J Child Orthop 2:169–175

Weber M, Siebert CH, Goost H, Johannisson R, Wirtz D (2002) Malleolus externus plasty for joint reconstruction in fibular aplasia: preliminary report of a new technique. J Pediatr Orthop B 11:1–11

Weber M, Schröder S, Berdel P, Niethard FU (2005) Register zur bundesweiten Erfassung angeborener Gliedmaßenfehlbildungen. Z Orthop 143:1–5

Austin T. Fragomen and S. Robert Rozbruch

Contents

A.T. Fragomen, MD (✉) • S.R. Rozbruch, MD
Limb Lengthening and Complex Reconstruction
Service, Hospital for Special Surgery, Weill Medical
College of Cornell University, New York, NY, USA
e-mail: fragomena@hss.edu; rozbruchsr@hss.edu

16.1 Introduction

Ankle distraction arthroplasty has been gaining popularity internationally as an alternative to fusion and prosthetic arthroplasty for the treatment of ankle arthritis. Many authors have reported success using this technique with improvement in functional outcome scores (Van Valburg et al. 1995, 1999; Saltzman and Buckwalter 1999; van Roermund et al. 2002; Marijnissen et al. 2002, 2003; Ploegmakers et al. 2005; Paley and Lamm 2005; Paley et al. 2008; Tellisi et al. 2009; Intema et al. 2011). Those that have seen positive clinical effects presume that there is a biological explanation behind these successes. It is known that mechanical loading of arthritic joints will lead to sclerosis and abnormal remodeling of the of subchondral bone (Arokoski et al. 2000; Lajeunesse 2004; Brandt et al. 2009). Further loading of the abnormal subchondral bone leads to increased damage of the underlying articular cartilage (Radin and Rose 1986). Many have postulated that unloading the joint will reverse the sclerosis of the subchondral bone, protect the remaining cartilage, and even allow for cartilage repair (Buckwalter and Mankin 1998; Saltzman and Buckwalter 1999). Adequate joint distraction directly unloads the mechanical stress from the arthritic joint (Fragomen et al., presented LLRS 2011). With the joint distracted, the repair process can then progress uninhibited by compressive forces normally present between the joint surfaces. Distraction also allows for intermittent pistonning within the joint during ambulation. This pistonning then creates intermittent joint fluid pressure that in turn stimulates the regenerating articular cartilage (Van Valburg et al. 1998). Most surgeons feel that joint distraction reduces pain through multiple processes. These include a change in subchondral sclerosis and a degree of articular cartilage reparative activity. Animal data has supported this contention and has even demonstrated hyaline cartilage formation in response to distraction (Kajiwara et al. 2005). Marijnissen et al. (2001) found modest increases in joint space and decrease in subchondral sclerosis seen in all postoperative x-rays. Recent studies also support the effects of distraction on subchondral and articular surface remodeling. Twenty-six patients undergoing ankle distraction arthroplasty for posttraumatic arthritis were evaluated preoperatively and at 1–2 years post surgery with CT and ankle arthritis scores. Clinical improvement was directly correlated with CT changes that demonstrated the disappearance of cystic areas originally present in the subchondral bone (Intema et al. 2011). Another study confirmed these findings and added further insight into joint changes induced by distraction. In an MR evaluation of pre- and post-op ankle distraction patients, authors found, consistently, that there was a decrease in subchondral bone thickness by 0.5 mm, an increase in joint space by 0.5 mm, and a decrease in the number and size of subchondral bone cysts after distraction treatment (Lamm and Gourdine-Shaw 2009).

16.2 Clinical Experience

We published a retrospective review of 25 patients who underwent ankle distraction from 1999 to 2006 (Tellisi et al. 2009). The mean patient age was 37.6 years: 16 male/7 female. Follow-up was 30-month post-frame removal (range 12–60 months). We were able to obtain follow-up on 23/25 patients. Adjuvant procedures were performed in some cases including Achilles tendon lengthening (5), ankle arthroscopy (4), open arthrotomy (1), and supramalleo-

lar tibial and distal fibular osteotomy to correct distal tibial deformity (6). Twenty-one patients (91 %) reported improved pain relief with those furthest post-ops experiencing the best results. Seventeen of twenty-three patients had significant improvement in pain and functional scores indicating a 74 % success rate. The average preoperative AOFAS score was 55 (range 29–82), and the average postoperative score was 74 (range 47–96). The difference between preoperative and postoperative scores was significant ($p = .005$). SF-36 scores showed modest improvement in all components. When the scores were analyzed for age, there was no significant difference between age groups, although the patients older than 60 trended toward greater improvement than younger patients. Two patients in the study went on to ankle fusion at last follow-up. Total ankle motion was maintained in all patients with improvement in the functional arc of motion in five patients who started with mild equinus contractures. Our clinical results are similar to those reported in the literature (Table 16.1). We feel that ankle distraction offers a promising solution for many people with ankle arthritis.

16.3 Surgical Technique

16.3.1 Overview

There are various techniques used to perform ankle distraction arthroplasty. Van Valburg et al. (1995) introduced the classic method using two tibial rings attached to the leg with two tensioned wires per ring. The foot ring was attached with four tensioned wires. This was a static external fixator (it has no hinges) with four rigid connections across the ankle joint. Distraction of 5 mm was performed gradually at 1 mm per day. Dutch authors also leave the external fixator in place for a minimum of 3 months but often more than 4 months (Van Valburg et al. 1995, 1999). The technique we use at our institute differs in many aspects. We use a streamlined external fixator (RAD frame, Small Bone Innovations, Morrisville, PA) with minimal points of fixation. The fixator is articulated allowing free range of motion at the

Table 16.1 Outcomes of ankle distraction arthroplasty

Author	Year	N (patients)	Good results (%)	Conclusion
Van Valburg et al.	1995	11	100	50 % increased joint space
Van Valburg et al.	1999	17	76	2 years to see benefits
Marijnissen et al.	2002	57	75	1 year to see benefits Randomized study favors DA
Ploegmakers et al.	2005	22	73	Good results at >7 year F/U
Paley et al.	2008	32	67	Recommend adjuvant procedures
Tellisi et al.	2009	25	74	91 % had some pain relief Hinged distraction preserves ankle ROM Patients >60 years old had good results
Lamm and Gourdine-Shaw	2009	3		MR showed increased joint space and decrease in subchondral cysts
Intema et al.	2011	26		Disappearance of subchondral cysts directly related to good clinical result

DA distraction arthroplasty, *ROM* range of motion

ankle joint. Like other authors, we recommend adjuvant procedures at the time of frame application, if indicated (Paley et al. 2008; Lamm and Gourdine-Shaw 2009). These include arthrotomy for osteophyte resection and microfracture, Achilles tendon lengthening, and supramalleolar osteotomy for malalignment. Ankle distraction is applied acutely in the operating room. Ankle range of motion starts early in the postoperative period. The frame is worn for a minimum of 10 weeks.

16.3.2 Preoperative Evaluation

Preoperative workup includes an alignment and mobility exam. Weight-bearing x-rays are used to establish the degree of arthritis and quantify malalignment. Osteophytes are also identified. MR is often used to recognize the location and degree of cartilage thinning and to localize subchondral cysts. The subtalar joint condition should also be evaluated to distinguish any contribution to the patient's overall pain.

A good candidate for ankle distraction includes any patient who has ankle arthritis and some meaningful joint mobility. Most patients are self-selected in that they have been offered ankle fusion and have forcefully refused arthrodesis. These patients want to maintain their ankle motion and decrease their pain, goals that ankle distraction can obtain. We have not identified, with significance, which patients are more likely to improve. An unpublished review was performed on our patients who achieved the most improvement in AOFAS scores after the distraction procedure. Pre- and postsurgical MR scans in these patients illuminated certain trends: these top-performing patients were between 30 and 40 years of age, had more intra-articular cartilage on pre-op MR scans, and had more mobility in the ankle joint presurgery. All of their MR scans demonstrated increases in joint space and disappearance of subchondral cysts consistent with previous studies (Lamm and Gourdine-Shaw 2009). Perhaps younger patients with more mobility and less arthritis are the ideal candidates, but our clinical series (Tellisi et al. 2009) indicated that patients over 60 years old fared best. Based on these findings, we do not use age, degree of arthritis, or absolute motion as inclusion criteria.

Contraindications are relative and include inflammatory arthritis, severe tibiotalar stiffness, and abnormal joint geometry. Our experience with rheumatoid arthritis (RA) has yielded a high failure rate with most patients requiring ankle fusion. RA is not a mechanical disease so it stands to reason that removing stress is not helpful. Patients who have severe stiffness of the ankle joint effectively have a fused ankle. They are wearing out the adjacent joints but continue to have tibiotalar joint pain. Ankle fusion will relieve their pain and not further compromise the adjacent joints. Advanced flattening of the talus, intra-articular pilon malunion with joint incongruence, and joint subluxation without realignment are probably best solved with ankle fusion.

16.3.3 Frame Application

The surgical technique we use for ankle distraction arthroplasty has been reported (Inda et al. 2003; Tellisi et al. 2009). Patients receive spinal anesthesia with IV sedation. The ipsilateral iliac crest is prepped and draped and 60 cc of bone marrow is aspirated from it. A pneumatic thigh tourniquet is used for the open portion of the surgery and is removed for the external fixator application. An anterior arthrotomy is created in most cases and anterior osteophytes are resected. Osteophytes that are accessible in the medial and lateral gutters are removed as well. All areas of visible cartilage degeneration are drilled or picked to produce microfractures of the subchondral bone. After the wound is closed, the tourniquet is deflated. The bone marrow aspirate is concentrated using any number of commercially available systems and is then injected into the ankle joint. (The injection of bone marrow aspirate concentrate into the ankle joint is a technique we use at our institute. There is no previous investigation analyzing the efficacy of this intervention; however, we are engaged in a prospective study evaluating this technique. Other centers that perform ankle distraction also inject adjuvant treatment into the joint including viscosupplementation, recombinant human growth hormone (rhGH), and platelet-rich plasma (PRP). We all feel that adding these additional interventions could be beneficial.) A circular external fixator, the Ring Fix system (Small Bone Innovations, Morrisville, PA), is applied to the ankle. The tibial ring is mounted to the distal tibia using two 6 mm hydroxyapatite coated, tapered half pins (Biomet, Parsippany, NJ). The pin sites are predrilled with a 4.8 mm drill bit and the blunt tipped pins are inserted by hand. The hinges are then aligned with the axis of rotation of the ankle by placing a wire along a line from the tip of the medial malleolus to the tip of the lateral malleolus. We then ensure that the center of the

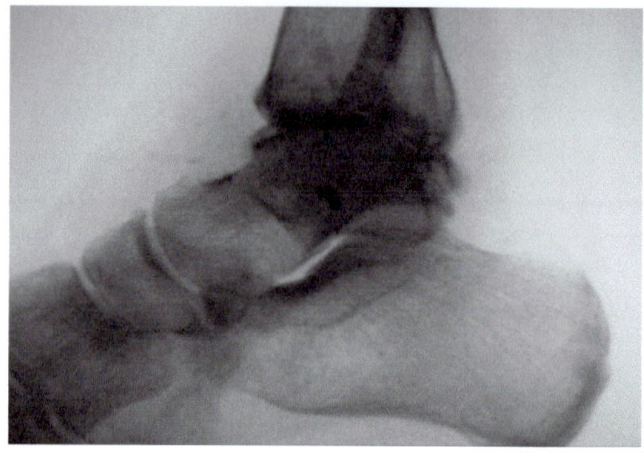

Fig. 16.1 A wire is inserted from the tip of the lateral malleolus to the tip of the medial malleolous through the talus. The position of the wire is checked on the lateral image. The hinges are then positioned along the axis of the wire. The wire is then removed

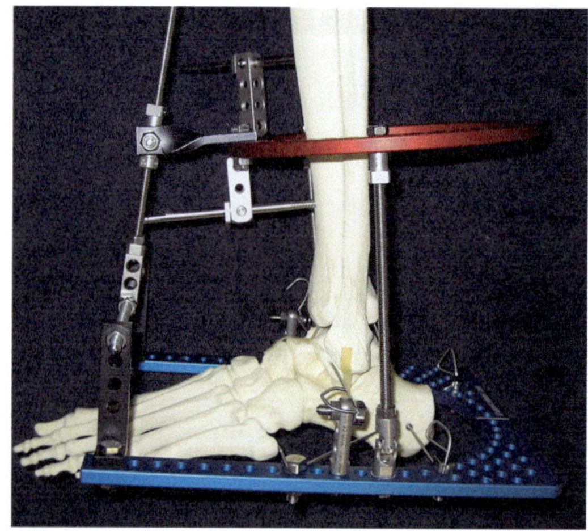

Fig. 16.2 The basic frame consists of a tibial ring with two tibial half pins and a foot ring with three tensioned foot wires

hinges rests against the ends of the wire. Final hinge position is confirmed on lateral fluoroscopy (Fig. 16.1). The foot ring is attached to the foot using three tensioned K-wires (Fig. 16.2). The typical pattern used is two crossing wires through the calcaneus and one wire through the talar neck (Fig. 16.3). The talus wire is important to prevent distraction through the subtalar joint. Distraction of 5 mm is applied acutely in the operating room. Further acute distraction is not applied acutely. For patients who have had previous surgery over the tarsal tunnel and may have

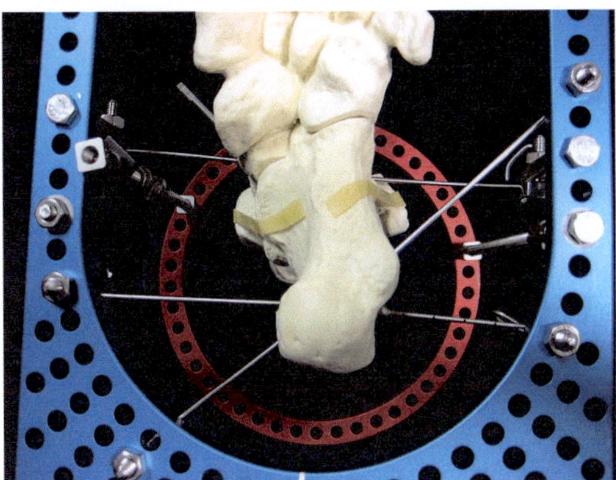

Fig. 16.3 A plantar view of the foot demonstrating the transverse olive wire inserted from lateral to medial, a crossed calcaneal wire, and the transverse talar neck wire

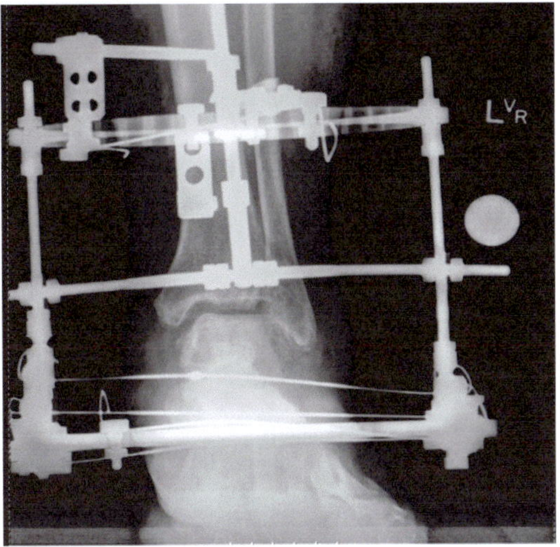

Fig. 16.4 A postoperative, AP, weight-bearing x-ray demonstrating a distracted tibiotalar joint space

scar tissue around the tibial nerve, we recommend gradual distraction. In these patients, acute distraction may cause neuropraxia. Similarly, if a patient has undergone an acute, simultaneous correction of an equinus contracture, the tibial nerve has already been stretched, and we recommend gradual distraction to prevent neuropraxia.

16.3.4 Postoperative Management

Patients are started on low molecular weight heparin that is continued for 3 weeks. They are encouraged to be weight bearing as tolerated starting postoperative day 1. The foot ring is locked in the neutral position. Ankle range of motion is started in the hospital by unlocking the anterior bar. A physical therapist and, ideally, a family member assist with ankle plantarflexion and dorsiflexion. Pin care is started postoperative day 2. We prescribe a once daily routine consisting of cleaning each pin site with a sterile cotton swab dipped in diluted hydrogen peroxide solution. The pin-skin junctions are then covered with a light gauze wrap. Showering is allowed 4 days after surgery provided there is no wound discharge. Neurologic status is checked immediately post surgery. If needed, further distraction is applied in the hospital before discharge to obtain 5 mm of joint space on x-ray. The ankle distraction space is rechecked at the first postoperative visit using weight-bearing x-rays, and additional

distraction is added as needed (Fig. 16.4). Sutures are removed at this visit as well. Postoperative follow-up is performed at regular intervals including 2, 6, and 10 weeks. The 10-week visit is the frame removal procedure. This is performed in the operating room under IV sedation. At this time the pin sites are prepped, the pins and wires are removed, the pin sites are debrided, and the ankle can be manipulated if necessary. Clean dressings are applied and the leg is paced into a walker boot. The patient is allowed weight bearing as tolerated ambulation and can use the boot as needed. Dressing removal and showering are allowed after 2 days. Follow-up visits are at 2 weeks, 6 weeks, 12 weeks, 6 months, 1 year, and then yearly after that. Weight-bearing ankle x-rays are obtained at each visit. An MR is obtained at 1-year follow-up for research purposes.

Authors have recommended that external fixators do not need to be removed in the operating room under anesthesia (Ryder and Gorczyca 2007). We cannot disagree more with this recommendation. Our technique calls for the use of hydroxyapatite-coated half pins which bind to the bone increasing extraction torque and decreasing pin loosening (Moroni et al. 2008). The pins often require significant force to remove which causes substantial pain even under light sedation. Pin sites bleed predictably and are better managed in the operating room setting. Sterile curettes are used to clean the pin sites, skin, and subcutaneous tissue. For these reasons, we recommend that the external fixators be removed under anesthesia in the operating room.

16.4 Current Recommendations and Trends

Ankle distraction arthroplasty is a procedure in evolution. It offers some clear benefits to most patients. There are very few complications making the risk-to-benefit ratio low favoring the surgical procedure. We feel that performing concomitant, adjuvant procedures is important to the success of the patient. If there are no osteophytes to resect, then we will refrain from arthrotomy. It is evident that recovery is faster and less painful without arthrotomy. The introduction of autologous stem cells to the ankle joint is experimental. It has been shown in an equine model that the addition of stem cells to classic microfracture for the treatment of a knee osteochondral defect demonstrated increased fill of defects, greater integration of repair cartilage with adjacent normal cartilage, and a higher content of type II collagen when compared with microfracture alone (Fortier et al. 2010). We may find that adding rhGH is more effective or that changing the method of stem cell introduction into the joint may be more efficacious. For example, the stem cells can be injected into the subchondral bone instead of into the joint (Jager et al. 2010). Joint distraction may help improve radiographic and clinical results in OATS (osteochondral autograft transplantation surgery) procedures (Belczyk et al. 2009) and in ACI (autologous chondrocyte implantation). Ankle arthrodiastasis may have a role in the prevention of posttraumatic arthritis. The ankle articular cartilage that has been traumatized by a shearing or compressive force (after bimalleolar dislocation or pilon fracture) may benefit from mechanical unloading in addition to anatomic reduction. This may require a combination of internal and external fixation which has not been problematic in our hands.

In a pending publication, we have looked at the critical amount of distraction needed to ensure that the joint surfaces will not have contact during normal ambulation. Our cadaver experiments have shown that an average amount of 4.4 mm of joint distraction is required to prevent contact between the articular surfaces. Therefore, the amount of ankle joint space needed (on average) on a weight-bearing x-ray is 4.4 mm+pre-op joint space.

In conclusion, joint distraction is an emerging technique that has a growing body of objective evidence to support the good clinical results that it provides. The indications for distraction arthroplasty are broadening and the technique continues to evolve. Other joints will likely benefit from this technique as well.

References

Arokoski J, Jurvelin J, Vaatainen U et al (2000) Normal and pathological adaptations of articular cartilage to joint loading. Scand J Med Sci Sports 10(4):186–198

Belczyk R, Stapleton J, Zgonis T et al (2009) A case report of simultaneous local osteochondral autografting and ankle arthrodiastasis for the treatment of a talar dome defect. Clin Podiatr Med Surg 26(2): 335–342

Brandt KD, Dieppe P, Radin E (2009) Etiopathogenesis of osteoarthritis. Med Clin North Am 93(1):1–24

Buckwalter JA, Mankin HJ (1998) Articular cartilage: degeneration and osteoarthritis, repair, regeneration, and transplantation. Instr Course Lect 47:487–504

Fortier LA, Potter HG, Rickey EJ et al (2010) Concentrated bone marrow aspirate improves full-thickness cartilage repair compared with microfracture in the equine model. J Bone Joint Surg Am 92(10):1927–1937

Inda D, Blyakher A, O'Malley M, Rozbruch SR (2003) Distraction arthroplasty for the ankle using the Ilizarov frame: techniques in foot & ankle surgery. Tech Foot Ankle Surg 2(4):249–253

Intema F, Thomas TP, Anderson DD et al (2011) Subchondral bone remodeling is related to clinical improvement after joint distraction in the treatment of ankle osteoarthritis. Osteoarthritis Cartilage 19: 668–675

Jager M, Hernigou P, Zilkens C et al (2010) Cell therapy in bone healing disorders. Orthop Rev (Pavia) 2(2):e20

Kajiwara R, Ishida O, Kawasaki K et al (2005) Effective repair of a fresh osteochondral defect in the rabbit knee joint by articulated joint distraction following subchondral drilling. J Orthop Res 23(4):909–915

Lajeunesse D (2004) The role of bone in the treatment of osteoarthritis. Osteoarthritis Cartilage 12 Suppl A: S34–S38

Lamm B, Gourdine-Shaw M (2009) MRI evaluation of ankle distraction: a preliminary report. Clin Podiatr Med Surg 26(2):185–191

Marijnissen A, Vincken K, Viergever M (2001) Ankle images digital analysis (AIDA): digital measurement of joint space width and subchondral sclerosis on standard radiographs. Osteoarthritis Cartilage 9:264–272

Marijnissen A, van Roermund P, van Melkebeek J et al (2002) Clinical benefit of joint distraction in the treatment of severe osteoarthritis of the ankle: proof of concept in an open prospective study and in a randomized controlled study. Arthritis Rheum 46(11):2893–2902

Marijnissen A, Van Roermund P, Van Melkebeek J et al (2003) Clinical benefit of joint distraction in the treatment of ankle osteoarthritis. Foot Ankle Clin 8(2):335–346

Moroni A, Cadossi M, Romagnoli M et al (2008) A biomechanical analysis of standard versus hydroxyapatite coated pins for external fixation. J Biomed Mater Res B Appl Biomater 86B(2):417–421

Paley D, Lamm BM (2005) Ankle joint distraction. Foot Ankle Clin 10(4):685–698

Paley D, Lamm B, Purohit R et al (2008) Distraction arthroplasty of the ankle- how far can you stretch the indications? Foot Ankle Clin 13:471–484

Ploegmakers J, van Roermund P, van Melkebeek J et al (2005) Prolonged clinical benefit from joint distraction in the treatment of ankle osteoarthritis. J Osteoarthritis Cartilage 13:582–588

Radin E, Rose R (1986) Role of subchondral bone in the initiation and progression of cartilage damage. Clin Orthop 21:34–40

Ryder S, Gorczyca J (2007) Routine removal of external fixators without anesthesia. J Orthop Trauma 21(8):571–573

Saltzman C, Buckwalter J (1999) Ankle arthritis: emerging concepts and management strategies. AAOS Instr Course Lect 48:233–240

Tellisi N, Fragomen A, Kleinmann D, Rozbruch SR (2009) Joint preservation of the osteoarthritic ankle using distraction arthroplasty. Foot Ankle Int 30(4):318–325

Van Roermund P, Marijnissen A, Lafeber F (2002) Joint distraction as an alternative for the treatment of osteoarthritis. Foot Ankle Clin 7(3):515–527

Van Valburg A, van Roermund P, Lammens J et al (1995) Can Ilizarov joint distraction delay the need for an arthrodesis of the ankle? A preliminary report. J Bone Joint Surg Br 77-B(5):720–725

Van Valburg A, van Roy H, Lafeber F et al (1998) Beneficial effects of intermittent fluid pressure of low physiological magnitude on cartilage and inflammation in osteoarthritis. An in vitro study. J Rheumatol 25(3):515–520

Van Valburg A, van Roermund P, Marijnissen A et al (1999) Joint distraction in treatment of osteoarthritis: a two-year follow-up of the ankle. Osteoarthritis Cartilage 7(5):474–479

Hindfoot Reconstruction by the Combined Technique

Levent Eralp, Mehmet Kocaoğlu, and İlker Eren

Contents

L. Eralp (✉)
Department of Orthopaedics and Traumatology,
Istanbul Universtiy, Istanbul, Turkey
e-mail: drleventeralp@gmail.com

M. Kocaoğlu, MD
Orthopedic Surgery Department,
Istanbul Memorial Hospital, Istanbul, Turkey
e-mail: drmehmetkocaoglu@gmail.com

İ. Eren
Department of Orthopaedics and Traumatology,
School of Medicine, Koç University, Istanbul, Turkey
e-mail: ilker.eren@gmail.com

Abbreviations

CEF   Circular type external fixator
K-wire Kirschner wire

17.1 Introduction

Numerous techniques have been introduced for ankle arthrodesis, for various etiologies. Each has its own advantages and disadvantages, requiring personalized treatment approach. Ankle arthrodesis with external fixators is a well-known technique. Ability to provide prolonged compression, segment transport, and lengthening are distinct advantages of Ilizarov (Thiryayi et al. 2010; Katsenis et al. 2005). However, long fixator time leads to complications (Paley 1990). Retrograde intramedullary nailing is also another well-known technique for ankle arthrodesis. They provide stable fixation, without fixator-related complications. But it is limited to patients without limb length discrepancy and segmental defects. Also nonunion due to lack of compression is another drawback of the device.

Utilization of external fixator with combination of intramedullary nail is a recently introduced advanced technique with securing the versatility of Ilizarov, avoiding its many complications (Eralp et al. 2007; Kocaoglu et al. 2006). Less fixator time leads to lower fixator-related complications and greatly improves patient comfort (Kocaoglu et al. 2004).

M. Kocaoğlu et al. (eds.), *Advanced Techniques in Limb Reconstruction Surgery*,
DOI 10.1007/978-3-642-55026-3_17, © Springer Berlin Heidelberg 2015

17.2   Indications

- Limb length discrepancy with concomitant unstable ankle joint due to neuropathic conditions (such as poliomyelitis, sciatic nerve damage or Charcot arthropathy)
- Bone loss within 1 cm of the articular surface of the ankle joint following trauma complicated by infection or segment loss, tumor resection, and bone deficiency due to radical debridement of osteomyelitis
- Bone loss due to debridement following infection at the site of a total ankle arthroplasty

17.3   Examination/Imaging

- This technique requires careful patient selection. The surgeon has to predict the possible bone gap resulting from resection or debridement accurately, so that an intramedullary nail and frame can be prepared preoperatively.
- This procedure has to be utilized as the second stage of osteomyelitis treatment. First stage is always debridement and antibiotherapy, with soft tissue reconstruction when necessary. Posttraumatic patients require meticulous vascular survey, regarding both physical examination and radiological assessment. Serious vascular impairment may render procedure contraindicated.
- Mentioned technique has advantages when there is concomitant ankle instability or deformity. It has to be stated if the deformity is flexible or rigid. Rigid deformities may require gradual correction before definitive arthrodesis.
- Preoperative planning with true size X-rays and standing orthoroentgenogram is mandatory. Intramedullary nail length and width has to be decided before, and additional locking holes have to be provided for more rigid fixation. When the lengthening or transportation is accomplished, regenerate has to be preserved with screws passing just proximally.
- As the procedure requires subtalar and tibiotalar arthrodesis, hindfoot has to be evaluated radiologically for any deformity or any deviation from normal anatomy.
- Magnetic resonance imaging is required before intervention for tumor and osteomyelitis. Most tumor patients require adjuvant chemo- or radiotherapy after resection. Immunosuppression and local soft tissue impairment due to radiotherapy may complicate an extremity for external fixation.

17.4   Positioning

- Patient has to be prepared on a radiolucent table with a sandbag under the ipsilateral buttock to prevent external rotation beyond neutral.
- A tourniquet will facilitate the exposure for tibiotalar and subtalar arthrodesis, which can be removed or deflated before intramedullary nailing and fixator application.

17.5   Instruments

- Intramedullary nail (authors prefer Orthopro 4G Tibial Nail, Izmir, Turkey)
- Circular type external fixator (CEF) (authors prefer CEF produced by Tasarimmed, Istanbul, Turkey)
- Flexible and rigid intramedullary reamers as well
- Gigli saw

17.6   Exposure for Subtalar and Tibiotalar Preparation

- Subtalar and tibiotalar joint is prepared through transmalleolar (transfibular) approach or subtalar approach alone.
- Transfibular approach provides a better visualization of both joints. The fibula is cut 1.5 cm above the joint line with an oblique osteotomy from proximal lateral to distal medial. Most distal medial tip of the osteotomy should be level with plafond. Removed distal fibula can be used as an autograft if necessary (Fig. 17.1).

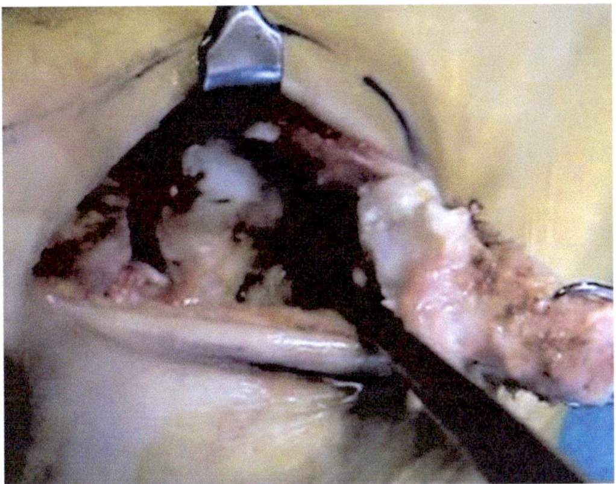

Fig. 17.1 Tibiotalar and subtalar joint dissection after transecting and elevating the fibula preserving distal attachment

- Anterior and posterior ligamentous structures are transected from the fibula (Fig. 17.1), preserving soft tissues around the talar neck to preserve vascular supply.
- Subtalar joint is accessible after removing fat pad (Fig. 17.1).

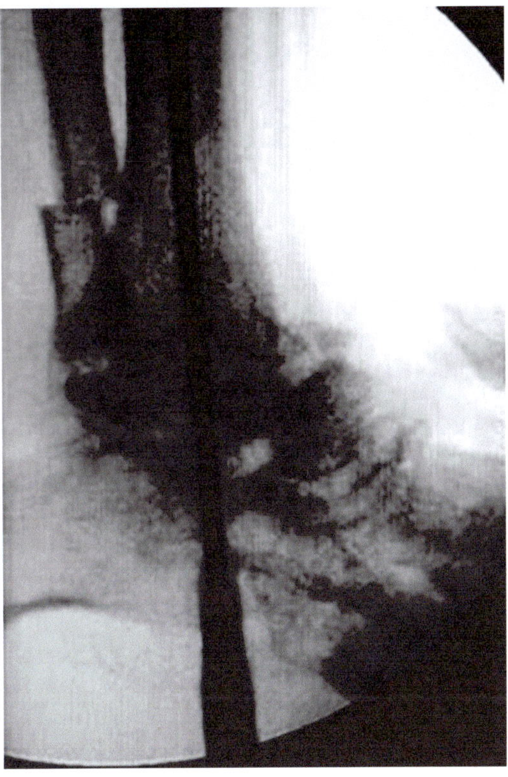

Fig. 17.2 Guidewire is inserted and reaming performed

17.7 Distal Tibial Reconstruction with Use of a Circular External Fixator and an Intramedullary Nail

- After preparing subtalar and tibiotalar joints, the foot is positioned in correct alignment (neutral to 5° of dorsiflexion in the sagittal plane, 5° of valgus in the frontal plane, and 5° of external rotation in the axial plane) for ankle arthrodesis. A threaded Kirschner wire is inserted through the calcaneus. Entry point of the wire and intramedullary nail is determined with image intensifier as the intersection of joint midline at frontal plane, with anterior 1/3 joint line at sagittal plane. Hole is enlarged with a cannulated drill over Kirschner wire and guidewire is inserted (Fig. 17.2). Reaming is performed over the guide in 0.5 mm increments. Medullary canal has to be reamed 2 mm over the diameter of the nail to be inserted.

- Corticotomy is performed at the planned level with a gigli saw. At least 6–8 cm bone should be preserved proximally.
- Intramedullary nail is inserted and nail is locked.
  - For bone segment transport without lengthening, both ends of the nail are locked (Fig. 17.3a).
  - For pure lengthening, just the distal end of the nail is locked (Fig. 17.3b).
  - Due to its proximal sagittal curvature (distal for this case as it is delivered retrograde), tibial intramedullary nail is preferred, which provides a dorsiflexion or plantar flexion effect to the ankle.
- Circular external fixator is prepared according to the procedure. For lengthening, one ring is placed proximal to the osteotomy and two rings distally (Fig. 17.3a). Proximal two rings are used for lengthening, while the distal ring and the foot ring compress the arthrodesis site.

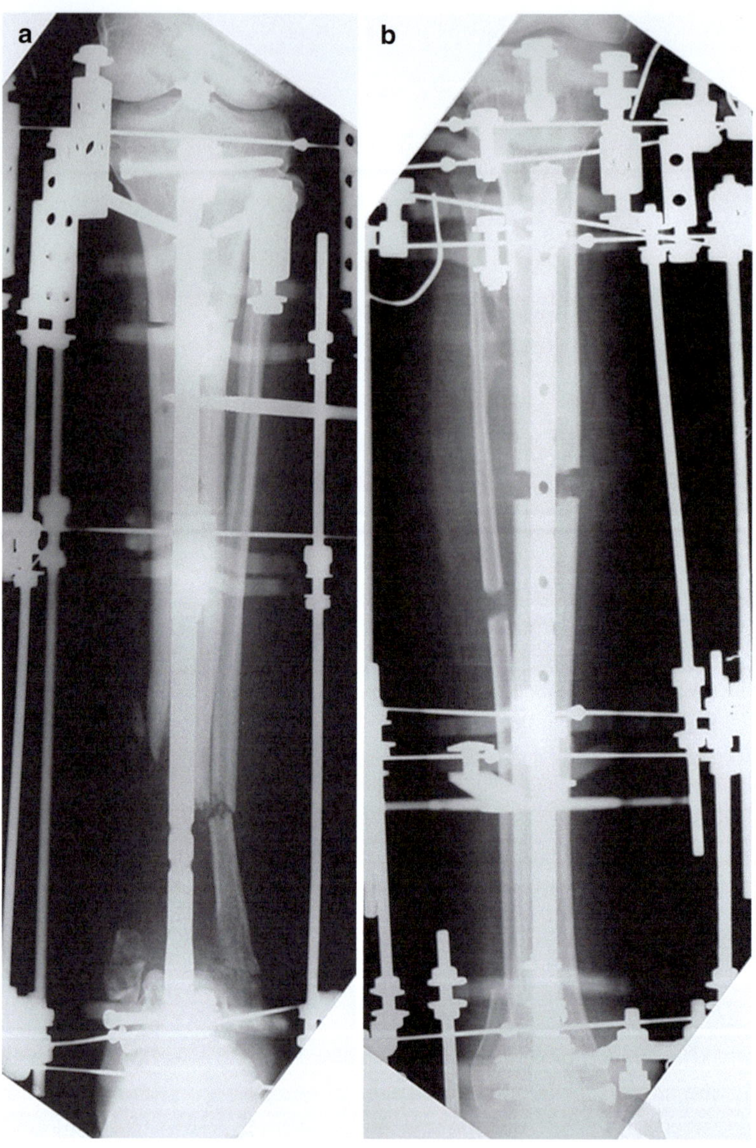

Fig. 17.3 (**a**) In case lengthening over nail is being performed, proximal holes are left unlocked. (**b**) For segment transport, both holes have to be locked

- Usually, there is enough bone present at the proximal tibia, just above the tip of the nail for the fixation. Both Schanz screws and Kirschner wires can be used. Rest of the fixation is achieved with wires, passing at least 1 mm away from intramedullary nail (Fig. 17.4). Foot ring is adapted with calcaneal Schanz screws or wires and metatarsal wires.
- In case of segment transport, two proximal rings secure the proximal tibia, while one ring transports segment. Just before the transported segment reaches docking site, autologous bone graft is packed and the nail locked just above with custom-made holes (Figs. 17.3b and 17.5).

17.8 Postoperative Care and Expected Outcomes

- Weight bearing is allowed immediately with two crutches, and range of motion exercises for the knee joint are started as soon as possible.
- Distraction is started at the seventh to tenth day postoperatively, at a rate of 1 mm/day divided into four equal increments.

- Patients should be screened for local and systemic signs of infection and with C-reactive protein levels for infection recurrence.
- During lengthening or transport, anteroposterior and lateral radiographs are obtained every 2 weeks and during consolidation once a month.
- When the desired lengthening or transport is achieved, the nail is locked and external fixator removed.

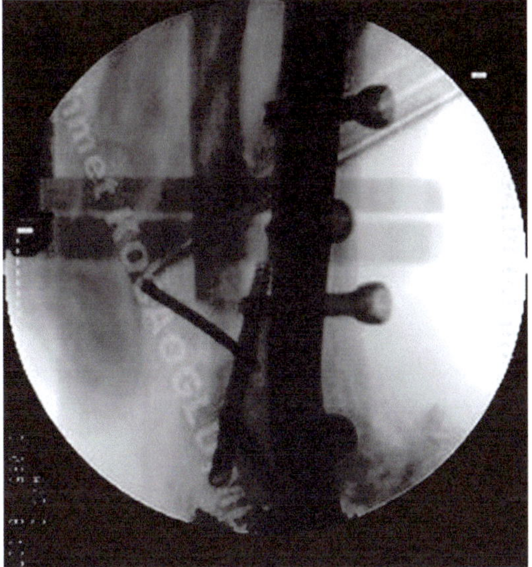

Fig. 17.4 As the Kirschner wires (K-wires) may be a source of infection, at least 1 mm safe zone should be left between the intramedullary nail and the wire

Pearls
- Intramedullary canal has to be overreamed by 2 mm then the diameter of the nail for easy gliding.
- There should be 1 mm of safe zone between pins, Schanz screws, and the intramedullary nail, to prevent secondary infection due to pin site problems.
- Poller screws can be utilized while reaming and insertion of the nail at the metaphyseal part of the distal tibia.

Pitfalls
- Prior to procedure, infection-free margins have to be achieved. Failure to do so will lead to more extensive bone loss, even panosteomyelitis and septic arthritis of adjacent joints.
- Failure to precisely determine the length and diameter of the intramedullary nail will lead

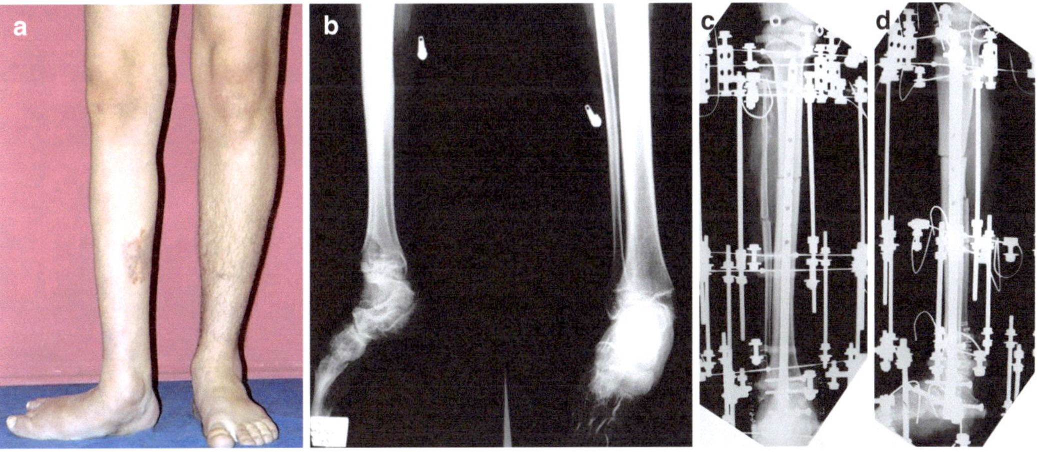

Fig. 17.5 (**a, b**) A 17-year-old male patient, diagnosed with ankle instability with shortening of the tibia, due to excision of neurofibrosarcoma arising from the sciatic nerve. Both lengthening and ankle arthrodesis planned. (**c, d**) Lengthening is achieved with Ilizarov circular external fixator, over an intramedullary nail which is delivered in a retrograde fashion. Note the custom-made locking holes on the AP and lateral views. Due to performed midfoot arthrodesis, Ilizarov frame extended distally to include foot as well. (**e–h**) End of the planned lengthening. Under general anesthesia, fixator removed and nail locked. To preserve foot arthrodesis, an above-knee plaster cast administered. (**i–l**) Union obtained both at the lengthening and ankle fusion site. A stable and plantigrade foot is achieved

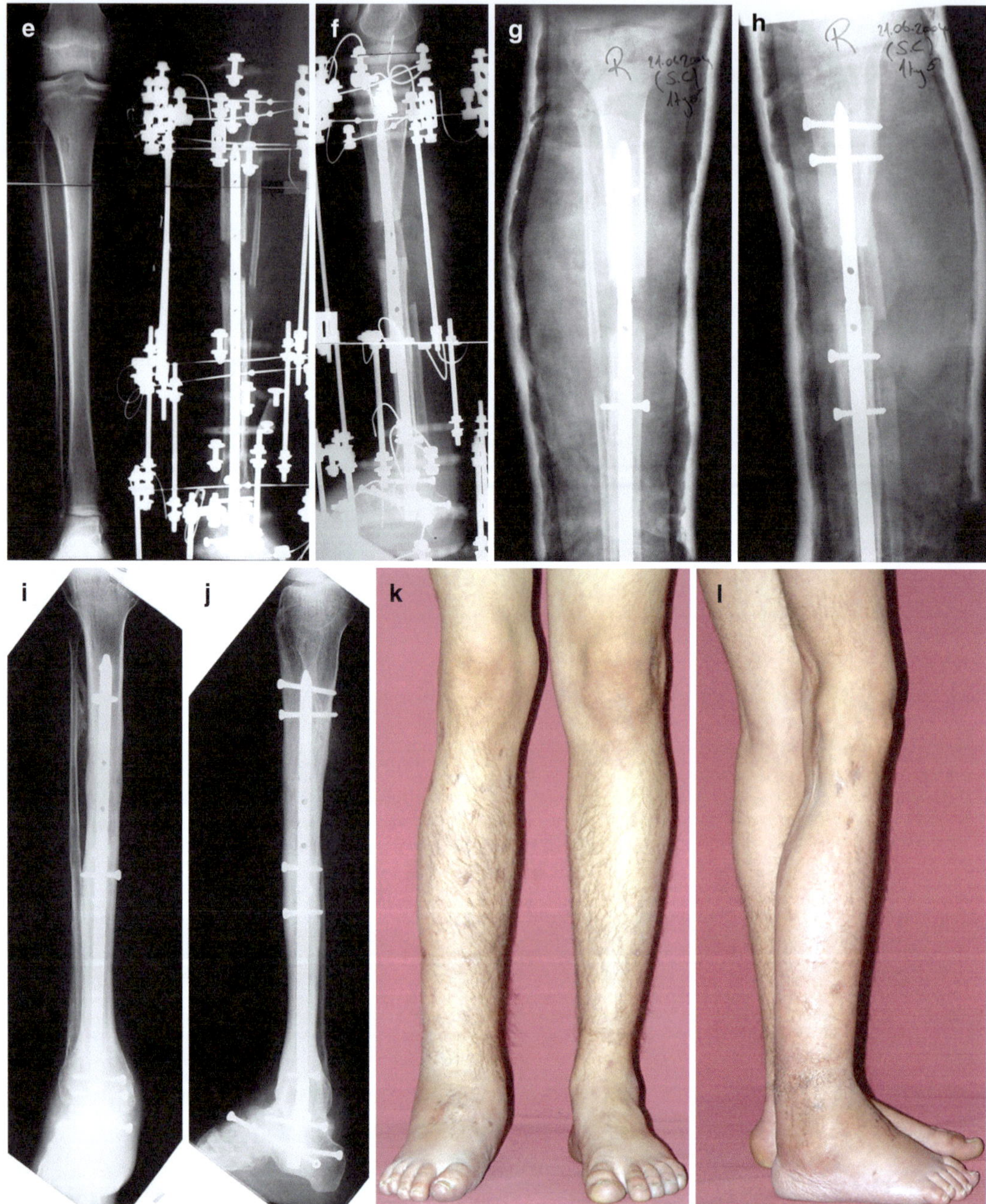

Fig. 17.5 (continued)

to many preoperative and postoperative complications. Meticulous planning is vital.

- Failure to place the circular external fixator parallel to intramedullary nail may arise problems while transporting or distracting bone such as inability to transport due to increased friction or inability to transport segment to the docking site, accurately.

Controversies

- This procedure is contraindicated when there is absence of calcaneus, noncompliance of patient, severe previous vascular injury, and Cierny-Mader host C patients.

References

Eralp L, Kocaoglu M, Yusof NM, Bulbul M (2007) Distal tibial reconstruction with use of a circular external fixator and an intramedullary nail. The combined technique. J Bone Joint Surg Am 89(10):2218–2224. doi:10.2106/JBJS.F.01579, 89/10/2218 [pii]

Katsenis D, Bhave A, Paley D, Herzenberg JE (2005) Treatment of malunion and nonunion at the site of an ankle fusion with the Ilizarov apparatus. J Bone Joint Surg Am 87(2):302–309, 87/2/302 [pii]

Kocaoglu M, Eralp L, Kilicoglu O, Burc H, Cakmak M (2004) Complications encountered during lengthening over an intramedullary nail. J Bone Joint Surg Am 86-A(11):2406–2411, 86/11/2406 [pii]

Kocaoglu M, Eralp L, Rashid HU, Sen C, Bilsel K (2006) Reconstruction of segmental bone defects due to chronic osteomyelitis with use of an external fixator and an intramedullary nail. J Bone Joint Surg Am 88(10):2137–2145. doi:10.2106/JBJS.E.01152, 88/10/2137 [pii]

Paley D (1990) Problems, obstacles, and complications of limb lengthening by the Ilizarov technique. Clin Orthop Relat Res 250:81–104

Thiryayi WA, Naqui Z, Khan SA (2010) Use of the Taylor spatial frame in compression arthrodesis of the ankle: a study of 10 cases. J Foot Ankle Surg 49(2):182–187. doi:10.1053/j.jfas.2009.05.015, S1067-2516(09)00218-X [pii]

Complex Foot Deformities: Correction with the Taylor Spatial Frame

18

Jeffrey L. Young, Bradley M. Lamm, and John E. Herzenberg

Contents

J.L. Young, MD • B.M. Lamm, DPM
J.E. Herzenberg, MD (✉)
Department of Orthopaedic Surgery,
Stanford University, International Center for Limb
Lengthening, Rubin Institute for Advanced
Orthopedics, Sinai Hospital of Baltimore,
2401 West Belvedere Avenue,
Baltimore, MD 21215, USA
e-mail: jlyoung@stanford.edu;
blamm@lifebridgehealth.org;
jherzenberg@lifebridgehealth.org

18.1 Indications

18.1.1 Indications

The Taylor Spatial Frame (TSF) (Smith & Nephew, Memphis, TN, USA) is a hexapod multiplanar circular external fixator (Eidelman and Katzman 2008). The indications for the TSF are similar to those of other multiplanar circular external fixators (e.g., Ilizarov) (Wukich and Belczyk 2006). These indications include:

- Gradual deformity correction, which minimizes the risks associated with acute correction (e.g., stretching of neurovascular structures) and also avoids closing wedge osteotomies that are required with acute correction.
- Feet with a compromised soft-tissue envelope from postsurgical scarring. The TSF provides correction and stability without extensive soft-tissue dissection.

18.1.2 Advantages

The TSF has several advantages over other multiplanar circular external fixators.

- With the TSF, the surgeon is able to define a virtual hinge and to correct both translation and rotation in the frontal, sagittal, and axial planes. Additionally, correction of multiple axes can occur simultaneously. This is helpful with foot deformities that involve deformity along multiple axes (e.g., planovalgus feet, equinovarus feet) (Floerkemeier et al. 2011).

- TSF and classical Ilizarov techniques can be combined. In some cases, single axis deformity correction may be less cumbersome with Ilizarov-type circular external fixation. For example, pure ankle equinus or pure metatarsus adductus may be more simply treated with Ilizarov techniques (Kirienko et al. 2004).

- External fixation methods of treatment offer the ability to assess the deformity during the correction process and to make changes as needed during the course of treatment. With the Ilizarov frame, changes sometimes require hardware modification, such as reconfiguring a hinge. With the TSF, the surgeon modifies the information in the TSF software program, which reprograms the deformity correction. The only hardware changes needed are occasional strut changes, which is a quick and simple office procedure.

18.2 Examination/Imaging

18.2.1 Assess the Deformity

Deformities such as ankle equinus or ankle calcaneus, hindfoot varus or hindfoot valgus, pes cavus, pes planus or rockerbottom, and forefoot adduction or forefoot abduction may occur in isolation or in combination. It is important to note the relationship among different segments of the foot. This information helps determine which osteotomy is required and which frame is necessary to achieve a plantigrade foot.

18.2.2 Assess the Joints

Ideally, joint-sparing procedures are preferred to joint-sacrificing procedures. For example, when the subtalar joint is supple, a U-osteotomy is contraindicated because subtalar joint mobility is sacrificed in this procedure. When stiff joints are painful, the surgeon should consider arthrodesis. The TSF may be helpful in severe deformity correction as a prelude to definitive arthrodesis.

18.2.3 Assess Muscle Function

Muscle imbalance and paralytic muscles may cause deformity. In this situation, tendon transfers following realignment procedures may help to maintain the correction. These are generally done staged rather than simultaneously.

18.2.4 Assess the Neurovascular Status

Insensate feet will require increased frame stability for protection. Check for sensation of the superficial peroneal nerve, the deep peroneal nerve, and the posterior tibial nerve. Also, assess for stocking paresthesia, commonly found in patients with diabetes. Assess the dorsalis pedis and posterior tibial pulses to determine the circulatory status of the foot. Reassess during surgery and during the correction process. Loss of sensation may indicate that correction is occurring too rapidly. In such cases, it might be necessary to slow, stop or reverse the correction. Surgical nerve decompression may be required.

18.2.5 Assess the Soft-Tissue Envelope

Scarring from previous surgical procedures makes soft-tissue dissection difficult and increases the risk of injury to neurovascular structures embedded in the scar tissue. Additionally, scar tissue is less compliant, which increases the risk of compression of the tarsal tunnel during deformity correction. In such cases, consider prophylactic tarsal tunnel decompression, prior to frame application (Lamm et al. 2006).

18.2.6 Radiographic Assessment

- Long leg standing radiographs can be used to assess limb length inequalities and limb alignment. Limb length discrepancies are commonly associated with complex foot deformities.

- Anteroposterior (AP) and lateral view radiographs of the ankle can be used to assess ankle joint orientation and the status of the joint. Common findings include flattop talus or ankle osteophytes. Lateral view radiographs obtained with the foot in maximum dorsiflexion and maximum plantar flexion help to assess the ankle range of motion.
- Hindfoot alignment (Saltzman) view radiographs can be used to assess the alignment of the calcaneus and the weightbearing axis of the hindfoot.
- AP and lateral view radiographs of the foot should be obtained, ideally with the patient bearing weight. For a non-ambulatory patient, simulated weightbearing radiographs can be obtained while the patient is seated. For severely deformed feet, obtain foot flat radiographs in which the plantar surface of the foot is placed on the ground and the images are obtained perpendicular to the foot, as opposed to the tibia. Important radiographic findings include diffuse osteopenia from non-weightbearing, as well as evidence of stress fractures from abnormal loading.

18.2.7 Common Radiographic Angles

- Figure 18.1
- Lateral Distal Tibial Angle (LDTA): Angle defined by the long axis of the tibia in the coronal plane and the distal tibial plafond. Normal is $89° \pm 4°$
- Anterior Distal Tibial Angle (ADTA): Angle defined by the long axis of the tibia in the sagittal plane and the distal tibial plafond. Normal is $80° \pm 2°$.
- Calcaneal Pitch Angle: Angle from the plantar surface of the foot to a line tangent to the inferior aspect of the calcaneal tuberosity on the lateral view. Normal is $17° \pm 6°$.
- Meary's Angle: Angle on the sagittal view of the foot defined by the long axis of the talus and the first metatarsal. Normal is $5° \pm 4°$.
- Hindfoot Alignment: The long axis of the calcaneus is approximately 1 cm lateral to the long axis of the tibia on the hindfoot alignment view.

- Plantigrade Line: A line perpendicular to the plantar surface of the standing foot, passing through the lateral process of the talus. This line should be colinear with the long axis of the tibia. The tibial line is normally 90° (range, 88–92°) relative to the floor.

- For sagittal planning of the hindfoot, the plantigrade line and the long axis of the tibia are the two most important lines.

18.3   Surgical Anatomy

- The osseous anatomy of the leg and foot are largely subcutaneous, facilitating pin and wire placement.
- Cutaneous nerves to avoid include the superficial peroneal nerve and the sural nerve. The superficial peroneal nerve lies on the anterolateral aspect of the distal tibia and across the dorsum of the foot. The sural nerve passes posterior and distal to the lateral malleolus.
- Posterior tibial nerve: This nerve is centrally located in the middle-third of the leg, between the deep and superficial posterior compartments. More distally, it travels more medially and passes posterior to the medial malleolus at the level of the ankle. There, the flexor retinaculum passes over the posterior tibial nerve, forming the tarsal tunnel. The tarsal tunnel is a site for potential nerve compression, especially with correction of hindfoot varus deformity or procurvatum deformity of the distal tibia. In these instances, prophylactic decompression should be considered. Distally, the posterior tibial nerve divides into three branches: the calcaneal nerve, the lateral plantar nerve, and the medial plantar nerve.
- Gastrocnemius soleus complex: These muscles resist ankle equinus and hindfoot valgus correction. Intramuscular lengthening of the gastrocnemius and soleus muscles allows lengthening and minimizes the risk of excessive of power loss.
- Plantar medial structures: The plantar fascia has significant tensile strength and can lead to

Fig. 18.1 (**a**) Common radiographic angles shown on a lateral view of the foot. (**b**) Common radiographic angles are shown on an axial view of the foot. *ADTA* anterior distal tibial angle, *JLCA* joint line congruence angle, *LDTA* lateral distal tibial angle, *PMA* plafond malleolar angle (Reprinted with permission from the Rubin Institute for Advanced Orthopedics, Sinai Hospital of Baltimore)

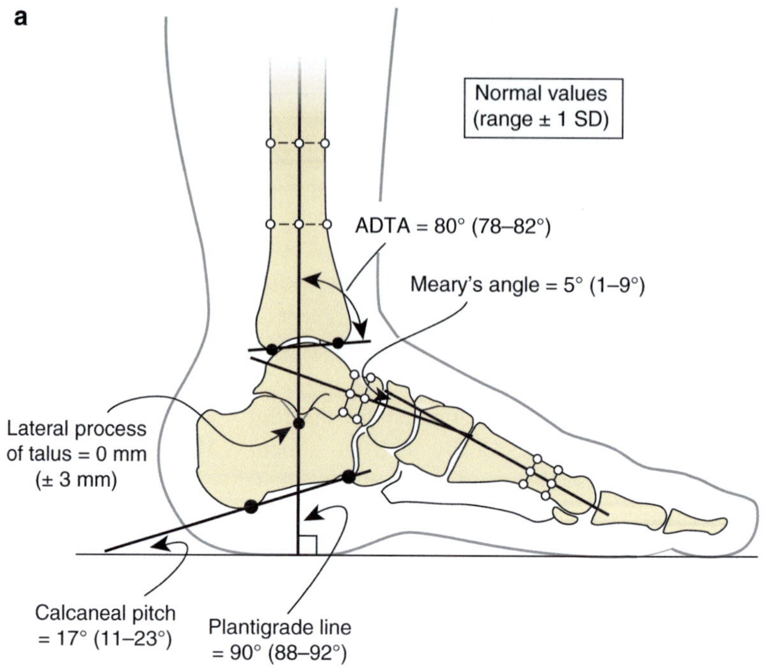

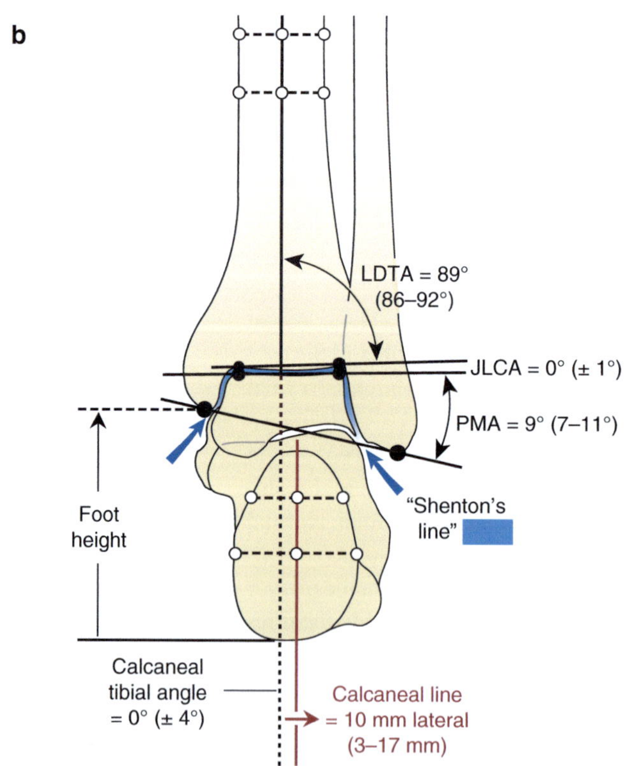

significant resistance against correction of cavus deformity. Consider release of the plantar fascia for a midfoot osteotomy. Flexor digitorum longus and flexor hallucis longus muscles may tighten during deformity correction and result in claw toes or metatarsal-phalangeal (MTP) joint subluxation. Consider intramuscular lengthening of both muscles, prophylactic pinning of the toes across the MTP joints, or aggressive splinting and stretching.

- Structure at risk (SAR): The spatialframe.com software program requires the surgeon to define the structure that will lengthen the quickest, thereby limiting the rate of correction. The structure at risk varies depending on the procedure and is defined by its position relative to the origin. For example, when correcting hindfoot varus, the structure at risk is the posterior tibial nerve as it passes through the tarsal tunnel. When correcting an equinus deformity, the structure at risk is the Achilles tendon. When correcting forefoot adduction through a midfoot osteotomy, the structure at risk is the medial edge of the osteotomy. A safe distraction rate is usually 1 mm/day, but this rate should be decreased if distraction is planned at multiple levels.

Pearls
- Prophylactic tarsal tunnel decompression is easier to perform prior to frame application. Once the frame is applied, access is limited.

18.4 Positioning

- Place the patient supine on a radiolucent table, with the foot approximately 30 cm from the end of the table to allow the surgeon room to work. Consider a bump under the ipsilateral hemipelvis to help maintain a patella-forward position. Verify the ability to obtain orthogonal views on the image intensifier prior to preparing the field and draping the extremity.

Pearls
- Place the bump below the sacrum and avoid direct compression of the sciatic nerve, especially for long procedures.

18.5 Procedure

18.5.1 Preoperative Planning

The goal of surgery is a plantigrade foot. Begin by defining the deformity and identify the center of rotation of angulation (CORA) (Fig. 18.2).

18.5.2 Osteotomies

- Decide if an osteotomy is required. For children older than 8 years of age who have less remodeling potential, consider an osteotomy. Nonetheless, successful deformity correction has been accomplished without osteotomies in children older than 8 years of age. Osteotomies are generally avoided in children <8 years of age.

18.5.2.1 Supramalleolar Osteotomy (SMO)

- Indicated for deformities in which the CORA is periarticular about the ankle. When the CORA and osteotomy are at different levels, a secondary translation at the osteotomy occurs with appropriate angular correction (Fig. 18.2e).
- Supramalleolar osteotomies allow for angular correction and lengthening.
- An SMO is performed either by drill corticotomy through a small anterior longitudinal incision or by percutaneously passing a Gigli saw around the tibia/fibula (Fig. 18.3).
- A restriction wire helps to prevent proximal migration of the Gigli saw, which commonly occurs due to the slope of the distal tibial metaphysis. Pass the Gigli saw at the desired level, then place a restriction wire just proximal to the Gigli saw (Fig. 18.2c).

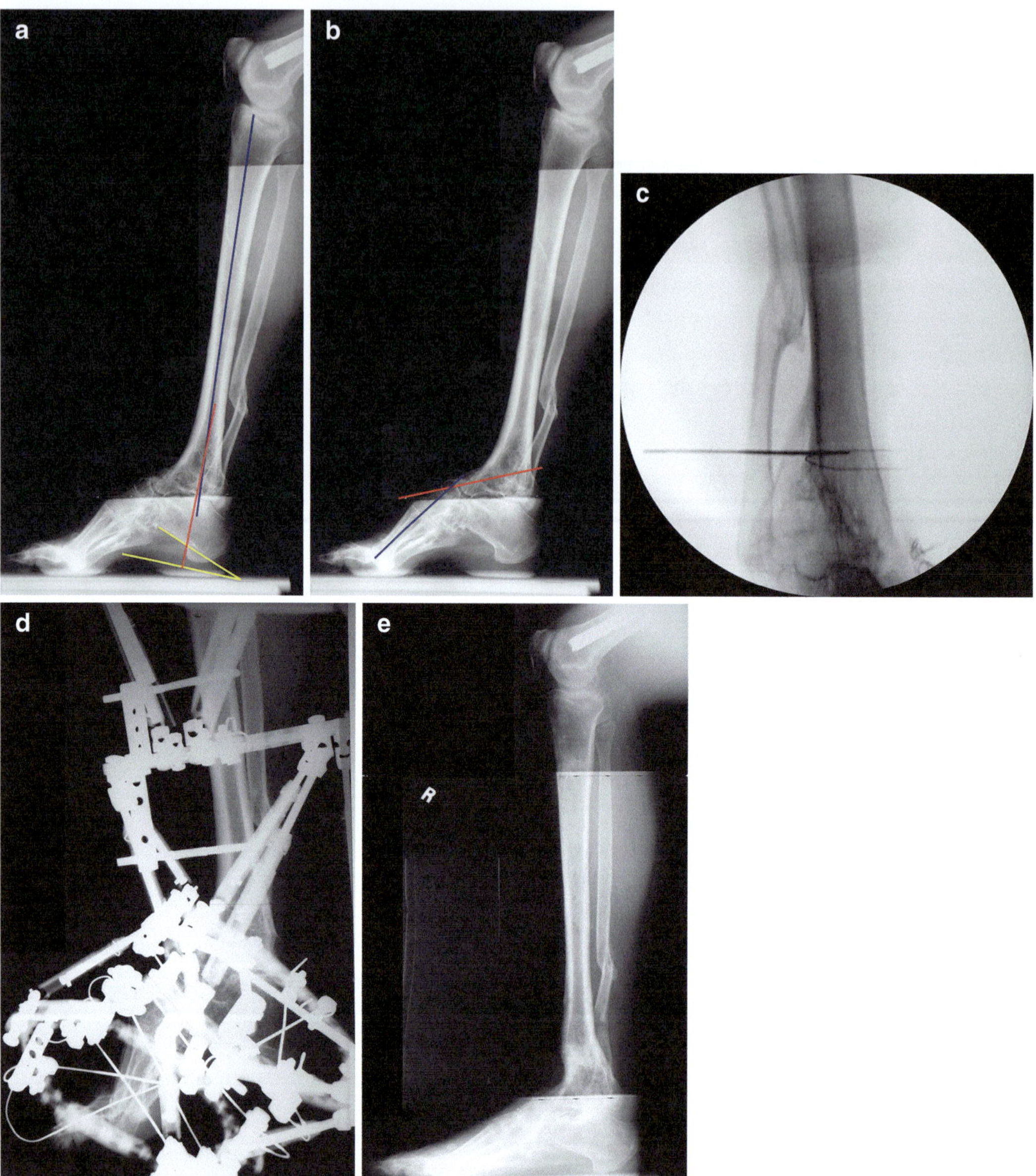

Fig. 18.2 A 50-year-old female presented with a history of a pilon fracture and subsequent ankle arthrodesis. (**a**) Lateral view radiograph shows preoperative planning for a supramalleolar osteotomy. The normal calcaneal pitch is drawn in *yellow*. A normal plantar angle of 90° is shown. The long axis of the tibia is shown in *blue*. The patient has a recurvatum deformity of 10° about the distal tibia. (**b**) Preoperative planning for midfoot osteotomy. Meary's angle is 30°. (**c**) The restrictor wire is a useful aide in controlling the level of the osteotomy. This wire prevents proximal migration of the Gigli saw. (**d**) A miter frame is shown. When combining a supramalleolar osteotomy and a midfoot osteotomy, apply a miter frame. (**e**) Final postoperative lateral view radiograph (Reprinted with permission from the Rubin Institute for Advanced Orthopedics, Sinai Hospital of Baltimore)

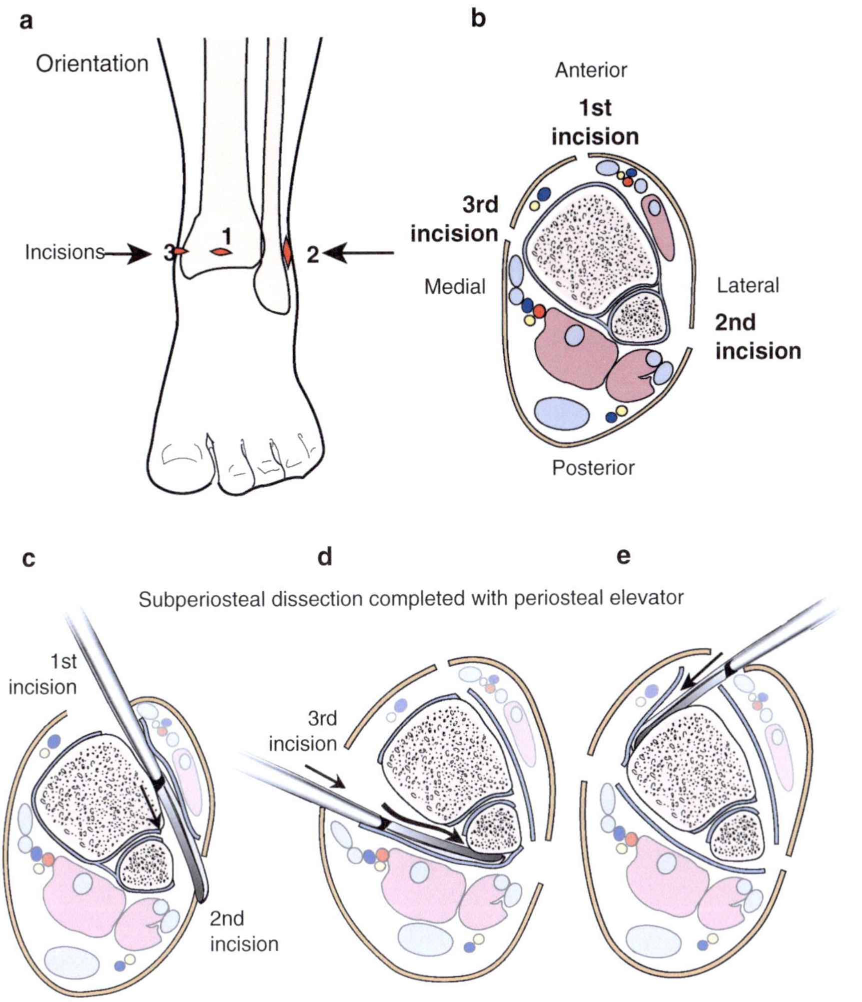

Fig. 18.3 Supramalleolar osteotomy illustration. (**a**, **b**) Percutaneous Gigli saw osteotomy in the supramalleolar region of the tibia and fibula. At this level, there is no space between the tibia and fibula through which to pass a suture. The Gigli saw is passed around both the tibia and the fibula, and both bones are cut together. Three small incisions are used: a transverse anterior incision, a longitudinal lateral incision, and a transverse medial incision. (**c**) First incision is a transverse anterior incision. The periosteum on the anterolateral aspect of the tibia and fibula is elevated. The second incision, a longitudinal lateral one, is made over the tip of the protruding elevator over the fibula. (**d**) Third incision is transverse medial incision. The periosteum is elevated on the posterior side of the tibia and fibula. (**e**) Then the periosteum is elevated on the anteromedial side of the tibia. (**f**) A long curved clamp is used to pass a suture from anterior to lateral. (**g**) Long end of the suture is divided. (**h–j**) Forceps and suture remnant removed. The Gigli saw is tied to the suture and pulled through from anterior to lateral. (**k**) Forceps, loaded with a second suture, is passed from the medial incision to the lateral one. (**l**, **m**) Long end of the second suture is divided. Forceps and suture remnant are removed. (**n**) Second suture is tied to the Gigli saw. (**o**) Suture and Gigli saw are pulled from the lateral incision to the medial one. (**p**) Gigli saw is used to cut the fibula and tibia from lateral to anteromedial. (**q**) The osteotomy is stopped midway through the tibia. Periosteal elevators are placed to protect the soft tissues. (**r**, **s**) Osteotomy is completed. The Gigli saw is cut and removed (Reprinted with permission from the Rubin Institute for Advanced Orthopedics, Sinai Hospital of Baltimore)

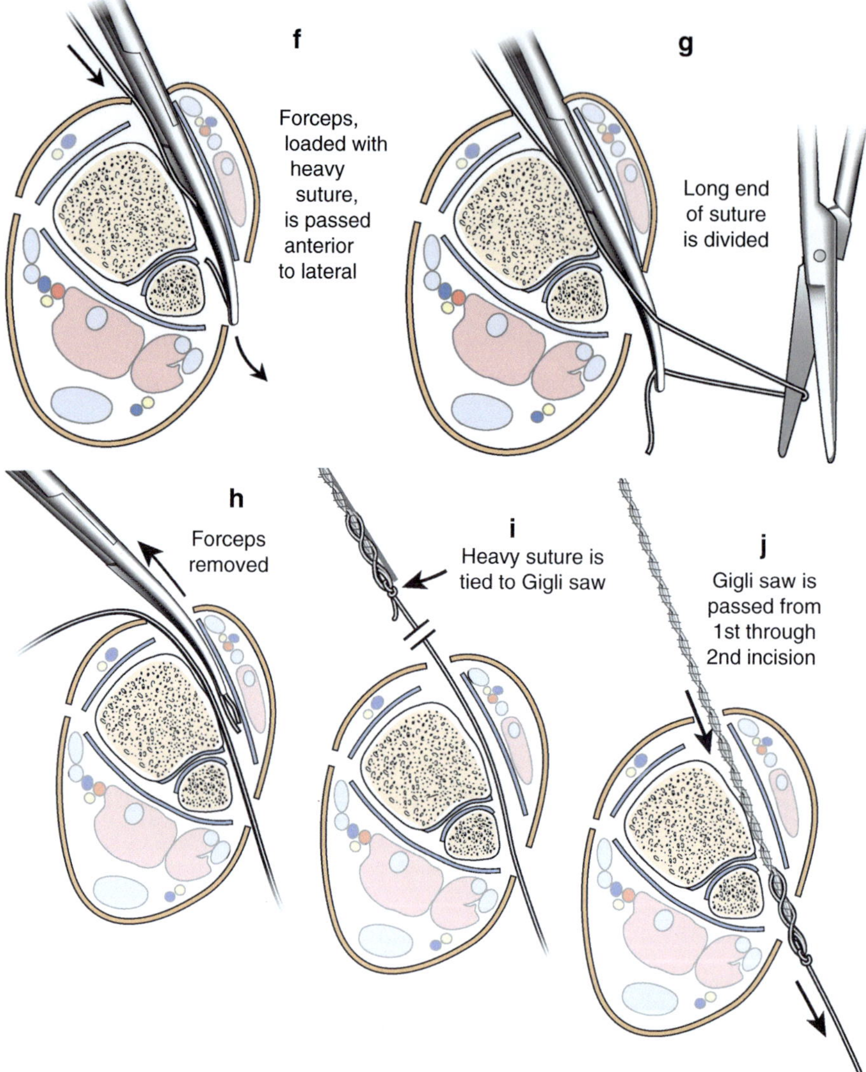

Fig. 18.3 (continued)

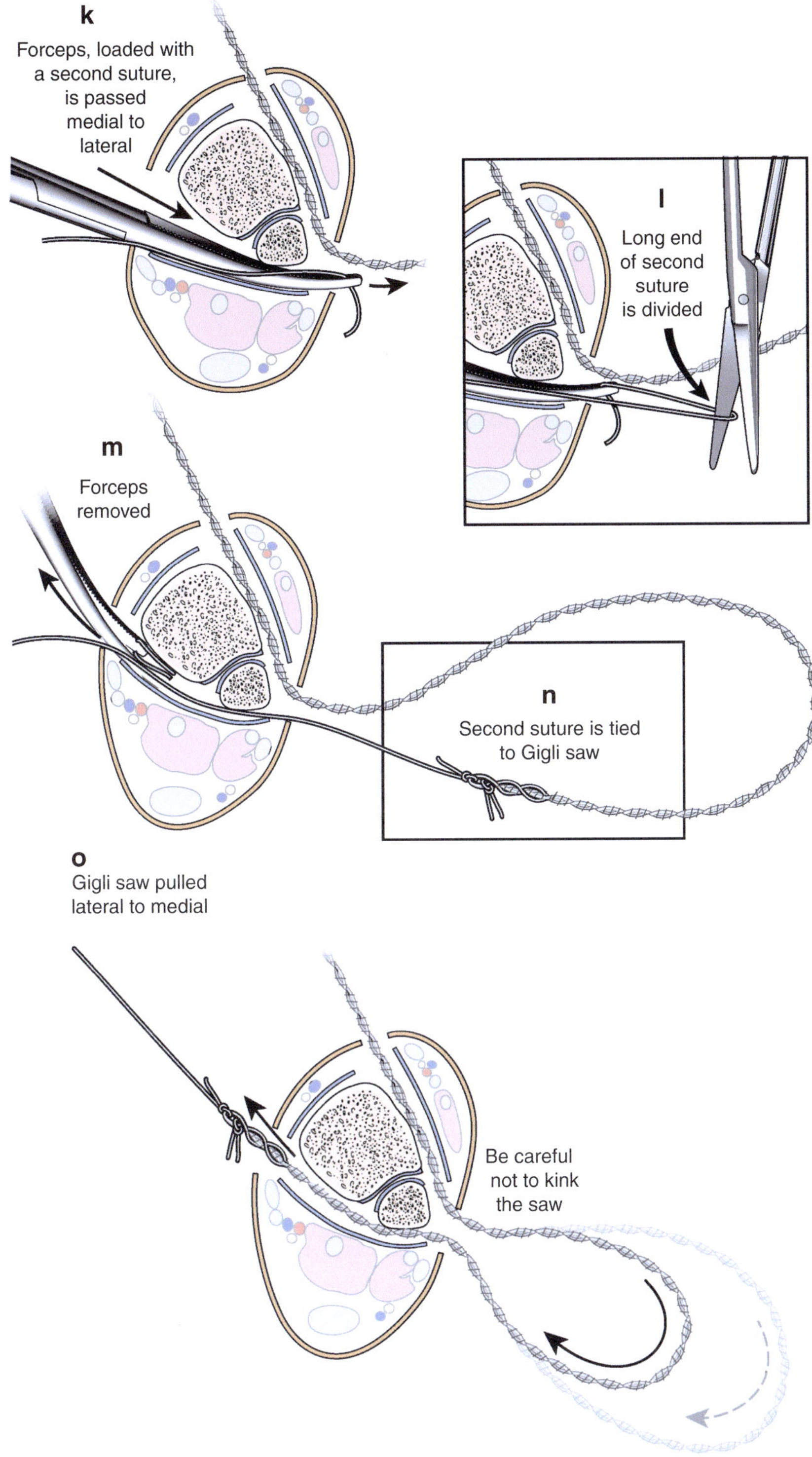

Fig. 18.3 (continued)

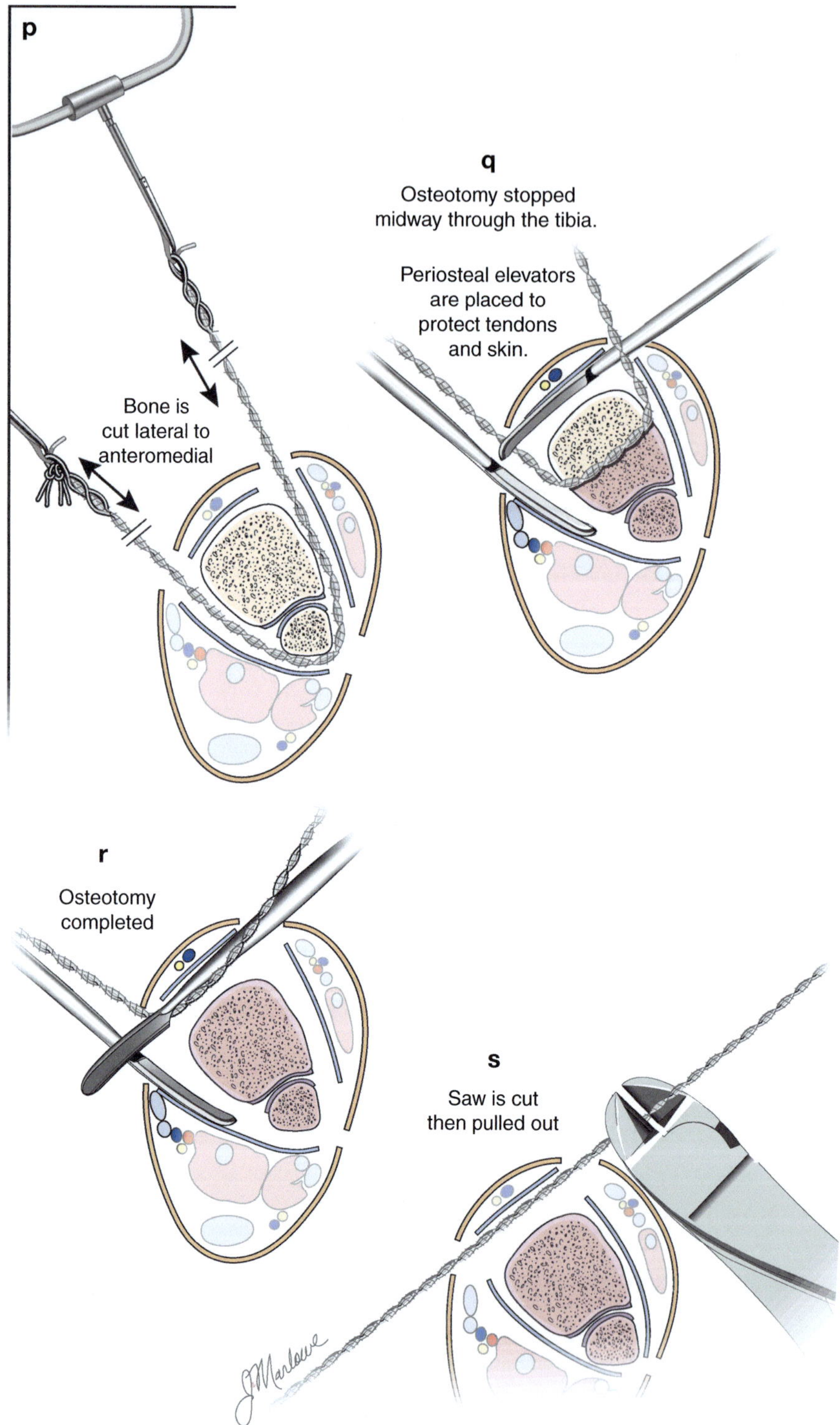

Fig. 18.3 (continued)

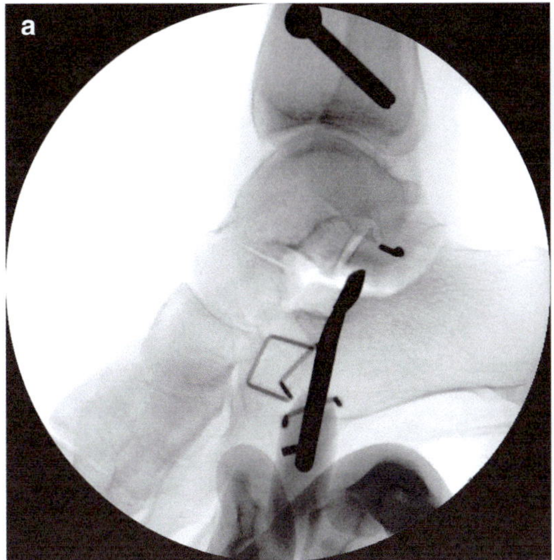
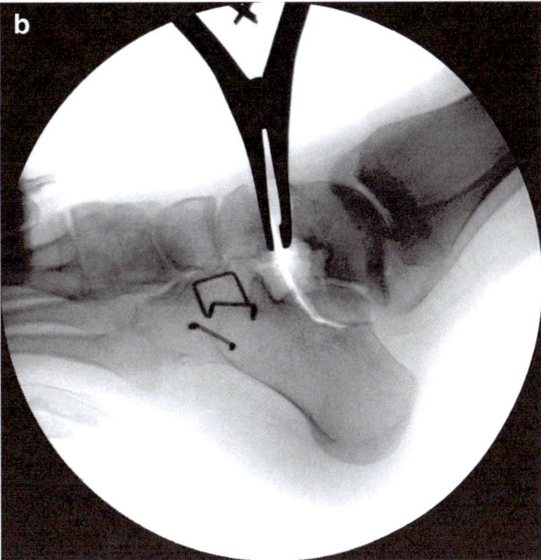

Fig. 18.4 (**a**) An olive wire captures the subtalar fragment and mounts proximally to allow distraction through the osteotomy and to prevent distraction through the subtalar joint. (**b**) Laminar spreaders are used to confirm completion of the osteotomy (Reprinted with permission from the Rubin Institute for Advanced Orthopedics, Sinai Hospital of Baltimore)

- This osteotomy allows the foot to move independent of the leg. Use a standard frame when performing an isolated SMO. Consider a Miter frame when SMO is combined with a midfoot osteotomy (Fig. 18.2d).

18.5.2.2 U-Osteotomy

- This osteotomy is indicated for deformities in which the CORA is at the level of the subtalar joint and the forefoot and hindfoot are well aligned. It is typically used in the setting of an equinus deformity with a flattop talus and is contraindicated when there is good subtalar joint movement.
- A U-osteotomy is performed through an Ollier's incision. Be mindful of the superficial peroneal nerve anteriorly and of the sural nerve posteriorly. Extensor digitorum brevis muscle is released from its origin and reflected anteriorly to expose the sinus tarsi.
- The osteotomy is performed under an image intensifier, across the talus neck, extending to the calcaneus, below the subtalar joint, and exiting posteriorly on the superior face of the calcaneal tuberosity. The subtalar fragment should be large enough to capture with a wire (Fig. 18.4a). This wire helps to ensure distraction across the osteotomy site and not across the subtalar joint. K-wires can be placed along the path of the intended osteotomy under image intensifier guidance. Then the path of these K-wires can be followed with the osteotome to make the osteotomy. The medial periosteum protects the posterior tibial neurovascular bundle. Laminar spreaders can be helpful in assessing completion of the osteotomy (Fig. 18.4b).
- This osteotomy allows the foot distal to the talus to be positioned independently so that a standard long bone frame can be applied (Fig. 18.5).
- The U-osteotomy creates two large bony surfaces with significant friction between fragments; therefore, programming at least 5–10 mm of distraction as a way station prior to deformity correction is required.
- There is also a risk for preconsolidation. We recommend that lengthening should begin around postoperative day 3.

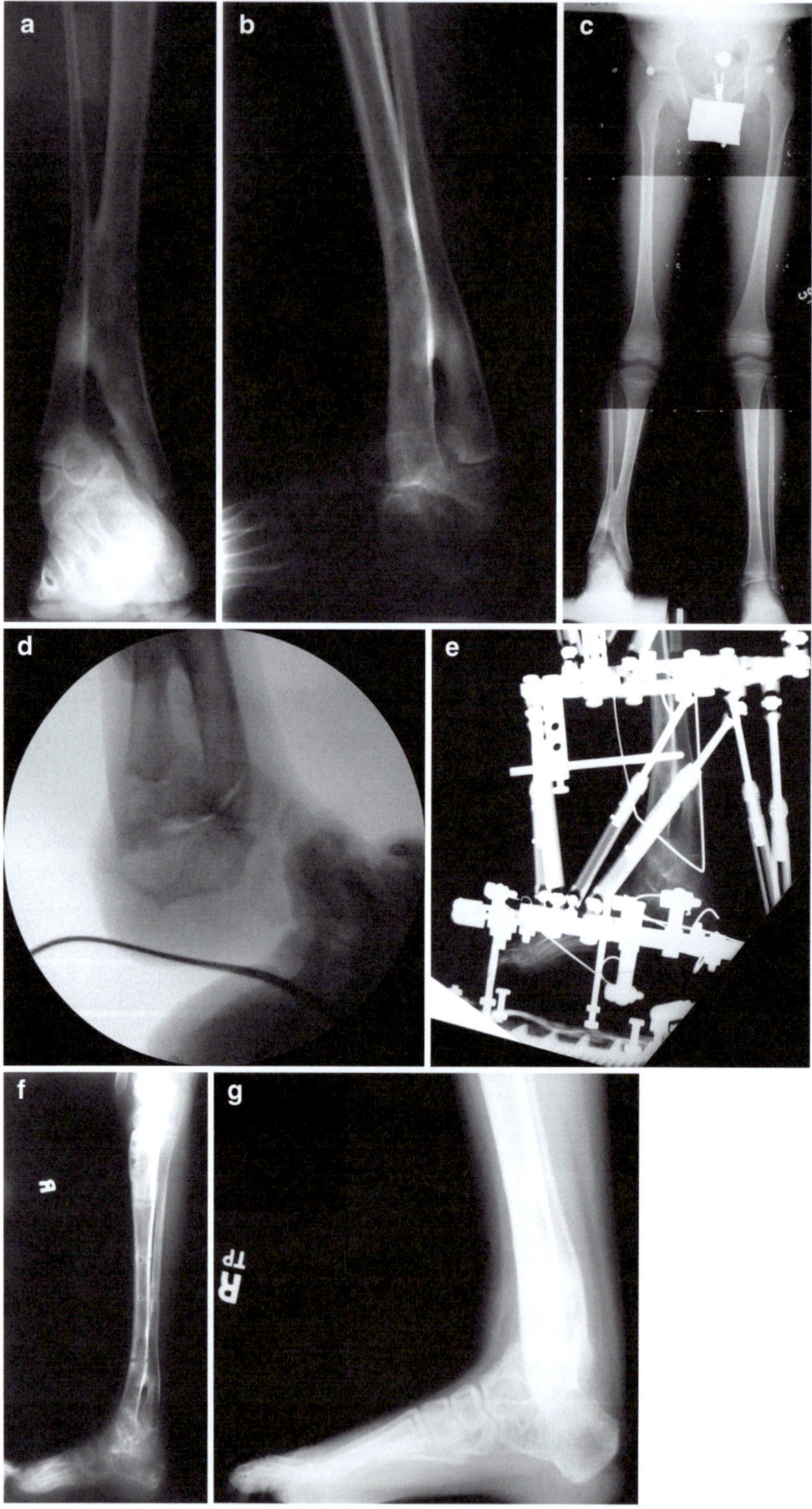

Fig. 18.5 U-osteotomy. (**a–c**) Preoperative anteroposterior (**a**), lateral (**b**), and long leg standing (**c**) radiographs. (**d**) Intraoperative image intensifier view shows the U-osteotomy. (**e**) Lateral view radiograph with standard TSF shows the regenerate bone. (**f**) Initial postoperative lateral view radiograph. (**g**) Lateral view radiograph of the right foot and ankle obtained 2 years postoperatively (Reprinted with permission from the Rubin Institute for Advanced Orthopedics, Sinai Hospital of Baltimore)

18.5.2.3 V-Osteotomy

- This osteotomy is indicated for deformities in which one CORA is present between the leg and hindfoot at the level of the subtalar joint and a second CORA exists between the forefoot and hindfoot, also at the level of the subtalar joint. In this situation, a V-osteotomy allows for independent manipulation of both the forefoot and hindfoot.
- The V-osteotomy consists of two osteotomies: one anterior and one posterior. It is performed through two separate incisions. The anterior osteotomy is a midfoot osteotomy, as described in Sect. 18.5.2.4. The posterior osteotomy is performed through an oblique incision on the medial or lateral side, over the calcaneal tuberosity. The posterior osteotomy crosses the body of the calcaneus. Take care to prevent injury of the neurovascular bundle on the medial side of the foot.
- The V-osteotomy creates three mobile fragments: the leg, the hindfoot, and the forefoot. A butt frame can be used in this situation. The butt frame can be cumbersome on small and even regular sized feet and result in a "ship-in-a-bottle" configuration. An alternative could be acute correction of the hindfoot. For pediatric feet, such a frame can be bulky; therefore, consider acute correction of the calcaneus or combining TSF methods with Ilizarov methods.
- Achilles tendon lengthening and plantar fascial release can help decrease resistance to deformity correction.

18.5.2.4 Midfoot Osteotomy

- This osteotomy is indicated for deformities in which the CORA is located in the midfoot but the hindfoot is well aligned.
- A midfoot osteotomy is best performed by percutaneous methods with a Gigli saw (Fig. 18.6). This osteotomy is performed at the level of the talocalcaneal neck, the navicular-cuboid, or the cuboid cuneiform. Do not perform the osteotomy at the base of the metatarsals because of the risk of injury to the digital neurovascular bundles.
- This osteotomy allows the forefoot to move independently. (Use a butt frame)

Pearls

These osteotomies are best reserved for adult feet.

- For a percutaneous SMO, pass the Gigli saw around the tibia and fibula prior to frame application. Initiate the osteotomy for the supramalleolar osteotomy, but do not complete the osteotomy before frame application or else the foot will become too unstable and difficult to work with during the remainder of the procedure.
- Supramalleolar osteotomies that are closer to the ankle heal faster, but there must be enough room for fixation of the distal fragment. If the osteotomy is more than 2–2.5 cm proximal to the ankle, expect slower healing rate.
- For a percutaneous midfoot osteotomy, pass the Gigli saw prior to frame application. In contrast to the SMO, complete the midfoot osteotomy before frame application. The forefoot will remain stable enough to work with during the remainder of the procedure.
- To perform a midfoot osteotomy, place one wire 5 mm proximal to and parallel to the osteotomy and another wire 5 mm distal to and parallel to the osteotomy. These wires help concentrate distraction forces on the midfoot osteotomy. Place these wires prior to frame application because the frame obscures visualization.
- To place a half pin in a tight space, first place a wire and then use a cannulated drill when the position of the wire is satisfactory.

18.5.3 Taylor Spatial Frame Selection

18.5.3.1 Basic TSF Principles

- Increasing the number of wires and half pins increases stability. Tensioned wires and single half pins have similar stability. Rings should be secured by at least three points of fixation.
- Operative mode choices in the TSF planning software include total residual or chronic modes. Always use total residual mode, which

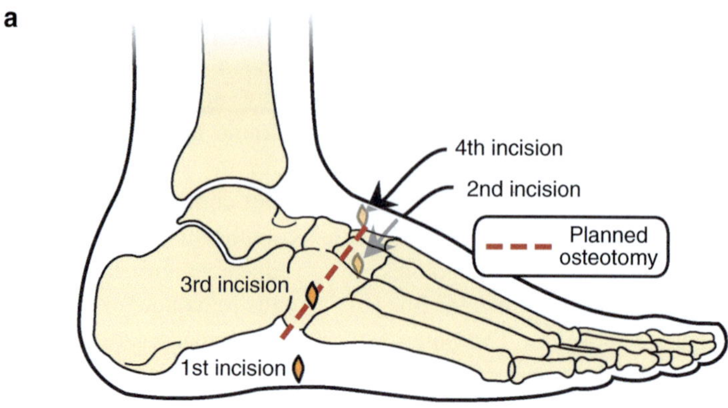

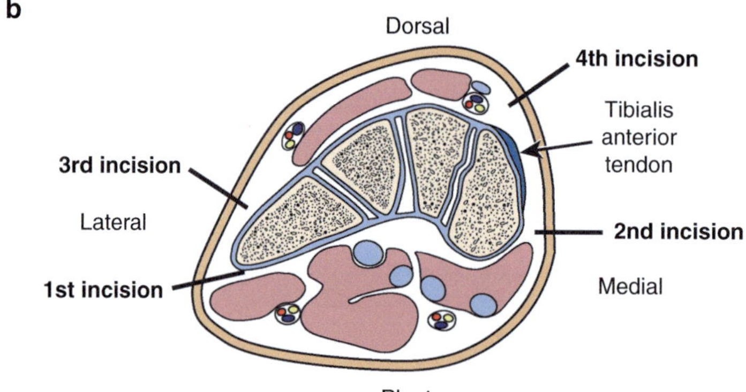

Fig. 18.6 Midfoot osteotomy illustration. (**a, b**) There are three levels in the midfoot at which a Gigli saw can be safely passed percutaneously: the talocalcaneal neck, cuboid-navicular bone, and cuboid cuneiform level. These illustrations show the cuboid cuneiform level. Four small incisions are used to pass the saw: plantar lateral, plantar medial, dorsolateral, and dorsomedial incisions. (**c, d**) First incision is a plantar lateral incision. The periosteum on the plantar aspect of the foot is elevated with a periosteal elevator. Because of the concavity of the transverse arch and the number of bones involved, the periosteal elevator often weaves in and out of the subperiosteal space. A plantar medial incision (second incision) is made. (**e, f**) A dorsolateral incision (third incision) is made. The periosteal elevator is used to create a tunnel underneath the long extensors of the dorsum of the foot. A fourth incision is made on the dorsomedial side. (**g**) Medial periosteum is elevated, which connects the dorsomedial and plantar medial incisions. (**h**) A suture is passed across the plantar aspect of the foot from lateral to medial (the reverse can also be done). The long end of the suture is cut. (**i, j**) Forceps and suture remnant are removed. The suture is tired to the Gigli saw. (**k**) Gigli saw is passed from medial to lateral under the foot. (**l**) Forceps, loaded with a second suture, is passed medially from the dorsomedial to the plantar medial incision. (**m**) Long end of the suture is divided. (**n, o**) Forceps and suture remnant are removed. A bend is created in the stiff end of the Gigli saw. (**p**) Gigli saw is passed medially from the plantar medial to the dorsomedial incision. (**q, r**) Process of passing a suture is repeated. In this case, the forceps, loaded with a heavy suture, is passed across the dorsal aspect of the foot from lateral to medial. The forceps and suture remnant are removed. The suture is divided and the long end is tied to the Gigli saw. (**s**) Gigli saw is passed from medial to lateral over the dorsal aspect of the foot. (**t**) Bone is cut medial to lateral, stopping at the cuboid. (**u, v**) Lateral periosteal bridge is elevated, and the cuboid is cut under the protection of the periosteal elevator. (**w**) Gigli saw is cut and then pulled out (Reprinted with permission from the Rubin Institute for Advanced Orthopedics, Sinai Hospital of Baltimore)

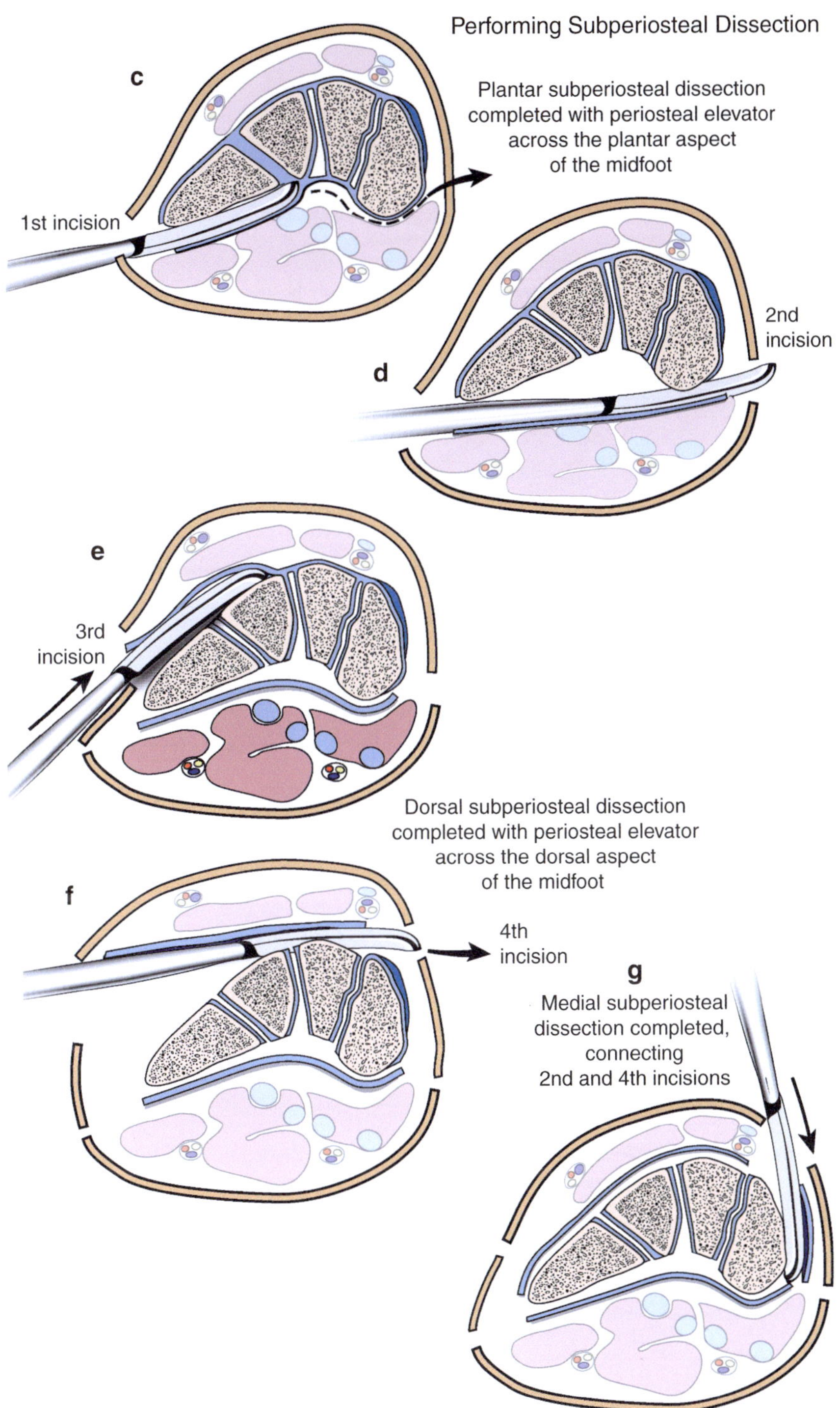

Fig. 18.6 (continued)

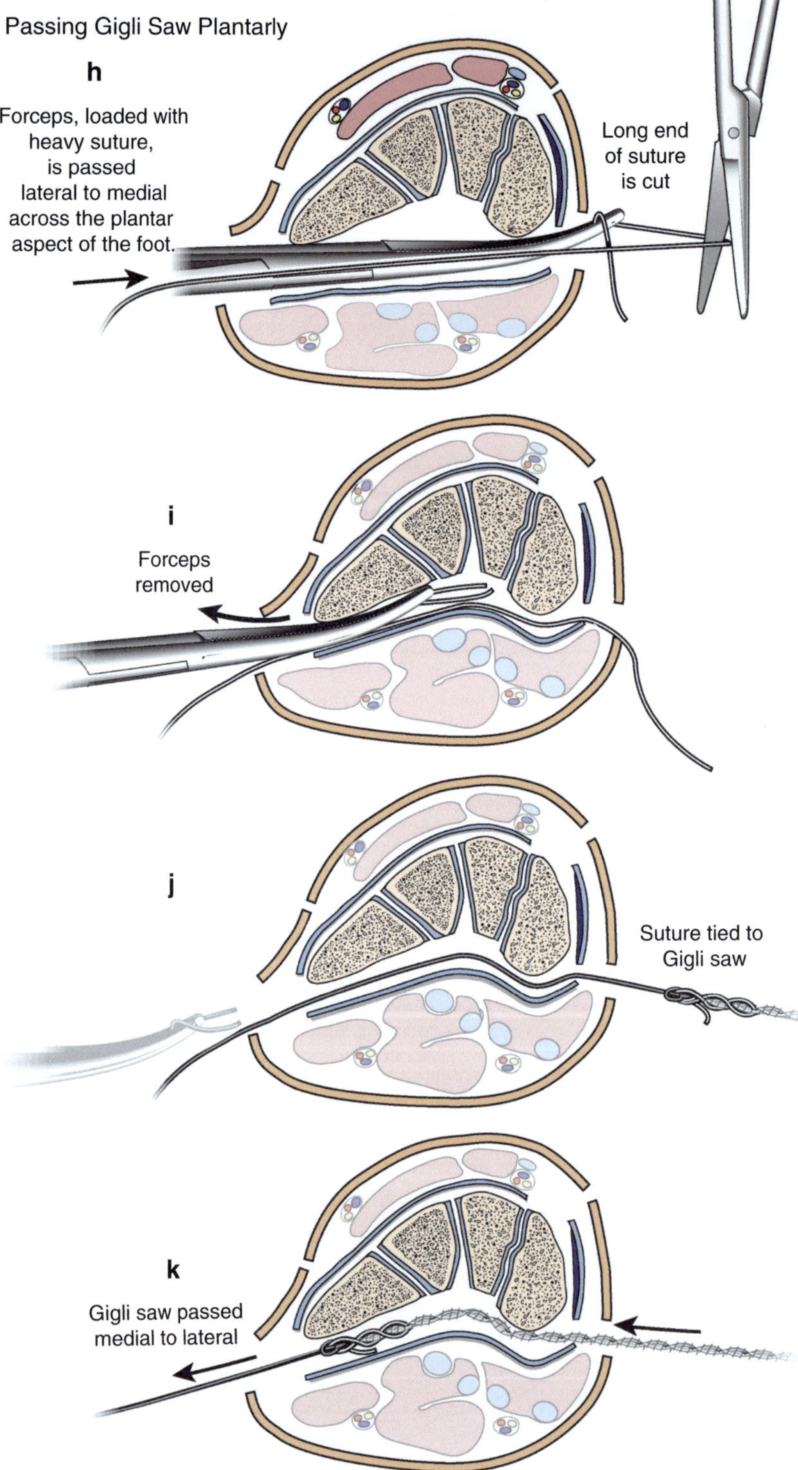

Fig. 18.6 (continued)

Passing Gigli Saw Medially

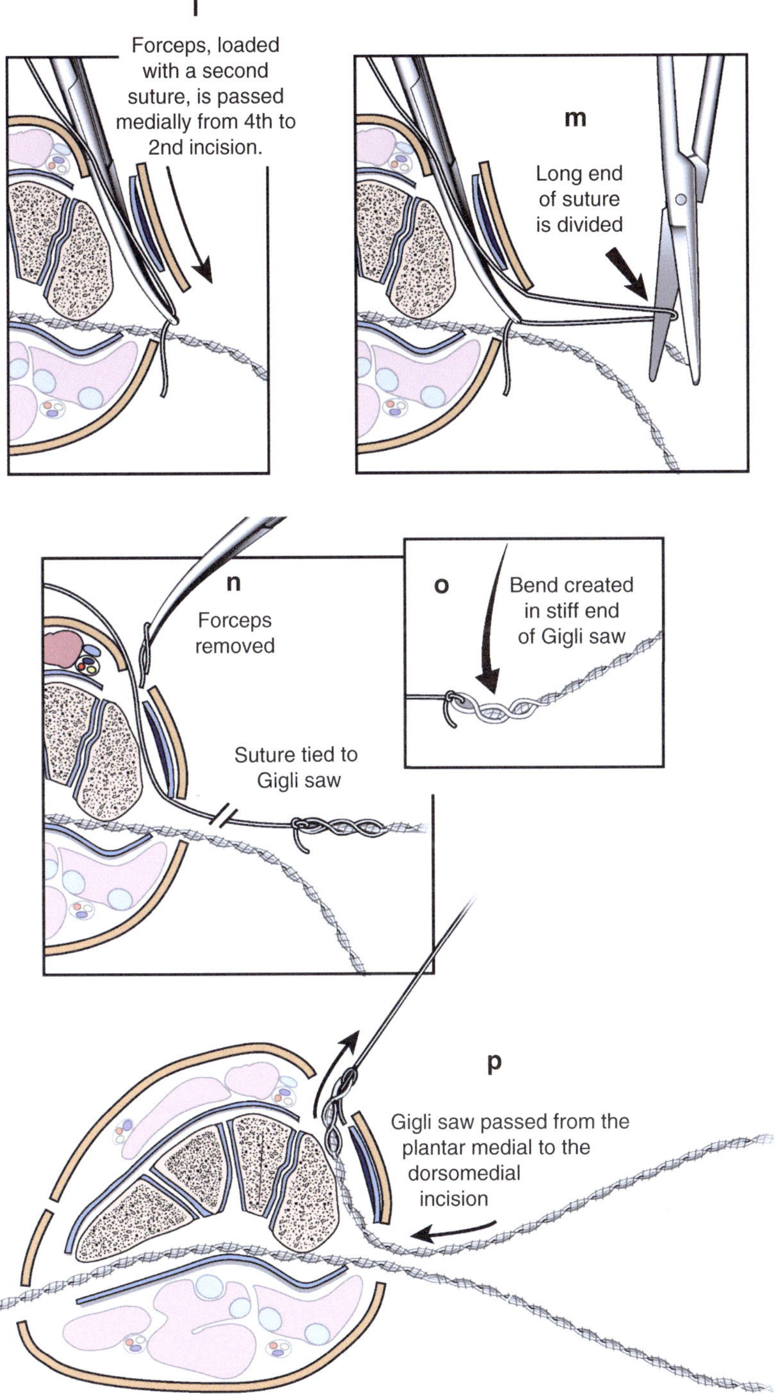

Fig. 18.6 (continued)

Passing Gigli Saw Dorsally

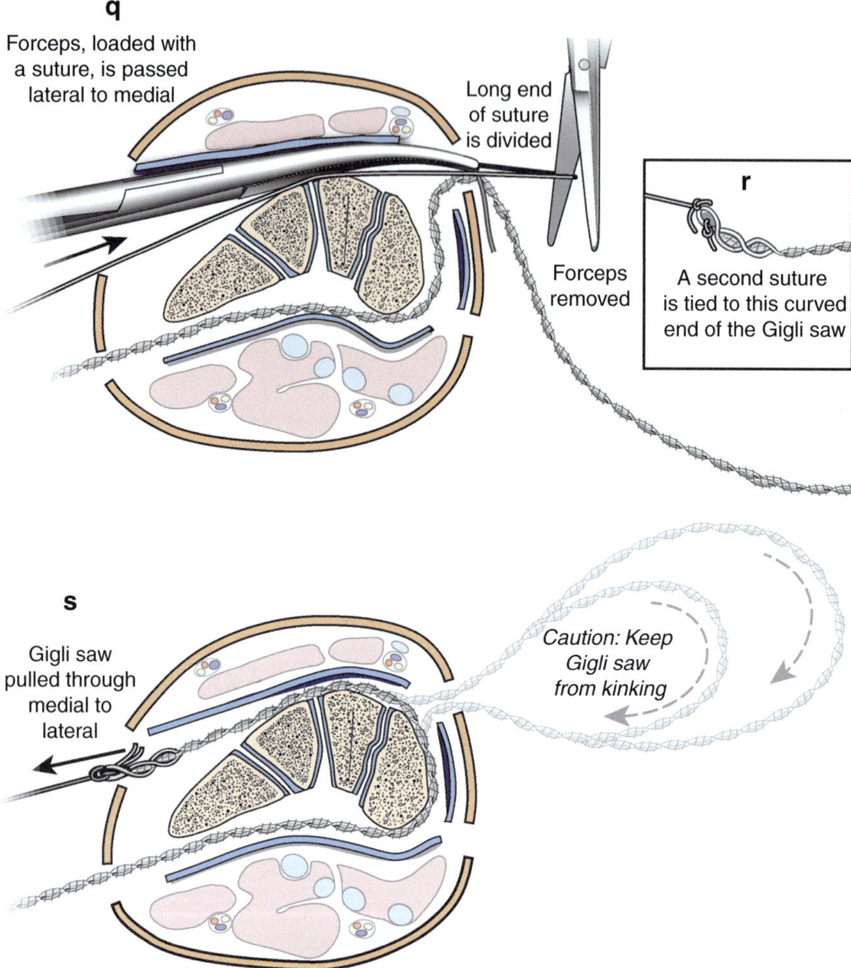

Fig. 18.6 (continued)

Performing the Osteotomy

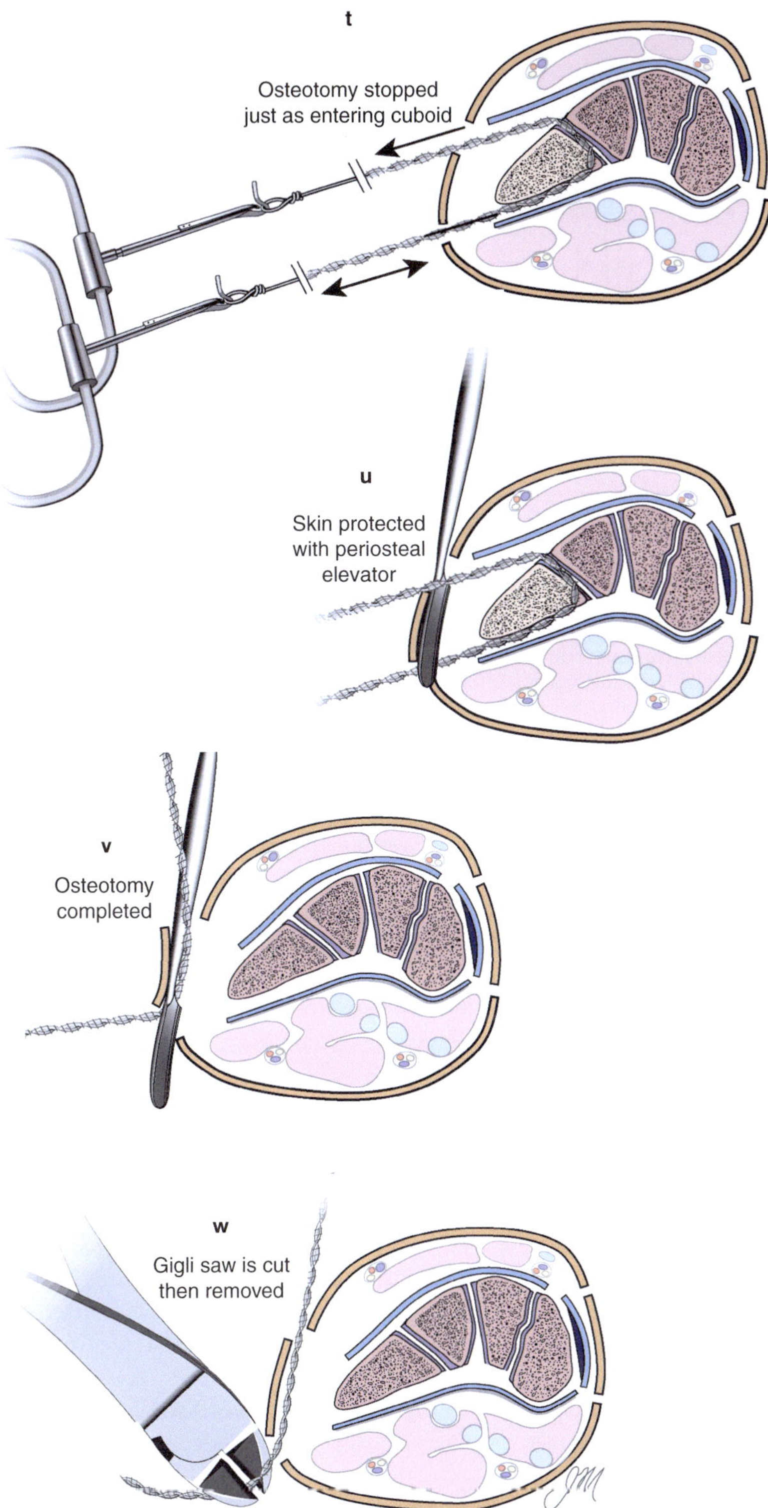

Fig. 18.6 (continued)

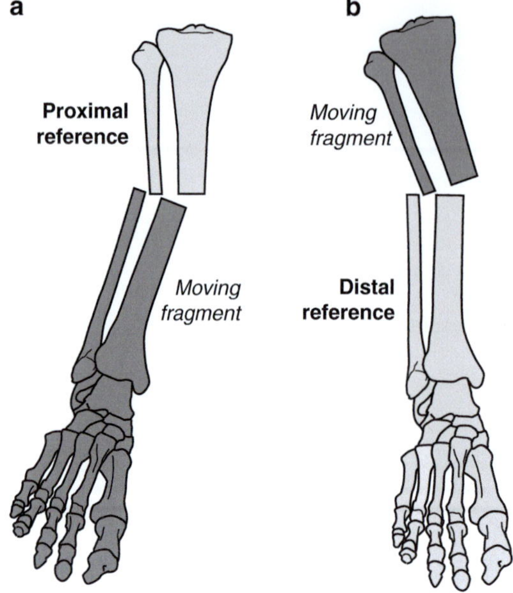

Fig. 18.7 Distal referencing versus proximal referencing. (**a**) In proximal referencing, translation and angulation are defined by the relationship of the distal fragment relative to the proximal fragment. (**b**) In distal referencing, translation and angulation are defined by the relationship of the proximal fragment relative to the distal fragment (Reprinted with permission from the Rubin Institute for Advanced Orthopaedics, Sinai Hospital of Baltimore)

takes the surgeon's input of initial deformity and mounting parameters and then allows the computer to determine a final frame configuration.

- Proximal or distal referencing can be chosen in most cases. In proximal referencing, translation and angulation are defined by the relationship of the distal fragment relative to the proximal fragment. In distal referencing, translation and angulation are defined by the relationship of the proximal fragment relative to the distal fragment. A deformity described by a proximal reference will have the same angulation as a deformity described by a distal reference, but the translation will be in opposite directions (Fig. 18.7).
- In the CORAsponding point method of TSF programming, the corresponding point is set to the CORA. In turn, the origin will always be located on the reference line, but away from the CORA by the defined amount of axial translation (Fig. 18.8).

18.5.3.2 Standard Long Bone Frame

- This frame consists of two rings with six TSF struts in between the rings (Fig. 18.9). The standard frame is used when the foot is being manipulated about the leg, such as with an SMO or a U-osteotomy.
- Place the proximal ring about the mid-diaphysis of the tibia. A reference wire is placed perpendicular to the long axis of the tibia. The ring is then suspended on the reference wire, and the reference wire is tensioned. Two or three additional half pins are applied to secure the proximal ring. When using a standard frame for a U-osteotomy, another wire needs to be placed through the subtalar fragment and secured to the proximal ring to ensure distraction occurs across the osteotomy.
- The distal ring is placed parallel to the plantar surface of the foot. Secure the ring with wires through the calcaneus and metatarsals. To capture the calcaneus, use two divergent counter-opposed olive wires. To tension the olive wires, lock the end of the olive wire with the olive to the frame and tension the opposite side. When passing wires through the metatarsals, avoid flattening the transverse metatarsal arch to capture all the metatarsals with a single wire, as this is unnecessary. Instead, pass one or two wires as shown in Fig. 18.10.
- When selecting "foot" as the correction area in the spatialframe.com planning software, choose the ankle type.
- Use distal referencing.
- Mounting parameters describe the position of the reference ring relative to the origin.
- Define the structure at risk by its relationship to the origin.

18.5.3.3 Miter Frame

- The miter frame is constructed from two full rings, one 2/3 ring, and twelve struts (Fig. 18.11a). Use this frame when combining an SMO with a midfoot osteotomy.
- The proximal ring goes around the mid-diaphysis of the tibia and is secured with two or three 6-mm half pins. For complex foot deformities in young children, use 4.5-mm half pins.

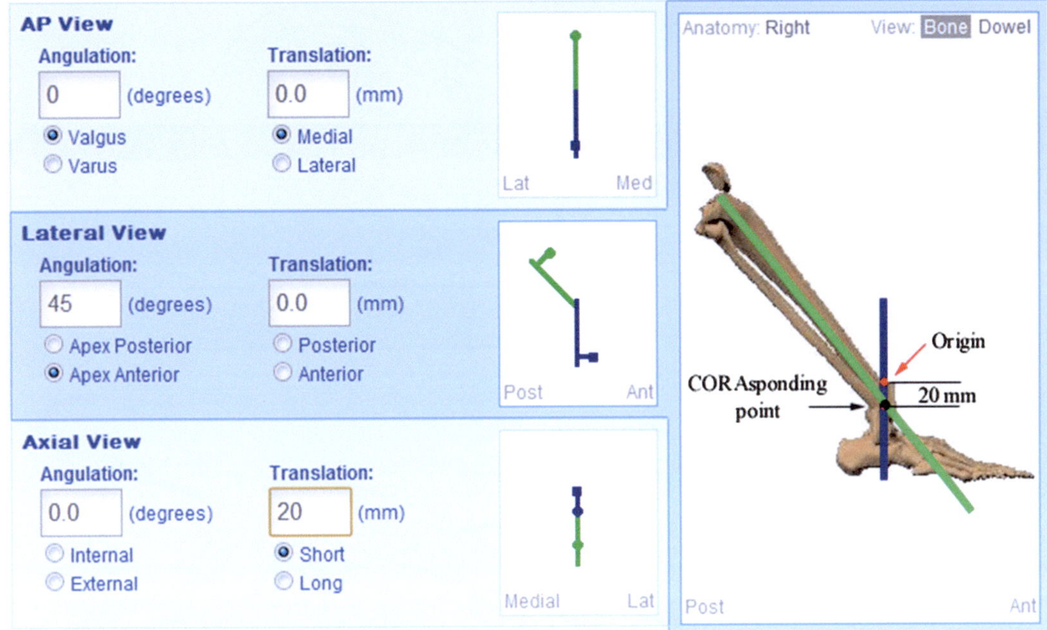

Fig. 18.8 CORAsponding point method, https://www.spatialframe.com

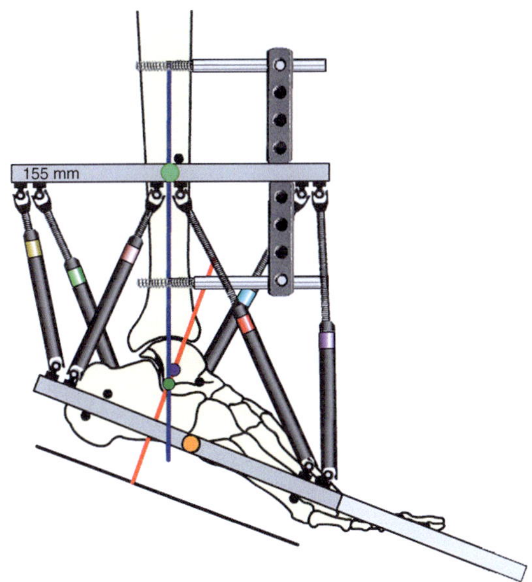

Fig. 18.9 Standard frame configuration (Reprinted with permission from the Rubin Institute for Advanced Orthopedics, Sinai Hospital of Baltimore)

- The distal ring is typically a full ring and is secured to the metatarsals by two or three tensioned 1/8 wires.
- Six struts are placed between each set of rings.
- Two separate programs are required in the spatialfram.com planning software. The hindfoot program uses the mid-diaphyseal region of the tibia and corrects the deformity between the leg and foot. The forefoot program uses the miter 6×6 ft correction type and corrects the relationship of the hindfoot and forefoot.
- The hindfoot program usually uses a proximal reference.
- The forefoot program uses a distal reference, which is the only option when using the miter frame program.
- For the forefoot program, the rotary frame angle for the mounting parameters is set to 180°. This places the master tab (where strut #1 and #2 come together on the more proximal ring) on the plantar aspect of the calcaneus.

- Use a 2/3 ring to secure the calcaneus. Two divergent counter-opposed olive wires or two divergent half pins are used to secure the calcaneus.

18.5.3.4 Butt Frame

- The butt frame is constructed from one standard ring and a U-ring or two U-rings placed around the hindfoot. One standard ring is

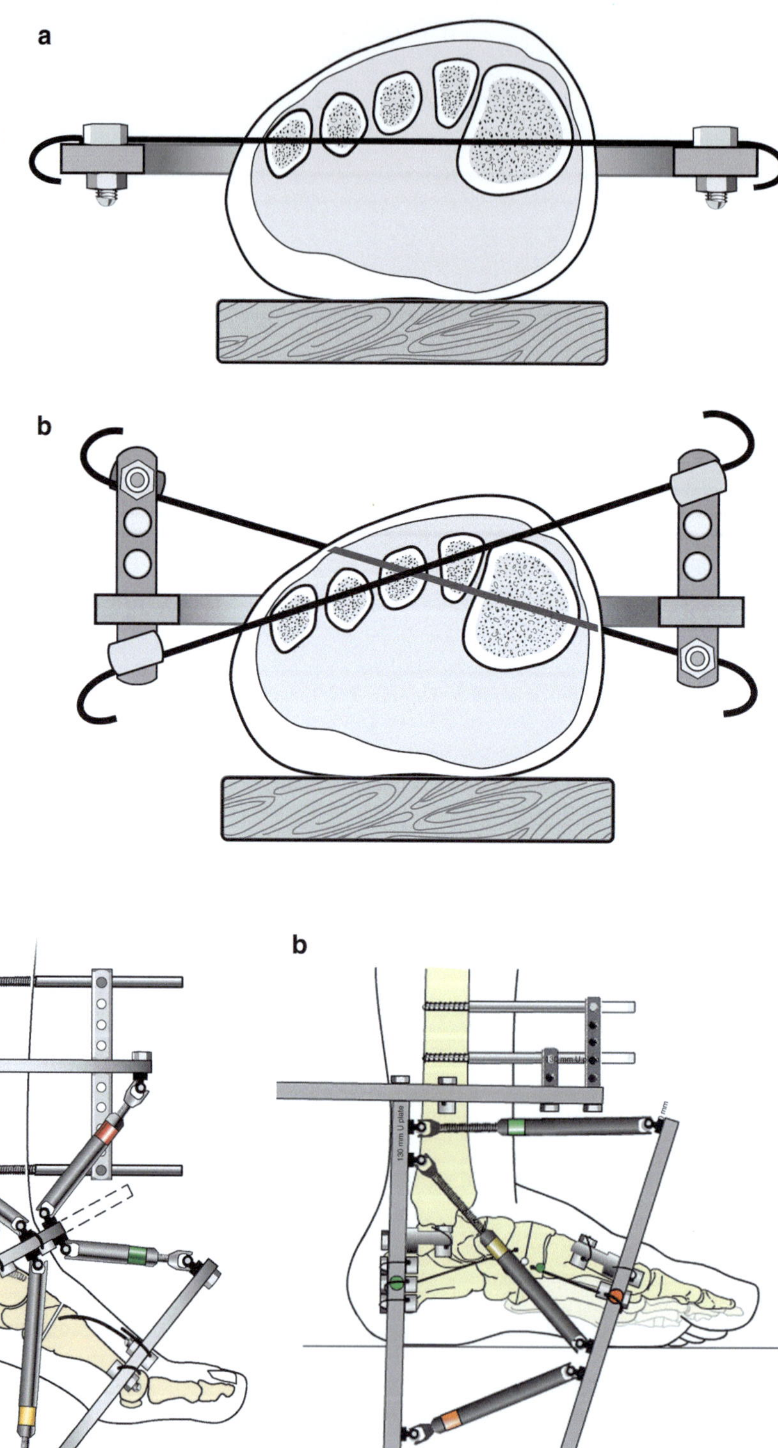

Fig. 18.10 Metatarsal wire configurations. One or two wires can be used to capture the metatarsals. In passing metatarsal wires, it is easiest to pass from the smaller bone to the larger bone. When applying a single metatarsal wire, as in (**a**), avoid flattening the metatarsal arch. When applying two metatarsal wires, as in (**b**), the wires are passed in a divergent pattern (Reprinted with permission from the Rubin Institute for Advanced Orthopedics, Sinai Hospital of Baltimore)

Fig. 18.11 Miter (**a**) and butt (**b**) frame configurations (Reprinted with permission from the Rubin Institute for Advanced Orthopedics, Sinai Hospital of Baltimore) placed about the forefoot, with six struts between (Fig. 18.11b). This configuration is particularly useful when a midfoot osteotomy is performed.

- One U-ring is secured about the distal tibia with a reference wire and two or three half pins. Alternatively, a standard ring may replace this proximal U-ring.
- The second vertical U-ring is secured perpendicular to the first U-ring. The foot is captured with counter-opposed olive wires through the calcaneus in the frontal plane. A smooth wire is placed transversely through the neck of the talus, proximal to the midfoot osteotomy.
- A full ring is placed about the metatarsals. It is secured with two divergent metatarsal wires and another wire placed just distal to the midfoot osteotomy. Toe wires may be incorporated into the distal metatarsal ring for more stability.
- Six struts attach the U-ring to a standard ring.
- Either proximal or distal referencing is used to match the radiographic images from which the deformity measurements are made. Usually, distal referencing is done, with the distal ring applied perpendicular to the forefoot.
- The rotary frame angle for the mounting parameters is set to 180° so that the master tab is located on the plantar aspect of the calcaneus.

- When correcting an angular deformity, especially when the osteotomy and CORA are at different levels, it is necessary to axially distract the fragments and disengage them prior to angular correction. The spatial frame program allows the user to prioritize axial translation correction in the deformity tab. Alternatively, a way station may be created by performing axial translation alone and then reprogramming for angular correction.
- To help place the foot ring parallel to the plantar surface of the foot, apply a flat surface such as a sterile cutting board to the plantar surface of the foot and use this flat surface as a reference. Additionally, wires can be placed first, followed by placement of the U-plate.
- For calcaneal wires, the lateral olive is placed perpendicular to the calcaneus and exits posterior to the neurovascular bundle. The medial olive wire is placed obliquely, targeting a point 1 cm proximal to the calcaneal-cuboid joint.
- For metatarsal wires, it is easiest to pass wires from a small target to a large target. Therefore, pass wires from the fifth metatarsal toward the first metatarsal.
- For the miter frame, check that the 2/3 ring selected for the calcaneus has a full complement of tabs. Some rings are chamfered on the ends and have only five holes instead of six.
- To remember the orientation of the struts for the miter frame and butt frame, imagine taking a tibial long bone frame, sliding it down the leg, and rotating 180°.
- Reference radiographs should be aligned with the reference ring.
- When applying a butt frame construct, shift the vertical ring as posterior as possible to allow more room for the TSF struts. Additionally, it is helpful to shift the metatarsal ring as far forward as possible.

18.6 Postoperative Care

18.6.1 Complications

18.6.1.1 Infections

- Infections are common, but oral antibiotics usually suffice. Most are pin site infections that rarely become osteomyelitis; however, serious cases do occur.
- Toxic shock syndrome and necrotizing fasciitis have been reported (Turker et al. 1992). These patients present ill with loss of appetite, decreased activity, and febrile. A diffuse rash may be present with toxic shock syndrome. Urgent attention is required, with urgent and aggressive resuscitation and initiation of empiric intravenous antibiotics.

18.6.1.2 Claw Toes and Metatarsal Phalangeal Joint Subluxation

- These complications occur when toe flexors become tight during lengthening and deformity correction. Prophylactic toe stretching exercises and the use of toe slings for passive stretches are helpful. Alternatively, the metatarsal-phalangeal joints can be pinned or flexor tendons can be lengthened by flexor tenotomy. Incorporating longitudinal toe wires in the distal ring increases the stability of the construct.

18.6.1.3 Premature Consolidation

- Premature consolidation is common in the foot, where the osteotomies have large cancellous surfaces. Distraction typically begins on postoperative day 3.
- When premature consolidation occurs, repeat the osteotomy.

Pearls

- Prophylactic toe fixation helps prevent claw toes and metatarsal-phalangeal joint subluxation. Additionally, this increases stability to forefoot fixation.

18.7 Special Frames

18.7.1 "PonseTaylor Method"

- The PonseTaylor method for clubfoot correction recapitulates the Ponseti sequence using the TSF (Fig. 18.12). It is useful in children aged 2–12 with recurrent clubfeet or previously operated clubfeet (Floerkemeier et al. 2011).
- Prior to TSF application, the foot is casted to correct the metatarsus adductus deformity.
- The method has two stages of correction and an optional third stage.
- During the first stage of the PonseTaylor method, the foot is rotated about the talus, correcting the forefoot adduction and hindfoot varus deformities.
- During the second stage of the PonseTaylor method, the foot is dorsiflexed to correct the equinus deformity.
- The optional third stage, sometimes called "PonseTaylor II," corrects residual cavus and the forefoot adduction deformity.

18.7.1.1 Preoperative Planning

- Preoperative planning should include assessment of deformity.
- Hindfoot varus should be overcorrected to approximately 20° valgus.
- Forefoot adduction should be overcorrected to approximately 40° of abduction/external rotation.
- Ankle equinus should be overcorrected to approximately 20–25° dorsiflexion.

18.7.1.2 Applying the TSF

- A standard long bone frame is applied. A tibial ring is placed about the mid-diaphysis of the tibia. The foot ring is mounted parallel to the plantar surface of the foot. The foot is

Fig. 18.12 The "PonseTaylor" method uses the TSF to recreate some principles of the Ponseti method to treat clubfoot. After a couple casts to correct the cavus deformity, Phase 1 addresses the forefoot adduction and hindfoot varus deformities. (**a**) PonseTaylor, Initial Phase 1: Axial, anteroposterior (*AP*), and lateral projections are shown, illustrating the application of a standard long bone frame. A tibial ring is placed about the mid diaphysis of the tibia. A foot ring mounted parallel to the plantar surface of the foot with two counter-opposed olive wires through the calcaneus and one or two smooth wires through the metatarsals. A distal tibia epiphysis wire prevents distraction across the distal tibia physis. A talar neck wire is passed from lateral to medial and secured to the proximal ring. (**b**) PonseTaylor, End of Phase 1: Axial, AP, and lateral projections are shown, illustrating the foot following correction of the external rotation and varus deformities. The goal of correction is approximately 20o valgus and 40o abduction/external rotation. Phase 2 addresses the equinus deformity. (**c**) PonseTaylor, Initial Phase 2: Hardware Modification: AP projections illustrating the transfer of the talar neck wire from the tibial ring to the foot ring. (**d**) PonseTaylor, Final Phase 2: Correction: Lateral and AP projections illustrate the position of the foot in the final corrected position, demonstrating correction of equinus, with over correction to 20o. Phase 3 addresses any residual forefoot adduction and cavus. (**e**) PonseTaylor, Initial Optional Phase 3: Hardware Modification: After building stable Ilizarov threaded rod constructs between the posterior and anterior halves of the foot ring, the foot ring cut using a Gigli saw to allow for lengthening on the medial side of the foot and shortening on the lateral side. (**f**) PonseTaylor Final Optional Phase 3: Correction: the foot and foot ring in the final corrected position, illustrating distraction of the medial foot. Laterally, the ring is allowed to compress to the patient's comfort

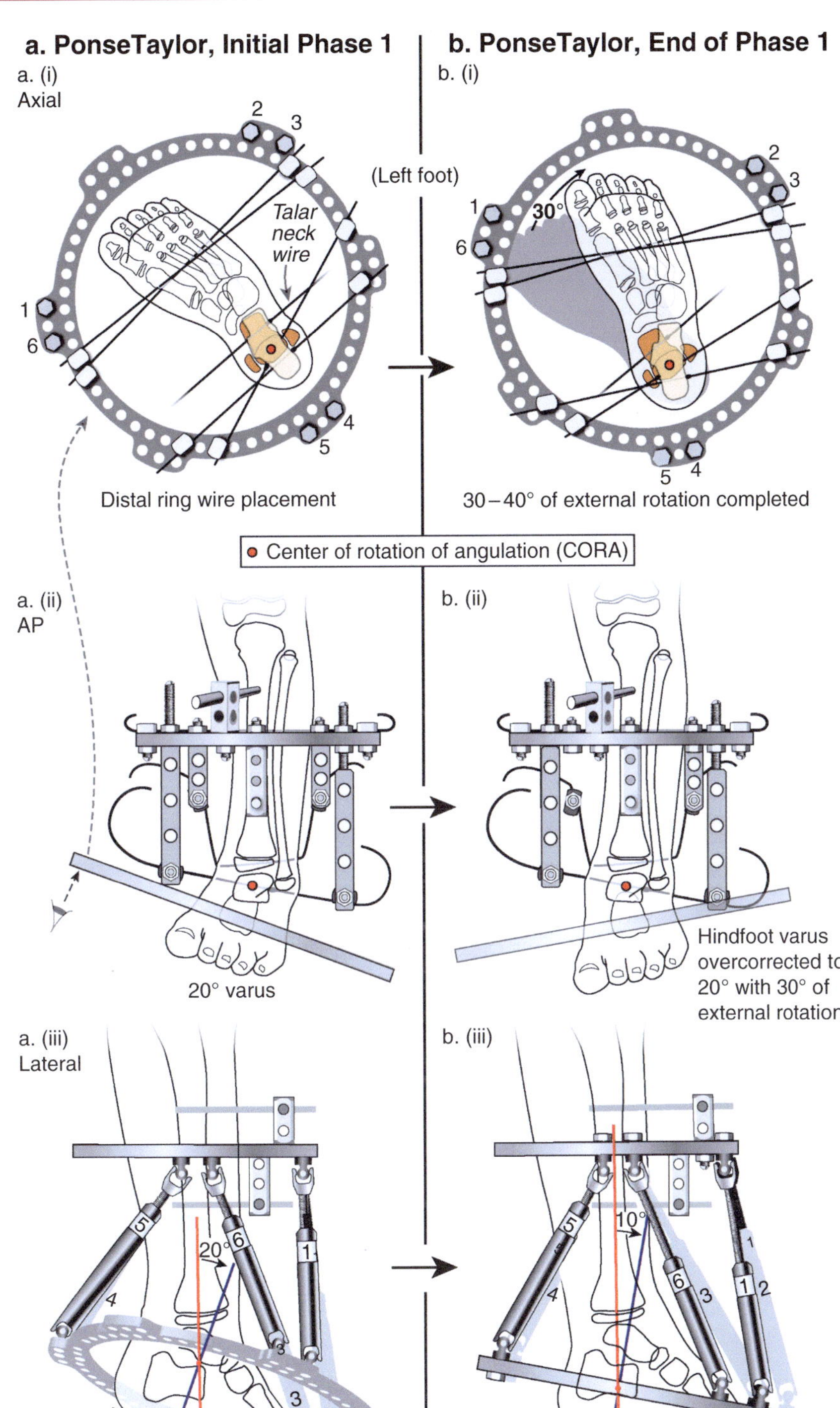
a. PonseTaylor, Initial Phase 1
a. (i)
Axial
2
3
(Left foot)
Talar
neck
wire
1
6
4
5
Distal ring wire placement
b. PonseTaylor, End of Phase 1
b. (i)
2
3
30°
1
6
5
4
30–40° of external rotation completed
● Center of rotation of angulation (CORA)
a. (ii)
AP
20° varus
b. (ii)
Hindfoot varus
overcorrected to
20° with 30° of
external rotation
a. (iii)
Lateral
5
20°
6
1
4
3
3
2
20° equinus
b. (iii)
5
10°
1
4
6
3
1
2
Residual equinus deformity of 10°

c. PonseTaylor, Initial Phase 2: Hardware Modification

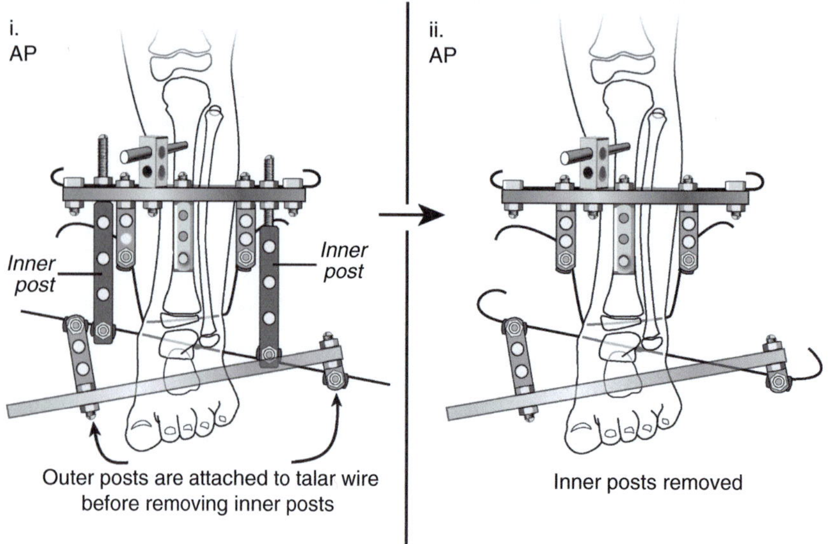

Outer posts are attached to talar wire before removing inner posts

Inner posts removed

d. PonseTaylor, Final Phase 2: Correction

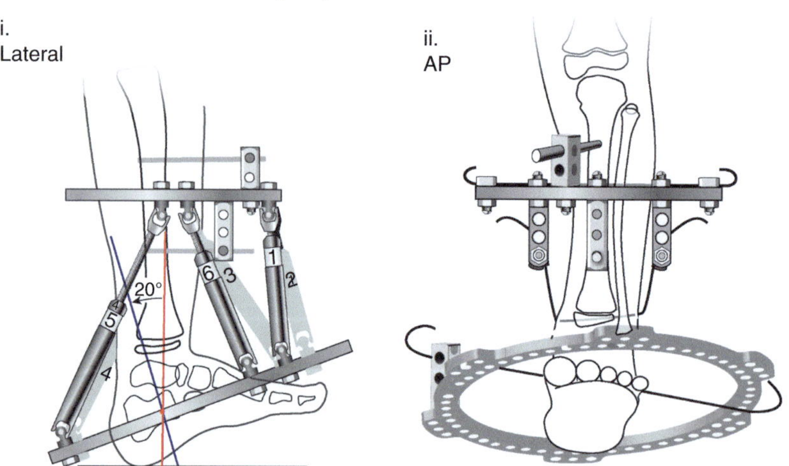

Equinus deformity overcorrected 20°

Fig. 18.12 (continued)

Fig. 18.12   (continued)

e. PonseTaylor, Initial Optional Phase 3: Hardware Modification

i.

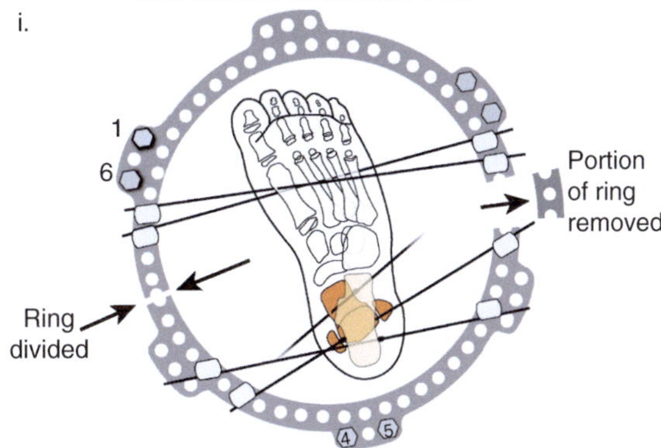

ii.
Distraction rods added

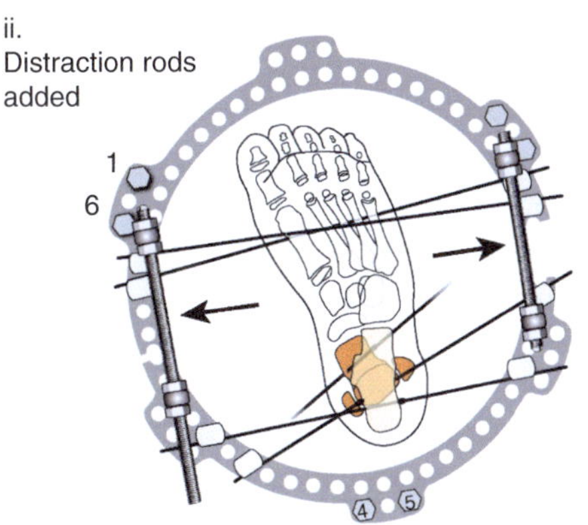

f. PonseTaylor, Final Optional Phase 3: Correction

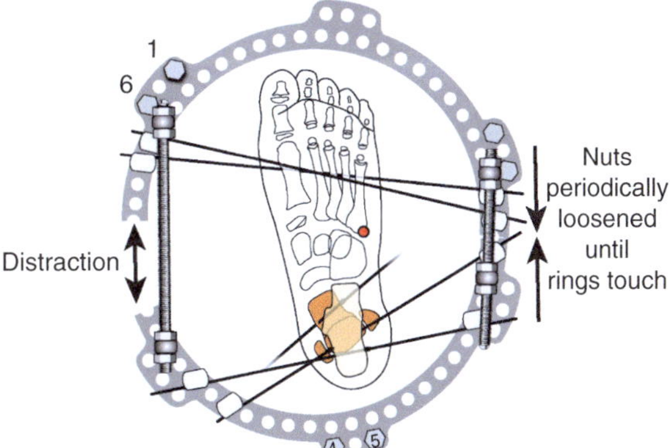

secured to the ring with two counter-opposed olive wires through the calcaneus and one or two smooth wires through the metatarsals.

- In choosing a foot ring, consider the location of the calcaneal wires as well as the metatarsal wires. Avoid selecting a ring in which the wires and struts interfere with placement of each other.

- In small children, it is reasonable to use a full standard circular ring around the foot. In older children and adults, an open foot ring or U-ring may be used.

- If the third stage of correction is needed (PonseTaylor II), then special care must be made in wire placement on the foot ring. In placing the calcaneal wires and metatarsal wires, orient the wires to allow for space between the forefoot segment and hindfoot segment, particularly on the convex (lateral) side.

18.7.1.3 Applying Special Wires

- To prevent physiolysis of the distal tibial physis during distraction of the ankle and subtalar joints, place a 1.8-mm wire in the distal tibial epiphysis. Bend the wire 90° like a stirrup on either side of the skin (medially and laterally) and attach the untensioned wire to the tibial ring proximally.

- Place an olive wire in the neck of the talus. The olive wire is placed from lateral to medial. This functions like the finger at the neck of the talus applying counterpressure during Ponseti casting.

- During the first stage of the PonseTaylor method, the foot is rotated about the talus. Therefore, the talar neck wire is secured off of drop plates to the proximal ring. This olive wire serves as the fulcrum, providing counterpressure to the lateral aspect of the talus while the foot is abducted and externally rotated. The two ends of the olive wire are left long to allow for modification during the second stage.

- During the second stage, the whole foot is dorsiflexed, including the talus. To facilitate the dorsiflexion of the talus, the talar neck wire is detached from the tibial ring and attached to the foot ring. This can be done in clinic in cooperative children or in the operating room

in less cooperative children. Uncurl both ends of the wire, attach it to the foot ring, tension the wire, and then disassemble the old vertical posts that attached it to the tibia.

18.7.1.4 TSF Programming

PonseTaylor Phase 1

- Phase 1 addresses the internal rotation and varus deformities. As the foot rotates about the talus, the origin is defined to be at the subtalar joint at the level of the lateral process in the lateral view and in the middle of the talus in the AP view. The total residual operating mode is chosen and a distal reference is used. As mentioned above, the goal of correction is approximately 20° valgus and 40° abduction external rotation. To prevent compression of the articular surfaces, the foot is additionally distracted 1 cm. For mounting parameters, the foot ring position is defined in terms of its location to the origin. The SAR is the posterior tibial nerve. It too is defined by its relative position to the origin. The safe distraction rate is approximately 1 mm/day.

PonseTaylor Phase 2

- Phase 2 corrects equinus. As mentioned above, the talar neck wire is detached from the tibial ring and attached to the foot ring to allow dorsiflexion of the whole foot. The deformity is defined still using a distal reference. Equinus is equivalent to a deformity in the lateral view, apex anterior.

- The goal of correction is overcorrection to at least 20° of dorsiflexion. Add additional distraction if needed. Reevaluate the mounting parameters.

- The origin is reassessed and is defined as the center of the talus on the lateral view. The Achilles tendon becomes the structure at risk when correcting equinus.

PonseTaylor Phase 3

- If additional forefoot adduction and cavus remain at the end of the second stage, the foot ring can be modified by using a Gigli saw.

- Prior to cutting the ring, build a stable Ilizarov threaded rod construct between the posterior and anterior halves of the foot ring, one medially and one laterally, to the foot for the purpose of differential distraction across the midfoot. Also, build a stable Ilizarov construct between the tibial ring and the posterior half of the foot ring with at least four threaded rods. Then, on the medial side, cut the ring at the level of the midfoot. On the lateral side, approximately two–three holes are cut from the ring. Medially, the foot is lengthened. Laterally, it is allowed to compress to the patient's comfort. This essentially converts the frame into a classical Ilizarov frame.

18.7.1.5 After Correction with the TSF

- Once correction is achieved, the foot is kept in the frame for an additional 4–6 weeks.
- As soon as the foot achieves a near plantigrade position, a foot plate is added to the frame and weightbearing is allowed.
- The total duration of treatment with external fixation is generally 3 months. Following removal of the frame, the foot is placed in a cast for 4 more weeks. Afterwards, the foot is placed into an ankle-foot orthosis with a plantar flexion stop. Then the patient begins physiotherapy for motion and strength.

Pearls

- In younger patients, preoperative casting may eliminate part of the deformity, such as metatarsus adductus. However, avoid prolonged casting preoperatively because disuse osteopenia might occur and weaken the fixation.
- When the need for the "PonseTaylor II" method is anticipated, make certain the forefoot wires and hindfoot wires are separated on the lateral side by at least three holes in the ring.

References

Eidelman M, Keren Y, Katzman A (2012) Correction of residual clubfoot deformities in older children using the Taylor spatial butt frame and midfoot Gigli saw osteotomy. J Pediatr Orthop 32(5):527–533

Floerkemeier T, Stukenborg-Colsman C, Windhagen H, Waizy H (2011) Correction of severe foot deformities using the Taylor spatial frame. Foot Ankle Int 32(2):176–182

Kirienko A, Villa A, Calhoun JH (2004) Ilizarov technique for complex foot and ankle deformities. Marcel Dekker, New York

Lamm BM, Standard SC, Galley IJ, Herzenberg JE, Paley D (2006) External fixation for the foot and ankle in children. Clin Podiatr Med Surg 23(1):137–166, ix

Turker R, Lubicky JP, Vogel LC (1992) Toxic shock syndrome in patients with external fixators. J Pediatr Orthop 12(5):658–662

Wukich DK, Belczyk RJ (2006) An introduction to the Taylor spatial frame for foot and ankle applications. Oper Tech Orthop 16(1):2–9

John Birch, Mikhail Samchukov,
Alexander Cherkashin, and Karl Rathjen

Contents

J. Birch, MD, FRCS(C) (✉) • M. Samchukov, MD •
A. Cherkashin, MD K. Rathjen, MD
Department of Orthopedics,
Texas Scottish Rite Hospital for Children,
2222 Welborn Street, Dallas, TX 75219, USA
e-mail: john.birch@tsrh.org;
mike@globalmednet.com;
alex.cherkashin@tsrh.org;
karl.rathjen@tsrh.org

19.1 Introduction

- Dubousset (1991) was the first to describe the use of circular fixation of the thoracic spine, lumbar spine, and pelvis using fine wires to achieve deformity correction and spinal stabilization in desperate deformities, particularly in patients with myelomeningocele who had failed more traditional spinal fusion techniques and whose health was seriously jeopardized by spinal instability with or without infection and inability to sit comfortably or stably. Only a few similar reports exist in the literature (Birch et al. 1997; Reyes-Sanchez et al. 2005).

- Seven patients have presented to us with severe spinal deformities recalcitrant or considered not amenable to traditional deformity correction, internal fixation, and fusion methods. All patients had upper lumbar or thoracic myelomeningocele, i.e., were paraplegic. Three patients had (infected) lumbar pseudarthrosis, two had severe lumbar hyperlordosis, one had progressive lumbar kyphosis with recurrent skin breakdown over the kyphotic area, and one had multiplanar spinal deformity with poor skin and lost the ability to sit comfortably in his wheelchair. Over the years, our fixation method has evolved, as well as has been adapted to the specific deformities to be addressed.

M. Kocaoğlu et al. (eds.), *Advanced Techniques in Limb Reconstruction Surgery*,
DOI 10.1007/978-3-642-55026-3_19, © Springer Berlin Heidelberg 2015

19.2 Objective

- The purpose of this chapter is to review the indications for the use of spinopelvic fixation and deformity correction, the evolution of our fixation strategies in these patients, preoperative planning and preparation, intraoperative management, and postoperative management based on our experience.
- We emphasize that these are highly complex procedures carried out on patients with very challenging clinical deformities and multiple medical problems. Careful preoperative preparation, intraoperative resourcefulness, and expert full-time postoperative nursing are essential to any potential successful outcome in these extraordinarily difficult cases.

19.3 Classification

- All patients were wheelchair-dependent with upper lumbar or thoracic level myelomeningocele, associated bowel and bladder paralysis, flail and insensate lower extremities, and shunted hydrocephalus.
- The nature of spinal deformity included:
  - Infected pseudarthrosis of the lumbar spine in three (two after previous attempted posterior spinal fusion to the pelvis with posterior segmental instrumentation and one spontaneous as a result of neglected tissue breakdown over a lumbar kyphosis with secondary spinal erosion).
  - Hyperlordosis of the spine in two resulting in difficulty sitting and perineal self-care (including self-catheterization). The rigid hyperlordosis was considered too extreme to anticipate adequate correction by traditional one- or two-stage anterior/posterior release and instrumentation.
  - One case of associated congenital lumbar kyphosis with recalcitrant skin breakdown and multiple episodes of recurrent deformity after previous spinal procedures.
  - One case of severe, complex three-dimensional spinal deformity interfering with comfortable sitting.

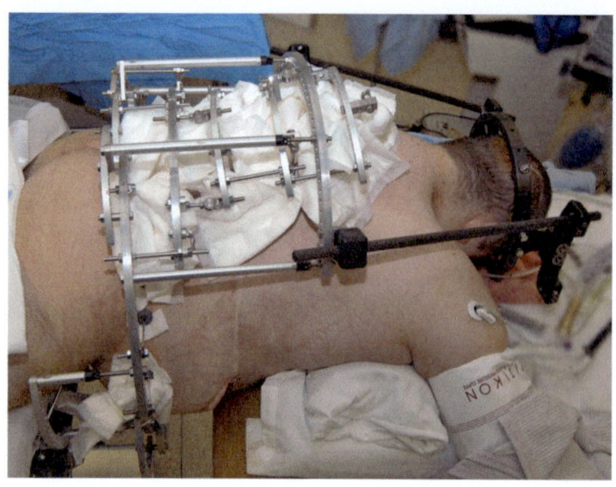

Fig. 19.1 Clinical photograph of patient with myelomeningocele, two-level infected pseudarthrosis of the lumbar spine, and morbid obesity. Fixation consists of pelvic wire and half-pin fixation, thoracic spinal fixation with pedicle half-pins, and a halo ring

19.4 Preoperative Planning

- Assessment that the clinical deformity/patient problem warrants this extensive and complicated treatment and is not amenable to simpler treatment methods.
- Imaging as described below to evaluate bone stock, shape, and size of the pelvis, lumbar spine, and thoracic spine where pedicle instrumentation is being considered.
- Actual fixation must be constructed so as to be adequate for the clinical situation. We have found (see Sect. 19.9 below) that hybrid fixation consisting of wires with or without half-pins in the pelvis and half-pin fixation at multiple levels in the thoracic spine provide adequate fixation for most purposes. We have also used transverse sacral and lower lumbar wires and halo fixation to the skull in specific cases where the additional fixation was feasible and desirable (Fig. 19.1).

19.5 Imaging

- Plain sitting AP and lateral radiographs of the spine are necessary to document the severity, nature, and location of spinal deformity.
- Axial CT of the intended area of fixation, specifically the lumbosacral spine and pelvis, and the thoracic spine in the intended area of

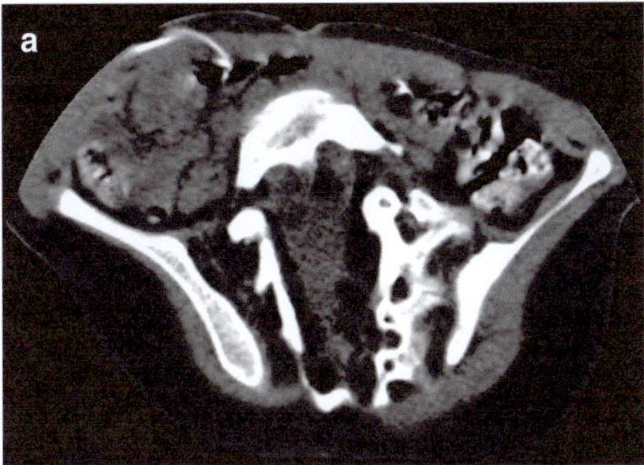

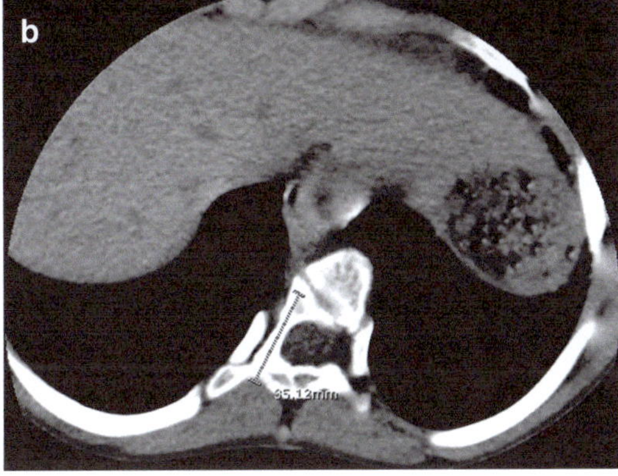

Fig. 19.2 (**a**, **b**) Axial CT of the intended areas of fixation is necessary to identify bone stock and shape in preparation for fixation. (**a**) Axial CT of the pelvis, for anticipated posterior-to-anterior open-wire fixation. (**b**) Axial CT of the thoracic spine at the level of intended posterior pedicle half-pin fixation

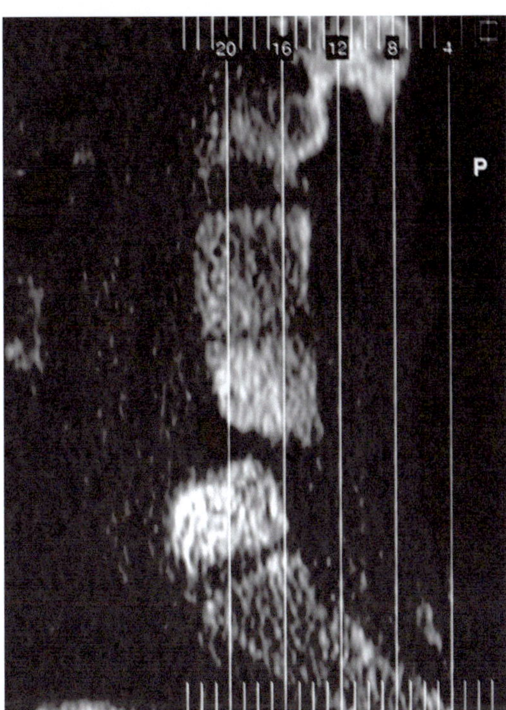

Fig. 19.3 Sagittal CT reconstruction of the lumbar spine identifying two-level lumbar pseudarthrosis and nature of residual sagittal deformity. Same patient as Fig. 19.1

thoracic pedicle fixation is essential (Fig. 19.2a, b). If necessary for the specific case, CT of the mid-lumbar spine with or without reconstructions may be helpful (Fig. 19.3).

- In patients with myelomeningocele and ventriculoperitoneal (VP) shunts, it is important to know the functional status of the shunt at the time of surgery. Patients who are shunt-dependent and being considered for residual spinal cord resection as part of the indicated spinal release must have a functioning shunt prior to that procedure.

19.6   Special Equipment Required

- Custom body rings or equivalent
- Extra length and diameter wires for large patients
- Special wire fixation bolts for larger-diameter wires
- Operating table setup as described below
- Special bed preparations as described below
- Dedicated staff to provide the full-time nursing care necessary during the prolonged hospitalization required to achieve a successful outcome in these extraordinarily challenging cases

19.7   Frame Construction

- We now use a custom ring or similar to fashion circular fixation of the pelvis, which will serve as the foundation to the entire construct (Fig. 19.4).
- The upper segment consists of a series of arches to which the thoracic pedicle half-pins are fixed as a block (Fig. 19.5).
- The pelvic ring and thoracic pedicle block are attached to each other in a manner required for the specific case: fixed in an acceptable position for patients with mobile-infected

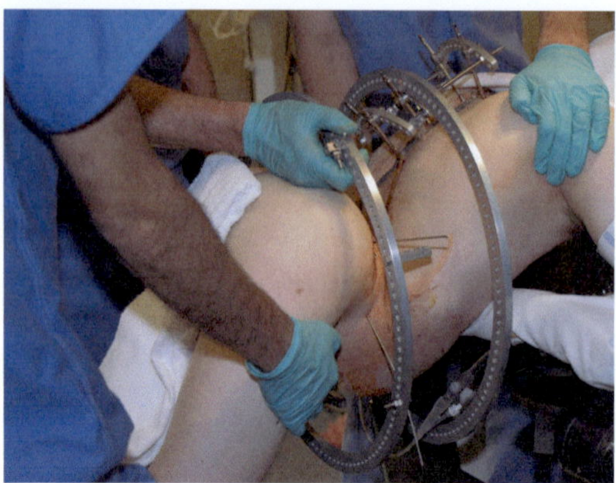

Fig. 19.4 A 360 mm custom-made aluminum ring, which we have used as both pelvic and "float" rings in our spinopelvic apparatus

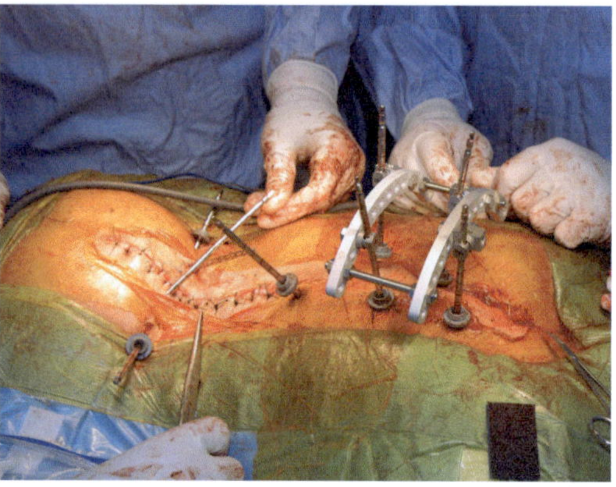

Fig. 19.5 Thoracic pedicle half-pins secured to an upper femoral arch

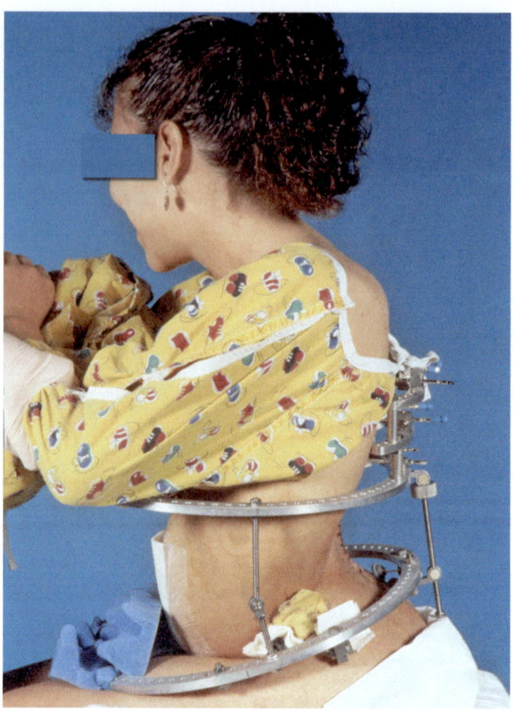

Fig. 19.6 Clinical photograph of a patient with hyperlordosis of the spine undergoing gradual correction of residual deformity. The upper segment consists of thoracic pedicle half-pins secured to arches, the lower segment of pelvic wires and half-pins secured to a full-body ring, and there is a "float" body ring between the two segments to facilitate hinge and motor connection between the segments

pseudarthrosis of the spine and with parallel hinges located under fluoroscopic control and "motors" used in either distraction or compress to effect gradual correction of hyperlordotic or kyphotic deformities (Fig. 19.6).

19.8 Intraoperative Patient Positioning

- Any initial indicated procedure (such as anterior and/or posterior spinal release or wound debridement) is carried out in a routine fashion per the surgeon's preference.

- For spinopelvic fixation, we position our patients prone between two operating tables, one to support the thorax and the other to support the legs from the lower pelvic area. The operating tables should be radiolucent to allow fluoroscopic imaging to aid in pedicle half-pin insertion. Split draping of the patient's upper and lower body segments will then allow circumferential access to the patient's pelvis and abdomen (Fig. 19.7).
- When we use anteriorly placed iliac half-pins to supplement pelvic fixation, we insert them first through anterior exposure of the pelvis (Fig. 19.8) and then turn the patient prone with re-prepping and draping as described above (Fig. 19.9).

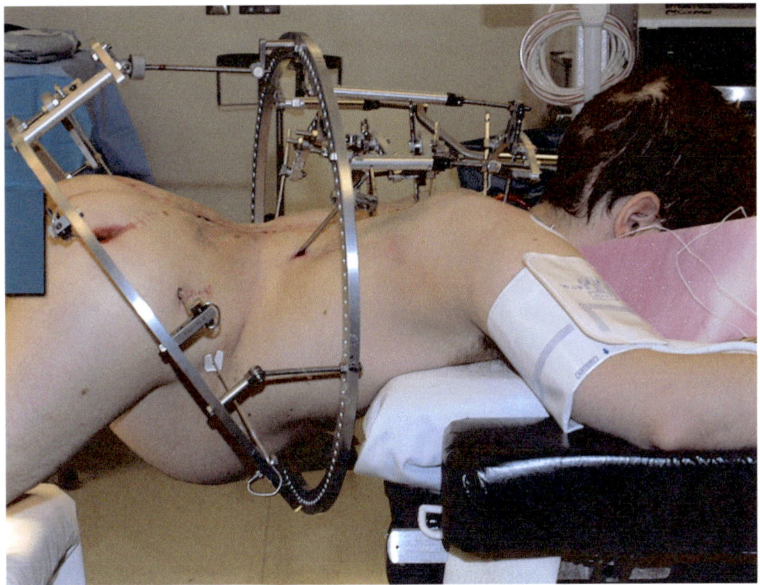

Fig. 19.7 Intraoperative patient positioning for spinopelvic fixation. Two operating tables are used, with the patient's thorax supported on one and the legs on a second table, allowing circumferential access to the pelvis and abdomen. Tabletops should be radiolucent to allow fluoroscopic imaging during fixation element insertion

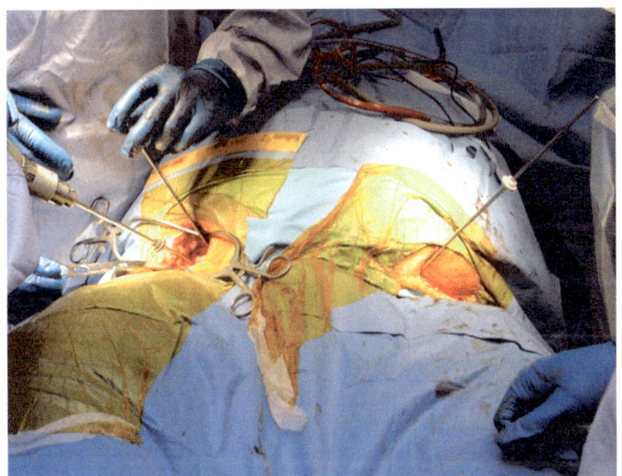

Fig. 19.8 In this patient (same patient as Figs. 19.1 and 19.3), pelvic fixation was supplemented by anteriorly inserted half-pins, which were inserted through an open incision, prior to positioning the patient as illustrated in Fig. 19.7

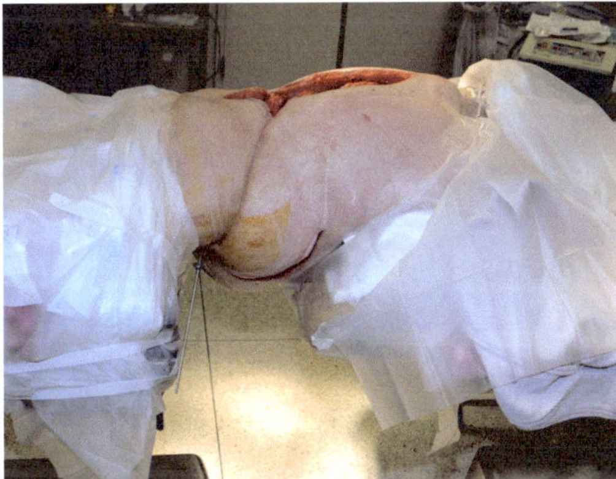

Fig. 19.9 Patient positioned prone as illustrated in Fig. 19.7, after insertion of anterior pelvic half-pins

19.9 Evolution of Our Technique of Spinal Fixation

- In the first report of thoraco-pelvic fixation of the spine in myelomeningocele by Shufflebarger and Dubousset 1991 (REF), fine-wire fixation secured to custom body

rings was used (Fig. 19.10). In this technique, pelvic fixation is achieved using wires placed in an open fashion from posterior to anterior in the iliac crests, avoiding exit within the pelvis, and transversely in the sacrum (under fluoroscopic control) (Fig. 19.11). Thoracic fixation consisted of transverse wires placed in an open fashion across the base of the spinous processes at as many levels as feasible (Fig. 19.10). These wires are inserted by first

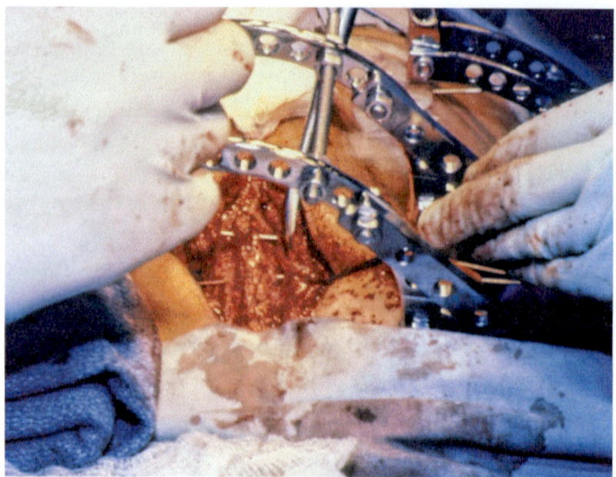

Fig. 19.10 Transverse process wires inserted in pairs across the base of the thoracic spinous processes and secured to body rings

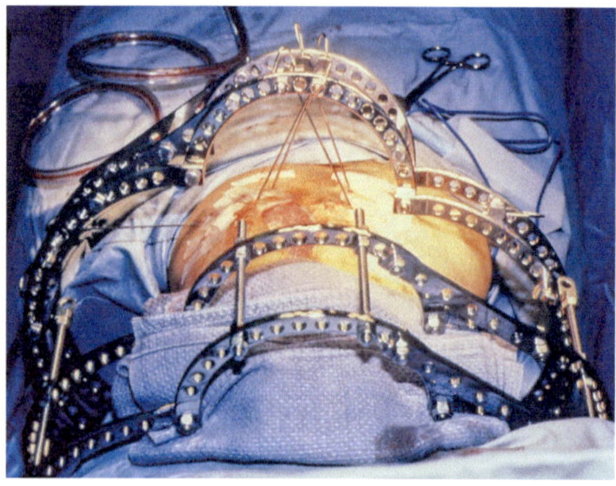

Fig. 19.11 Illustration of wires inserted in the ilium (under direct vision, from posterior to anterior after exposure of the outer iliac crest), and transversely through the body of S1

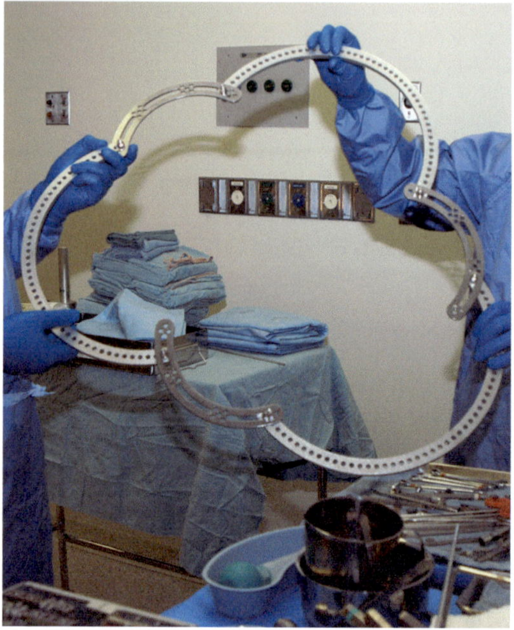

Fig. 19.12 "Cloverleaf" pelvic "ring" fashioned from segments of a 360 mm full-body ring connected by arches. Used for pelvic fixation in patient illustrated in Fig. 19.1

exposing the thoracic spine posteriorly and mobilizing the skin and subcutaneous tissue from the posterior thorax. Then, from a point near the posterior axillary line, wires are inserted transcutaneously transversely under direct vision from one side of the thorax to the other, taking care to keep the wires from entering the chest and guiding them across the base of the spinous process for bony purchase. The wires are then tensioned to the body rings. The thoracic and pelvic rings were then connected so as to reduce and stabilize the kyphotic lumbar pseudarthrosis.

- We have used custom-made 300–360 mm. full rings (Fig. 19.4) for the pelvic fixation (or modification of the same in one case of extreme size) (Fig. 19.12) in each case, to serve as the "foundation" to the construct. The nature of fixation to the thoracic segment (with or without a mid-trunk "float" ring or extension to a halo) is determined by the nature of the spinal deformity and the purpose of treatment. It is important that the pelvic ring be tilted superiorly from posterior to anterior to allow comfortable sitting without requiring excessive reclining of the patient and of sufficient size to guarantee no abdominal wall/soft tissue encroachment.
- The weakest and most challenging aspect of this fixation method is the insertion and use of the transverse spinous process wires. Therefore, for all of our subsequent cases, we replaced these wires with posteriorly inserted half-pins placed in the pedicles of the thoracic spine under direct vision with the aid of intraoperative fluoroscopy. The number of and size

of such pins is at the discretion of the surgeon, based on the size of the pedicles; for most of our cases, we use either 4–5 mm half-pins placed bilaterally in at least three levels of the thoracic spine, secured to arches (Fig. 19.5), which are in turn secured to the pelvic ring or "float" ring, as the spinal deformity requires (Fig. 19.6). This form of fixation is much more secure and less obtrusive to the patient, particularly with respect to arm function and comfort, than transverse wires secured to a full ring.

- We have supplemented wire fixation of the iliac crest and sacrum with half-pins inserted into the region of the posterior superior iliac spine or anteriorly into the iliac crest.

19.10 Treatment Strategies Adapted to Specific Spinal Deformities

Patients fell into three main categories of deformity/clinical problems:

- *Hyperlordosis* interfering with comfortable sitting and perineal self-care (including intermittent catheterization). The hyperlordosis resulted in weight-bearing on the upper thighs in the sitting position and the perineum being directed posteriorly out of vision for the patients (both females) so that self-catheterization was difficult to impossible. The purpose of intervention was to allow gradual correction of residual hyperlordosis after anterior and posterior spinal release, using circular external fixation.
- *Technique*:
  - Intraoperatively: same day, anterior thoracoabdominal spinal release, posterior spinal release, and external fixation of the spine and pelvis. At the index procedure, bone graft was placed in the intervertebral disc spaces and along the exposed residual posterior spinal elements to facilitate fusion.
  - Postoperatively: gradual posterior distraction around hinges placed at the anterior

vertebral body to effect gradual correction of the lordotic spine. The patients were maintained in the corrected position to allow spontaneous fusion of the spine.

- *Infected pseudarthrosis of the spine.* Three patients presented with infected pseudarthrosis of the lumbar spine, two after attempted spinal fusion and instrumentation for spinal deformity and one spontaneously after neglect resulting in soft tissue breakdown followed by spinal column erosion.
- *Technique.* In all cases, residual spinal implants (if any) were removed, and the wound thoroughly debrided. The spine was then immobilized by upper (spinal) and lower (distal spine and pelvis) fixation and stabilization until soft tissue and bony healing.
- *Recalcitrant kyphotic deformity and complex spinal deformity cases* (one each) were treated in a fashion similar to that used for the patients with hyperlordotic deformity of the spine, consisting of appropriate anterior and posterior spinal release/osteotomy, spinopelvic fixation, and postoperative manipulations of the external fixation elements to effect gradual correction of the deformity.

19.11 Postoperative Management

- Expert, competent, and enthusiastic nursing care are essential to successful outcome in these extraordinarily challenging cases. All of our patients have remained hospitalized for the duration of their treatment in spinopelvic fixation (90–175 days).
- Specific arrangements for comfortable lying are required, because of the presence of the pelvic ring and the thoracic posterior arches. We have used two bed adaptations to good effect: mounting a patient-size rectangular foam block on plywood with a "cutout" to match the fixation (Fig. 19.13) and a "Roho cushion™" and pillows to support the patient.
- Patients sit most comfortably in a semi-reclined position in a reclining wheelchair, to prevent excessive contact between the anterior thighs

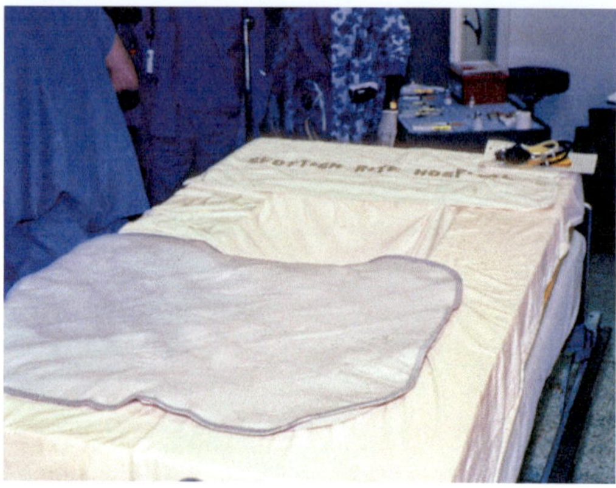

Fig. 19.13 Foam block glued to plywood, with a shallow cutout to allow the patient to rest supine or prone without undue pressure on the apparatus

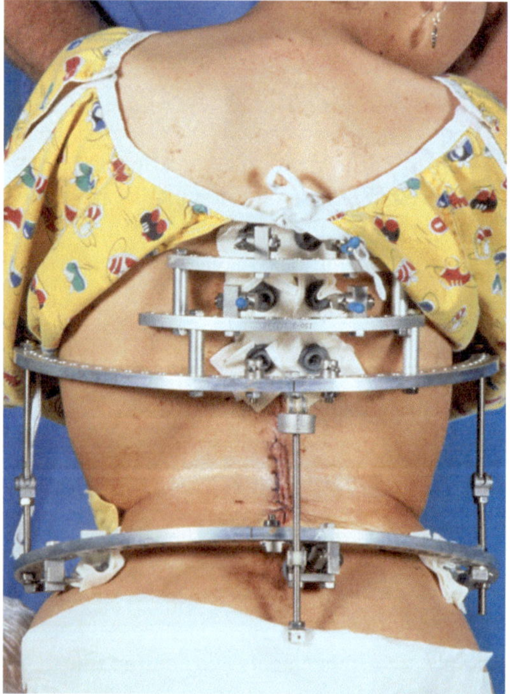

Fig. 19.14 Standard pin-site care, consisting of 2×2 gauze pressed to the skin with rubber stoppers and daily cleansing, is employed for these patients

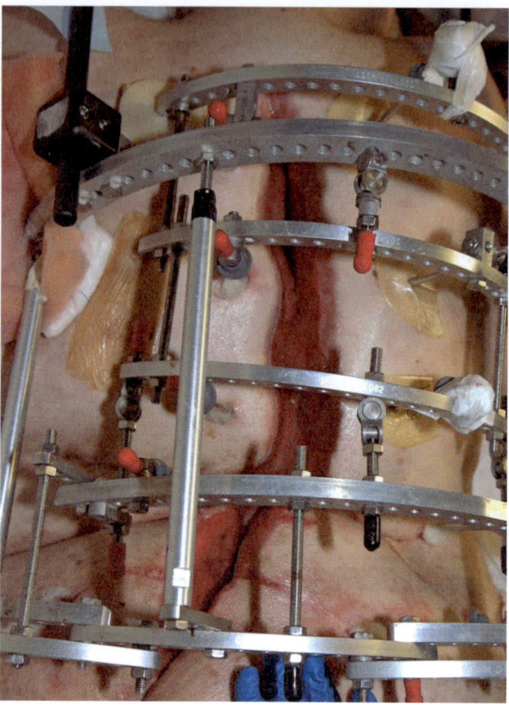

Fig. 19.15 Patient illustrated in Fig. 19.1 with obesity and large anterior and posterior wounds used to debride the deep infection. Vacuum-assisted wound device (VACs) used under the spinopelvic fixation

- We have used a pin-site care routine similar to that for extremity fixation, with 2×2 gauze held by rubber stoppers (applied to the wires/half-pins at the time of surgery) (Fig. 19.14), and daily cleansing with saline or peroxide after showering.
- One patient with obesity and massively infected, two-level pseudarthrosis of the lumbar spine requiring anterior and posterior drainage during initial treatment was treated with vacuum-assisted sponge (VACs) dressings of his anterior and posterior wounds, with excellent healing (Fig. 19.15).

and the pelvic ring. A custom insert support for their back/apparatus may be fashioned from foam, as necessary. Multi-person assist or patient transport lift (such as a Hoyer™ lift) may be required to accomplish transfers from bed to chair/wheelchair/toilet.

19.12 Patient Outcomes

- The two patients with hyperlordosis of the spine achieve adequate correction of the deformity to allow comfortable sitting and self-catheterization (Fig. 19.16a–d).

- The three patients with infected pseudarthroses of the spine had complete resolution of their infection, solid fusion of the affected spinal segment, and adequate correction of residual spinal deformity (Fig. 19.17a–c).
- One patient with recalcitrant lumbar kyphosis and chronic skin breakdown lost pelvic fixation after 6 weeks, and the external fixation had to be removed. However, the patient's spine healed with adequate correction of the kyphosis so that no further treatment was required.
- One patient with complex spinal deformity had satisfactory improvement of the deformity (Fig. 19.18a–d).

19.13 Complications

- One patient had early loss of pelvic fixation requiring premature removal of the entire apparatus.
- Our index patient (the only one with transverse wire fixation of the thoracic spine via spinous processes) translated coronally along the wires at the time of fixator removal. However, no adverse effect was noted. This problem as well as the inconvenience of the lateral placement of the wires led us to replace this type of fixation by thoracic pedicle half-pins.

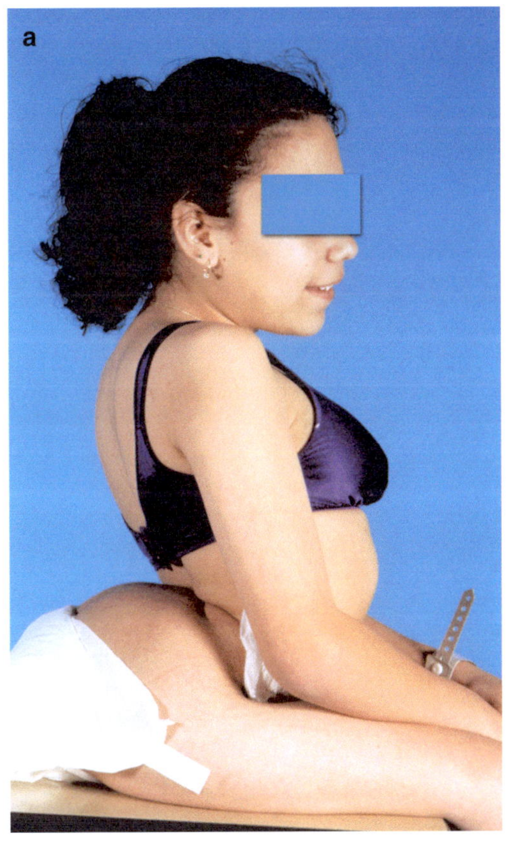
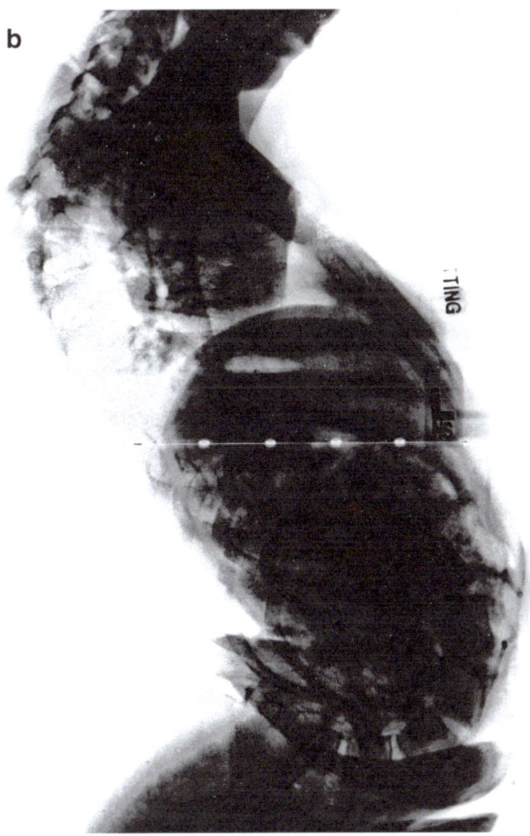

Fig. 19.16 (**a–d**) Patient with hyperlordosis of the lumbar spine preventing perineal self-care. Patient was able to assume self-care after correction of the hyperlordosis. (**a**) Preoperative photograph, sitting. (**b**) Preoperative sitting lateral radiograph of the spine. (**c**) Postoperative photograph, sitting. (**d**) Postoperative sitting lateral radiograph of the spine, 5-year outcome

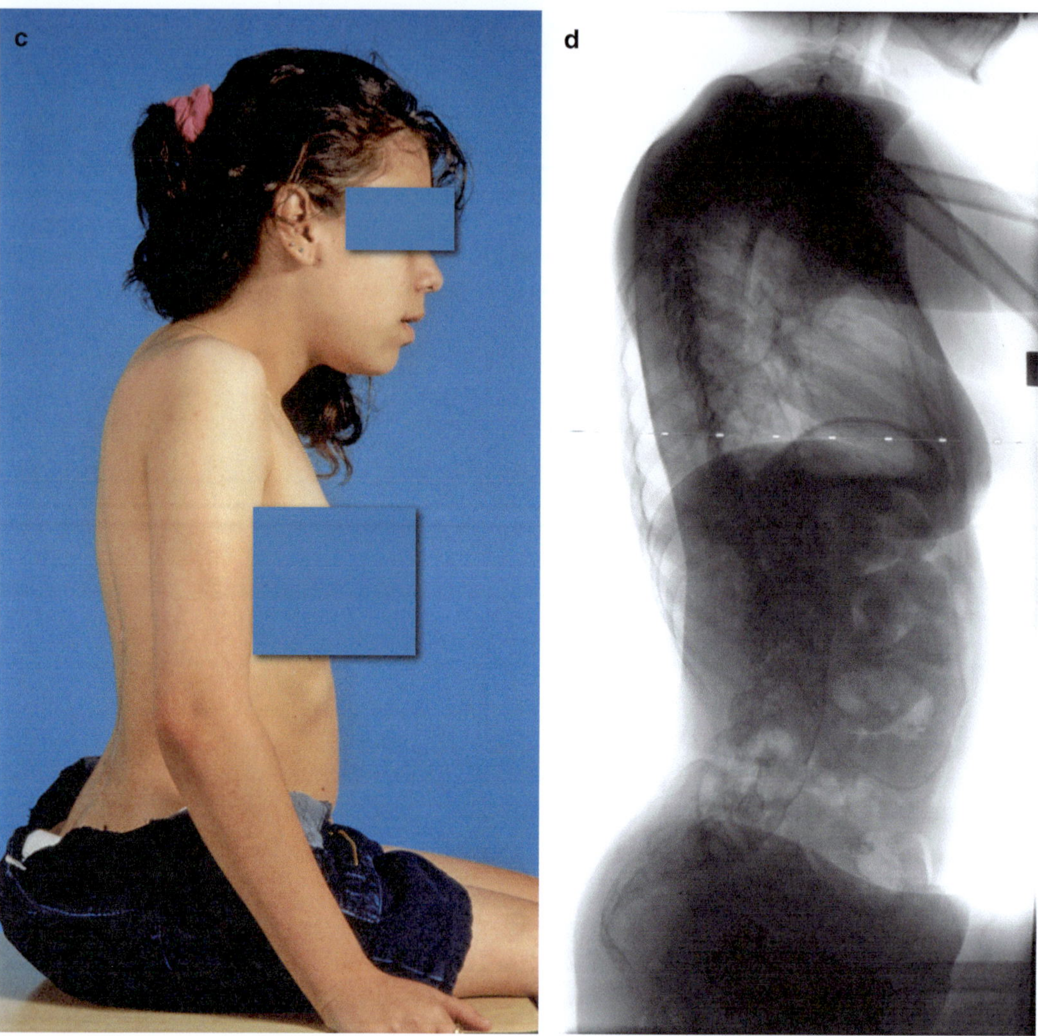

Fig. 19.16 (continued)

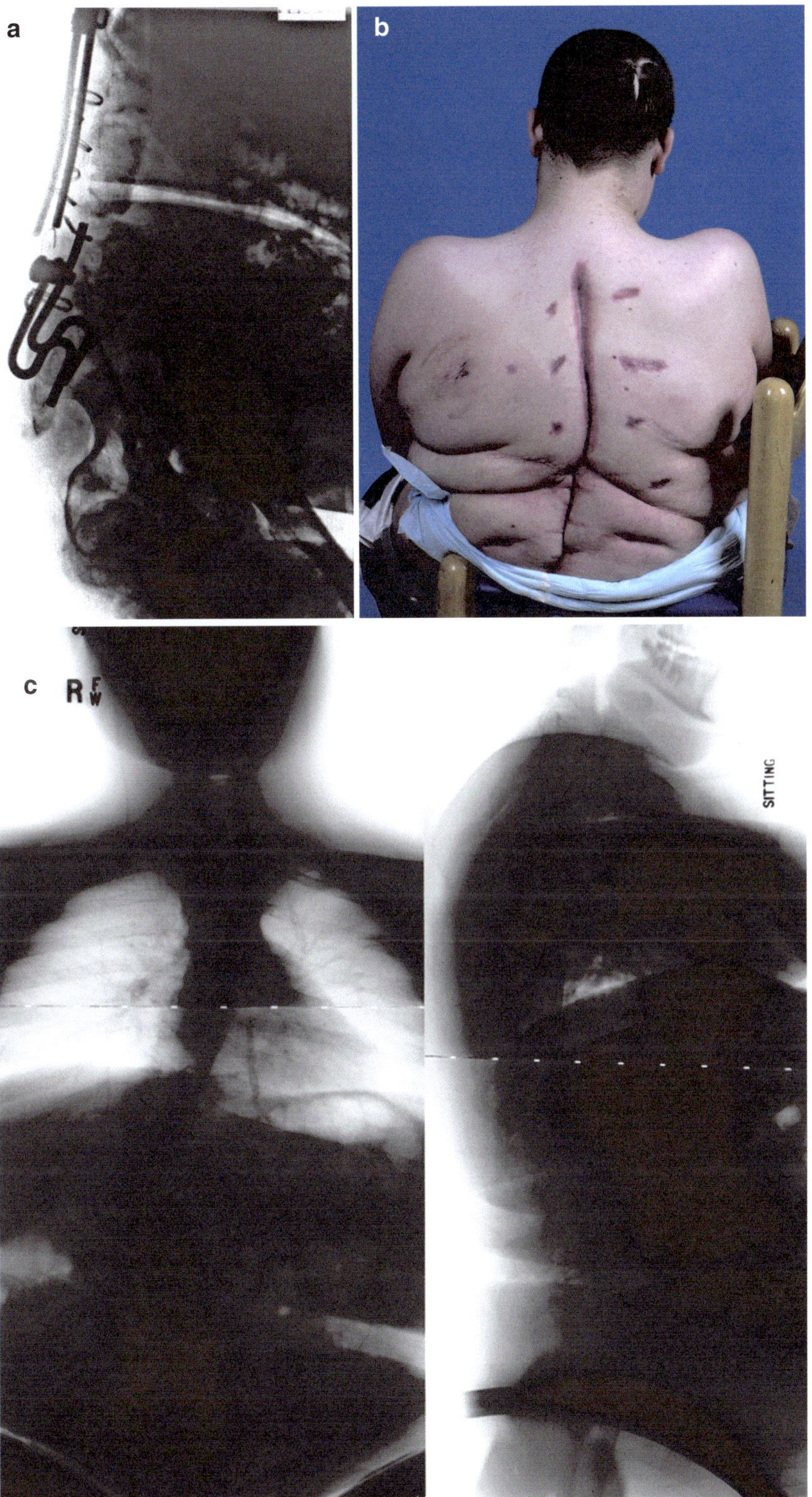

Fig. 19.17 (**a–c**) Patient with postoperative infected non-union of the lumbar spine. Same patient as Fig. 19.1. (**a**) Preoperative radiograph of mobile lumbar spine with broken spinal implants. The patient has massive abscess poste-riorly and in the retroperitoneal space and is systemically ill. Postfixation appearance illustrated in Figs. 19.1 and 19.17. (**b**) Clinical appearance after wound healing and spontaneous spinal fusion. (**c**) Radiographic appearance

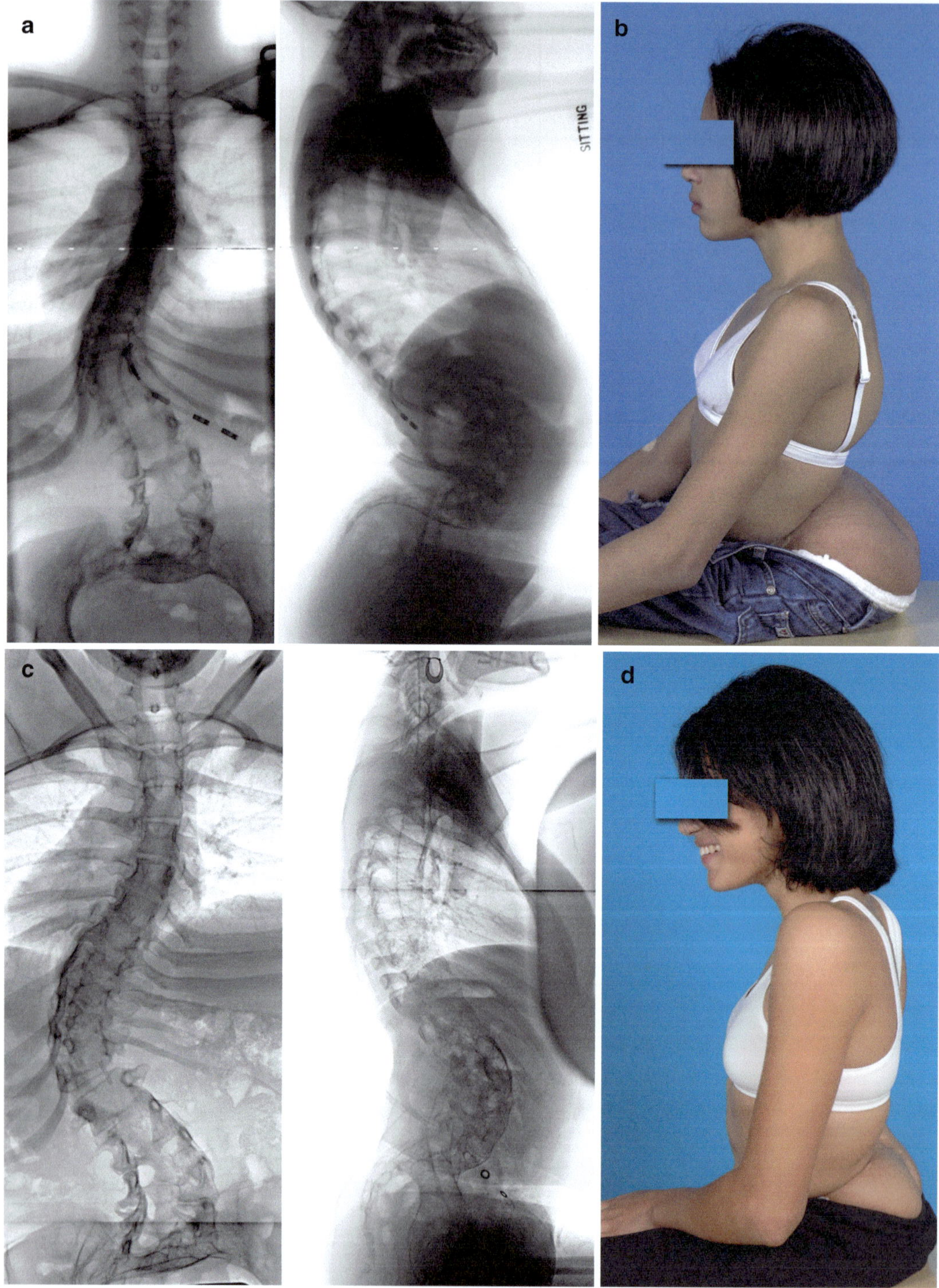

Fig. 19.18 (**a–d**) Patient with complex spinal deformity and myelomeningocele. (**a**) Preoperative radiograph. (**b**) Preoperative photograph. (**c**) Postoperative radiograph. (**d**) Postoperative photograph

Conclusions

- Otherwise insoluble spinal deformities can be successfully treated by carefully planned fixation of the thoracic spine and pelvis using custom body rings and imaginative fixation, with or without gradual postoperative correction of residual deformity.
- Extraordinary nursing support is required to care for these patients adequately.

Bibliography

Birch JG, Samchukov ML, Richards BS, Karol LA, Ross JD (1997) Modified ilizarov apparatus for the management of severe spinal deformities in children. A report of four cases. In: 7th ASAMI North America Annual Meeting, San Francisco, paper 48

Dubousset J (1991) La technique d'Ilizarov. Procede de sauvetage en chirurgie du rachis. Rev Chir Orthop Suppl 177:144

Reyes-Sanchez A, Rosales LM, Miramontes V (2005) External fixation for dynamic correction of severe scoliosis. Spine J 5:418–442

Sink EL, Karol LA, Sanders J, Birch JG, Johnston CE, Herring JA (2001) Efficacy of perioperative halogravity traction in the treatment of severe scoliosis in children. J Pediatr Orthop 21(4):519–524

Pelvic Inlet Reconstruction for Obstruction Associated with Lumbosacral Agenesis Utilizing Distraction Osteogenesis and Circular External Fixation

Mikhail Samchukov, John Birch, and Alexander Cherkashin

Contents

M. Samchukov, MD (✉) • J. Birch, MD, FRCS(C)
A. Cherkashin, MD
Department of Pediatric Orthopedics, Texas Scottish
Rite Hospital for Children, 2222 Welborn Street,
Dallas, TX 75219, USA
e-mail: mike@globalmednet.com;
john.birch@tsrh.org; alex.cherkashin@tsrh.org

20.1   Introduction

- Lumbosacral agenesis or caudal regression syndrome is a severe congenital anomaly characterized by the absence of some portion of the sacrum and lumbar spine. In contrast to myelomeningocele, however, these patients rarely have central nervous system anomalies such as hydrocephalus or Arnold-Chiari malformation and typically have well-preserved or completely intact lower extremity sensation, even when significant motor, bowel, and bladder paralysis are present (Adra et al. 1994; Boemers et al. 1994; Boulas 2009; Caird et al. 2007; Cama et al. 1996; Emami-Naeini et al. 2012; Garcia et al. 2001; Guidera et al. 1991; Junquera et al. 2006; Harlow et al. 1995; Phillips et al. 1982; Van and Fourie 1984; Wilmshurst et al. 1999).

- One complication of this disorder is the development of progressive obstruction of the pelvic inlet, which in severe cases may require colostomy due to severe deformity of the

M. Kocaoğlu et al. (eds.), *Advanced Techniques in Limb Reconstruction Surgery*,
DOI 10.1007/978-3-642-55026-3_20, © Springer Berlin Heidelberg 2015

pelvis with the absence of a sacrum and the inward growth of the acetabula.

- To ambulate, patients with lumbosacral agenesis may require spinopelvic stabilization, extension-producing releases, osteotomies at the hips and knees, and extensive orthotic support.

20.2 Classification

- Caudal regression syndrome was first classified by Renshaw who proposed four types of lumbosacral agenesis (Renshaw 1978):
  - Type I is either total or partial unilateral sacral agenesis with intact pelvic ring and lumbosacral junction.
  - Type II includes partial sacral agenesis with a partial but bilaterally symmetric defect, stable articulation between the ilia, and normal but hypoplastic first sacral vertebra.
  - Type III is a variable lumbar and total sacral agenesis with the ilia articulating with the sides of the lowest present vertebra.
  - Type IV comprises variable lumbar and total sacral agenesis with the caudal end plate of the lowest vertebra resting above either fused ilia or an iliac amphiarthrosis.
- In more recent classification introduced by Guille, the spinal deformity was divided into three types (Guille et al. 2002):
  - In type A, there is either a slight gap between the ilia or the ilia are fused in the midline, one or more lumbar vertebrae are absent, and the caudal aspect of the spine articulates with the pelvis in the midline maintaining the vertical alignment of the spine.
  - In type B, the ilia are fused together, some of the lumbar vertebrae are absent, and the most caudal lumbar vertebra articulates with one of the ilia, and the most caudal aspect of the spine shifted away from the midline.
  - In type C, there is total agenesis of the lumbar spine, the ilia are fused together, and there is a visible gap between the most caudal intact thoracic vertebra and the pelvis.

20.3 Objective

- The purpose of this chapter is to report the management and outcome of an adolescent female with severe lumbosacral agenesis and pelvic inlet obstruction.
- The main objective is to demonstrate that a pelvic inlet reconstruction using distraction osteogenesis and circular external fixation can provide pelvic expansion and allow self-catheterization, reversal of a colostomy, and normal sexual life and produce a stable long-term result.

20.4 Patient

- The patient was a 15-year-old female with lumbosacral agenesis who presented with a history of subacute obstruction of the pelvis requiring an emergency colostomy 3 years previously.
- She was born of a normal pregnancy and delivered at term with morphologic features of severe caudal regression syndrome including a single fused ilium with a disassociation between the lumbar spinal remnant and the pelvis, bowel and bladder paralysis, and symmetric lower extremity deformities including stiff equinovarus feet, stiff flexed knees, and stiff dislocated hips.
- Although lower extremity sensation was intact, she had no significant motor movement in the lower extremities. No spina bifida was present, and no hydrocephalus ever developed.

20.5 Clinical Examination

- The patient had the classic fully manifested form of lumbosacral agenesis (Renshaw type IV, Guille type C) with short stature and marked disproportion between the thorax and the pelvis.
- Her major problem was spinopelvic instability and gradual closing of the pelvis, which narrowed very severely. The patient had no bladder control, but her primary urinary complaints

were that she leaked urine and was unable to self-catheterize because of pain. Furthermore, digital examination of the vagina was not possible because of bony obstruction of the introitus.

- As with most patients with type IV lumbosacral agenesis, she had developed progressive spinopelvic kyphosis and scoliosis. Her hips had severe restriction of motion and were in a position of flexion-abduction contracture. She also had fixed equinovarus deformities of the feet.

- No other malformation or impairment was detected on clinical examination.

20.6 Imaging

- Radiographs at the time of presentation demonstrated the absence of lumbar vertebral bodies below L2, total absence of the sacrum, fused ilia, and lumbopelvic disassociation with a visible gap between the most caudal intact thoracic vertebra and the pelvis (Figs. 20.1 and 20.2).

- CT scan with 3D reconstruction confirmed the severity of the pelvic inlet obstruction which had developed with growth (Fig. 20.3).

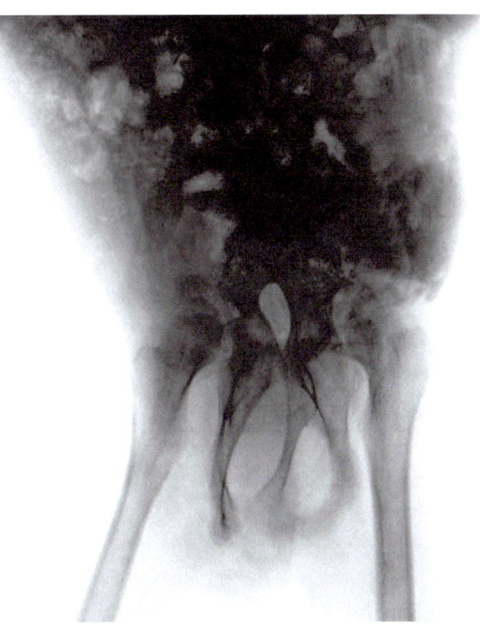

Fig. 20.2 Preoperative AP radiograph of the pelvis. There has been virtual approximation of the acetabula with pelvic inlet obstruction

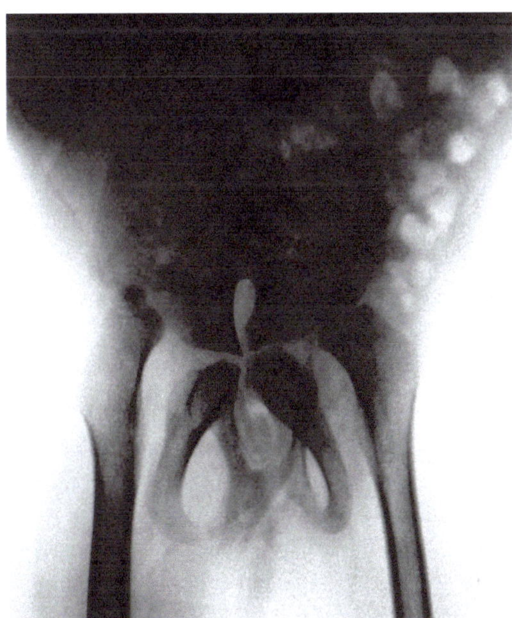

Fig. 20.1 AP pelvic radiograph demonstrating severe (Renshaw type IV, Guille type C) lumbosacral agenesis with the absence of the lower lumbar spine and the fused ilia

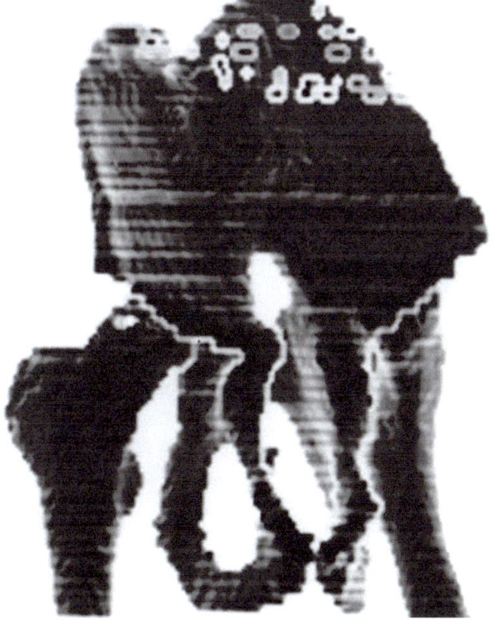

Fig. 20.3 Preoperative CT with 3D reconstruction illustrating the nature and severity of the bony deformity

20.7 Treatment Options

- The treatment of patients with Renshaw type IV and Guille type C caudal regression syndrome must be individualized and performed by a multidisciplinary team involving pediatrician, general surgeon, orthopedic surgeon, physiotherapist, and social worker. The pathologies that require special attention are orthopedic deformities and bladder and bowel continence, along with preservation of renal function.
- To improve functional performance and provide maximum autonomy to the patient in sitting and standing positions, two types of surgical intervention have been suggested including fixation of the spine and correction of the lower limb deformities (Gregoire and Zerdani 2001). Knee flexion and foot deformities may be corrected by surgical releases or by shortening corrective osteotomy followed by orthotic support.
- Stabilization of the residual spine to the pelvis may be indicated for the patient with severe lumbopelvic instability. Lumbopelvic arthrodesis can be achieved using internal rod or plate fixation with bone grafting between the pelvis and spine (Rieger et al. 1990; Winter 1991; Dumont et al. 1993).
- In some cases with severe spine deformities, the use of external fixation has been suggested using LRS monolateral system or Ilizarov circular external fixation frame (Dubousset 1991; Birch et al. 1997; Reyes-Sanchez et al. 2005; Griffet et al. 2011).
- Because of the significant physiological functional impairments in our patient caused by pelvic inlet obstruction, we decided to perform a pelvic inlet reconstruction through a posterior vertical midline iliac osteotomy followed by gradual distraction posteriorly using Ilizarov circular external fixation frame (Fig. 20.4).

20.8 Preoperative Planning

- Preoperative planning was essential to pelvic inlet reconstruction and included defining the level and direction of the iliac osteotomy; designing a functioning circular external fixation assembly, identifying the technique of bone segment fixation and monitoring of new bone formation in the distraction gap; calculating the amount of posterior pelvic widening and the rate and rhythm of distraction; and defining the duration of consolidation period and criteria for removal of external fixation.
- CT scan with 3D reconstruction of the pelvis was beneficial in construction of a custom specialized circular external fixation frame.

20.9 Frame Construction

- The apparatus consisted of four 240-mm diameter Ilizarov 5/8 rings assembled in pairs approximately 5 cm apart. In each pair, two parallel external supports were connected to each other by two vertically positioned threaded rods (Fig. 20.5a).
- Both pairs were interconnected at their most anterior points by a single vertically positioned threaded rod permitting rotation of those partial ring pairs relative to each other in the horizontal plane. In order to shift the axis of rotation posteriorly so that the symphysis pubis acted as the true axis of rotation without distraction, the most anterior holes of the 5/8 rings connected to the vertically placed threaded rod were modified into 3-hole slots (Fig. 20.4c).
- This connection allowed the constructed frame to be opened like a book around the anterior vertical threaded rod by distraction of posteriorly placed horizontal threaded rods (Fig. 20.5b).

20.10 Patient Positioning

- For the initial surgical procedure, the patient was placed prone between two operating tables, one to support the thorax and the other to support the legs. The pelvis and abdomen were draped circumferentially in the surgical field. This positioning allowed circumferential access to the patient's pelvic and thorax.
- It was important to maintain the full circumferential access to the pelvis throughout the surgical procedure for radiographic control, osteotomy, wire insertion, and frame application.

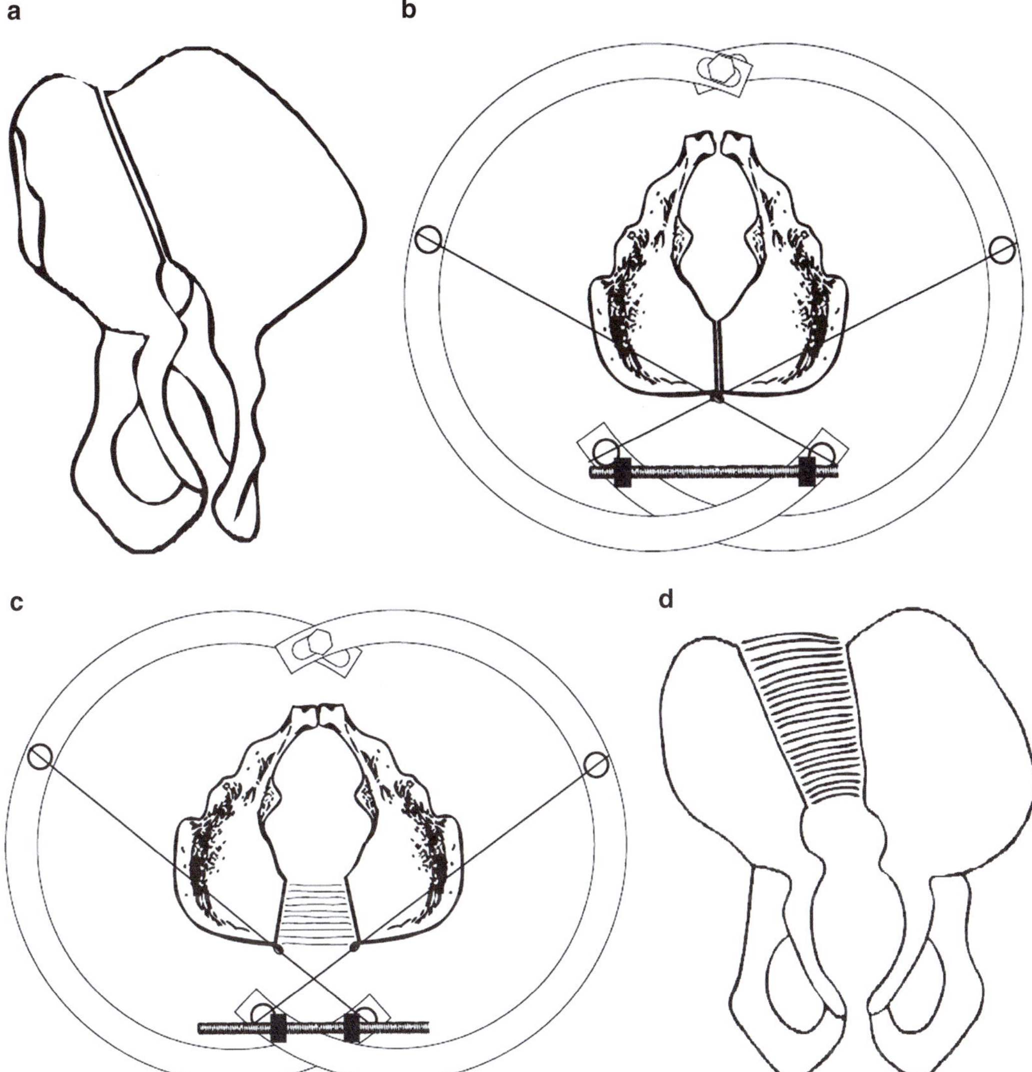

Fig. 20.4 Diagrams of the pelvic inlet reconstruction using circular external fixation and distraction osteogenesis technique: (**a**) vertical osteotomy of the fused ilia performed through a posterior approach; (**b**) two pairs of 1.8-mm diameter olive wires inserted in a cross-fixing fashion and attached to a proper pair of the 5/8 rings; (**c**) gradual horizontal distraction resulted in gradual bone separation posteriorly simultaneously with angular rotation around the symphysis; (**d**) the pelvic inlet is restored by creating bone distraction regenerate posteriorly and angularly rotating the ilia around the symphysis pubis

20.11 Osteotomy

- The single fused ilium was approached through a midline posterior incision and exposed subperiosteally (Fig. 20.6a, b).
- A vertical osteotomy of the fused ilia was performed using an osteotome, curettes, and rongeur (Fig. 20.6c).

20.12 Frame Application

- Two pairs of 1.8-mm diameter olive-stopper wires were inserted in a cross-fixing fashion, two for each hemi-iliac wing (Fig. 20.7). All four wires were inserted in a posteromedial to anterolateral projection and attached to their respective pair of the 5/8 rings (Fig. 20.8a).

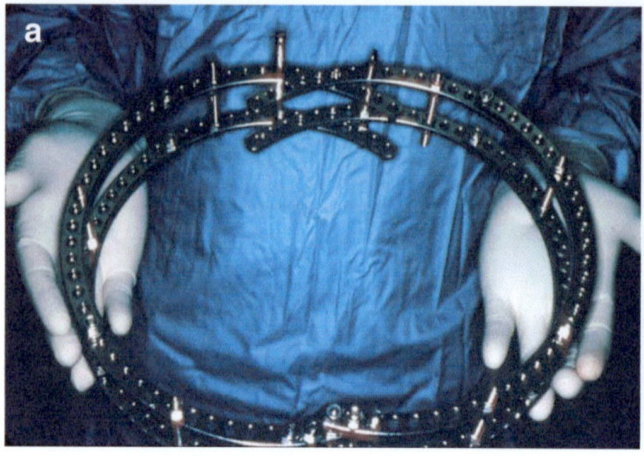
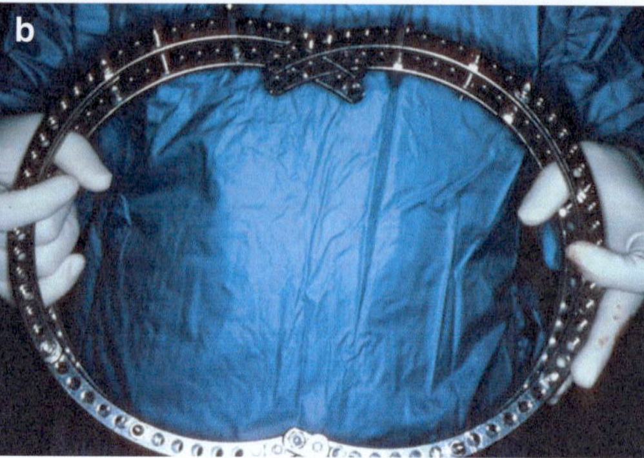

Fig. 20.5 Preoperative construction of the circular external fixator: (**a**) frame consisted of four 240-mm diameter Ilizarov 5/8 rings assembled in pairs and interconnected anteriorly by a single vertically positioned threaded rod; (**b**) the constructed frame can be opened like a book around the anterior vertical threaded rod by distraction of posteriorly placed horizontal threaded rods

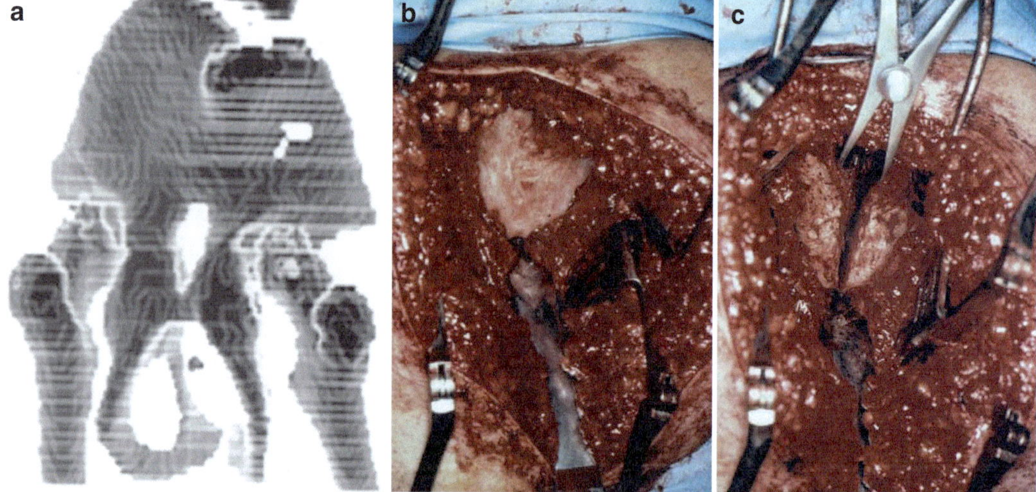

Fig. 20.6 Vertical osteotomy of the fused ilia: (**a**) preoperative CT with 3D reconstruction illustrating fused ilia posteriorly; (**b**) intraoperative photograph of the posterior exposure; (**c**) intraoperative photograph of the vertical osteotomy of the fused iliac wings

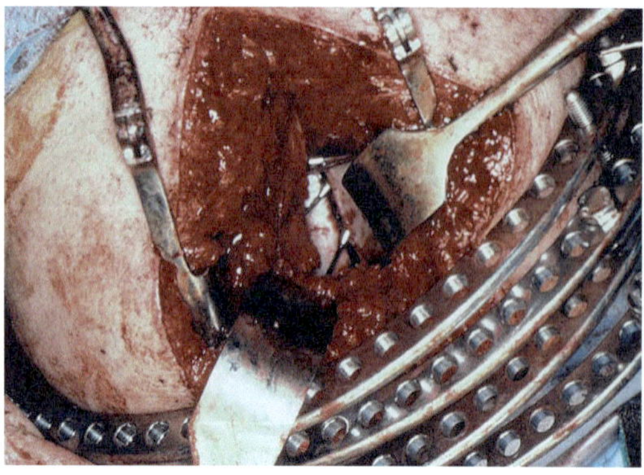

Fig. 20.7 Intraoperative photograph demonstrating two pairs of olive wires inserted under direct vision from posteromedial to anterolateral through the osteotomy site

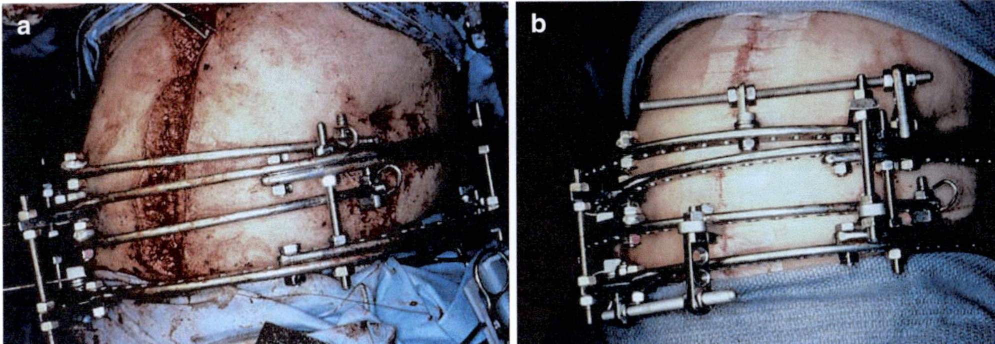

Fig. 20.8 Circular frame application: (**a**) four cross wires attached to a proper pair of the 5/8 rings; (**b**) external supports connected by two threaded rods posteriorly for gradual horizontal distraction

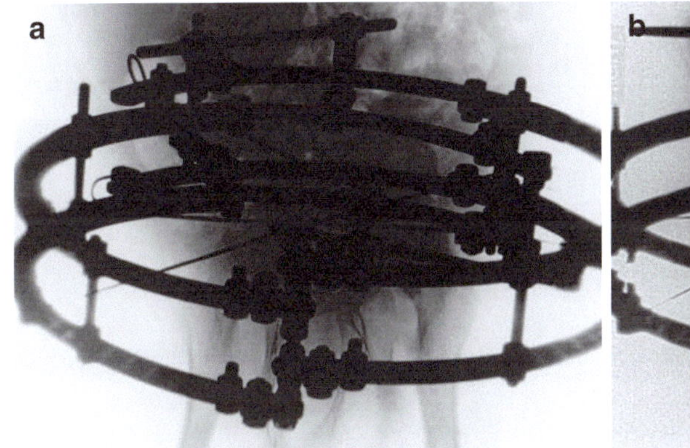
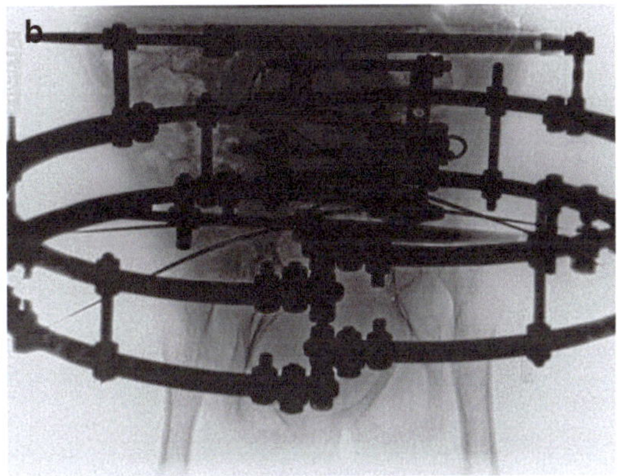

Fig. 20.9 Postoperative radiographs demonstrating gradual bone segment separation posteriorly simultaneously with angular rotation against the symphysis pubic: (**a**) pelvic x-ray at the beginning of distraction; (**b**) pelvic x-ray at the end of distraction

- The pre-constructed frame was centralized on the pelvis and aligned in the coronal and sagittal planes using the midline iliac osteotomy posteriorly and symphysis pubic anteriorly as anatomical reference landmarks.
- The apparatus was positioned in such a way that 3.0–4.0 cm of space was maintained between the soft tissue and the internal surface of the frame. The wires were rigidly secured to the frame and tensioned appropriately.
- The pairs of the anteriorly hinged external supports were connected by two threaded rods posteriorly for gradual horizontal distraction (Fig. 20.8b). For smooth frame rotation, threaded distraction rods were attached to the frame using male posts and nylon insert nuts.
- At this point, the wound was closed and well-padded dressing was applied around the wires to minimize movement of the soft tissues.

20.13 Gradual Distraction

- Gradual horizontal distraction between the two 5/8 ring pairs was commenced on the fifth postoperative day at the rate of 0.25 mm four times per day (Fig. 20.9a). The applied distraction forces resulted in gradual bone segment separation posteriorly simultaneously with an angular rotation around the symphysis pubis (Fig. 20.9b).

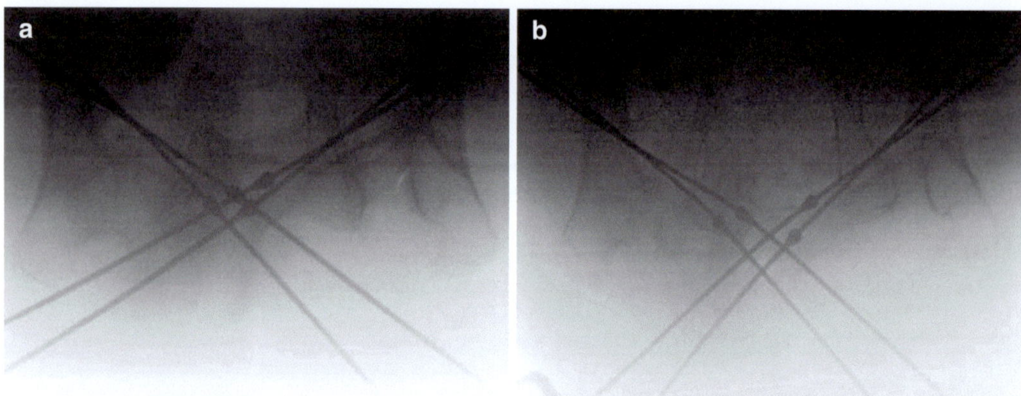

Fig. 20.10 Postoperative radiographs demonstrating changes in the distance between the opposing olive stoppers used to monitor the distraction gap: (**a**) pelvic x-ray at the beginning of distraction; (**b**) pelvic x-ray at the end of distraction

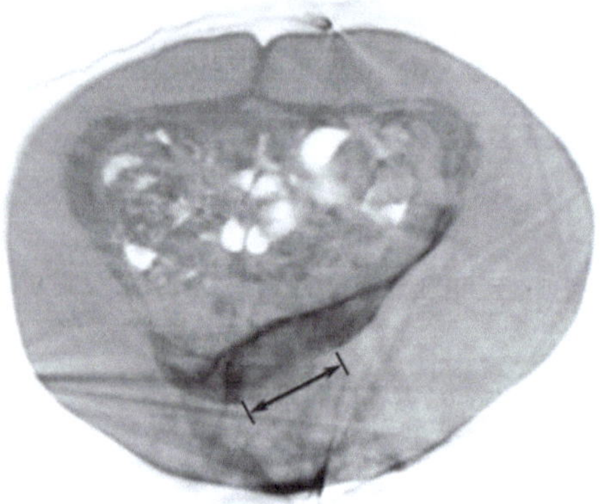

Fig. 20.11 Postoperative CT illustrating 6-cm distraction gap between the iliac wings posteriorly

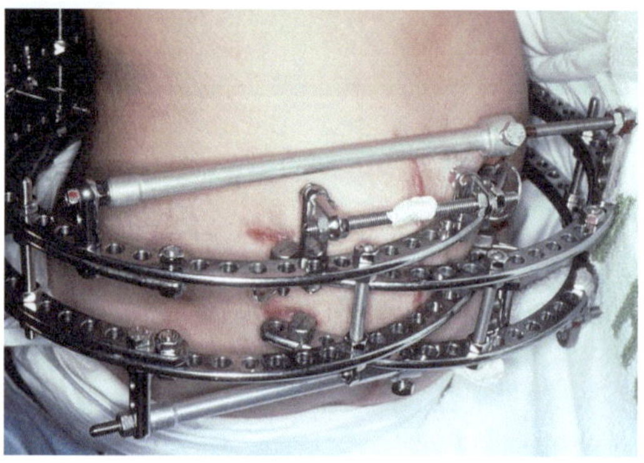

Fig. 20.12 Postoperative photograph illustrating threaded distraction rods replacement by more rigid telescopic distraction rods

- The distance between the opposing olive stoppers on the radiographs was used to monitor the distraction gap (Fig. 20.10a, b). Distraction was continued until the desired distraction gap was achieved between the iliac wings posteriorly. The total distraction period was 8 weeks and resulted in 6 cm of posterior widening of the pelvic inlet (Fig. 20.11). During the distraction period, patient was able to walk with crutches, sit, and look after her colostomy.

20.14 Frame Adjustments and Modifications

- Due to significant wire movement in the horizontal plane during pelvic widening, soft tissue tension around the wires was periodically released to eliminate pain and prevent pin tracks infection.
- The frame assembly was checked regularly and adjusted as needed. In order to continue distraction and maintain frame stability during consolidation period, threaded distraction rods were replaced by more rigid telescopic distraction rods after first 4 weeks of distraction (Fig. 20.12).

20.15 Consolidation Period

- The frame was removed after 3-month consolidation period.
- Reestablishment of adequate pelvic inlet was confirmed by x-ray, CT scan, and pelvic examination under anesthesia (Figs. 20.13 and 20.14). Rectal and vaginal examinations

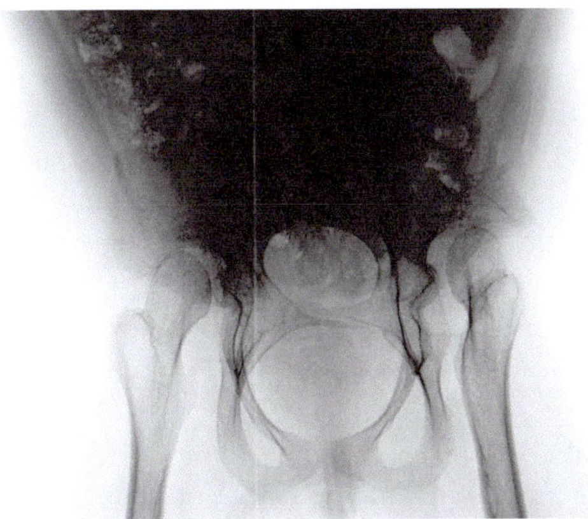

Fig. 20.13 Radiograph after frame removal demonstrating pelvic inlet reconstruction and actively remodeling posterior distraction bone regenerate

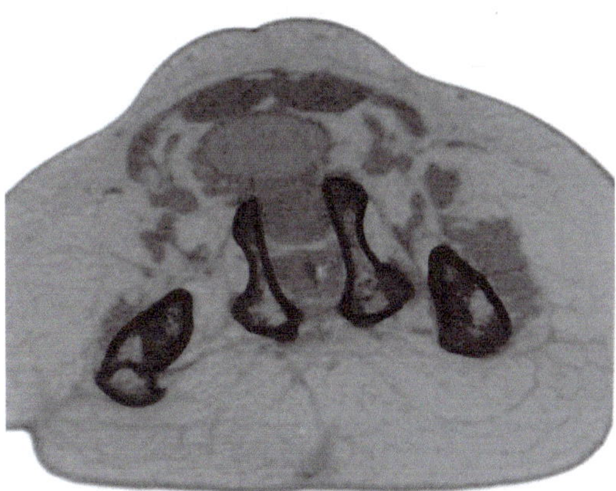

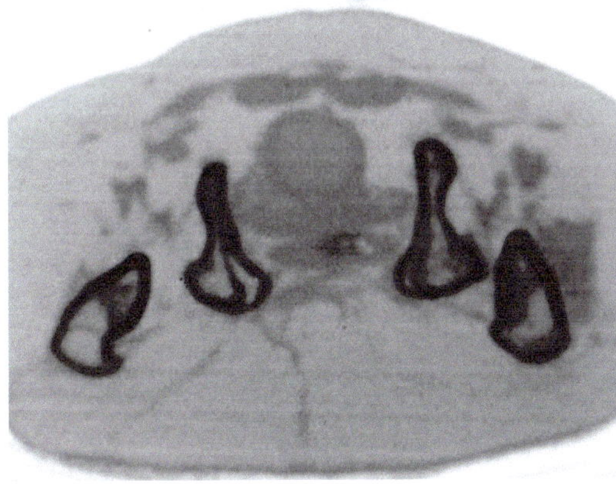

Fig. 20.14 Comparative preoperative (*top*) and post-frame removal (*bottom*) CT scans confirming adequate pelvic widening and reestablishment of the pelvic inlet

revealed the adequate pelvic widening, sufficient for colostomy take down and presumptive normal sexual function.

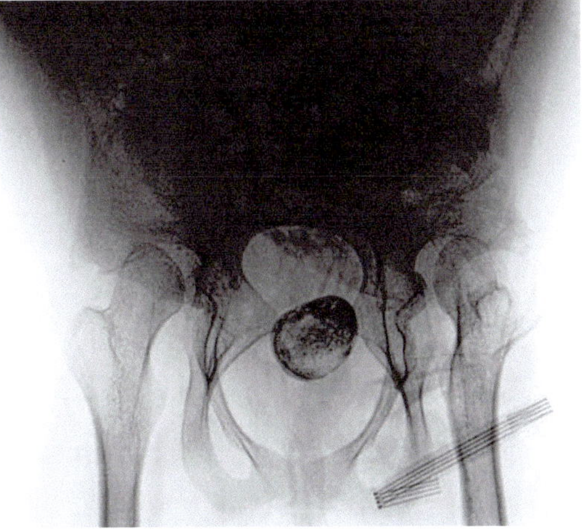

Fig. 20.15 Radiograph 2 years after frame removal illustrating tremendously improved pelvic inlet and remodeled newly formed bone in the distraction gap

20.16 Complications

- Transient dysesthesia in the left buttock and leg of undetermined etiology resolved spontaneously during the treatment.

20.17 Two-Year Follow-Up

- Radiographs 2 years after frame removal (Fig. 20.15) showed tremendously improved pelvic inlet and remodeled newly formed bone in the distraction gap (Birch et al. 1992).
- Patient showed improvement of sitting tolerance with no pain. She was independently ambulatory with underarm crutches, a swing-through gait, without lower extremity braces in regular shoes.
- In addition to her ability to participate in self-catheterization program, she had normal sexual function. Possible bladder stimulation followed by intermittent catheterization or artificial sphincter and colostomy revision were discussed at that time.

20.18 Long-Term Outcome

- The patient was examined 19 years after frame removal at 34 years of age.

- Radiographic appearance of the pelvic reconstruction showed a fairly remarkable preservation of the distraction gap and confirmed maintenance of the pelvic inlet (Fig. 20.16).

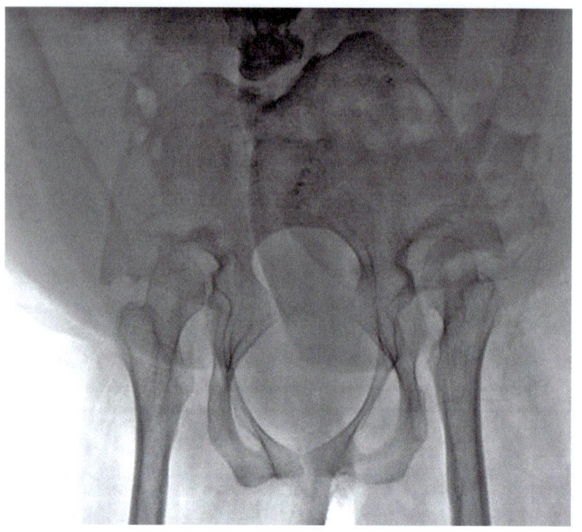

Fig. 20.16 Radiograph 19 years after frame removal demonstrating remarkable preservation of the distraction gap and confirming maintenance of the pelvic inlet

- She has retained the ability to ambulate with crutches. There is a pseudoarticulation between the lumbar spine and the pelvis with 60° of motion allowing both sitting and standing positions (Fig. 20.17).
- Patient has her original colostomy (no complications since 1993) and did not request its reversal due to anticipated need to wear diapers. She takes Ditropan for bladder control, does not use diapers or catheterize, has been able to remain content of urine by medicinal management only, and uses a regular toilet.
- The patient is very happy with her social life. She was married twice and conceived three children naturally; all were delivered 4–6 weeks preterm by elective cesarean section. All children are extremely intelligent with no physical impairment of any kind.
- The patient does experience low back pain of unknown etiology treated symptomatically and has episodes of pyelonephritis. No other specific abnormalities are noted except for

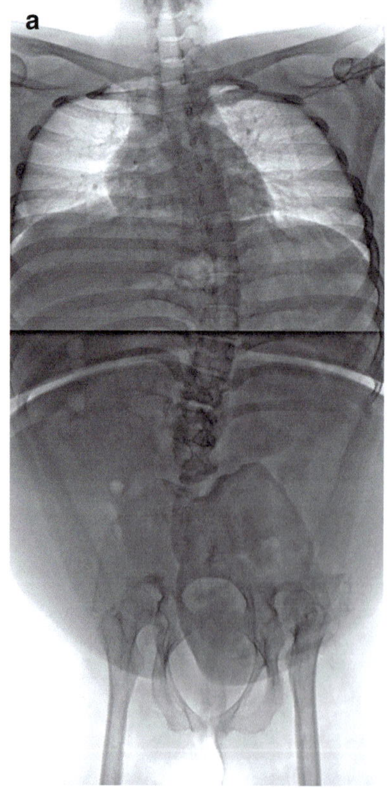
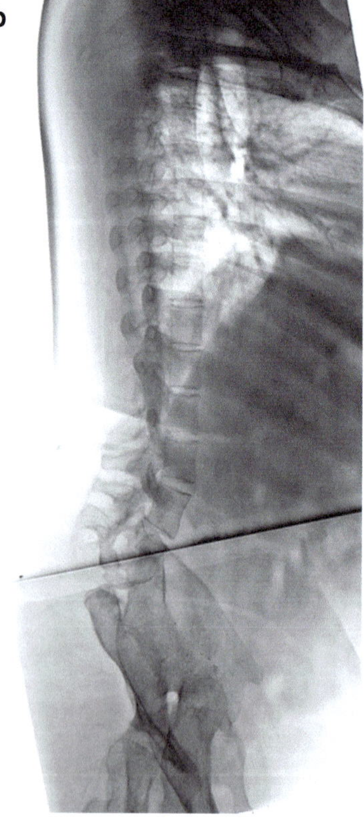

Fig. 20.17 Radiograph 19 years after frame removal illustrating pseudoarticulation between the lumbar spine and the pelvis: (**a**) AP radiograph; (**b**) ML radiograph

that related to the distorted anatomy and the fixed dislocation of both hips.

Conclusion

- This unique method of pelvic inlet reconstruction using circular external fixation and distraction osteogenesis may be indicated for patients with profound lumbosacral agenesis in occasional, carefully considered cases of pelvic obstruction.

References

Adra A, Coerdero D, Mejides A et al (1994) Caudal regression syndrome: etiopathogenesis, prenatal diagnosis, and perinatal management. Obstet Gynecol Surv 49(7):508–516

Birch JG, Samchukov ML, Stabell RS (1992) Pelvic inlet reconstruction for obstruction associated with lumbosacral agenesis using ilizarov apparatus: a case report. Bull Hosp Joint Dis Orthop Inst 52(1):39

Birch JG, Samchukov ML, Richards BS, Karol LA, Ross JD (1997) Modified ilizarov apparatus for the management of severe spinal deformities in children. A report of four cases. In: 7th ASAMI North America Annual Meeting, San Francisco, paper 48

Boemers T, van Gool J, de Jong T et al (1994) Urodynamic evaluation of children with caudal regression syndrome (caudal dysplasia sequence). J Urol 151:1038–1040

Boulas MM (2009) Recognition of caudal regression syndrome. Adv Neonatal Care 9(2):61–69

Caird MS, Hall JM, Bloom DA et al (2007) Outcome study of children, adolescents, and adults with sacral agenesis. J Pediatr Orthop 27:682–685

Cama A, Palmieri A, Capra V et al (1996) Multidisciplinary management of caudal regression syndrome (26 cases). Eur J Pediatr Surg 6(Suppl 1):44–45

Dubousset J (1991) La technique d'Ilizarov. Procede de sauvetage en chirurgie du rachis. Rev Chir Orthop Suppl 177:144

Dumont CE, Damsin JP, Forin V, Carlioz H (1993) Lumbosacral agenesis. Three cases of reconstruction using Cotrel-Dubousset or L-rod instrumentation. Spine 18(9):1229–1235

Emami-Naeini P, Nejat F, Rahbar Z et al (2012) Urological manifestation of sacral agenesis. J Pediatr Urol 8:181–186

Garcia T, Liborio R, Pais R et al (2001) Caudal regression syndrome. Lumbo-sacral agenesis. Acta Med Port 14(1):83–88

Gregoire A, Zerdani S (2001) Lumbo-sacral agenesis. Clinical analysis and treatment relating to 4 observations. Pediatr Med Chir 23(2):89–98

Griffet J, Leroux J, El Hayek T (2011) Lumbopelvic stabilization with external fixator in a patient with lumbosacral agenesis. Eur Spine J 20(Suppl 2):161–165

Guidera KJ, Raney E, Ogden JA et al (1991) Caudal regression: a review of seven cases, including the mermaid syndrome. J Pediatr Orthop 11:743–747

Guille JT, Benevides R, DeAlba CC et al (2002) Lumbosacral agenesis: a new classification correlating spinal deformity and ambulatory potential. J Bone Joint Surg Am 84:32–38

Harlow CL, Partington MD, Thieme GA (1995) Lumbosacral agenesis: clinical characteristics, imaging, and embryogenesis. Pediatr Neurosurg 23(3):140–147

Junquera JMA, Sugranes JC, Calvo RM et al (2006) Evolution urologica de pacientes con agenesia de sacro: 20 anos de seguimiento. Arch Esp Urol 56(6):595–600

Phillips WA, Cooperman DR, Lindquist TC et al (1982) Orthopedic management of lumbosacral agenesis. Long-term follow-up. J Bone Joint Surg Am 64:1282–1294

Renshaw TS (1978) Sacral agenesis. A classification and review of twenty-three cases. J Bone Joint Surg Am 60:373–383

Reyes-Sanchez A, Rosales LM, Miramontes V (2005) External fixation for dynamic correction of severe scoliosis. Spine J 5:418–426

Rieger MA, Hall JE, Dalury DF (1990) Spinal fusion in a patient with lumbosacral agenesis. Spine 12:1382–1384

Van H, Fourie IJ (1984) Sacral agenesis and neurologic bladder dysfunction. A case report and review of the literature. S Afr Med J 65:55–56

Wilmshurst JM, Kelly R, Borzyskowski M (1999) Presentation and outcome of sacral agenesis: 20 years' experience. Dev Med Child Neurol 41:806–812

Winter RB (1991) Congenital absence of the lumbar spine and sacrum: one-stage reconstruction with subsequent two-stage spine lengthening. J Pediatr Orthop 11(5):666–670

21

Pelvic Support Osteotomy (PSO): Indications, Limits and Complications

Maurizio Catagni, Francesco Guerreschi, Luigi Lovisetti, and Haridimos Tsibidakis

Contents

M. Catagni (✉)
Department of Orthopaedic Surgery,
Alessandro Manzoni Hospital, Lecco, Italy
e-mail: maurizio@catagni.it

F. Guerreschi
Department of Orthopaedic Surgery, Lecco Hospital,
Lecco, Italy

L. Lovisetti
Divisione di Ortopedia e Traumatologia A,
Ospedale S. Anna, Como, Italy

H. Tsibidakis
Department of Orthopaedic Surgery
and Traumatology, Lecco, Italy

21.1   Introduction

Alteration in anatomy and function is a common characteristic in many pathologies regarding the hip joint, congenital or acquired, and therapeutic solutions are difficult to find.

Pelvic support osteotomies have a long tradition in orthopaedic surgery and trace back to the first half of the twentieth century; their aim is to reorient the biological tissues to improve gait and to offer pelvic support (Rozbruch et al. 2005; Manzotti et al. 2003).

Pelvic osteotomies have been described and performed by several authors for hip stabilization by medial shifting of the anatomic axis compared to the mechanical axis of the femur (Milch 1989). In particular, Schanz, Milch and Charry proposed proximal femoral support osteotomies to resolve problems of instability and abnormal gait. These osteotomies cause an excessive valgus of the mechanical axis alignment and ignore the coexistent leg length discrepancy. The goal of these procedures was an abduction osteotomy in the subtrochanteric region of the femur, providing a method of stabilization for the proximal femur with a good range of motion of the hip. Bouvier, in 1838, performed subtrochanteric osteotomy aiming at pelvic support in congenital dislocation of the hip (Stack and George 1959). Kirmission, in 1894, suggested femoral osteotomy for the treatment of non-reducible dislocation with the aim to correct the frequent presence

M. Kocaoğlu et al. (eds.), *Advanced Techniques in Limb Reconstruction Surgery*,
DOI 10.1007/978-3-642-55026-3_21, © Springer Berlin Heidelberg 2015

433

of adduction contracture (Kirmission 1894; Shepherd 1960). Von Baeyer, in 1918, made a subtrochanteric osteotomy to increase tension of the pelvic-femoral muscles and support better the pelvis (Milch 1989). Adolf Lorenz proposed a bifurcation osteotomy to correct deformity and to restore stability during weight bearing modified later on by Schanz and Hass (Shepherd 1960; Lorenz 1919). The disadvantage of these early attempts of hip's stabilization by osteotomy was the significant additional leg length discrepancy, and no attempt at normalizing the lower limb mechanical axis was made with the consequence of abnormal mechanical forces on the knee resulting in valgus angulation.

Gavril Ilizarov was the first to perform a proximal femur valgus osteotomy combined with a lengthening–varus osteotomy located distally, in order to restore physiological force distribution at the knee and ankle joint and to balance leg length (Ilizarov 1983; Ilizarov and Samchukov 1988).

21.2 Indications

The pelvic support osteotomy is a surgical procedure for the salvage of damaged hips of patients in whom arthrodesis or hip arthroplasty is not indicated (Callaghan et al. 1985). It is an appropriate procedure in adolescents or young adults who have painless limping, restriction of hip motion and early-onset fatigue to walking as a consequence of hip damages after neonatal septic arthritis; the sequelae of neonatal septic arthritis have been classified by Hunka et al.(1982). While the less severely affected varieties of types I to III are amenable to the more usual hip reconstruction procedures (either pelvic or femoral osteotomies or both), types IV and V, in which a greater part of the true hip is destroyed, are indicated for PSO.

Other diseases taking advantage of PSO are severe hip dysplasia and neglected congenital dislocations or those where the treatment failed and those presenting neuromuscular disorders (in case of polio, myelomeningocele, and cerebral palsy and epiphysiolysis) (Rozbruch et al. 2005).

Finding the solution to these problems is not easy. In addition it is frequently necessary to be able to adapt treatment considering age, sex and individual life expectation.

A similar situation is observed in failed treatment of traumatic hip dislocation with hip instability or after a Girdlestone arthroplasty, with joint instability that allows proximal migration of the femur during loading, decreasing the gluteal lever arm with a final Trendelenburg gait (Schiltenwolf et al. 1996). The limp although initially is painless becomes painful, and walking tolerance decreases with time (Schiltenwolf et al. 1996; Kocaoglu et al. 2002).

21.3 Methods

The technique described by Ilizarov is essentially the union of two different operations (Shepherd 1960; Ilizarov 1983):

1. A valgus subtrochanteric osteotomy for pelvic support. The level of the osteotomy is located at the correspondence of the lower profile of the obturator foramen; then the distal part of the femur must be angulated in a relative abduction (range 45–90° due to the preoperative ROM).
2. An osteotomy of the distal femur to perform limb lengthening and axial deformity correction of the lower limbs.

This procedure can be performed, thanks to the great versatility of the Ilizarov fixator, which allows correction of any residual axial deformity as well during the treatment studying the gait with full loading.

The two osteotomies produce a kind of "lightning-shaped" femur that, as a final result, stabilizes the hip and realigns the mechanical axis.

The ROM of the hip is intact or lightly reduced but retensioning the pelvitrochanteric muscles leads to a better abduction and a simultaneous improvement or disappearance of Trendelenburg sign.

Photo 21.1 3D computerized tomography of a patient with pelvic support osteotomy

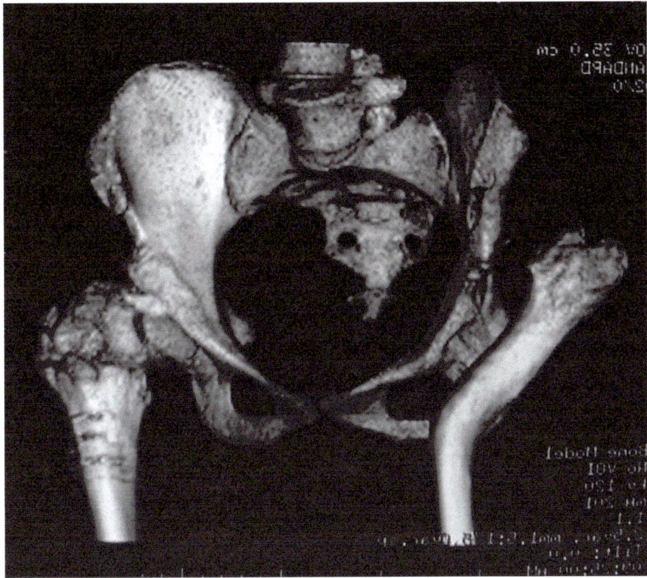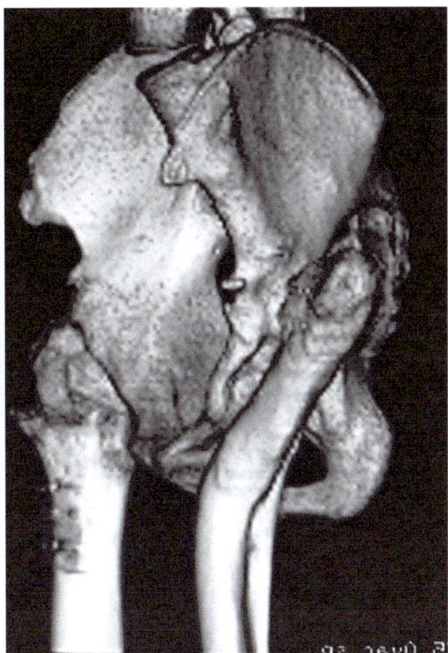

The reason of the improvement of stability is due to the increment of the surface of support between the femur and pelvis soft tissues (Photo 21.1) and to the retension of the gluteus caused by translation of the trochanteric region laterally to the iliac crest.

At the end of the treatment, the limb length discrepancy is eliminated and a normal alignment of the knee joint is obtained.

The aesthetic aspect of PSO is very satisfactory because the soft tissue of the thigh hides the double angulation of the femur and the proximal valgus correction of the subtrochanteric osteotomy moves laterally the gluteal region offering a better clinical aspect with respect to the one before surgery (hypotonic hip). In the end, a better abduction of the hip improves personal hygiene and sexual activity.

21.4   Preoperative Planning

To determine the right position of proximal osteotomy is necessary to perform both static and dynamic hip x-rays:

1. Orthostatic x-rays in bipodalic weight bearing – to evaluate the static axis of the lower limbs (Fig. 21.1).
2. Dynamic x-rays with monopodalic bearing on the pathological limb – to evaluate Trendelenburg sign and the shortening of the proximal femur during weight bearing (Fig. 21.2); a second dynamic x-ray is taken in maximum adduction with patient in the supine position.

With these x-rays, we can plan the level of the osteotomy (distal part of the obturator foramen) and the correction's angle.

The planning is completed with the evaluation of the varus and lengthening correction of the distal femur. A transparent copy of the x-ray with monopodalic bearing is used, and a subtrochanteric cut is made (>20–30° with respect to the pelvis projection in the monopodalic bearing x-ray); then two lines are drawn: one passing by the medial part of the osteotomy and the centre of the knee and a second one passing by the tibia's axis; the angle obtained corresponds to the one necessary to obtain the alignment of the mechanical axis of the lower

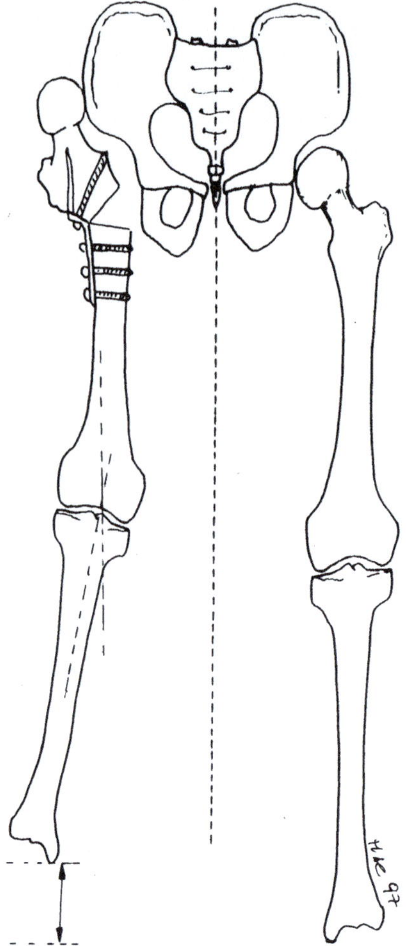

Fig. 21.1 Osteotomy planning in standing position

limb (Figs. 21.3 and 21.4). This preoperative planning could be helpful, but the final decisions of the various corrections are performed during treatment.

21.5 Operative Technique

In the original operative technique described by Ilizarov, the whole fixation was performed with K-wires connected to half rings in the proximal part of the femur and full rings in the distal part.

In 1986 this fixation was modified using new arches (type Catagni-Cattaneo) (Catagni et al. 1996) and pin fixation (Fig. 21.5).

Thanks to these modifications, specific beds were no more used and patients could sit normally (impossible with the original fixation).

Transfixion of femoral artery and sciatic nerve is also avoided, as wire track infections are also reduced.

The use of pin instead of K-wires reduces pain in patients and permits a complete ROM of the hip, avoiding flexion contractions that where often seen using the original apparatus. These contractions in flexion prevent correct evaluation of the mechanic axis because patients could not have a normal full weight-bearing stand.

Also only a pin-based fixation is used on the distal part, with the exception of a single K-wire (Fig. 21.6).

21.6 Operation

The pre-assembled frame consists of two 90° arches proximally set at the estimated angle of valgus osteotomy, a floating ring and two full rings distal to hinges to allow lengthening and varus rotation of the distal femur. Generally the arches and rings will be parallel at the end of the procedure, although this is not necessary if the individual anatomy dictates otherwise.

The frame is pictured in Figs. 21.7 and 21.8. The patient is placed on a fracture table to allow circumferential access to the thigh and a surgical assistant access between the legs. The leg is supported just distal to the knee with the foot free, to allow full knee motion during surgery.

Three K-wires are placed in the proximal femur corresponding to the intended level of the proximal arch, proximal osteotomy and distal arch, and an intraoperative x-ray is obtained. Such wire is used just for references and an x-ray is taken.

Figs. 21.2 and 21.3
Dynamic planning with
monopodalic bearing on the
pathological limb

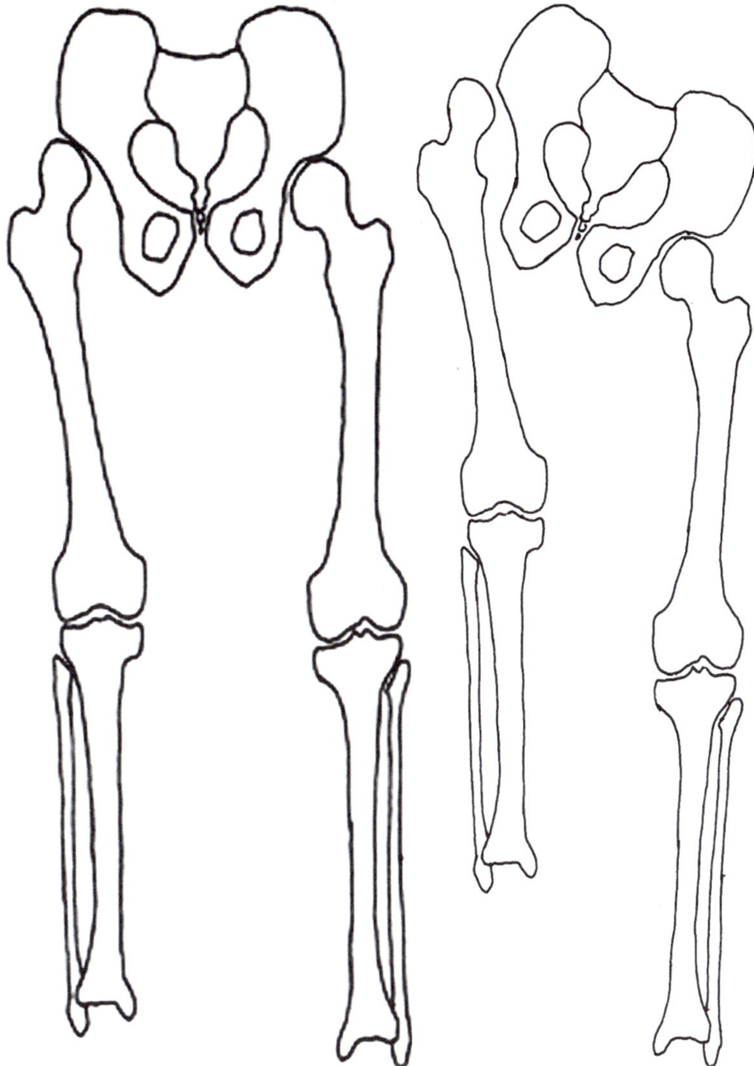

The proximal intertrochanteric 5 mm half-pin is placed at the predetermined angle to the skin. The leg is maximally adducted during insertion of this pin to avoid soft-tissue contact between the two arches. The frame is suspended with a transverse 1.8 mm wire in the distal ring, parallel to the knee joint. The remaining wires and half-pins are inserted. The proximal femoral osteotomy is performed through a lateral incision. Standard osteotomy technique with minimal soft-tissue disruption is used. A 4/5 cm incision is used to allow palpation of the bone ends; impaling the distal and lateral cortices of the proximal fragment into the intramedullary canal of the distal fragment can increase stability. After connecting and stabilizing the proximal arches, the distal osteotomy is performed with Gigli saw. A final intraoperative x-ray is obtained to control the fixation and alignment (Figs. 21.9, 21.10, 21.11, 21.12, and 21.13).

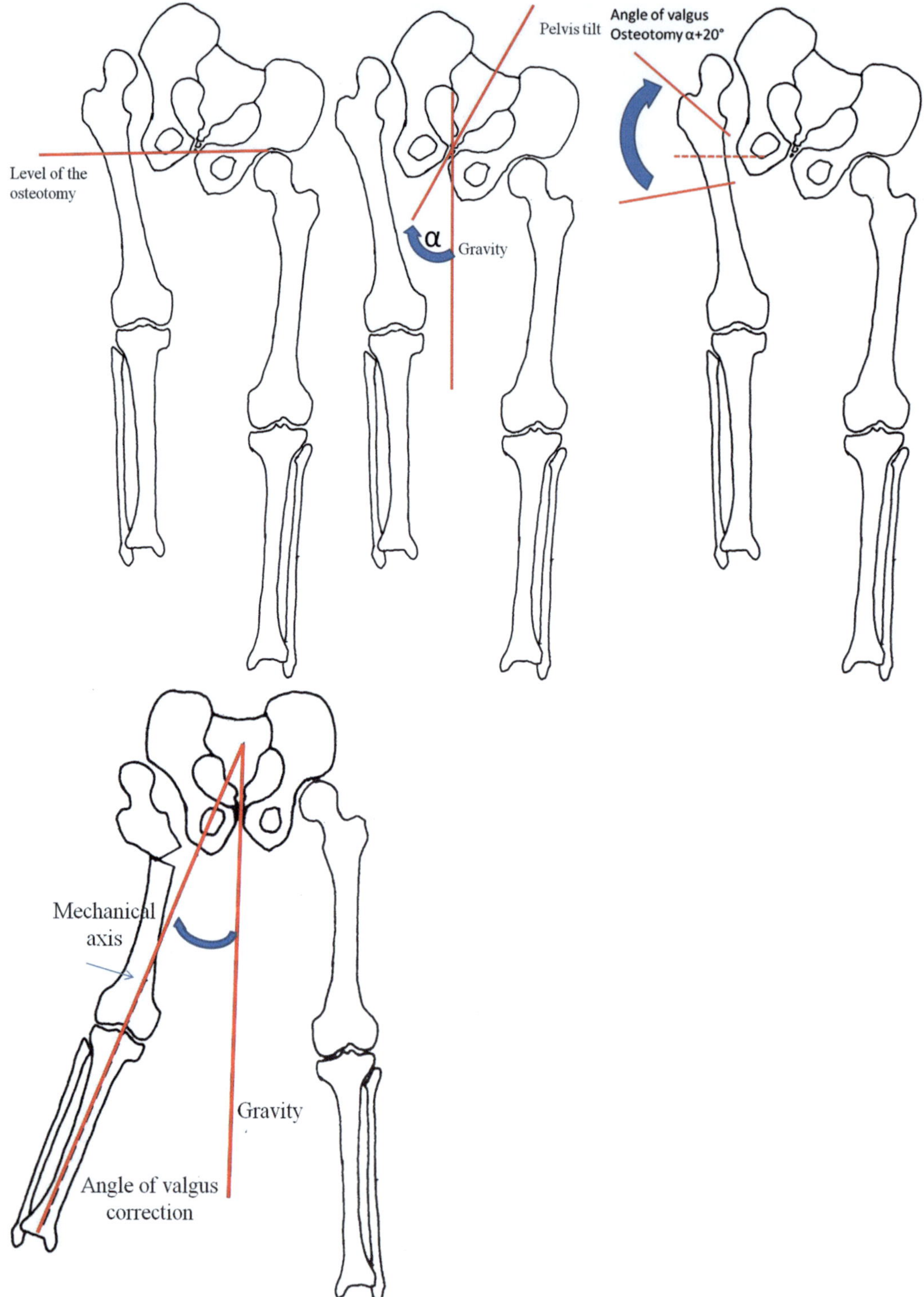

Figs. 21.4, 21.5, 21.6, and 21.7 With these x-rays, we can plan the level of the osteotomy

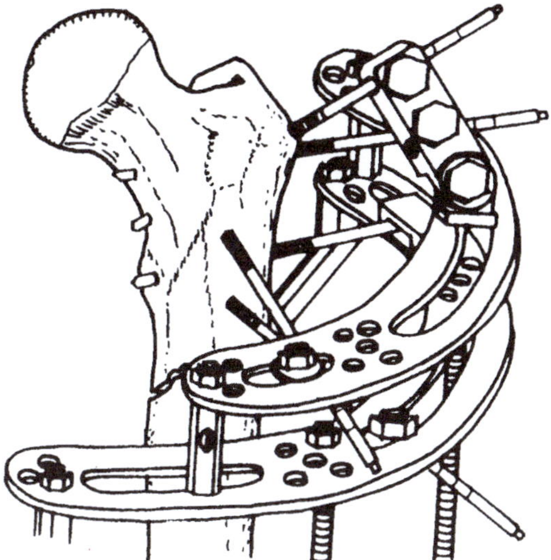

Fig. 21.8 Overview of the proximal part of the frame

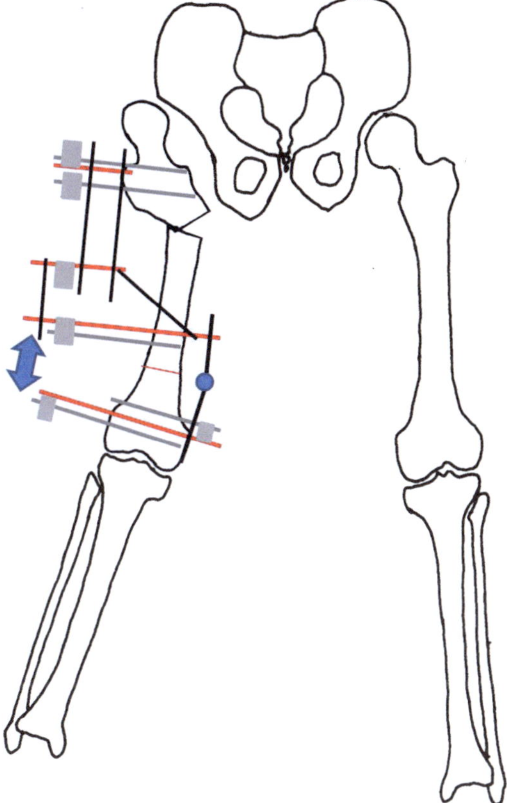

Fig. 21.10 Frame placed and correction performed

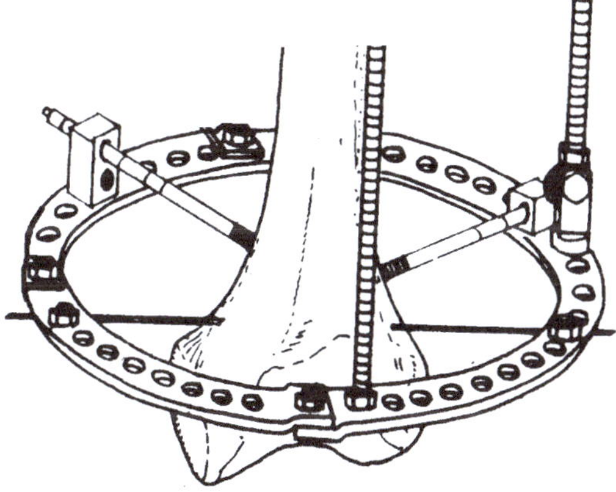

Fig. 21.9 Overview of the distal part of the frame

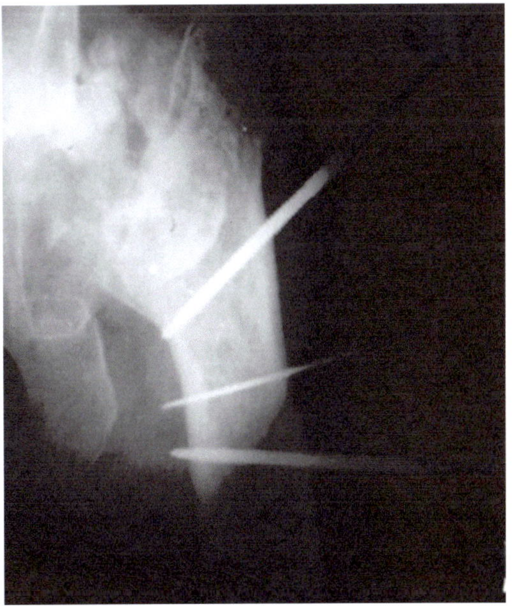

Fig. 21.11 Half-pin placement in x-ray

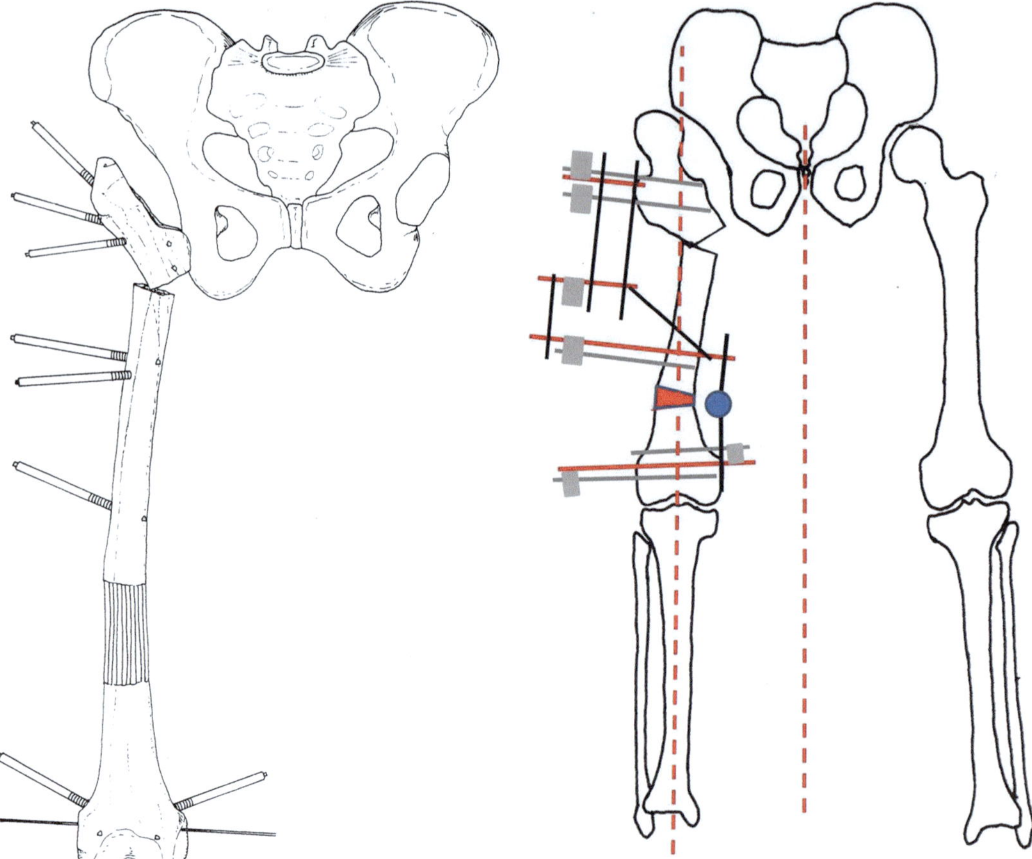

Fig. 21.12 Half-pin placement and lengthening

Fig. 21.13 Distal varus and proximal valgus alignment shown

21.7 Post-op Care

Weight bearing is allowed as tolerated, usually beginning partial weight bearing in 2/3 days. The dynamic nature of Ilizarov apparatus allows "fine-tuning" of proximal and distal angles. When the angle of the proximal osteotomy is satisfactory, compression is applied between the arches. Lengthening begun distally, 1/4 mm four times a day starting at the 5/7 postoperative day. Varus angulation of the distal femur is created near the end of lengthening, using the hinges between the two distal rings (Catagni and Cattaneo 1986; Cattaneo et al. 1990; Catagni 1992). Mechanical axis and leg length are "fine-tuned" after the patient has undergone weight

bearing. Physical therapy is used to strengthen the hip abductors and adductors and to maintain hip and knee motion. After appropriate length and alignment are obtained, the frame is left in a static mode until satisfactory healing of the osteotomy and regenerate allows frame removal. The distal transverse wire can be removed at the end of lengthening to facilitate knee motion.

Sometimes, it is necessary to lengthen the apparatus by fixation of the tibia and use appropriate hinges to allow movements and prevent subluxation or stiffness of the knee that can occur in cases of great femoral dysmetria that leads to a great distal femoral lengthening and axial correction.

In the worst cases we apply the apparatus not only to prevent problems on the knee but also to perform tibial lengthening in the metaphyseal region to reduce:

1. The correction forces on the femur
2. Stiffness of the knee
3. The time of treatment

It is proved that the healing of a trifocal lengthening is shorter than a bifocal one, and a 2\3 cm discrepancy of lengthening between knees is well tolerated both aesthetically and mechanically.

21.8 Complications

The most frequent complication is the pin's tract infection, mostly around the distal pins and during the distraction phase. *Fracture regenerate* that occurred after frame removal, *premature consolidation*, *delayed consolidation* and *residual limb length discrepancy are also complications.*

Most of the patients had knee stiffness after frame removal due to prolonged external fixation time. We found that knee range of motion showed progressive improvement during the 6-month period following frame removal.

Tendency to knee valgus and external rotatory subluxation at the joint, during lengthening, can be observed. This complication was even expected in the poliomyelitis patients or in the patient who showed knee instability during preoperative evaluation.

21.9 Presentations

21.9.1 Case Report of Septic Arthritis

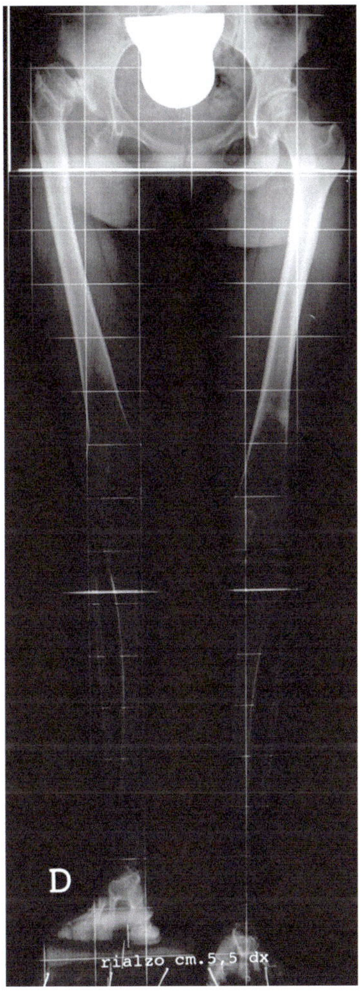

Fig. 21.14 Dynamic x-rays

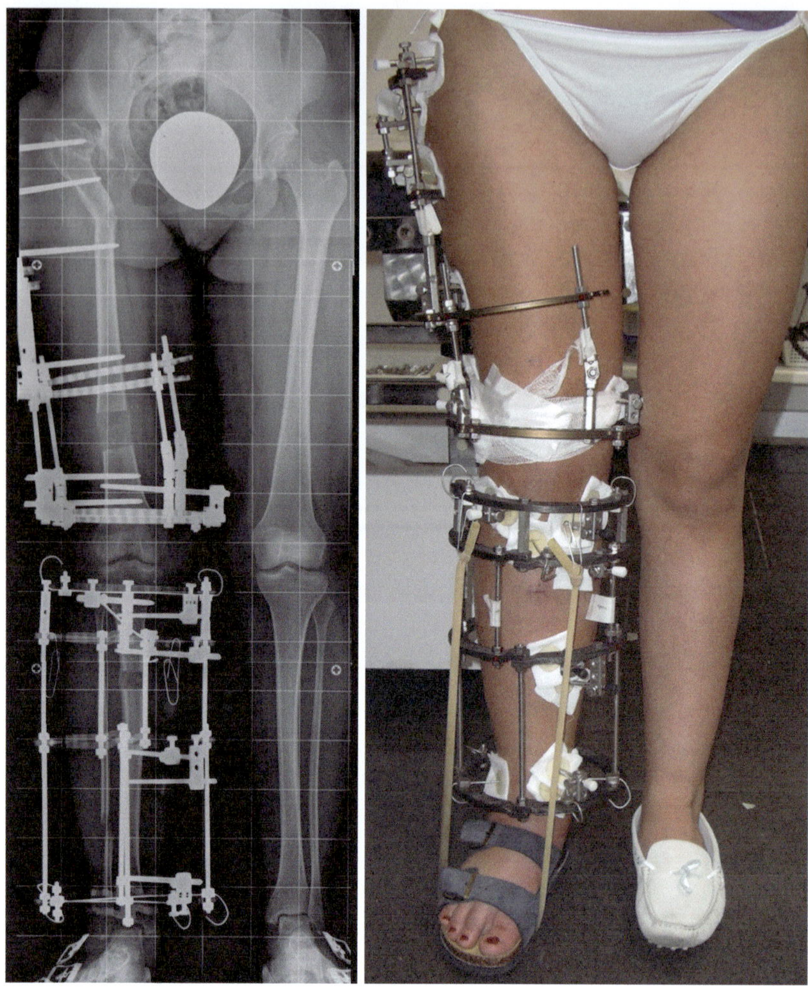

Figs. 21.15 and 21.16 X-rays during the treatment and photos of the frame

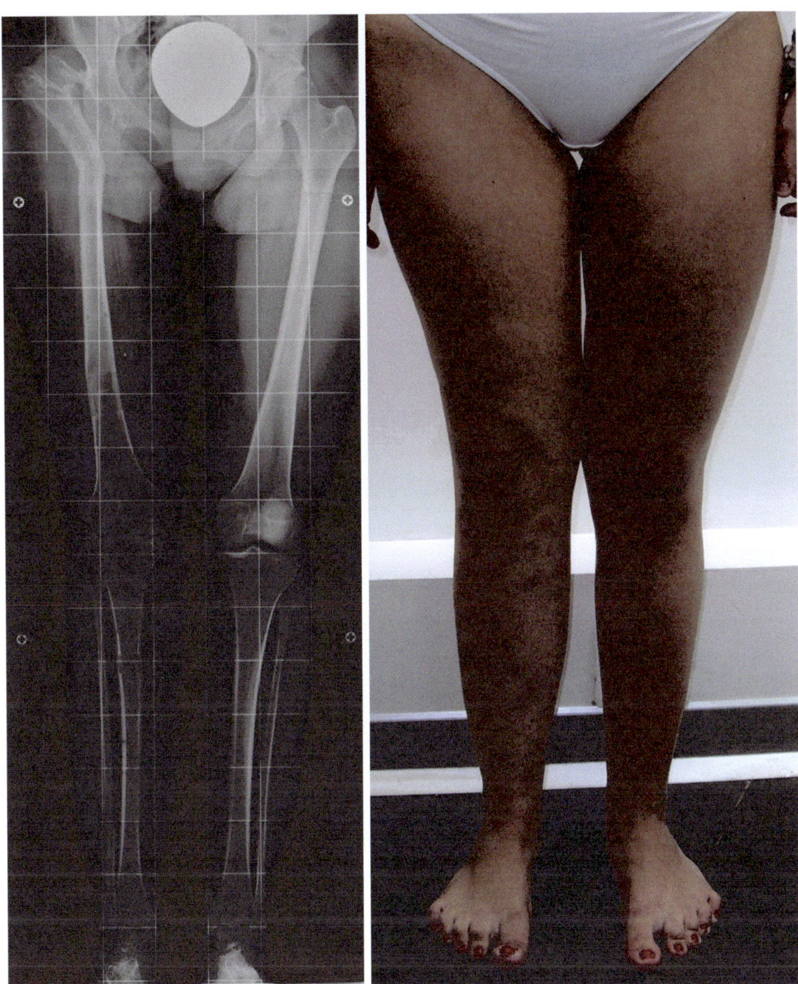

Figs. 21.17 and 21.18 X-rays after the treatment and photos of the patient

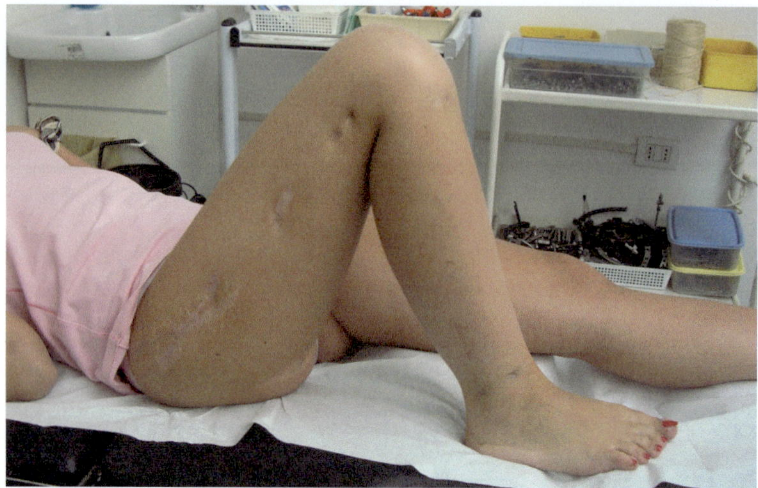

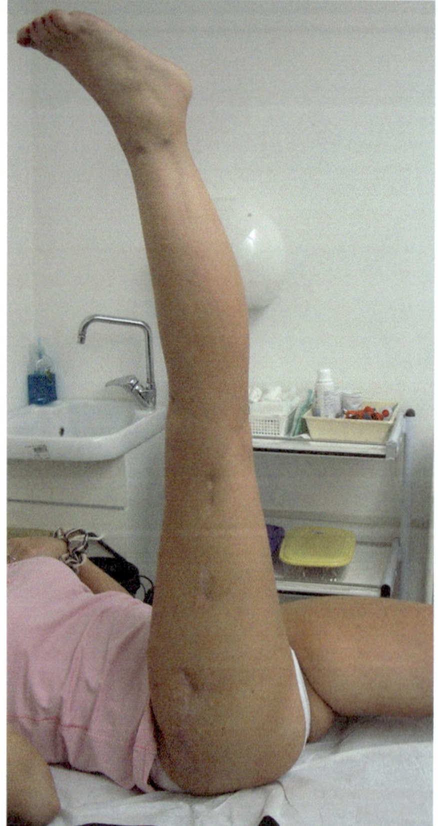

Figs. 21.19 and 21.20 Photos of the patient's ROM of the hip and knee

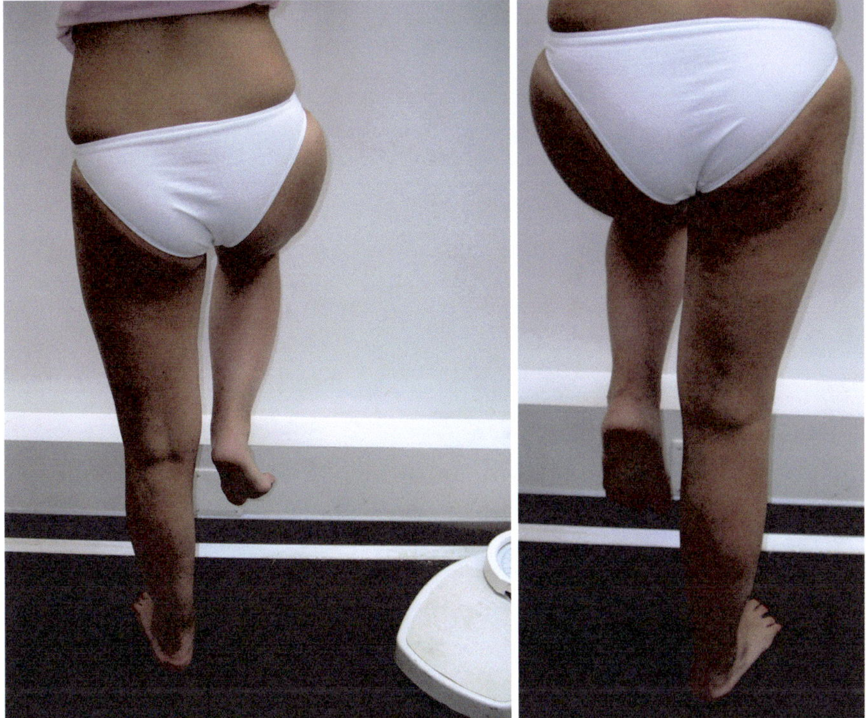

Figs. 21.21 and 21.22 Trendelenburg sign after treatment

21.9.2 Case of Neglected Dislocations

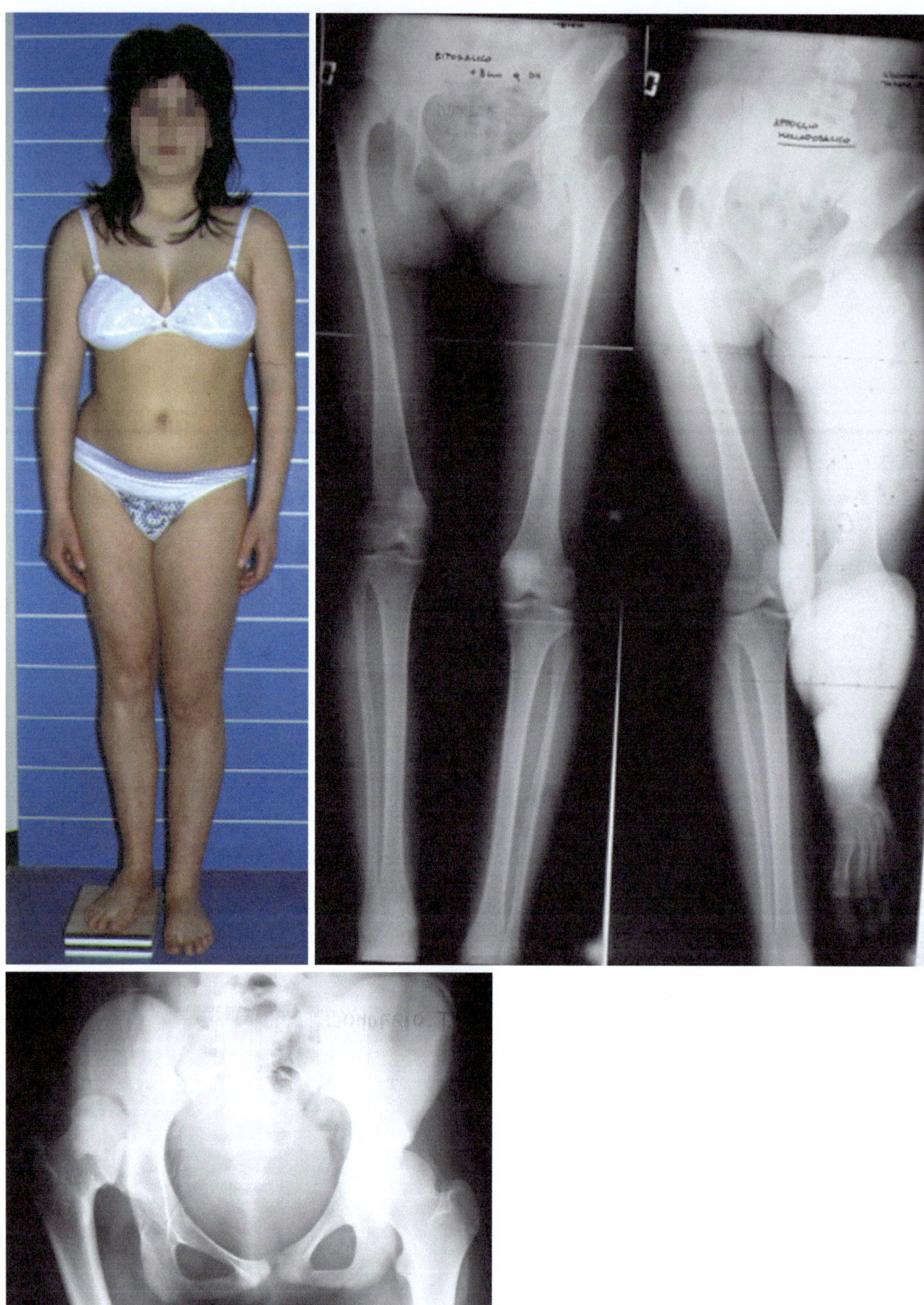

Figs. 21.23, 21.24, and 21.25 Dynamic x-rays

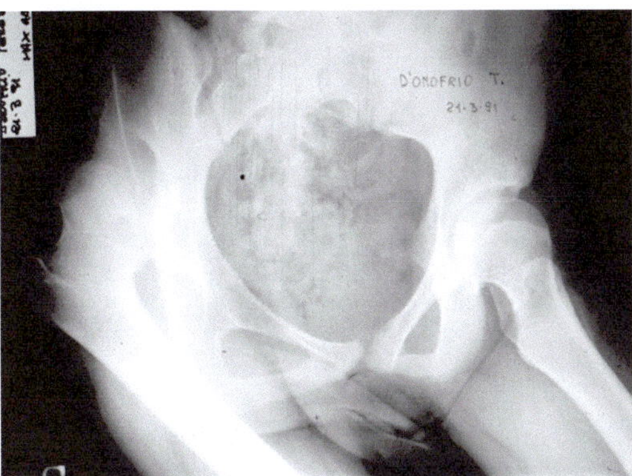

Fig. 21.26 Dynamic x-ray in maximum adduction with patient in the supine position

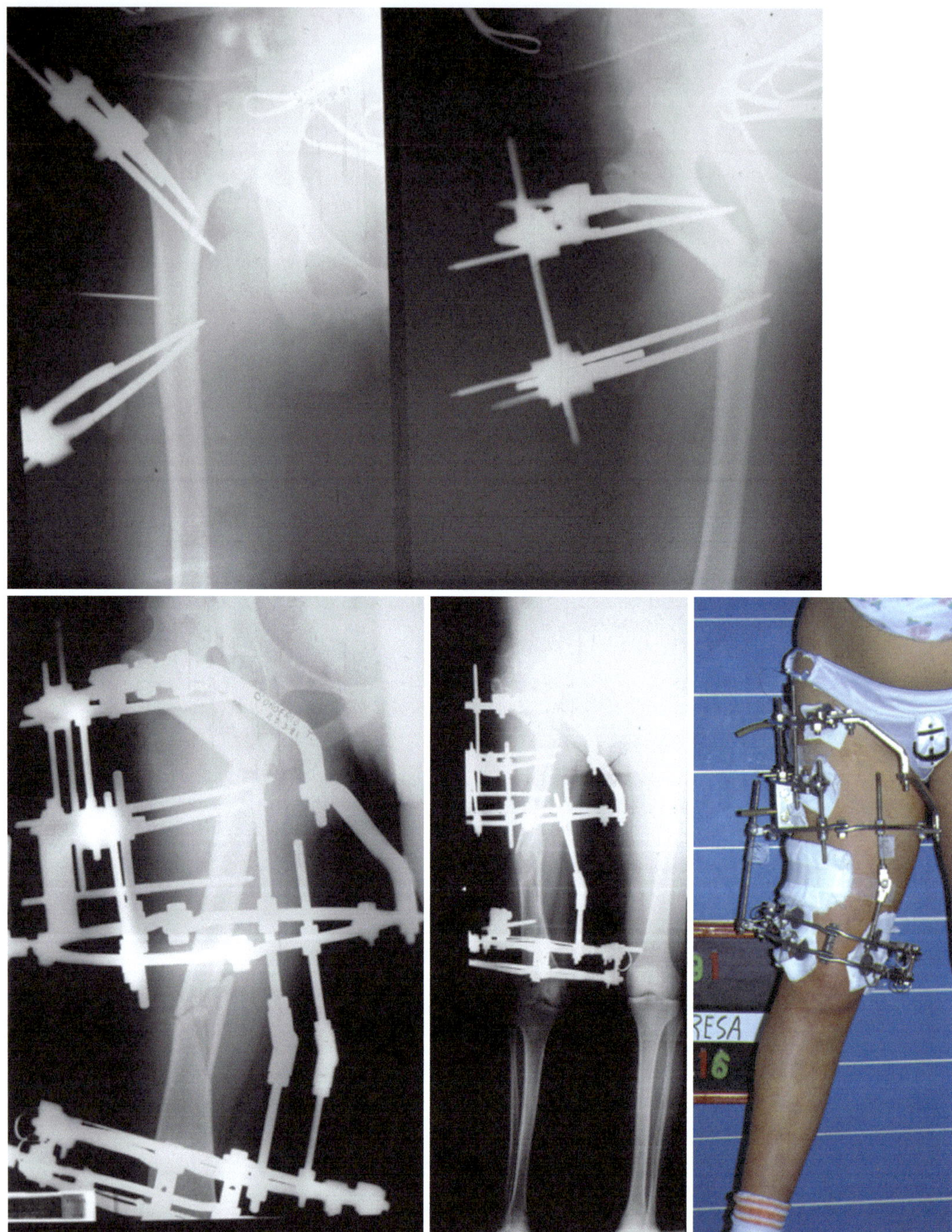

Figs. 21.27, 21.28, 21.29, and 21.30 X-rays during the treatment and photos of the patient

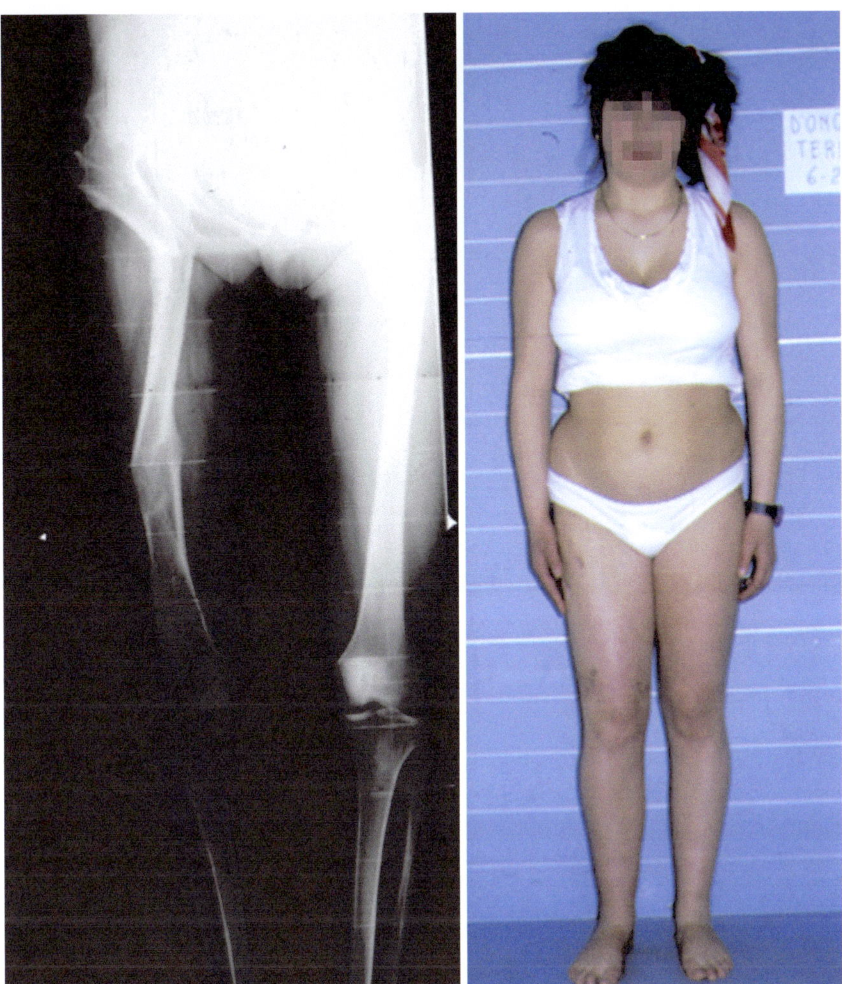

Figs. 21.31 and 21.32 X-rays after the treatment and photos of the patient

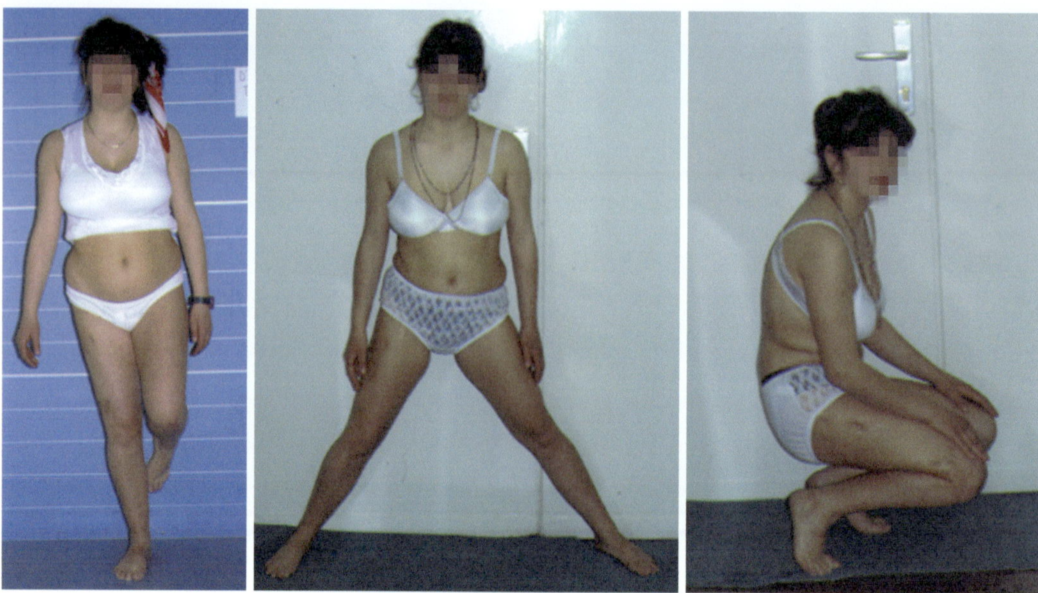

Figs. 21.33, 21.34, and 21.35 Photos of the patient's ROM of the hip and knee and Trendelenburg sign after treatment

The Ilizarov hip reconstruction stands out from other salvage procedures mainly by the improved functional outcome. Total hip arthroplasty, in contrast, which is demanded by some authors (Kim et al. 2003; Lai et al. 2001), is—predominately in children and adolescents—afflicted with a high risk of complications (Davlin et al. 1990; Garvin et al. 1991) and does not counteract the insufficiency of the gluteus muscles in a proper fashion. According to Inan et al., who examined the influence of pelvic support osteotomies in congenital dislocated hips on the gluteus medius muscle, the mentioned procedure even restores abductor muscle length and volume (Inan et al. 2005).

Hence, it is our opinion that the indication for total hip arthroplasty in chronically dislocated hips should be preserved for adulthood if positive effects of the pelvic support osteotomy subside and symptoms reoccur. Since paralysis of the important muscles around the hip may increase the risk of prosthesis instability, total hip arthroplasty would not be a valuable future alternative in this case.

However, novel prosthesis designs with modular stems are available, offering advanced options for anatomical reconstruction, even in complex situations (Benazzo et al. 2007).

The expectations of the patient population of today are for interventions to resolve lameness (Choi et al. 2005). A recommendation for observation only is not readily accepted. While arthrodesis remains a good solution for a degenerate, unstable, and painful joint, it is more likely to be used for smaller joints in the limb. An arthrodesis of the hip provides stability and complete pain relief but it has adverse effects on the lower back, contralateral hip and knee (Sponseller et al. 1984; Callaghan et al. 1985). Currently two appropriate treatment options for a deficient or unstable hip are total joint replacement and a pelvic support osteotomy (Choi et al. 2005; Kocaoglu et al. 2002; El-Mowafi 2005).

Total joint replacement of a deficient hip is technically difficult with a significant complication rate of excessive shortening, sciatic or femoral nerve palsy, fracture of the femoral shaft, and early postoperative dislocation and aseptic loosening (El-Mowafi 2005; Inan and Bowen 2005). When correctly and successfully performed, it improves range of motion, gait symmetry and efficiency and provides excellent pain relief

(El-Mowafi 2005; Paavilainen et al. 1993). However, even with current surgical techniques and prosthesis designs, a total hip replacement in young patients is still controversial (Aksoy and Musdal 2000). An active lifestyle can subject the joint replacement to high mechanical stresses rendering a likelihood of early implant loosening (Kocaoglu et al. 2002; Paavilainen et al. 1993; Inan and Bowen 2005; Berry 1999). Revision of a total hip arthroplasty in a patient with previous hip deficiency is often more difficult than a standard revision operation (El-Mowafi 2005).

After diffusion of the Ilizarov method in Europe since the early 1980s, interest in the pelvic support osteotomy was renewed. The Ilizarov technique, allowed to solve the problems of the knee valgus and limb shortening, determined these osteotomies.

The aim of these osteotomies is to eliminate the Trendelenburg sign, mediated by the axle load and lower limb muscles' pelvitrochanteric retension, and also to improve the abduction and hip extension.

The pelvic support osteotomy constitutes an alternative treatment method for a young adult with an unstable hip. The principles of the pelvic support osteotomy are to perform an abduction and extension effect in the femur at the level of the ischium to increase the range of abduction, support the femur on the pelvis, reduce lumbar lordosis and increase the distance from the pelvis to the greater trochanter, which tightens the gluteus medius and prevents Trendelenburg limp (Bombelli 1993).

Alleviation of the pain was the most significant functional outcome of the treatment. It was also noted that limping could be improved. In 1993 Bombelli demonstrated that an apparent lengthening may occur by over abduction of the distal femoral fragment (Bombelli 1993). This excessive abduction causes genu valgum, increases the shearing stresses on the knee joint and may cause knee pain and low back pain. Catagni (1998) claimed that unilateral subtrochanteric valgus extension osteotomy causes considerable leg length discrepancy and secondary genu valgum induced by excessive valgus.

The preoperative considerations involve a careful clinical and radiological assessment together with a discussion of alternative surgical solutions. Surgical planning is based on data obtained from clinical and x-ray assessment; both will provide the surgeon with answers to (a) the level of the proximal osteotomy; (b) the amount of valgus, extension and derotation at the proximal osteotomy; (c) the level of the distal osteotomy; and (d) the amount of varus and lengthening at the distal osteotomy.

In case of inveterate dislocations, the result remains unchanged over time without pain problems and stable function. In dysplasia, where there is a kind of articulation, function is improved, but after 10–12 years pain and functional limitation appears and necessity of using a prosthesis is mandatory. However this decision is difficult to take, and surgeons' goal is to avoid arthroplasty in young age (Cattaneo et al. 1996). The aim is to perform a total hip replacement in one step when the osteotomy is made in a high hip and the medullar canal maintains its anatomy (Thabet et al. 2012). Performing the medialization of the greater trochanter permits stem implant.

Otherwise this procedure can be performed in two steps when osteotomy is located in a low level and alignment of the femur's medullary canal is obtained by intramedullary nailing followed by prosthesis implantation (Figs. 21.46, 21.47, and 21.48).

The outcome of septic arthritis or infected prostheses; the result remains broadly stable over time. However, in rare cases and after years when the risk of infection is eliminated, placing a new prosthesis could be a good solution.

In conclusion, if there is no joint, the result does not change over time but not in cases of permanent presence of articular contact between the head and soft tissues of the pelvis.

The Ilizarov hip reconstruction is a wellaccepted operative salvage procedure in chronically dislocated hips of adolescents for providing stability, gait improvement and leg length equalization. As it also considers the realignment of the knee joint and permits equalization of the concomitant leg length discrepancy, usually, external systems have been required up to now.

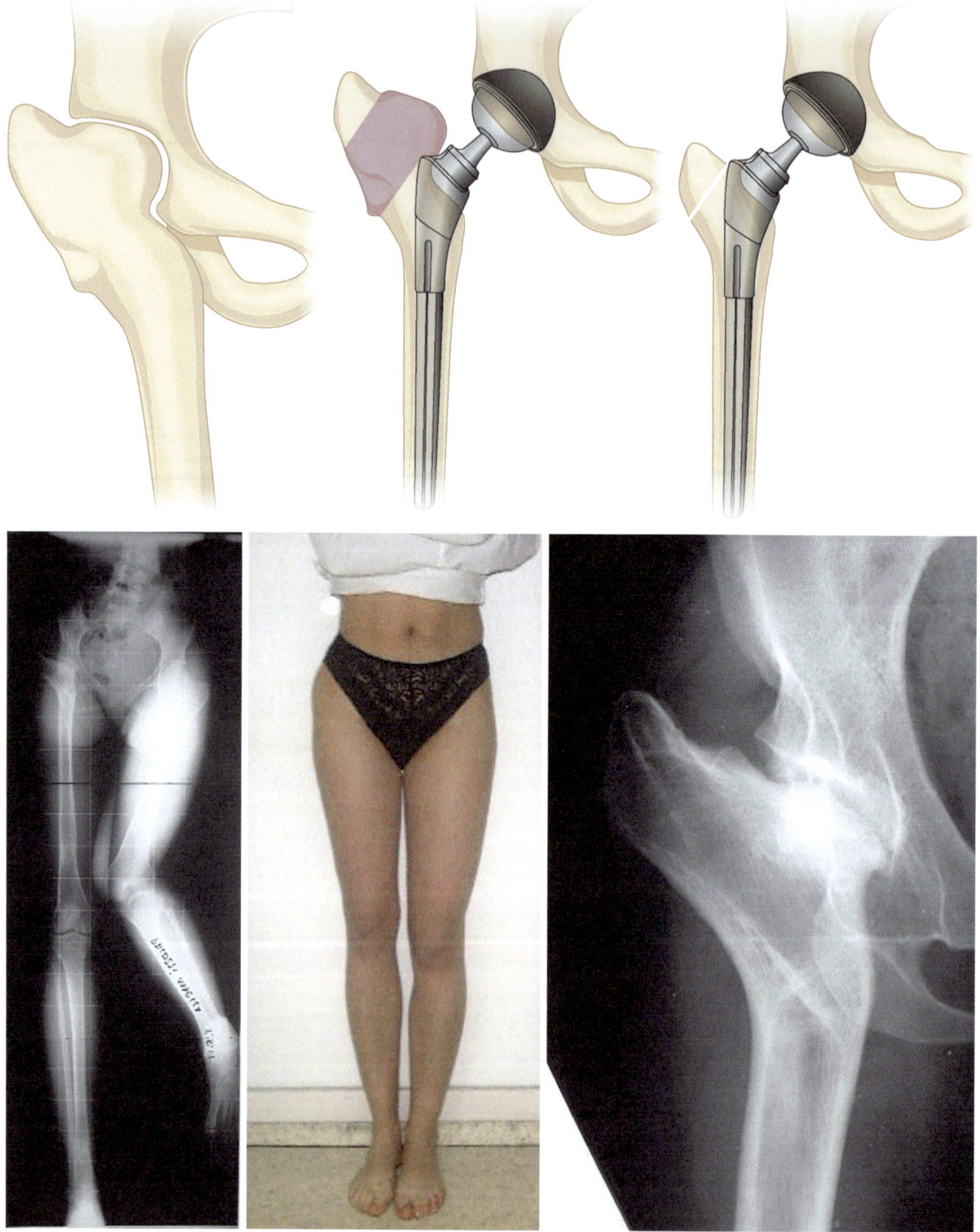

Figs. 21.36, 21.37, 21.38, 21.39, 21.40, 21.41, 21.42, 21.43, 21.44, and 21.45 Hip dysplasia with evolution in hip arthritis after 15 years

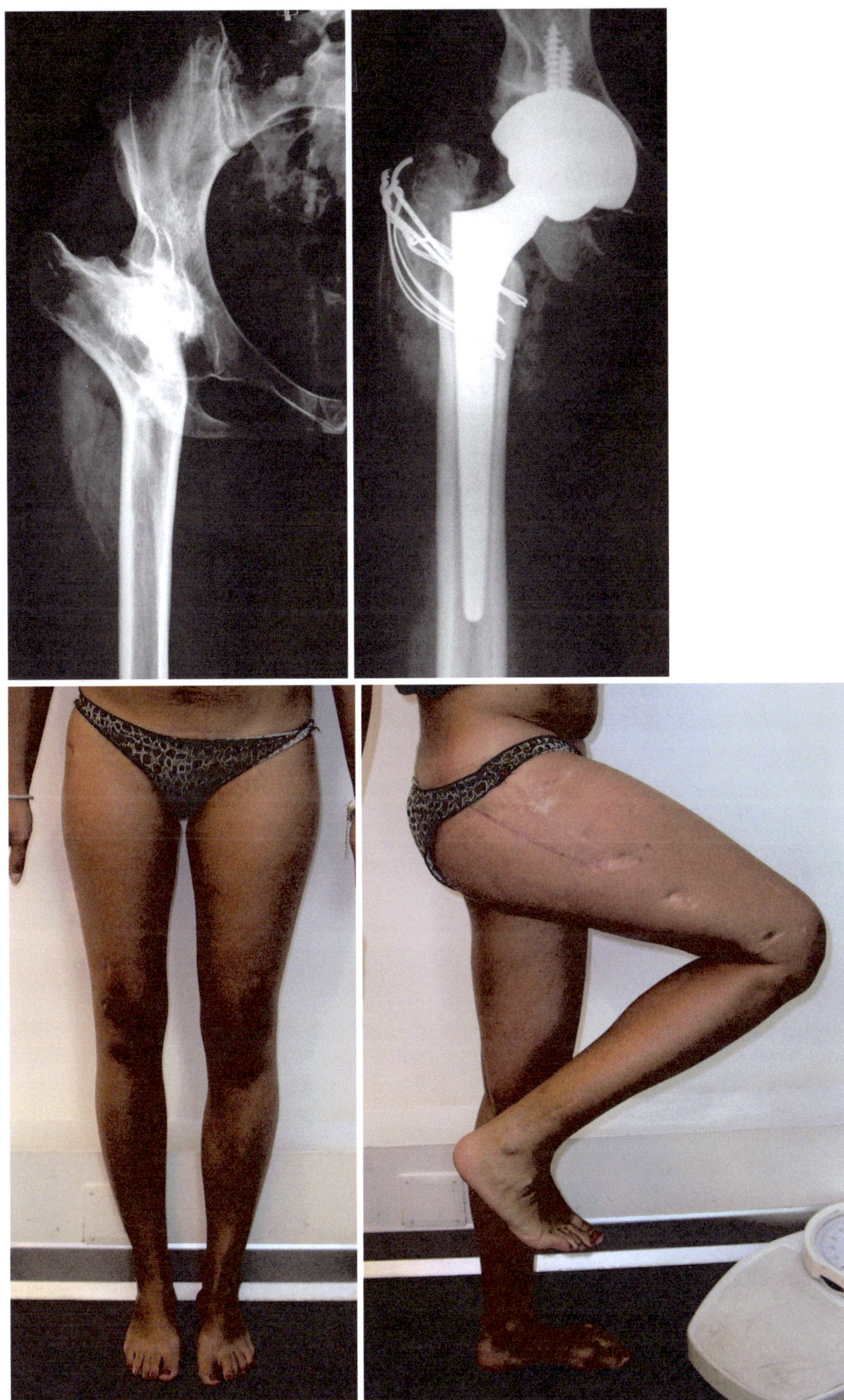

Figs. 21.36, 21.37, 21.38, 21.39, 21.40, 21.41, 21.42, 21.43, 21.44, and 21.45 (continued)

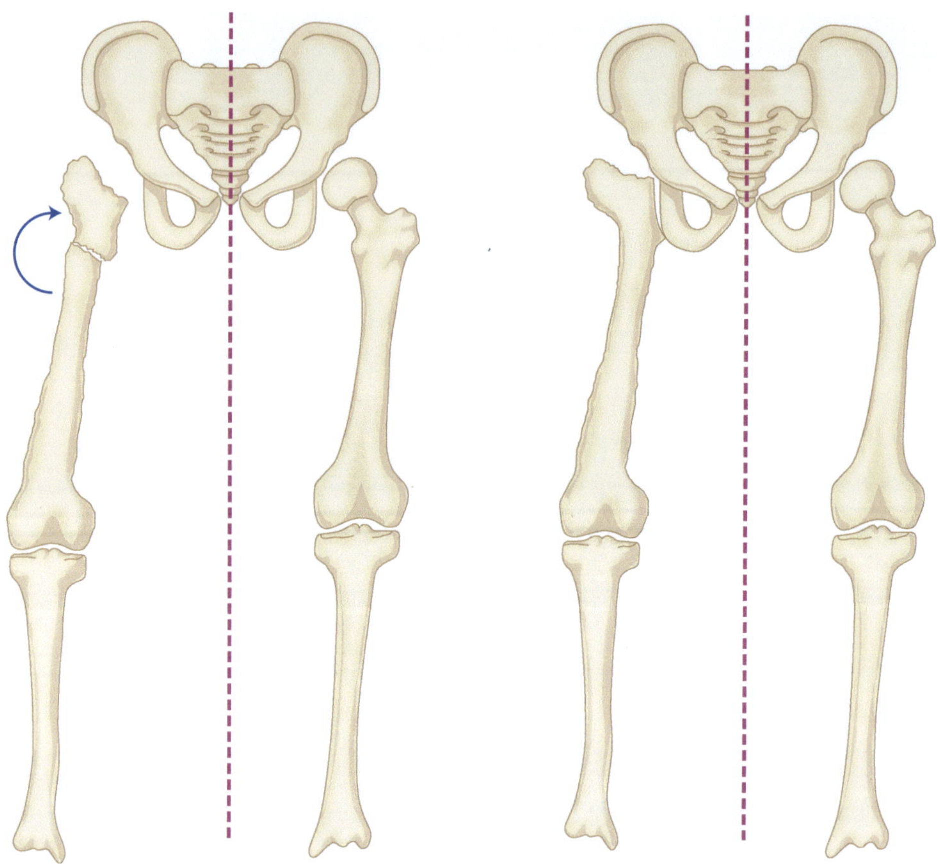

Fig. 21.46 Correction of proximal femur alignment

Fig. 21.47 Correction of proximal femur alignment

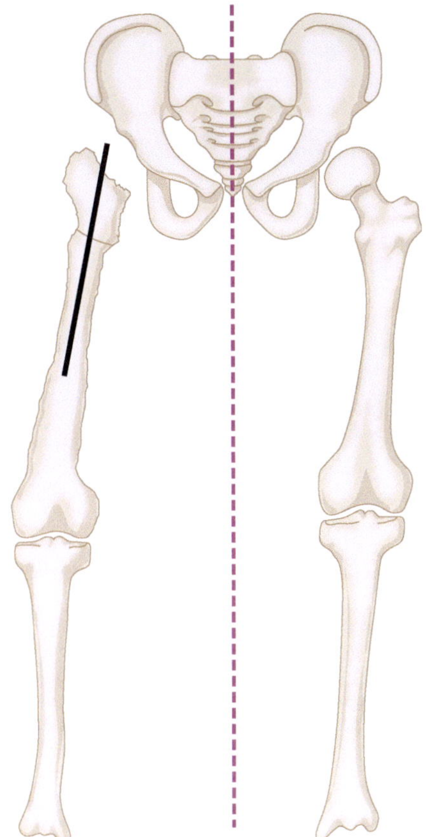

Fig. 21.48 Correction of proximal femur alignment

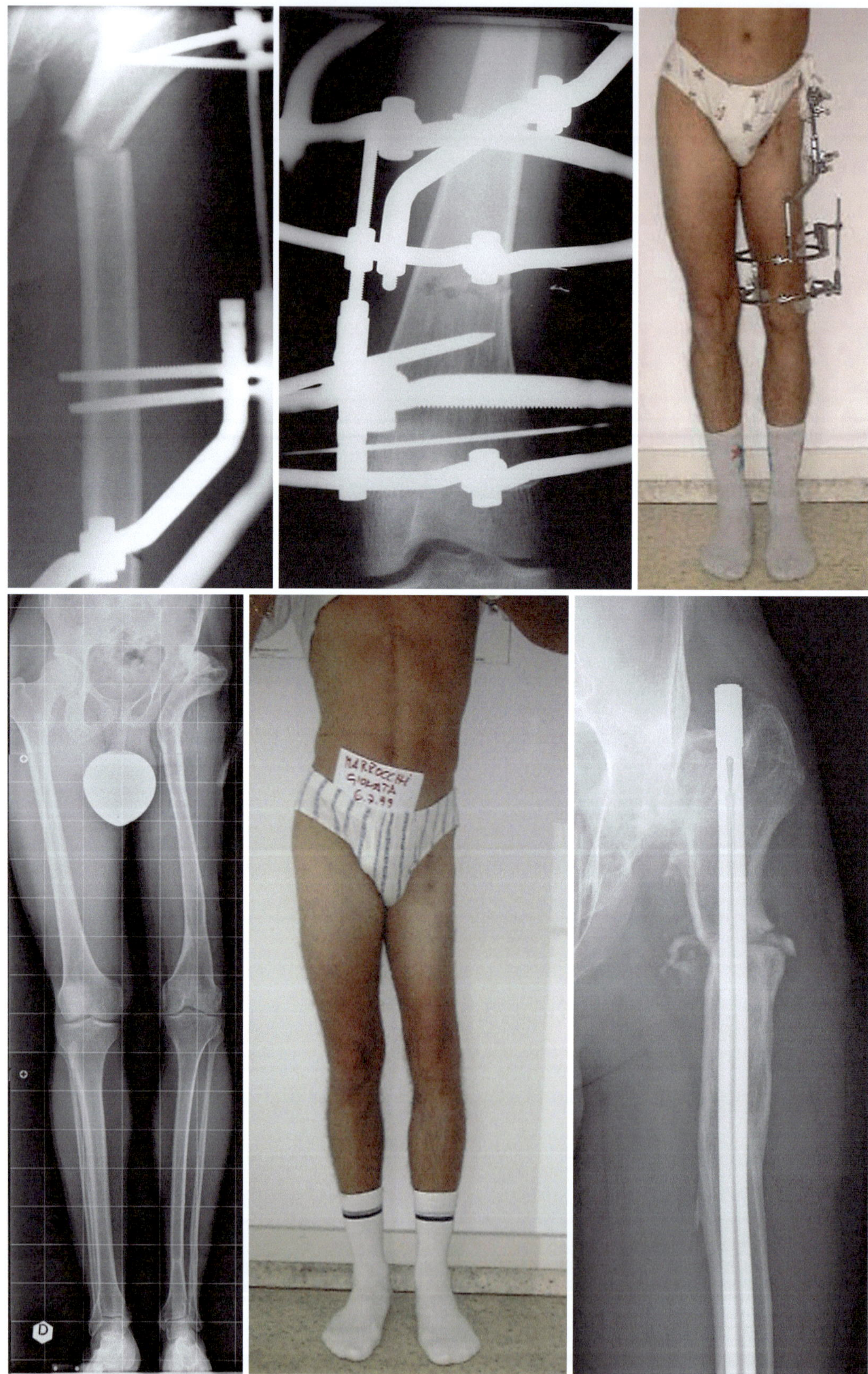

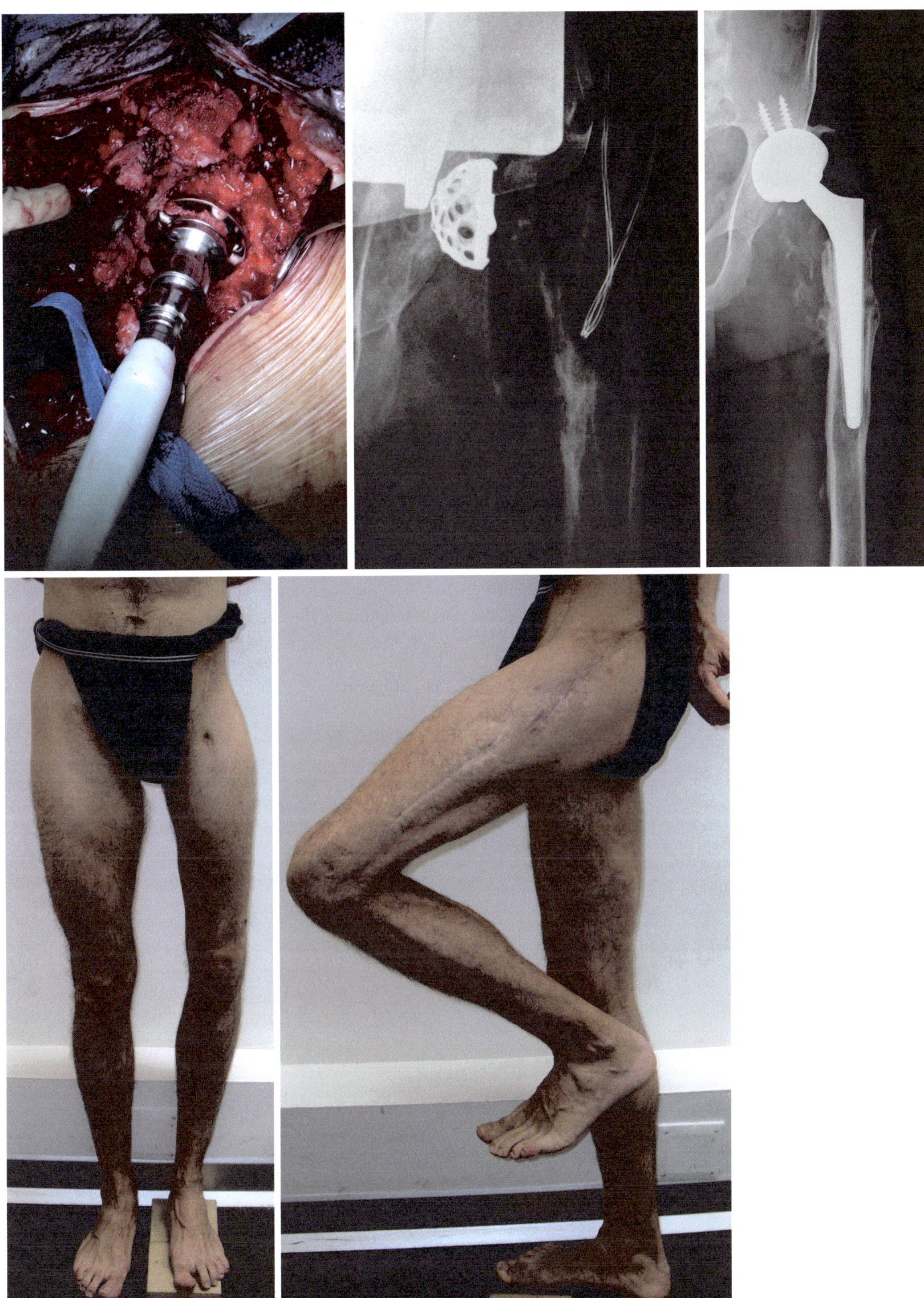

Figs. 21.49, 21.50, 21.51, 21.52, 21.53, 21.54, 21.55, 21.56, 21.57, 21.58, and 21.59 (continued)

Figs. 21.49, 21.50, 21.51, 21.52, 21.53, 21.54, 21.55, 21.56, 21.57, 21.58, and 21.59 Hip subluxation in dysplasia: arthritis evolution in 15 years

Especially in limb lengthening, the advantages of fully implantable techniques such as low complication rates and fast rehabilitation are well known and described consistently in the recent literature (Krieg et al. 2008; Leidinger et al. 2006).

The experience highlighted at our centre (Catagni et al. 1998) showed that the method of Ilizarov for the hip reconstruction (with a hybrid system) seems to be free from serious general complications and is able to improve the function of the affected limb avoiding progression of these pathologies. This procedure may be useful in young patients in whom a prosthetic intervention could not ensure the absence of significant stress and functional deterioration over time.

Bibliography

Aksoy MC, Musdal Y (2000) Subtrochanteric valgus-extension osteotomy for neglected congenital dislocation of the hip in young adults. Acta Orthop Belg 66(2):181–186

Benazzo F, Cuzzocrea F, Stroppa S, Ravasi F, Dalla Pria P (2007) Modular stems in DDH. Hip Int 17(Suppl 5):S138–S141

Berry DJ (1999) Total hip arthroplasty in patients with proximal femoral deformity. Clin Orthop Relat Res 369:262–272

Bombelli R (1993) Structure and function in normal and abnormal hips: how to rescue mechanically jeopardized hips. Springer, Berlin

Callaghan JJ, Brand RA, Pedersen DR (1985) Hip arthrodesis. A long-term follow-up. J Bone Joint Surg Am 67(9):1328–1335

Catagni MA (1992) Current trends in the treatment of simple and complex bone deformities using the Ilizarov method. Instr Course Lect 41:423–430

Catagni M, Cattaneo R (1986) Osteogenesi in distrazione nei grandi allungamenti degli arti. In: Atti del I Congresso ASAMI, Firenze, pp 102–109

Catagni MA, Malzev V, Kirienko A, Bianchi-Maiocchi A (1996) Advances in Ilizarov apparatus assembly: fracture treatment, pseudarthroses, lengthening, deformity correction. Medicalplastic, Milan

Catagni M, Malzev V, Kirienko A (1998) Treatment of disorders of the hip joint. In: Maiocchi A (ed) Advances in Ilizarov apparatus assembly. Medi Surgical Video, Milan

Cattaneo R, Benedetti G, Villa A, Catagni M, Argnani F, Stefini S (1990) Gli allungamenti nei diversi distretti degli arti inferiori: esperienze a confronto. Metodo di Ilizarov Suppl vol XVI, GIOT (2):105–118

Cattaneo R, Catagni M, Guerreschi F (1996) Il metodo di Ilizarov nel trattamento dei fallimenti delle protesi dell'anca. Giornale Italiano di Ortopedia e Traumatologia Suppl vol XXII

Choi IH, Shin YW, Chung CY, Cho TJ, Yoo WJ, Lee DY (2005) Surgical treatment of the severe sequelae of infantile septic arthritis of the hip. Clin Orthop Relat Res 434:102–109

Davlin LB, Amstutz HC, Tooke SM, Dorey FJ, Nasser S (1990) Treatment of osteoarthrosis secondary to congenital dislocation of the hip. Primary cemented surface replacement compared with conventional total hip replacement. J Bone Joint Surg Am 72(7):1035–1042

El-Mowafi H (2005) Outcome of pelvic support osteotomy with the Ilizarov method in the treatment of the unstable hip joint. Acta Orthop Belg 71(6):686–691

Garvin KL, Bowen MK, Salvati EA, Ranawat CS (1991) Long-term results of total hip arthroplasty in congenital dislocation and dysplasia of the hip. A follow-up note. J Bone Joint Surg Am 73(9):1348–1354

Hunka L, Said SE, MacKenzie DA, Rogala EJ, Cruess RL (1982) Classification and surgical management of the severe sequelae of septic hips in children. Clin Orthop Relat Res 171:30–36

Ilizarov GA (1983) Transosseous osteosynthesis. Springer, New York

Ilizarov GA, Samchukov ML (1988) Reconstruction of the femur by the Ilizarov method in the treatment of arthrosis deformans of the hip joint. Ortop Travmatol Protez (6):10–13

Inan M, Bowen RJ (2005) A pelvic support osteotomy and femoral lengthening with monolateral fixator. Clin Orthop Relat Res 440:192–198

Inan M, Alkan A, Harma A, Ertem K (2005) Evaluation of the gluteus medius muscle after a pelvic support osteotomy to treat congenital dislocation of the hip. J Bone Joint Surg Am 87(10):2246–2252. doi:10.2106/jbjs.d.02727

Kim YH, Oh SH, Kim JS (2003) Primary total hip arthroplasty with a second-generation cementless total hip prosthesis in patients younger than fifty years of age. J Bone Joint Surg Am 85-A(1):109–114

Kirmission E (1894) De' l'osteotomie sous-trochante'rienne ap-plique'e a certains cas de luxation conge'nitale de la hanche. (flexion de la cuisse avec adduction conside'rable). Rev d'Orthop :137

Kocaoglu M, Eralp L, Sen C, Dincyurek H (2002) The Ilizarov hip reconstruction osteotomy for hip dislocation: outcome after 4–7 years in 14 young patients. Acta Orthop Scand 73(4):432–438. doi:10.1080/000 16470216308

Krieg AH, Speth BM, Foster BK (2008) Leg lengthening with a motorized nail in adolescents : an alternative to external fixators? Clin Orthop Relat Res 466(1):189–197. doi:10.1007/s11999-007-0040-3

Lai KA, Lin CJ, Jou IM, Su FC (2001) Gait analysis after total hip arthroplasty with leg-length equalization in women with unilateral congenital complete dislocation of the hip–comparison with untreated patients. J Orthop Res 19(6):1147–1152. doi:10.1016/s0736-0266(01)00032-8

Leidinger B, Winkelmann W, Roedl R (2006) Limb lengthening with a fully implantable mechanical distraction intramedullary nail. Z Orthop Ihre Grenzgeb 144(4):419–426. doi:10.1055/s-2006-942169

Lorenz A (1919) Ueber die Behandlung der irreponiblen angeborenen Huftluxationen und der Schenkelhalspseudoarthrosen mittels Gabelung (Bifurkation des oberen Femurendes). Wien Klin Wchnschr (XXXII)

Manzotti A, Rovetta L, Pullen C, Catagni MA (2003) Treatment of the late sequelae of septic arthritis of the hip. Clin Orthop Relat Res 410:203–212. doi:10.1097/01.blo.0000063782.32430.37

Milch H (1989) The "pelvic support" osteotomy. 1941. Clin Orthop Relat Res 249:4–11

Paavilainen T, Hoikka V, Paavolainen P (1993) Cementless total hip arthroplasty for congenitally dislocated or dysplastic hips. Technique for replacement with a straight femoral component. Clin Orthop Relat Res 297:71–81

Rozbruch SR, Paley D, Bhave A, Herzenberg JE (2005) Ilizarov hip reconstruction for the late sequelae of infantile hip infection. J Bone Joint Surg Am 87(5):1007–1018. doi:10.2106/jbjs.c.00713

Schiltenwolf M, Carstens C, Bernd L, Lukoschek M (1996) Late results after subtrochanteric angulation osteotomy in young patients. J Pediatr Orthop B 5(4):259–267

Shepherd MM (1960) A further review of the results of operations on the hip joint. J Bone Joint Surg Br 42-B:177–204

Sponseller PD, McBeath AA, Perpich M (1984) Hip arthrodesis in young patients. A long-term follow-up study. J Bone Joint Surg Am 66(6):853–859

Stack JK, George K (1959) Pelvic support osteotomy for certain fracture complications of the hip. Am J Surg 97(5):644–648

Thabet AM, Catagni MA, Guerreschi F (2012) Total hip replacement fifteen years after pelvic support osteotomy (PSO): a case report and review of the literature. Musculoskelet Surg 96(2):141–147. doi:10.1007/s12306-011-0178-8

Index

M. Kocaoğlu et al. (eds.), *Advanced Techniques in Limb Reconstruction Surgery,*
DOI 10.1007/978-3-642-55026-3, © Springer Berlin Heidelberg 2015

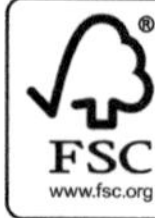